PHARMACEUTICAL MICROBIOLOGY

Pharmaceutical Microbiology

EDITED BY

W. B. HUGO
BPharm PhD FRPharmS
Formerly Reader in Pharmaceutical Microbiology
University of Nottingham

AND

A. D. RUSSELL
Bpharm DSc PhD FRPharmS FRCPath
Professor of Pharmaceutical Microbiology
University of Wales Cardiff
Cardiff

SIXTH EDITION

b

**Blackwell
Science**

© 1977, 1980, 1983, 1987, 1992, 1998 by
Blackwell Science Ltd
Editorial Offices:
Osney Mead, Oxford OX2 0EL
25 John Street, London WC1N 2BL
23 Ainslie Place, Edinburgh EH3 6AJ
350 Main Street, Malden
  MA 02148 5018, USA
54 University Street, Carlton
  Victoria 3053, Australia
10, rue Casimir Delavigne
  75006 Paris, France

Other Editorial Offices:
Blackwell Wissenschafts-Verlag GmbH
Kurfürstendamm 57
10707 Berlin, Germany

Blackwell Science KK
MG Kodenmacho Building
7–10 Kodenmacho Nihombashi
Chuo-ku, Tokyo 104, Japan

First published 1977
Second edition 1980
Third edition 1983
Reprinted 1986
Fourth edition 1987
Reprinted 1989, 1991
Italian Edition 1991
Fifth edition 1992
Reprinted 1993, 1994, 1995
Sixth edition 1998

Set by Setrite Typesetters Ltd,
Hong Kong
Printed and bound in Great Britain by
MPG Books Ltd, Bodmin, Cornwall

DISTRIBUTORS

  Marston Book Services Ltd
  PO Box 269
  Abingdon, Oxon OX14 4YN
  (*Orders*: Tel: 01235 465500
      Fax: 01235 465555)

USA
  Blackwell Science, Inc.
  Commerce Place
  350 Main Street
  Malden, MA 02148 5018
  (*Orders*: Tel: 800 759 6102
        781 388 8250
      Fax: 781 388 8255)

Canada
  Login Brothers Book Company
  324 Saulteaux Crescent
  Winnipeg, Manitoba R3J 3T2
  (*Orders*: Tel: 204 224-4068)

Australia
  Blackwell Science Pty Ltd
  54 University Street
  Carlton, Victoria 3053
  (*Orders*: Tel: 3 9347 0300
      Fax: 3 9347 5001)

A catalogue record for this title
is available from the British Library

ISBN 0-632-04196X

Library of Congress
Cataloging-in-publication Data
Pharmaceutical microbiology
edited by W.B. Hugo and A.D. Russell.
  —6th ed.
      p.   cm.
  Includes bibliographical references and
  index.
  ISBN 0-632-04196-X
  1. Pharmaceutical in microbiology.
  2. Anti-infective agents.
  I. Hugo, W.B. (William Barry)
  II. Russell, A.D. (Allan Denver),
  1936–
  QR46.5.P48   1998
  615′.1′01579—dc21
97-31976
CIP

Contents

Contributors, vii

Preface to the Sixth Edition, ix

Preface to the First Edition, x

Part 1 Biology of Microorganisms

1 Bacteria, 3
W. B. Hugo

2 Yeasts and moulds, 35
J. R. Dickinson

3 Viruses, 53
D. J. Stickler

4 Principles of microbial pathogenicity and epidemiology, 75
P. Gilbert

Part 2 Antimicrobial Agents

5 Types of antibiotics and synthetic antimicrobial agents, 91
A. D. Russell

6 Clinical uses of antimicrobial drugs, 130
R. G. Finch

7 Manufacture of antibiotics, 149
S. A. Varian

8 Mechanisms of action of antibiotics, 162
P. A. Lambert

9 Bacterial resistance to antibiotics, 181
E. G. M. Power

10 Chemical disinfectants, antiseptics and preservatives, 201
E. M. Scott & S. P. Gorman

11 Evaluation of non-antibiotic antimicrobial agents, 229
W. B. Hugo & A. D. Russell

12 Mode of action of non-antibiotic antibacterial agents, 256
W. B. Hugo

13 Resistance to non-antibiotic antimicrobial agents, 263
A. D. Russell

14 Fundamentals of immunology, 278
J. R. Furr

15 The manufacture and quality control of immunological products, 304
F. W. Sheffield

16 Vaccination and immunization, 321
P. Gilbert & D. G. Allison

Part 3 Microbial Aspects of Pharmaceutical Processing

17 Ecology of microorganisms as it affects the pharmaceutical industry, 339
E. Underwood

18 Microbial spoilage and preservation of pharmaceutical products, 355
E. G. Beveridge

19 Contamination of non-sterile pharmaceuticals in hospital and community environments, 374
R. M. Baird

20 Principles and practice of sterilization, 385
S. P. Denyer & N. A. Hodges

21 Sterile pharmaceutical products, 410
M. C. Allwood

22 Factory and hospital hygiene and good manufacturing practice, 426
S. P. Denyer

23 Sterilization control and sterility assurance, 439
S. P. Denyer & N. A. Hodges

24 Production of therapeutically useful substances by recombinant DNA technology, 453
S. B. Primrose

25 Additional applications of microorganisms in the pharmaceutical sciences, 469
A. D. Russell

Index, 493

Contributors

D. G. ALLISON BSc, PhD, *Lecturer in Pharmacy, School of Pharmacy and Pharmaceutical Sciences, University of Manchester, Manchester*

M. C. ALLWOOD BPharm, PhD, MRPharmS, *Professor of Clinical Pharmaceutics, Pharmacy Academic Practice Unit, School of Health and Community Studies, University of Derby, Mickleover, Derby*

R. M. BAIRD BPharm, PhD, MRPharmS, *Research Fellow of the Daphne Jackson Memorial Fellowships Trust, School of Pharmacy and Pharmacology, University of Bath, Bath*

E. G. BEVERIDGE BPharm, PhD, MRPharmS, MIBiol, CBiol, MIQA, *Principal Lecturer in Pharmaceutical Microbiology, School of Health Sciences, University of Sunderland, Sunderland*

S. P. DENYER BPharm, PhD, MRPharmS, *Professor of Pharmaceutical and Applied Microbiology and Head, Department of Pharmacy, University of Brighton, Moulsecoomb, Brighton*

J. R. DICKINSON BSc, PhD, *Senior Lecturer in Yeast Molecular Biology, School of Pure & Applied Biology, University of Wales Cardiff, Cardiff*

R. G. FINCH MB, ChB, FRCP, FRCPath, FFPM, *Consultant Physician in Microbial Diseases, City Hospital NHS Trust, Nottingham, and Professor of Infectious Diseases, Division of Microbiology and Infectious Diseases, Faculty of Medicine, Queen's Medical Centre, University of Nottingham, Nottingham*

J. R. FURR MPharm, PhD, MRPharmS, *Lecturer in Pharmaceutical Microbiology, Welsh School of Pharmacy, University of Wales Cardiff, Cardiff*

P. GILBERT BSc, PhD, *Senior Lecturer in Pharmacy, School of Pharmacy and Pharmaceutical Sciences, University of Manchester, Manchester*

S. P. GORMAN BSc, PhD, MPSNI, *Professor of Pharmaceutical Microbiology, School of Pharmacy, Medical Biology Centre, Queen's University of Belfast, Belfast*

N. A. HODGES BPharm, PhD, MRPharmS, *Principal Lecturer in Pharmaceutical Microbiology, University of Brighton, Moulsecoomb, Brighton*

W. B. HUGO BPharm, PhD, FRPharmS, *Formerly Reader in Pharmaceutical*

Microbiology, University of Nottingham. Present address: 618 Wollaton Road, Nottingham

P. A. LAMBERT BSc, PhD, DSc, *Senior Lecturer in Microbiology, Department of Pharmaceutical Sciences, Aston University, Aston Triangle, Birmingham*

E. G. M. POWER BSc, PhD, *Lecturer in Microbiology, Department of Microbiology, United Medical and Dental Schools, St. Thomas' Hospital, Lambeth Palace Road, London*

S. B. PRIMROSE BSc, PhD, *Vice-President, European Operations, Azurr Environmental, Winnersh Triangle, Wokingham, Berks*

A. D. RUSSELL BPharm, DSc, PhD, FRPharmS, FRCPath, *Professor of Pharmaceutical Microbiology, Welsh School of Pharmacy, University of Wales Cardiff, Cardiff*

E. M. SCOTT BSc, PhD, MPSNI, *Senior Lecturer in Pharmaceutics, School of Pharmacy, Medical Biology Centre, Queen's University of Belfast, Belfast*

F. W. SHEFFIELD MB, ChB, *The Limes, Wilcot, Pewsey, Wiltshire. Formerly Head of the Division of Bacterial Products, National Institute for Biological Standards & Control, South Mimms, Hertfordshire*

D. J. STICKLER BSc, MA, DPhil, *Senior Lecturer in Microbiology, School of Pure & Applied Biology, University of Wales Cardiff, Cardiff*

E. UNDERWOOD BSc, PhD, *Nutritional Product & Process Development Manager, SMA Nutrition, Taplow, Maidenhead*

S. A. VARIAN BSc, PhD, *Fermentation Extraction Operations Manager, Glaxo Wellcome Operations, Ulverston, Cumbria*

Preface to the Sixth Edition

We were delighted to be asked to produce a sixth edition of *Pharmaceutical Microbiology* and we thank the publishers for their considerable input. With the willing cooperation of our co-authors, we have been able to update and modify our text. Several chapters are under new authorship in an attempt to produce a fresh approach. Some chapters have been streamlined but others expanded to take into account the rapid changes and progress being made in certain areas. A new chapter on vaccination and immunization has been introduced to act as a link with the updated chapters on the principles of immunity and the production of immunological products. The chapter on antibiotic assays has been deleted from this edition because it was considered not only that few developments had taken place in this field during the past few years but also that the topic had been comprehensively dealt with in the previous edition.

We hope that this edition will satisfy the needs of pharmacy students, now that the pharmacy degree has been extended to 4 years, and that it will also be of value to pharmacy graduates in hospital, industry and general practice as well as to microbiologists working in the pharmaceutical industry.

W. B. Hugo
A. D. Russell

Preface to the First Edition

When we were first approached by the publishers to write a textbook on pharmaceutical microbiology to appear in the spring of 1977, it was felt that such a task could not be accomplished satisfactorily in the time available.

However, by a process of combined editorship and by invitation to experts to contribute to the various chapters this task has been accomplished thanks to the cooperation of our collaborators.

Pharmaceutical microbiology may be defined as that part of microbiology which has a special bearing on pharmacy in all its aspects. This will range from the manufacture and quality control of pharmaceutical products to an understanding of the mode of action of antibiotics. The full extent of microbiology on the pharmaceutical area may be judged from the chapter contents.

As this book is aimed at undergraduate pharmacy students (as well as microbiologists entering the pharmaceutical industry) we were under constraint to limit the length of the book to retain it in a defined price range. The result is to be found in the following pages. The editors must bear responsibility for any omissions, a point which has most concerned us. Length and depth of treatment were determined by the dictate of our publishers. It is hoped that the book will provide a concise reading for pharmacy students (who, at the moment, lack a textbook in this subject) and help to highlight those parts of a general microbiological training which impinge on the pharmaceutical industry.

In conclusion, the editors thank most sincerely the contributors to this book, both for complying with our strictures as to the length of their contribution and for providing their material on time, and our publishers for their friendly courtesy and efficiency during the production of this book. We also wish to thank Dr H. J. Smith for his advice on various chemical aspects, Dr M. I. Barnett for useful comments on reverse osmosis, and Mr A. Keall who helped with the table on sterilization methods.

W. B. Hugo
A. D. Russell

Part 1
Biology of Microorganisms

Pharmaceutical microbiology is one of the many facets of applied microbiology, but very little understanding of its posed and potential problems will be achieved unless the basic properties of microorganisms are understood.

This section considers, in three separate chapters, the anatomy and physiology of bacteria, fungi and yeasts, and viruses, together with a survey of the characters of individual members of these groups likely to be of importance to the applied field covered by this book. Additional information is provided about more rapid methods for detecting bacteria. The final chapter in this section (Chapter 4) considers the principles of microbial pathogenicity and epidemiology.

The treatment is perforce brief, but it is hoped that the material will give an understanding of the essentials of each group which may be amplified as required from the bibliographic material listed at the end of each chapter.

1 Bacteria

1	**Introduction**		5.6.5	Bioluminescence
2	**Structure and form of the bacterial cell**		**6**	**Properties of selected bacterial species**
2.1	Size and shape		6.1	Gram-positive cocci
2.2	Structure		6.1.1	*Staphylococcus*
2.2.1	Cell wall		6.1.2	*Streptococcus*
2.2.2	Cytoplasmic membrane		6.1.3	*Diplococcus* (now *Streptococcus*)
2.2.3	Cytoplasm		6.2	Gram-negative cocci
2.2.4	Appendages to the bacterial cell		6.2.1	*Neisseria* and *Branhamella*
2.2.5	Capsules and slime		6.3	Gram-positive rods
2.2.6	Pigments		6.3.1	*Bacillus*
2.3	The bacterial spore		6.3.2	*Clostridium*
2.3.1	The process of spore formation		6.3.3	*Corynebacterium*
2.3.2	Spore germination and outgrowth		6.3.4	*Listeria*
2.3.3	Parameters of heat resistance		6.4	Gram-negative rods
			6.4.1	*Pseudomonas*
3	**Toxins**		6.4.2	*Vibrio*
			6.4.3	*Yersinia* and *Francisella*
4	**Reproduction**		6.4.4	*Bordetella*
4.1	Binary fission		6.4.5	*Brucella*
4.2	Reproduction involving genetic exchange		6.4.6	*Haemophilus*
			6.4.7	*Escherichia*
4.2.1	Transformation		6.4.8	*Salmonella*
4.2.2	Conjugation		6.4.9	*Shigella*
4.2.3	Transduction		6.4.10	*Proteus (Morganella, Providencia)*
			6.4.11	*Serratia marcescens*
5	**Bacterial growth**		6.4.12	*Klebsiella*
5.1	The growth requirements of bacteria		6.4.13	*Flavobacterium*
5.1.1	Consumable determinants		6.4.14	*Acinetobacter*
5.1.2	Environmental determinants		6.4.15	*Bacteroides*
5.1.3	Culture media		6.4.16	*Campylobacter*
5.2	Energy provision		6.4.17	*Helicobacter*
5.3	Identification of bacteria		6.4.18	*Chlamydia*
5.3.1	Selective and diagnostic media		6.4.19	*Rickettsia*
5.3.2	Examples of additional biochemical tests		6.4.20	*Legionella*
			6.5	Acid-fast organisms
5.4	Measurement of bacterial growth		6.5.1	*Mycobacterium*
5.4.1	Mean generation time		6.6	Spirochaetes
5.5	Growth curves		6.6.1	*Borrelia*
5.6	Quicker methods for detecting bacteria		6.6.2	*Treponema*
5.6.1	Microscopy		6.6.3	*Leptospira*
5.6.2	Flow cytometry			
5.6.3	Microcalorimetry		**7**	**Further reading**
5.6.4	Electrical conductivity			

1 Introduction

Bacteria share with the blue–green algae a unique place in the world of living organisms. Formerly classified with the fungi, bacteria were considered as primitive members of

Table 1.1 The main features distinguishing prokaryotic and eukaryotic cells

Feature	Prokaryotes	Eukaryotes
Nucleus	No enclosing membrane	Enclosed by a membrane
Cell wall	Peptidoglycan	Cellulose
Mitochondria	Absent	Present
Mesosomes	Present	Absent
Chloroplasts	Absent	Present

the plant kingdom, but they are now called *prokaryotes*, a name which means primitive nucleus. All other living organisms are called *eukaryotes*, a name implying a true or proper nucleus. This important division does not invalidate classification schemes within the world of bacterial, animal and plant life.

This subdivision is not based on the more usual macroscopic criteria; it was made possible when techniques of subcellular biology became sufficiently refined for many more fundamental differences to become apparent. Some of the criteria differentiating eukaryotes and prokaryotes are given in Table 1.1.

Recently, a third class must be added to the bacteria and blue–green algae. Organisms in this class have been named the Archaebacteria; they differ from bacteria and blue–green algae in their wall and membrane structure and pattern of metabolism. They are thought by many to be the first living organisms to have appeared on earth.

2 Structure and form of the bacterial cell

2.1 Size and shape

The majority of bacteria fall within the general dimensions of 0.75–4 μm. They are unicellular structures which may occur as cylindrical (rod-shaped) or spherical (coccoid) forms. In one or two genera, the cylindrical form may be modified in that a single twist (vibrios) or many twists like a corkscrew (spirochaetes) may occur.

Another feature of bacterial form is the tendency of coccoid cells to grow in aggregates. Thus, there exist assemblies (i) of pairs (called diplococci); (ii) of groups of four arranged in a cube (sarcinae); (iii) in a generally unorganized array like a bunch of grapes (staphylococci); and (iv) in a chain like a string of beads (streptococci). The aggregates are often so characteristic as to give rise to the generic name of a group, e.g. *Diplococcus* (now called *Streptococcus*) *pneumoniae*, a cause of pneumonia; *Staphylococcus aureus*, a cause of boils and food poisoning; and *Streptococcus pyogenes*, a cause of sore throat.

Rod-shaped organisms occasionally occur in chains either joined end to end or branched.

2.2 Structure

Three fundamental divisions of the bacterial cell occur in all species: cell wall, cell or cytoplasmic membrane, and cytoplasm.

Extensive chemical studies have revealed a basic structure of alternating *N*-acetylglucosamine and *N*-acetyl-3-*O*-1-carboxyethyl-glucosamine molecules, giving a polysaccharide backbone. This is then cross-linked by peptide chains, the nature of which varies from species to species. This structure (Fig. 1.1) possesses great mechanical strength and is the target for a group of antibiotics which, in different ways, inhibit the biosynthesis occurring during the cell growth and division (Chapter 8).

This basic peptidoglycan (sometimes called murein or mucopeptide) also contains other chemical structures which differ in two types of bacteria, Gram-negative and Gram-positive. In 1884, Christian Gram discovered a staining method for bacteria which bears his name. It consists of treating a film of bacteria, dried on a microscope slide, with a solution of a basic dye, such as gentian violet, followed by application of a solution of iodine. The dye complex may be easily washed from some types of cells which, as a result, are called Gram-negative whereas others, termed Gram-positive, retain the dye despite alcohol washing. These marked differences in behaviour, discovered by chance, are now known to be a reflection of different wall structures in the two types of cell. These differences reside in the differing chemistry of material attached to the outside of the peptidoglycan (Fig. 1.2).

In the walls of Gram-positive bacteria, molecules of a polyribitol or polyglycerol-phosphate are attached by covalent links to the oligosaccharide backbone; these entities

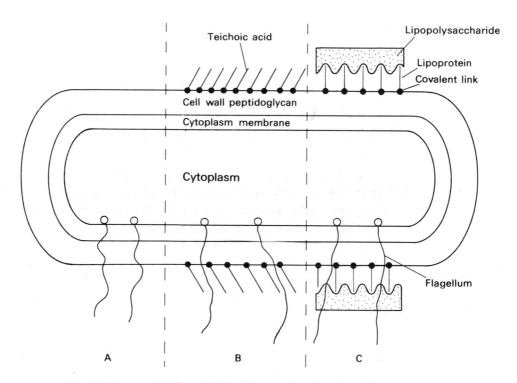

Fig. 1.1 Diagram of the bacterial cell. A, the generalized structure of the bacterial cell; B, Gram-positive structure; C, Gram-negative structure.

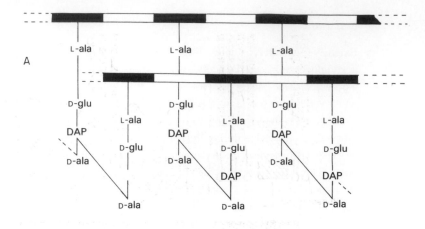

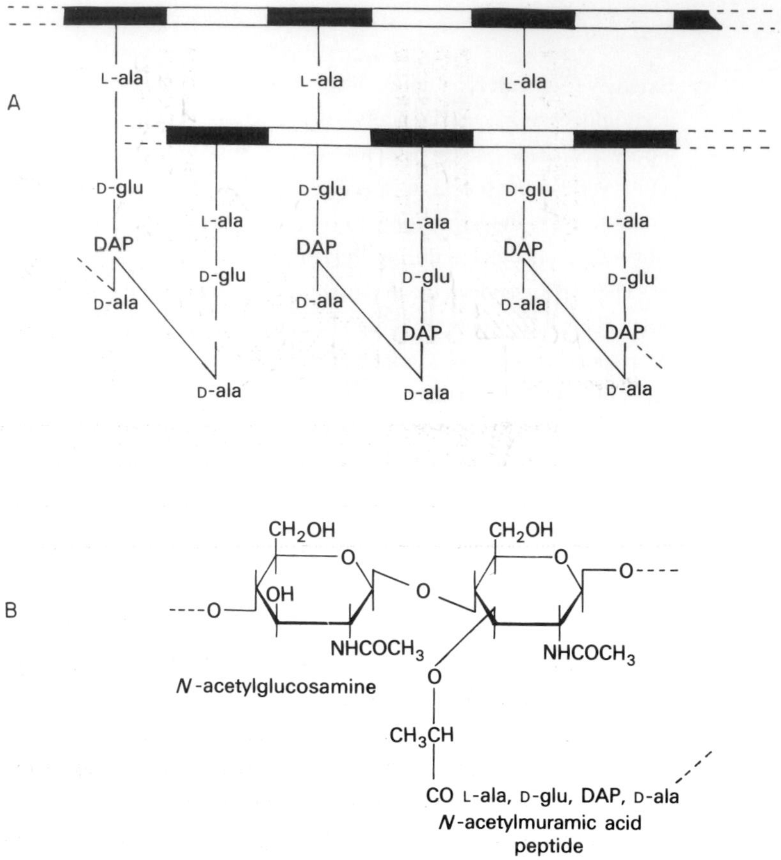

Fig. 1.2 A, peptidoglycan of *Escherichia coli*. ■, *N*-acetylmuramic acid; □, *N*-acetylglucosamine. B, repeating unit of peptidoglycan of *E. coli*. L-ala, L-alanine; D-glu, D-glutamine; DAP, diaminopimelic acid; D-ala, D-alanine.

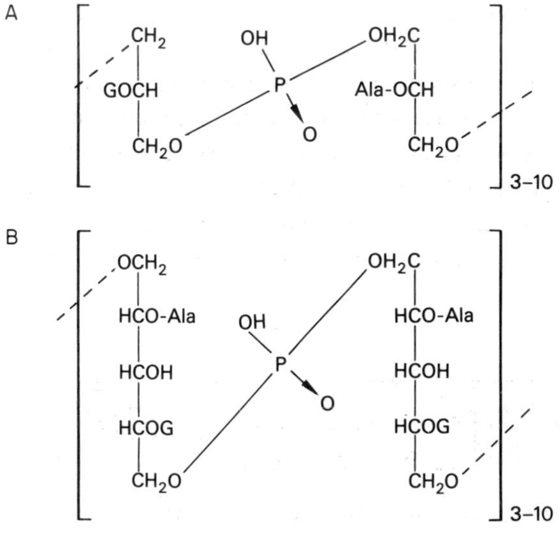

Fig. 1.3 A, glycerol teichoic acid; B, ribitol teichoic acid; G, glycosyl; Ala, D-alanyl.

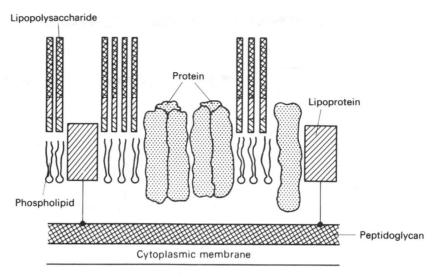

Fig. 1.4 Diagram showing detailed structure of the envelope of Gram-negative bacteria.

are teichoic acids (Fig. 1.3A, B). The glycerol teichoic acid may contain an alanine residue (Fig. 1.3A). Teichoic acids do not confer additional rigidity on the cell wall, but as they are acidic in nature they may function by sequestering essential metal cations from the media on which the cells are growing. This could be of value in situations where cation concentration in the environment is low.

The Gram-negative cell envelope (Fig. 1.4) is even more complicated; essentially, it contains lipoprotein molecules attached covalently to the oligosaccharide backbone and in addition, on its outer side, a layer of lipopolysaccharide (LPS) and protein attached by hydrophobic interactions and divalent metal cations, Ca^{2+} and Mg^{2+}. On the inner side is a layer of phospholipid (PL).

The LPS molecule consists of three regions, called lipid A, core polysaccharide and O-specific side chain (Fig. 1.5). The O-specific side chain comprises an array of sugars that are responsible for specific serological reactions of organisms, which are used in identification. The lipid A region is responsible for the toxic and pyrogenic (fever-producing) properties of this group (see Chapter 18).

The complex outer layers beyond the peptidoglycan in the Gram-negative species, the outer membrane, protect the organism to a certain extent from the action of toxic chemicals (see Chapter 13). Thus, disinfectants are often effective only at concentrations higher than those affecting Gram-positive cells and these layers provide unique protection to the cells from the action of benzylpenicillin and lysozyme.

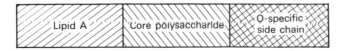

Fig. 1.5 Lipopolysaccharide structure in Gram-negative bacteria.

Part of the LPS may be removed by treating the cells with ethylenediamine tetra-acetic acid (EDTA) or related chelating agents (Chapter 12).

The proteins of the outer membrane, many of which traverse the whole structure, are currently the subject of active study. Some of the proteins consist of three subunits, and these units with a central space or pore running through them are known as porins. They are thought to act as a mechanism of selectivity for the ingress or exclusion of metabolites and antibacterial agents (see Chapter 8).

2.2.2   *Cytoplasmic membrane*

The chemistry and structure of this organelle have been the subject of more than a century of research, but it is only during the last 20 years that some degree of finality has been realized.

Chemically, the membrane is known to consist of phospholipids and proteins, many of which have enzymic properties. The phospholipid molecules are arranged in a bimolecular layer with the polar groups directed outwards on both sides. The structures of some phospholipids found in bacteria are shown in Fig. 1.6. Earlier views held that the protein part of the membrane was spread as a continuous sheet on either side of the

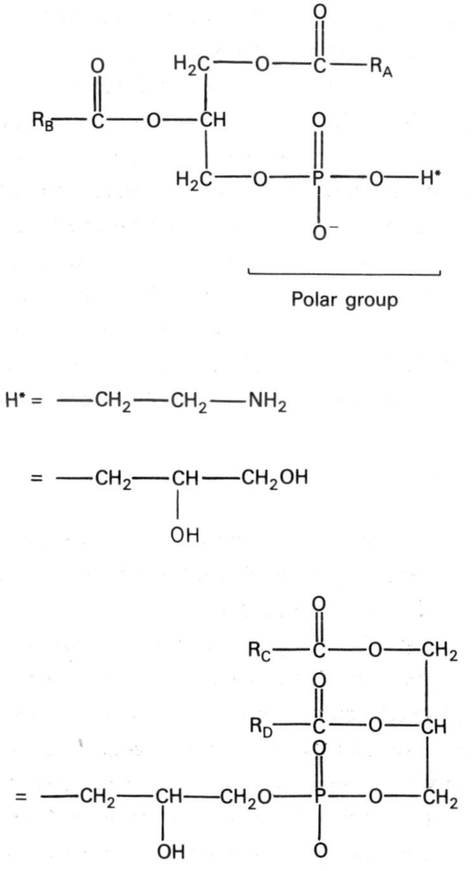

Fig. 1.6 The structure of some phospholipids found in *E. coli*. A, the structure of phosphatidic acid. H* of this structure is replaced by grouping B–D to give the following phospholipids: B, phosphatidylethanolamine; C, phosphatidylglycerol; D, diphosphatidylglycerol (cardiolipin). R_A.COO and R_B.COO are fatty acid residues.

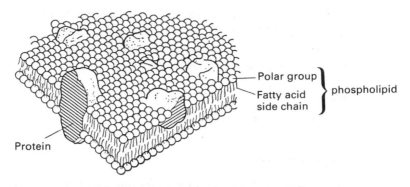

Polar group
Fatty acid
side chain
} phospholipid

Protein

Fig. 1.7 Membrane structure.

phospholipid bilayer. The current view is that protein is distributed in local patches in the bilayer, the mosaic structure (Fig. 1.7).

Unlike the wall, which has great mechanical strength, determines the characteristic shape of the cell and is metabolically inert, the membrane is structurally a very delicate organelle and is highly active metabolically.

The membrane acts as a selective permeability barrier between the cytoplasm and the cell environment; the wall acts only as a sieve to exclude molecules larger than about 1 nm. Certain enzymes, and especially the electron transport chain, that are located in the membrane are responsible for an elaborate active transport system which utilizes the electrochemical potential of the proton to power it.

An interesting experiment serves to illustrate the differing mechanical strengths of the wall and membrane. The wall of some Gram-positive bacteria may be partially dissolved by treatment of cells with lysozyme or in the case of Gram-negative cells with EDTA plus lysozyme. Upon doing this, cells so treated burst due to the fact that the cytoplasm contains a large number of solutes giving it an effective osmotic pressure of 608–2533 kPa (6–25 atm). Water enters the cell, now no longer protected by the peptidoglycan, causing the naked protoplast to swell and burst. If this experiment is conducted in a medium containing 0.33 M sucrose, a non-penetrating solute, the osmotic pressure inside and outside the protoplast is equalized, thus no bursting occurs, and forms free of cell wall (protoplasts) may be observed in the medium.

2.2.3   *Cytoplasm*

The cytoplasm is a viscous fluid and contains within it systems of paramount importance. These are the nucleus, responsible for the genetic make-up of the cell, and the ribosomes, which are the site of protein synthesis. In addition are found granules of reserve material such as polyhydroxybutyric acid, an energy reserve, and polyphosphate or volutin granules, the exact function of which has not yet been elucidated. The prokaryotic nucleus or bacterial chromosome exists in the cytoplasm in the form of a loop and is not surrounded by a nuclear membrane. Bacteria carry other chromosomal elements: episomes, which are portions of the main chromosome that have become isolated from it, and plasmids, which may be called miniature chromosomes. These are small annular pieces of DNA which carry a limited amount of genetic information, often associated with the expression of resistance to antimicrobial agents (Chapters 9 and 13).

Despite the differences in nuclear structures between prokaryotes and eukaryotes, the genetic code, i.e. the combination of bases which does for a particular amino acid in the process of protein synthesis, is the same as it is in all living organisms.

2.2.4 Appendages to the bacterial cell

Three types of thread-like appendages may be found growing from bacterial cells: flagella, pili (fimbriae) and F-pili (sex strands).

Flagella are threads of protein often $12\,\mu m$ long which start as small basal organs just beneath the cytoplasmic membrane. They are responsible for the movement of motile bacteria. Their number and distribution varies. Some species bear a single flagellum, others are flagellate over their whole surface.

Pili are responsible for haemagglutination in bacteria and also for intercellular adhesiveness giving rise to clumping. At present, a clear role for these structures has not been formulated.

F-pili or sex strands are part of a primitive genetic exchange system in some bacterial species. Part of the genetic material may be passed from one cell to another through the hollow pilus, thus giving rise to a simple form of sexual reproduction.

2.2.5 Capsules and slime

Some bacterial species accumulate material as a coating of varying degrees of looseness. If the material is reasonably discrete it is called a capsule, if loosely bound to the surface it is called slime.

Recently a phenomenon of resistance to biocide solutions has been recognized (see also Chapters 9 and 13) in which bacteria adhere to a container wall and cover themselves with a carbohydrate slime called a glycocalyx; thus, doubly protected (wall and glycocalyx), they have been found to resist biocide attack.

Bacillus anthracis, the causative organism of anthrax, possesses a capsule composed of polyglutamic acid; the slime layers produced by other organisms are of a carbohydrate nature.

An extreme example of slime production is found in *Leuconostoc dextranicum* and *L. mesenteroides* where so much carbohydrate, called dextran, may be produced that the whole medium in which these cells are growing becomes almost gel-like. This phenomenon has caused pipe blockage in sugar refineries and is deliberately encouraged for the production of dextran as a blood substitute (Chapter 25).

2.2.6 Pigments

Some bacterial species produce pigments during their growth which give the colonies a characteristic colour.

Thus, *Staphylococcus aureus* produces a golden yellow pigment, *Serratia marcescens* a bright red pigment. There appears to be no valid function for these pigments but they may afford the cell some protection from the toxic effects of sunlight.

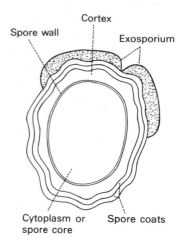

Fig. 1.8 Diagram of a transverse section of a bacterial spore.

2.3   The bacterial spore

In a few bacterial genera, notably *Bacillus* and *Clostridium*, a unique process takes place in which the vegetative cell undergoes a profound biochemical change to give rise to a structure called a spore or endospore (Fig. 1.8). This process is not part of a reproductive cycle, but the bacterial endospore is highly resistant to adverse environments such as lack of moisture or essential nutrients, toxic chemicals and radiations and high temperatures. Because of their heat resistance all sterilization processes have to be designed to destroy the bacterial spore.

2.3.1   The process of spore formation

In general, an adverse environment, and in particular the absence or limited presence of one component, induces spore formation. Examples of such components are alanine, Zn^{2+}, Fe^{2+}, PO_3^{3-} and, in the case of the aerobic (oxygen-requiring) *Bacillus* species, oxygen. Equally, certain substances, for instance Ca^{2+} and Mn^{2+}, have to be present for the process of spore formation to proceed to completion.

If the conditions for spore formation are fulfilled the sequence of events shown in Fig. 1.9 occurs.

The essential genetic material of the original vegetative bacterium is retained in the core or protoplast; around this lies the thick cortex which contains the murcin or peptidoglycan already encountered as a cell wall component (see Fig. 1.2). The outer coats which are protein in composition are distinguished by their high cysteine content. In this respect they resemble keratin, the protein of hair and horn.

Another feature of the spore is the presence of pyridine 2,6-dicarboxylic acid (DPA) (Fig. 1.10) occurring as a complex with calcium, which at one time was implicated in heat resistance. The isolation of heat-resistant spores containing no Ca-DPA has refuted this hypothesis.

The reason for heat resistance is thought to lie in the fact that the core or spore cytoplasm becomes dehydrated during sporulation. The mechanism for this dehydration

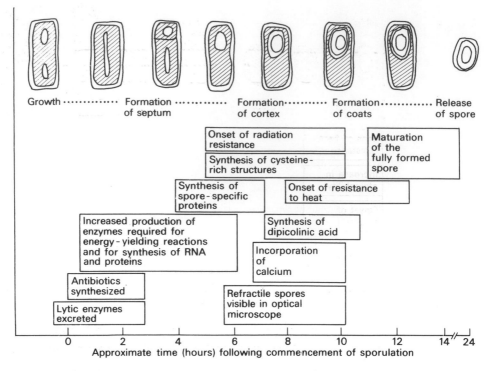

Fig. 1.9 Changes occurring during spore formation. The position and length of the boxes represent the approximate time and duration of the various activities.

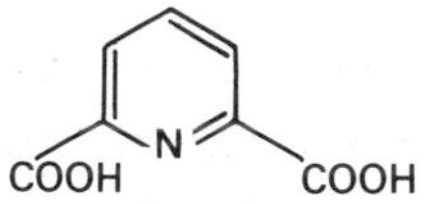

Fig. 1.10 Pyridine 2,6-dicarboxylic acid, dipicolinic acid (DPA).

is the mechanical expulsion of water by the expansion of the peptidoglycan network which comprises the cortex—the expanded cortex theory.

Dehydration of the core by means of concentrated sucrose solution also results in heat resistance.

The tough keratin-like spore coats probably help to protect the spore core or protoplast from the harmful effects of chemicals. Radiation resistance has not been fully explained.

The same generally impervious properties make spores difficult to stain by simple stains. However, if a slide preparation of spores is warmed with a stain the spores are dyed so effectively that dilute acid will not wash out the colour. This is the basis of the acid-fast stain for spores.

2.3.2   *Spore germination and outgrowth*

In nature, spores can revert to the vegetative form by a process called either 'germination' or 'germination and outgrowth'. The process of germination may be triggered by specific

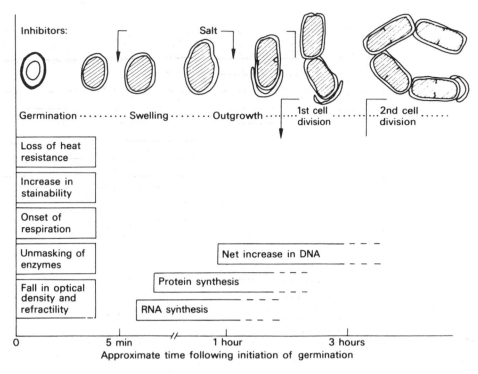

Fig. 1.11 Spore germination, outgrowth and division of the outgrown cells.

germination stimulants, such as L-alanine or glucose, by the physical processes of shaking with small glass beads, or by sublethal heating (e.g. at 60°C for 1 hour). Outgrowth and subsequent growth depends on the presence of the necessary nutrients for the particular organism concerned. The stages of germination and outgrowth, and also the action of inhibitors of the process, are shown in Fig. 1.11.

2.3.3   *Parameters of heat resistance*

The existence and possible presence of bacterial spores determines the parameters, i.e. time and temperature relationships, of thermal sterilization processes which are used extensively by the food and pharmaceutical industry. These are defined below (see also Chapters 20 and 23).

1 *D*-value (decimal reduction time, DRT) is the time in minutes required to destroy 90% of a population of cells. The *D*-value has little relevance to the sterilization of medicines for injection, surgical instruments or dressings, where a process designed to kill all living spores must be developed. The *D*-value is used extensively in the food industry.

2 The F_0-value is a process-describing unit expressed in terms of minutes at 121.1°C (originally 250°F) or a corresponding time–temperature relationship to produce the same complete spore-killing effect.

3 The *z*-value is the increase in temperature (°C) to reduce the *D*-value to one-tenth.

3   Toxins

Although bacteria are associated with the production of disease, only a few species are disease-producing or pathogenic.

The mechanism whereby the bacteria produce the disease with its attendant symptoms is often due to the cells' ability to produce specific poisons, toxins or aggressins (Chapter 14). Many of these are tissue-destroying enzymes which can damage the cellular structure of the body or destroy red blood cells. Others (neurotoxins) are highly specific poisons of the central nervous system, for example the toxin produced by *Clostridium botulinum* is, weight for weight, one of the most poisonous substances known.

4   Reproduction

4.1   Binary fission

The majority of bacteria reproduce by simple binary fission; the circular chromosome divides into two identical circles which segregate at opposite ends of the cell. At the same time, the cell wall is laid down in the middle of the cell, which finally grows to produce two new cells each with its own wall and nucleus. Each of the two new cells will be an exact copy of the original cell from which they arose and no new genetic material is received and none lost.

4.2   Reproduction involving genetic exchange

For many years, it was thought that binary fission was the only method of reproduction in bacteria, but it is now known that there are three methods of reproduction in which genetic exchange can occur between pairs of cells, and thus a form of sexual reproduction is exhibited. These processes are transformation, conjugation and transduction. Further details of these processes as they affect antibiotic resistance will be found in Chapter 9.

4.2.1   *Transformation*

In 1928, long before the role of DNA, the genetic code and the mechanics of genetics and gene expression were known, Griffith found that a culture of *Streptococcus pneumoniae* deficient in capsular material could be made to produce normal capsulated cells by the addition of the cell-free filtrate from a culture in which a normal capsulated strain had been growing. The state of knowledge at that time was insufficient for the great significance of this experiment to be realized and developed. It was not until 16 years later that the material in the culture filtrate responsible for the re-establishment of capsulated cells was shown to be DNA.

4.2.2   *Conjugation*

Conjugation, discovered in 1946, is a natural process found in certain bacterial genera and involves the active passage of genetic material from one cell to another by means of the sex pili (p. 10). However, despite the resemblance of this process to the complete genetic exchange found in eukaryotes, it is not possible to designate male and female bacteria. Bacteria which are able to effect transfer contain in their genetic make-up a fertility factor and are designated F⁺ strains. These are able to transfer part, and in some cases all, of their genetic material to F⁻ strains.

It should be realized that this is an extremely brief and incomplete account of conjugation. The importance of bacterial conjugation in antibiotic resistance will be considered later (Chapter 9).

4.2.3 *Transduction*

Viruses are discussed more fully elsewhere (Chapter 3). However, there are certain groups of viruses, called bacteriophages (phages), which can attack bacteria. This attack involves the injection of viral DNA into bacterial cells which then proceed to make new virus particles and destroy cells. Some viruses, known as temperate viruses, do not cause this catastrophic event when they infect their host, but can pass genetic material from one cell to another.

In summary, then, conjugation is a natural process representing the early stages in a true sexually reproductive process. Transformation involving autolysis of the culture with loss of genetic material, and transduction arising out of an infective process, are secondary processes which are not known to occur in eukaryotes; nevertheless, they must have taken their part in microbial evolution.

5 Bacterial growth

The preceding account has been concerned with the single bacterial cell and the information has been obtained by various forms of microscopy and by chemical analysis. Further bacteriological information has been, and is being, obtained by observing bacteria in very large numbers either as a culture in liquid growth medium or as colonies on a solid growth medium. Under these circumstances bacteria can be seen but the behaviour of aggregates is really a statistical average behaviour of its individuals. A somewhat fanciful analogy is that whereas a molecule of a chemical substance is invisible, molecules in mass, i.e. a chemical specimen, are visible and macroscopic properties are determinable.

5.1 The growth requirements of bacteria

The determinants of microbial growth are described as consumable and environmental.

5.1.1 *Consumable determinants*

The consumables represent the essential food or nutritional requirements. Conventionally they include sugars, starches, proteins, vitamins, trace elements, oxygen, carbon dioxide and nitrogen; but bacteria are probably the most omnivorous of all living organisms and to the above list may be added plastic, rubber, kerosene, naphthalene, phenol and cement. One is left feeling that there is no substance which is immune to microbial attack. It is easy, too, to overlook the importance of water; bacteria cannot grow without water and, besides a milieu in which to thrive, water also provides hydrogen as part of reaction sequences for the metabolism of the substrates.

Some bacteria have very simple growth requirements, and the following medium (expressed as $g\,l^{-1}$) will support the growth of a wide range of species: glucose, 20; $(NH_4)_2HPO_4$, 0.05. On the other hand, some species may need the addition of some 20 amino acids and perhaps 8–10 vitamins or growth factors (thiamine or vitamin B_1 is an example of the latter) before growth will occur, and it follows that these requirements have to be present in natural environments also. Between the extremes of the nutritionally non-exacting and the nutritionally highly exacting, a whole range of intermediate requirements are found.

The requirements of a microorganism for an amino acid or vitamin can be used to determine the amount of that substance in foods or pharmaceutical products by growing the organism in a medium containing all the essential requirements and measured doses of the substance to be determined.

Mention has been made of gases as part of the bacterial consumables list. Some bacteria cannot grow unless oxygen is present in their immediate atmosphere; in practical terms this means that they grow in air. Such organisms are called obligate aerobes. Another group is actually inhibited in the presence of oxygen, this gas behaving almost as an intoxicant, and such bacteria are known as obligate anaerobes. A large number of species can grow both in the presence and absence of oxygen and these are termed facultative bacteria. These organisms, however, make much better use of foodstuffs, i.e. their consumables, when growing in air. A fourth group is named microaerophilic: these grow best in the presence of oxygen at slightly lower concentrations than that found in air. Special techniques are needed to grow anaerobic bacteria which, briefly, consist of cultivation in oxygen-free atmospheres or growth in culture media containing a reducing agent; sometimes a combination of both methods is used.

5.1.2   *Environmental determinants*

The main environmental determinants of microbial growth are pH and temperature. The availability of water may be lowered when certain solutes are present in high concentration; thus, concentrated salt and sugar solutions may either slow down or prevent growth.

Most bacteria grow best at pH values of 7.4–7.6, on the alkaline side of neutrality, but some bacterial species are able to grow at pH 1–2 or 9–9.5, although they are exceptional.

Bacteria also show a wide range of growth temperatures. Those organisms which cause disease in man and other mammals, and in consequence have been extensively studied, grow best at the temperature of the mammalian body, i.e. 37–39°C. However, viable microorganisms have been recovered from hot springs, the polar seas and submarine volcanic fissures (thermal vents), and there are bacteria which can grow in domestic refrigerators. Bacteria which grow best at 15–20°C are called psychrophiles, at 25–40°C mesophiles, and at 55–75°C thermophiles.

The growth of bacteria, as with other living organisms, can be inhibited or prevented. Antiseptics, disinfectants, antibiotics and chemotherapeutic agents are the names given to special chemicals developed to combat infection. They are discussed in later chapters.

Culture media

Mention has already been made of the wide variety of consumable nutrients which may be required by bacteria, and also how some bacteria can grow in simple aqueous solution containing an energy source, such as glucose, and a few inorganic ions.

For the routine cultivation of bacteria, a cheap source of all likely nutrients is desirable, and it should also be remembered that even bacteria whose minimum requirements are very simple grow far better on more highly nutritious media.

The media usually employed are prepared from protein by acid or enzymic digestion. Typical sources are muscle tissue (meat), casein (milk protein) and blood fibrin. Their digestion provides a supply of the natural amino acids and, because of their origin as living tissue, they will also contain vitamins or growth factors and mineral traces. Solutions of these digests, with the addition of sodium chloride to optimize the tonicity, comprise the common liquid culture media of the bacteriological laboratory. If it is required to study the characteristic colony appearance of cultures, the above media may be solidified by a natural carbohydrate gelling agent, agar, which is derived from seaweed.

In addition, a vast array of special culture media have been developed containing chemicals which by either their selective inhibitory properties or characteristic changes act as selective and diagnostic agents to pick out and identify bacterial species from specimens containing a mixture of microorganisms. The examination of faeces for pathogens is a good example.

As stated in section 5.1.1, some bacteria will not grow in the presence of oxygen. These anaerobes may be grown by placing cultures in an oxygen free atmosphere, or adding a reducing agent such as cooked meat or sodium thioglycollate to the media.

5.2   Energy provision

The growth requirements outlined above express themselves in growth itself through the less tangible but fundamental necessity of energy which is provided by metabolism. Not all metabolic reactions, however, provide energy; esterase activity is an example of one that does not.

The energy provision by carbohydrate metabolism has been extensively studied from the beginning of this century, chiefly in an attempt to understand the basic biochemistry of alcohol production from carbohydrate. However, many laboratory culture media contain only nitrogenous compounds and their metabolism is of importance as it clearly provides energy for growth and maintenance.

In addition, living cells need a system of energy storage and this is provided by 'bond energy', strictly the free energy of hydrolysis of a diphosphate bond in the compound adenosine triphosphate (ATP).

Energy-yielding reactions and energy-storage systems form a common pattern found in all living systems and may be depicted thus:

$$\text{Reactant} \rightarrow \text{products} + \text{energy} \begin{array}{l} \nearrow \text{stored} \\ \searrow \text{utilized as produced.} \end{array}$$

A fundamental characteristic of the overall reaction is that it proceeds by a series of steps, each catalysed by a separate enzyme. This ensures gentle and not explosive release of energy and also provides a useful set of intermediates for the biosynthetic reactions which are concomitant to growth.

It is the complexity of the array of enzymes, coenzymes and intermediates which at first sight provides a daunting barrier to those wishing to try to understand cellular energetics.

As stated in section 5.1.1, some bacteria derive energy from food sources without the use of oxygen, whereas others are able to use this gas. The pathway of oxygen utilization itself is also a stepwise series of reactions and thus the overall picture emerges of cellular metabolism characterized by multistep reactions.

Although bacteria (the prokaryotes) differ in many fundamental ways from all other living organisms (see Table 1.1), their metabolic pathways do not. The handling of carbohydrates by the Embden–Meyerhof pathway and the Krebs citric acid cycle and many of the reactions of the metabolism of nitrogen-containing compounds are common to both eukaryotes and prokaryotes. The enzymes and coenzymes for handling molecular oxygen are also strikingly similar in both classes. A full treatment of these pathways is given in the former editions of this book and in textbooks of biochemistry and microbial chemistry.

5.3   Identification of bacteria

The varying metabolic activities of bacteria and their response to immediate environmental factors have been exploited in the design of special diagnostic and selective media. Recipes for these run into many hundreds; such media are used in hospital and public health laboratories for identifying organisms found in samples believed to be contaminated by them, and as an aid to diagnosis and treatment. In addition they are used to detect contaminants in pharmaceutical products (*British Pharmacopoeia* 1993). A few examples will be given to illustrate the principle.

5.3.1   *Selective and diagnostic media*

MacConkey's medium. This was introduced in 1905 to isolate Enterobacteriaceae from water, urine, faeces, foods, etc. Essentially, it consists of a nutrient medium with bile salts, lactose and a suitable indicator. The bile salts function as a natural surface-active agent which, while not inhibiting the growth of the Enterobacteriaceae, inhibits the growth of Gram-positive bacteria which are likely to be present in the material to be examined.

Escherichia coli and *Klebsiella pneumoniae* subsp. *aerogenes* produce acid from lactose on this medium, altering the colour of the indicator, and also adsorb some of the indicator which may be precipitated around the growing cells. The organisms causing typhoid and paratyphoid fever and bacillary dysentery do not ferment lactose, and colonies of these organisms appear transparent.

Many modifications of MacConkey's medium exist; one employs a synthetic surface-active agent in place of bile salts.

Bismuth sulphite agar. This medium was developed in the 1920s for the identification of *Salmonella typhi* in water, faeces, urine, foods and pharmaceutical products. It consists of a buffered nutrient agar containing bismuth sulphite, ferrous sulphate and brilliant green.

Escherichia coli (which is also likely to be present in material to be examined) is inhibited by the concentration (0.0025%) of brilliant green used, while *Sal. typhi* will grow luxuriantly. Bismuth sulphite also exerts some inhibitory effect on *E. coli*.

Salmonella typhi, in the presence of glucose, reduces bismuth sulphite to bismuth sulphide, a black compound; the organism can produce hydrogen sulphide from sulphur-containing amino acids in the medium and this will react with ferrous ions to give a black deposit of ferrous sulphide (Table 1.2).

Selective media for staphylococci. It is often necessary to examine pathological specimens, food and pharmaceutical products for the presence of staphylococci, organisms which can cause food poisoning as well as systemic infections.

In media selective for enterobacteria a surface-active agent is the main selector, whereas in staphylococcal medium sodium and lithium chlorides are the selectors; staphylococci are tolerant of 'salt' concentrations to around 7.5%. Mannitol salt, Baird–Parker (BP) and Vogel–Johnson (VJ) media are three examples of selective staphyloccocal media. Beside salt concentration the other principles are the use of a selective carbon source, mannitol or sodium pyruvate together with a buffer plus acid–base indicator for visualizing metabolic activity and, by inference, growth. BP medium also contains egg yolk; the lecithin (phospholipid) in this is hydrolysed by staphylococcal (esterase) activity so that organisms are surrounded by a cleared zone in the otherwise opaque medium. The *United States Pharmacopeia* (1990) includes a test for staphylococci in pharmaceutical products, whereas the *British Pharmacopoeia* (1993) does not.

Selective media for pseudomonads. These media depend on the relative resistance of pseudomonads to the quaternary ammonium disinfectant cetrimide. In some recipes the antibiotic nalidixic acid (Chapter 5) is added, to which pseudomonads are also resistant.

Table 1.2 Appearance of bacterial colonies on bismuth sulphite agar

Organism	Appearance
Salmonella typhi *Salmonella enteritidis* *Salmonella schotmülleri*	Black with blackened extracolonial zone
Salmonella paratyphi *Salmonella typhimurium* *Salmonella choleraesuis*	Green
Shigella flexneri *Shigella sonnei*	Brown
Other shigellae *Escherichia coli*	No growth

Selective media for legionellas and listerias. Such have been devised.

Media for fungi. Most fungi encountered as contaminants in pharmaceutical products will grow on media similar to that used to grow bacteria. Growth is favoured, however, if the proportion of carbohydrate is increased in relation to that of nitrogenous constituents.

Thus, media for the cultivation of fungi often contain additional glucose, malt, sucrose or wort. The optimum pH for mould growth is usually on the acid side of neutrality and so the pH of culture media for moulds is usually 5–6. This, while entirely suitable for most common moulds, at the same time discourages bacterial growth and thus renders the medium selective. Examples of such media are Sabouraud maltose or dextrose agar, malt extract agar and soya tryptone agar.

The optimum temperature varies widely from species to species but in general the common moulds will grow better at 22–25°C than most human pathogenic and commensal bacteria. It is customary, therefore, to incubate mould cultures at lower temperatures than bacterial cultures.

A comprehensive account of culture media may be found in the Oxoid manual (see references).

5.3.2   *Examples of additional biochemical tests*

The differing ability to ferment sugars, glycosides and polyhydric alcohols is widely used to differentiate the Enterobacteriaceae and in diagnostic bacteriology generally. The test is usually carried out by adding the reagent aseptically to sterilized peptone water and a suitable indicator, contained in a 5-ml bottle closed with a rubber-lined screw cap and containing a small inverted tube filled with the medium. Acid production is indicated by a change in colour of the indicator, and gas production by gas collecting in the inverted tube.

It is possible to buy ingenious testing devices which consist of a plastic strip containing cavities in which dried reagents are placed. Such a strip may contain some 50 different tests and is used by depositing in the cavity a culture medium containing a suspension of bacteria from the colony to be investigated. The strip is then incubated. This is the API system (API Laboratory Products, Basingstoke, Hants). Another useful device consists of a plastic tube with a number of compartments of about $1.2\,cm^3$, each containing agar medium. These are inoculated by means of a still wire run through their centre; this enables some 11 tests to be carried out. It is known as the Enterotube.

5.4   **Measurement of bacterial growth**

The quantification of the growth response to the total environment may be determined by counting the bacterial population to see if it changes with the passage of time. The most direct method is literally to count the bacterial cells placed on a calibrated microscope slide. This slide has a grid of 0.05-mm squares ruled on it and is so arranged that when a microscope slide is placed in position on two ledges raised by 0.02 mm, a known volume ($0.00005\,mm^3$) is spread over each square. From the counts per unit of known volume, the total count may be calculated. This method cannot distinguish between living and dead bacteria, however, and to determine the number of living bacteria in a culture it is necessary to perform what is known as a viable count. In this method, an aliquot of the culture, suitably diluted, is mixed with, or placed on the surface of, a suitable solid culture medium and the mixture incubated. Viable colonies appear in or on the medium and are counted. It will be realized here that a single bacterium in the original culture being plated is assumed to give rise to a single viable colony—this may not always be true, and aggregates of two or more cells may give rise to a single colony. Ideally, this situation should be avoided, but in order to present some notion of scientific correctness or semantic perfection, the viable count may be referred to as the number of colony-forming units (cfu) rather than as 'number of bacteria'.

A third method of determining the changes in a viable population is to take advantage of the fact that bacteria in suspension scatter or absorb light. By shining a light beam through a bacterial suspension and calculating changes in light intensity by allowing the emergent beam to fall on a photoelectric cell connected to a galvanometer, the bacterial population observed as light-scattering or light-absorbing units may be determined. This method is rapid but it counts both living and dead bacteria and, for that matter, non-bacterial particles. A calibration curve relating bacterial numbers to galvanometer reading must be produced for each experimental circumstance.

Great care, skill and understanding are required to determine the state of a bacterial population whether growing, stationary or dying.

In addition to these time-honoured methods, newer techniques involving bio-luminescense, fluorescent dyes (epifluorescence) and physical methods such as impedance, calorimetry and flow cytometry have been developed. A feature being sought in these methods is rapidity: see section 5.6.

5.4.1   *Mean generation time*

The time interval between one cell division and the next is called the generation time. When considering a growing culture containing many thousands of cells, a mean generation time is usually calculated.

If a single cell reproduces by binary fission, then the number of bacteria n in any generation will be as follows:

1st generation $n = 1 \times 2$ $= 2^1$
2nd generation $n = 1 \times 2 \times 2$ $= 2^2$
3rd generation $n = 1 \times 2 \times 2 \times 2 = 2^3$
yth generation $n = 1 \times 2^y$ $= 2^y$

For an initial inoculum of n_0 cells, as distinct from one cell, at the yth generation the cell population will be:

$$n = n_0 \times 2^y$$

This equation may be rewritten thus:

$$\log n = \log n_0 + y \log 2$$

whence

$$y = \frac{\log n - \log n_0}{\log 2} = \frac{\log n - \log n_0}{0.3010}$$

where y is the number of generations that have elapsed in the time interval between determining the viable count n_0 and the population reaching n.

If this time interval is t, then the mean generation time G is given by the expression:

$$G = \frac{t}{y} = \frac{t}{\dfrac{\log n - \log n_0}{0.3010}} = \frac{t \times 0.3010}{\log n - \log n_0}$$

5.5   Growth curves

When a sample of living bacteria is inoculated into a medium adequate for growth, the change in viable population with time follows a characteristic pattern (Fig. 1.12).

The first phase, A, is called the lag phase. It will be short if the culture medium is adequate, i.e. not necessarily minimal, and is at the optimum temperature for growth. It may be longer if the medium is minimal or has to warm up to the optimum growth temperature, and prolonged if toxic substances are present; other things being equal, there is a relationship between the duration of the lag phase and the amount of the toxic inhibitor.

In phase B it is assumed that the inoculum has adapted itself to the new environment and growth then proceeds, each cell dividing into two. Cell division by binary fission may take place every 15–20 minutes and the increase in numbers is exponential or logarithmic, hence the name log phase. Phase C, the stationary phase, is thought to occur as a result of the exhaustion of essential nutrients and possibly the accumulation

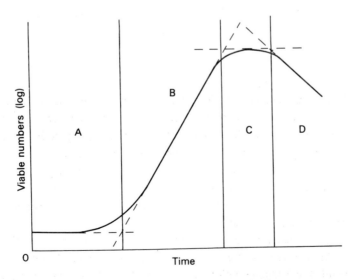

Fig. 1.12 Typical bacterial growth curve: A, lag phase; B, log phase; C, stationary phase; D, phase of decline.

of bacteriostatic concentrations of wastes. Growth will recommence if fresh medium is added to provide a new supply of nutrients and to dilute out toxic accumulations.

In phase D, the phase of decline, bacteria are actually dying due to the combined pressures of food exhaustion and toxic waste accumulation.

5.6 Quicker methods for detecting bacteria

The methods for determining bacterial contamination both quantitatively and qualitatively which have been outlined in sections 5.3, 5.4 and 5.5 have the general disadvantage that they involve an incubation period of 15–72 hours before a reliable answer is obtained.

In the case of pharmaceutical quality control, and in many other spheres, methods which give an answer in a shorter time are being investigated, evaluated and in some cases used. Some of these quicker or rapid methods will be referred to in this section.

5.6.1 *Microscopy*

It had been found that if bacteria are stained with acridine orange and examined under fluorescent microscopy, viable, as distinct from dead, cells fluoresce with an orange–red hue. This basic observation has been adapted to an ingenious method of determining bacterial content and may be completed within 1 hour.

The method, known as the direct epifluorescent filtration technique (DEFT), consists of filtering the liquid to be tested through a membrane filter, staining the filter with the acridine orange and examining the filter under a fluorescent microscope. The organisms may be counted, thus rendering the technique quantitative. This method has been used to determine microbial contaminants in intravenous fluids and was able to detect organisms at a level of 25/ml. DEFT presents difficulties if the fluid to be examined is viscous, although this may be overcome by dilution. Water-soluble solids may be dissolved before difficulties with water-immiscible, viscous liquids and water-insoluble solids.

5.6.2 *Flow cytometry*

This technique together with the Coulter counting technique depends upon a simple but ingenious device. A potential difference is maintained in a circuit which includes a tube with a small orifice submerged in a conducting liquid (Fig. 1.13).

If a liquid containing particulate matter, blood cells, bacteria or suspensions of inanimate matter is passed down the tube, when a particle passes through the orifice a change in resistance in the circuit occurs and the change may be recorded by the usual detection or print-out devices. Both the number of particles per unit of time and their size may be determined.

There are certain points to be borne in mind, however, with this method:

1 In the counting of bacteria, both dead and living cells will be counted and sized although prestaining with a dye and a sophistication of the instrumentation has been investigated.

2 A further possible disadvantage is that the orifice may become blocked during use.

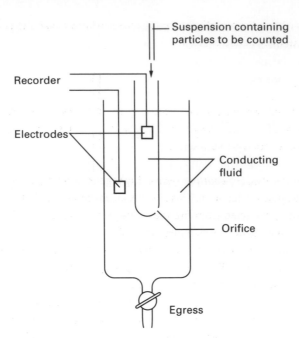

Recorder

Electrodes

Suspension containing
particles to be counted

Conducting
fluid

Orifice

Egress

Fig. 1.13 Principle of electronic
particle counter: Coulter counter.

3 If the bacterial content of an inanimate suspension, i.e. a medicine such as milk of magnesia, is being examined both bacteria and magnesium hydroxide particles will be detected, although here again methods of distinguishing the two types of particle have been developed.

5.6.3.

Microcalorimetry

This method depends on the fact that bacteria like all living organisms produce heat when they metabolize. Because of the small amount of heat produced, especially sensitive calorimetric devices are required hence the name microcalorimetry. The specimen to be evaluated is diluted with a nutrient medium and, if microorganisms are present and can metabolize, heat is produced and can be measured. An interesting offshoot of this technique is the fact that differing organisms produce different heat outputs and this may provide a means of identification. Microcalorimetry may enable organisms to be detected and possibly identified in 3 hours.

5.6.4

Electrical conductivity

When organisms grow in a liquid media their metabolic products can create a change in the conductivity of the media, a fact noted in 1898. Research has shown that colony numbers of about 10/ml are required to produce a measurable conductivity change. The actual changes in the media may be measured also by changes in impedance (resistance to an alternating current) or the change in its electrical capacity. As with all techniques it has certain limitations. If the level of initial contamination of a product is low, incubation of a sample in a suitable broth will be necessary to increase the organism content to nearer 10/ml. This will add to the time of the test. Another limitation lies in

the detection of non-fermentative microorganisms whose metabolic activity pro
little change in media conductivity.

<table>
<tr><td>5.6.5</td><td>*Bioluminescence*</td></tr>
</table>

5.6.5   *Bioluminescence*

It has long been known that certain insects (e.g. the beetles known as fire flies) and two or three genera of bacteria possess the ability to emit light; this property has been utilized in quality control and research.

The use of the fire fly light-emitting system. Light generation depends on the oxidation of a substance known as luciferin. This is a fatty aldehyde such as dodecanal. An enzyme called luciferase, extracted from fire flies, catalyses the oxidation. The reaction also requires ATP. Thus, light emission measures ATP.

The detection of bacteria by this method depends on the fact that they, like all living material, contain ATP but here arises a potential problem.

When determining the bacterial content of, for example, foods, clinical material and even water, elaborate techniques are required to eliminate non-bacterial ATP. Also, the sample being tested has to undergo an extraction process to remove ATP from any bacteria present. The problem of non-microbial ATP is not likely to be met in the examination of pharmaceuticals and toilet goods, however.

Comprehensive kits are available to analysts, bacteriologists and research workers to perform the determination of ATP. They include, or are backed by, special light-measuring equipment (luminometers) to estimate light emission and follow its extinction.

The use of luminous bacteria. A naturally occurring light-emitting bacterium, *Photobacterium fischeri*, was used as early as 1942 to assay antibiotics, the end-point being taken as the extinction of light as viewed visibly.

With the advent of genetic engineering it has been possible to insert the light-emitting genes of a natural bioluminescent organism, the so-called *lux* cluster into organisms more relevant to medicine and public health, e.g. *Escherichia coli, Salmonella typhimurium, Listeria* spp. and *Mycobacterium smegmatis* amongst others. The extinction of light in these organisms is used to mark the end-point in an estimation of biocide activity and thermal stress to quote two examples of the application of this method.

Rapid methods have great appeal in microbial quality control and certain areas of research, but it should always be borne in mind, especially in quality control, that rigorous testing of the method should be carried out in comparison to accepted methods.

Rapid and quicker methods have an extensive literature and mainly review-type publications are given at the end of the chapter.

6   Properties of selected bacterial species

In this section, no attempt will be made to follow the modern classification system; the reader is referred to the works of Bergey (Buchanan & Gibbons 1974), Cowan and Steel (Cowan 1993) and Logan (1994) for an overview of classification.

Gram-positive cocci

Staphylococcus

The spheres grow characteristically in aggregates which have been likened to a bunch of grapes. The organisms are non-motile and non-sporing; they can grow aerobically or anaerobically. *Staphylococcus aureus* produces a golden yellow pigment. It is a cause of skin lesions such as boils, and can affect bone tissue in the case of staphylococcal osteomyelitis. It produces a toxin which, if ingested with food in which the organism has been growing, can give rise to food poisoning. A common manifestation of its infection is the production of pus, i.e. the organism is pyogenic. Other common conditions associated with staphylococcal infections are styes, impetigo and conjunctivitis.

6.1.2

Streptococcus

These also are non-sporing, spherical organisms which grow characteristically in chains like strings of beads, and can grow aerobically or anaerobically.

Streptococcus pyogenes can be an extremely dangerous pathogen; it produces a series of toxins, including an erythrogenic toxin which induces a characteristic red rash, and a family of toxins which destroy the formed elements of blood.

Typical diseases caused by *Strep. pyogenes* are scarlet fever and acute tonsillitis (sore throat), and the organism is a dangerous infective agent in wounds and in blood poisoning after childbirth (puerperal sepsis). Rheumatic fever and acute inflammation of the kidney are serious sequelae of streptococcal infection. Invasive streptococcal infection can cause necrosis of subcutaneous tissue (necrotizing fasciitis) together with other serious systemic pathologies.

6.1.3

Diplococcus (now Streptococcus)

As the name implies, these organisms grow in pairs, otherwise they are similar to streptococci and are now referred to as streptococci. *Streptococcus pneumoniae* is the causal agent of acute lobar pneumonia and also of meningitis, peritonitis and conjunctivitis. This organism can also initiate an invasive infection.

6.2 Gram-negative cocci

6.2.1

Neisseria and Branhamella

The Gram-negative pathogenic cocci belong to the genus *Neisseria*. The cells are slightly curved rather than true spheres and have been likened to a kidney bean in shape. They often occur in pairs and embedded in pus cells. *Neisseria gonorrhoeae* is the causal organism of the venereal disease gonorrhoea. The organism can also affect the eyes, causing a purulent ophthalmia. *Neisseria meningitidis* is a cause of cerebrospinal fever or meningococcal meningitis. *Branhamella catarrhalis* (formerly *N. catarrhalis*) is a harmless member of the genus and is often isolated from sputum.

6.3 Gram-positive rods

The genera of importance in this group are *Bacillus, Clostridium* and *Corynebacterium*.

6.3.1 *Bacillus*

Members of this genus are widespread in air, soil and water, and in animal products such as hair, wool and carcasses. It occurs characteristically as a large rod with square ends; it is aerobic and spore-forming. The most dangerous member of the group, *B. anthracis*, is the causal organism of anthrax. *Bacillus cereus* has been implicated during recent years as a cause of food poisoning, *B. polymyxa* is the source of the antibiotic polymyxin, *B. brevis* of tyrothricin and *B. subtilis* and *B. licheniformis* of bacitracin.

6.3.2 *Clostridium*

Clostridia are anaerobic, spore-forming rods. The genus contains a number of dangerous pathogens.

Clostridium septicum, Cl. perfringens (*welchii*) and *Cl. novyi* (*oedematiens*) cause serious damage to tissue if they are able to develop in wounds where the oxygen supply is limited. Tissue may be destroyed, and carbon dioxide produced from muscle glycogen gives rise to the condition known as gas gangrene.

Clostridium botulinum secretes an extremely toxic nerve poison and ingestion of food in which this organism has grown is fatal. Cooking rapidly destroys the poison but cold meats, sausages and pâtés that contain the organism and that are eaten uncooked are possible sources of botulism. *Clostridium tetani* also produces a powerful central nervous system poison and gives rise to the condition known as lockjaw or tetanus. *Clostridium sporogenes* is a non-pathogenic member of the genus and is sometimes used as a control organism for anaerobic culture media in sterility testing (although the *European Pharmacopoeia* specifies *Cl. sphenoides*: Chapter 23).

Clostridium difficile, described in older texts as of little significance as a pathogen if present in the gut, may, after therapy with antibiotics such as clindamycin or ampicillin, remain uninhibited, grow and produce toxins which give rise to a serious condition known as pseudomembranous colitis. The organism will usually succumb to vancomycin.

6.3.3 *Corynebacterium*

Corynebacterium diphtheriae, which is non-sporing, is the causal organism of diphtheria, a disease which has largely been eradicated by immunization (Chapter 16).

Gardnerella vaginalis (previously named *C. vaginale* or *Haemophilus vaginalis*), although often part of the normal flora of the vagina, can be a cause of vaginitis. It has been suggested that the condition is expressed in association with anaerobes. It responds to treatment with metronidazole (Chapter 5).

6.3.4 *Listeria*

Listeria monocytogenes has been known as a pathogen since the 1920s. It has achieved prominence and some notoriety lately as a contaminant in dairy products. It occurs as a non-sporing Gram-positive coccobacillus or rod-shaped organism, and is able to survive and multiply at low temperatures. Thus, it is essential that freezer cabinets in retail outlets should be maintained at temperatures low enough to prevent growth of the organism.

Ingestion of *L. monocytogenes* can cause abortion in humans and animals and in the case of listeriosis a prime characteristic is an increase in monocytes.

Listeriosis may be treated with a combination of ampicillin and gentamicin.

6.4 Gram-negative rods

6.4.1 *Pseudomonas*

Pseudomonas aeruginosa (*pyocyanea*) has, in recent years, assumed the role of a dangerous pathogen. It has long been a troublesome cause of secondary infection of wounds, especially burns, but is not necessarily pathogenic. With the advent of immuno-suppressive therapy following organ transplant, systemic infections including pneumonia have resulted from infection by this organism. It has also been implicated in eye infections resulting in the loss of sight.

Pseudomonas aeruginosa is resistant to many antibacterial agents (Chapters 9, 13) and is biochemically very versatile, being able to use many disinfectants as food sources.

6.4.2 *Vibrio*

Vibrio cholerae (*comma*) is often seen in the form of a curved rod (or a comma), hence its alternative specific name. It is the causal organism of Asiatic cholera. This disease is still endemic in India and Burma, and was in the UK until the nineteenth century, the last epidemic occurring in 1866. It is a water-borne organism and infection may be prevented in epidemics by boiling all water and consuming only well-cooked foodstuffs. *Vibrio parahaemolyticus* occurs in sea water and has been implicated in food poisoning following consumption of raw fish. It accounts for more than half the cases of food poisoning in Japan, where raw fish, suchi, is an important dietary item. Food poisoning from this organism also occurs in the UK.

6.4.3 *Yersinia and Francisella*

Yersinia pestis (formerly *Pasteurella pestis*) is the causal organism of plague or the Black Death which ravaged the UK at various times, the Great Plague occurring in 1348. It infects the lymphatic system to give bubonic plague, the more usual form, or the respiratory system, giving the rapidly fatal pneumonic plague.

Francisella tularensis (formerly *Pasteurella tularensis*) causes tularaemia in humans, a disease endemic in the American Midwest and contracted from infected animals.

6.4.4 *Bordetella*

Bordetella pertussis is the causal organism of whooping-cough, a disease which has been largely eradicated by a successful immunization programme (Chapter 16).

6.4.5   *Brucella*

This genus is found in many domesticated animals and in some wild species.

Brucella abortus is a cause of spontaneous abortion in cattle. In humans it causes undulant fever, i.e. a fever in which temperature undulates with time. *Brucella melitensis* infects goats; it causes an undulant fever called Malta fever, which is common in people living in Mediterranean countries where large flocks of goats are kept.

Brucella suis is found in pigs; it too manifests itself in humans as undulant fever and occurs frequently in North America.

6.4.6   *Haemophilus*

Haemophilus influenzae owes its specific name to the fact that it was thought to be the causal organism of influenza (now known to be a virus disease) as it was often isolated in cases of influenza. It is the main cause of infantile meningitis and conjunctivitis and is one of the most important causes of chronic bronchitis.

6.4.7   *Escherichia*

Escherichia coli and the organisms listed below (sections 6.4.8–6.4.12) are members of a group of microorganisms known as the enterobacteria, so called because they inhabit the intestines of humans and animals. Many selective and diagnostic media and differential biochemical reactions are available to isolate and distinguish members of this group, as they are of great significance in public health.

Escherichia coli is a cause of enteritis in young infants and the young of farm animals, where it can cause diarrhoea and fatal dehydration. It is a common infectant of the urinary tract and bladder in humans, and is a cause of pyelitis, pyelonephritis and cystitis.

6.4.8   *Salmonella*

Salmonella typhi is the causal organism of typhoid fever, *Sal. paratyphi* causes paratyphoid fever, whilst *Sal. typhimurium, Sal. enteritidis* and very many other closely related organisms are a cause of bacterial food poisoning.

6.4.9   *Shigella*

Shigella shiga, Sh. flexneri, Sh. sonnei and *Sh. boydii* are the causes of bacillary dysentery.

6.4.10   *Proteus (Morganella, Providencia)*

Proteus vulgaris and *Pr. morganii* can infect the urinary tract of humans. They are avid decomposers of urea, producing ammonia and carbon dioxide. These organisms occasionally cause wound infection. Some species have the generic name *Morganella* or *Providencia*.

6.4.11   *Serratia marcescens*

This very small organism, 0.5–1.0 μm long, has been used to test bacterial filters. It is not to be regarded as non-pathogenic, although infections arising from it are rare.

6.4.12   *Klebsiella*

Klebsiella pneumoniae subsp. *aerogenes* is found in the gut and respiratory tract of man and animals, and in soil and water. It may be distinguished from *E. coli* by a pattern of biochemical tests (Table 1.3). It can give rise to acute bronchopneumonia in humans but is not a common pathogen.

6.4.13   *Flavobacterium*

Various species of this characteristically pigmented genus occur in water and soil and can contaminate pharmaceutical products.

6.4.14   *Acinetobacter*

This genus has the same distribution and the same opportunities for causing contamination as *Flavobacterium*. These organisms are not pigmented.

6.4.15   *Bacteroides*

The characteristic of this genus is that its members are anaerobes. They occur in the alimentary tract of humans and animals and have been associated with wound infections, especially after surgery. *Bacteroides fragilis* is a frequently encountered member of the genus.

6.4.16   *Campylobacter*

Campylobacters are thin, Gram-negative organisms which are in essence rod-shaped but often appear in culture with one or more spirals or as 'S' and 'W' (gull-winged) shaped cells. They are microaerophilic or anaerobic and move by means of a single polar flagellum. They are unable to grow below 30°C.

Table 1.3 Comparison of *E. coli* and *K. pneumoniae* subsp. *aerogenes*

	Indole	MR	VP	Citrate	44°C
E. coli	+	+	−	−	−
K. pneumoniae subsp. *aerogenes*	−	−	+	+	+

Campylobacter jejuni has emerged during the last few years as a major cause of enteritis in humans and is mainly transmitted by contaminated food, in other words it is a food-poisoning microorganism.

6.4.17 Helicobacter

This genus, originally grouped with the campylobacters (section 6.4.16), is now considered a separate genus. *Helicobacter pylori* is of interest as a cause of peptic ulcer.

6.4.18 Chlamydia

The diseases associated with chlamydias (e.g. psittacosis) were at one time thought to be due to what were regarded as large viruses.

Chlamydias, however, are bacteria and have been shown to possess a cell wall containing muramic acid (section 2.2.1), to contain ribosomes of the bacterial (prokaryotic) type, to reproduce themselves by binary fission and to be inhibited by antibiotics active against bacteria.

They are coccoid-shaped organisms and the feature which at one time consigned them to the virus class was the fact that they would only reproduce in living tissue.

Chlamydia psittaci is the causal organism of psittacosis or ornithosis and occurs mainly in the parrot family (hence psittacosis), but it is now known to be found in other avian species (hence ornithosis). It is often found in persons who work in pet shops selling parrots and budgerigars, and can be fatal.

Chlamydia trachomatis can cause a variety of diseases in humans, for example trachoma, conjunctivitis and non-gonococcal urethritis. It is sensitive to the rifampicins, the tetracyclines and erythromycin.

6.4.19 Rickettsia

This group of microorganisms shares with chlamydias the property of growing only in living tissue. Rickettsiae occur as small ($0.3 \times 0.25\,\mu$m) rod-shaped or coccoid cells. They can be stained by special procedures. Division is by binary fission. They may be cultivated in the blood of laboratory animals or in the yolk sac of the embryo of the domestic fowl, and it is by this method that the organism is grown to produce vaccines.

Infection with rickettsiae gives rise to a variety of typhus infections in humans, the intermediate carriers being lice, fleas, ticks or mites. Rickettsiae can occur without harm to these arthropod hosts.

Amongst the diseases caused by rickettsiae are epidemic typhus, trench fever and murine typhus, caused by *R. prowazeki*, *R. quintana* and *R. typhi*, respectively. Q-fever is caused by *Coxiella burneti*.

6.4.20 Legionella

Few people can have failed to have heard of Legionnaires' disease or legionellosis.

The causal organism of this disease, which must have existed undetected from time immemorial, was isolated and verified in 1977 and called *L. pneumophila*.

It causes an influenza-like fever which is accompanied by pneumonia in 90% of cases and which was usually diagnosed as atypical or viral pneumonia.

Legionella pneumophila is a rod-shaped, Gram-negative organism which grows on a conventional laboratory medium provided the concentrations of cysteine and iron are optimal. The organism will grow on a medium of sterilized tap water. This is in keeping with its known habitat of water supplies, especially water maintained in storage tanks, and must rely on the correct nutrients being present in the water.

The organism is sensitive to the antibiotic erythromycin (Chapter 5).

In addition to *L. pneumophila*, 16 other species of *Legionella* of proven pathogenicity have been described.

6.5 Acid-fast organisms

These comprise a group of organisms which, like the Gram-positive and Gram-negative groups, have been named after a staining reaction.

Due to a waxy component in the cell wall these organisms are difficult to stain with ordinary stain solutions, the hydrophobic nature of the wall being stain repellent; however, if the bacterial smear on the slide is warmed with the stain, the cells are dyed so strongly that they are not decolorized by washing with dilute acid, hence the term acid-fast. Many bacterial spores exhibit the phenomenon of acid fastness.

6.5.1 *Mycobacterium*

Mycobacterium tuberculosis is the causal organism of tuberculosis in humans. Allied strains cause infections in animals, e.g. bovine tuberculosis and tuberculosis in rodents. Due to the waxy nature of the cell wall this organism will resist desiccation and will survive in sputum. Tuberculosis has been largely eliminated by immunization and chemotherapy.

Mycobacterium leprae is the cause of leprosy.

6.6 Spirochaetes

Spirochaetes have a unique shape, structure and mode of locomotion. They are not stained easily by normal staining methods and thus cannot be designated either Gram-negative or Gram-positive. They are best observed by dark-ground illumination. They are slender rods in the form of spirals, like a corkscrew, and may be as long as $500\,\mu$m. Examples of spirochaete genera follow.

6.6.1 *Borrelia*

Borrelia recurrentis causes a relapsing fever in humans. *Borrelia vincenti* is the cause of Vincent's angina in humans, an ulcerative condition of the mouth and gums. *Borrelia burgdorferi* is the causal organism of the tick-borne Lyme disease.

Treponema

Treponema pallidum is the causal organism of syphilis. *Treponema pertenue* causes the tropical disease called yaws.

Leptospira

Leptospira icterohaemorrhagiae is the cause of a type of jaundice in humans called Weil's disease. The disease is carried by rats and is encountered in sewer workers. Other species of *Leptospira*, with hosts ranging from domestic animals such as the pig to wild animals such as opossums and jackals, give rise to a variety of fevers encountered locally or widely across the world.

Note: All organisms are potential pathogens in ill or immunologically compromised patients.

7 Further reading

Buchanan R.E. & Gibbons N.E. (eds) (1974) *Bergey's Manual of Determinative Bacteriology*, 8th edn. Baltimore: Williams & Wilkins.

Collee J.G., Duguid J.P., Fraser A.G. & Marmion B.P. (1989) *Mackie & McCartney's Practical Microbiology*, 13th edn. Edinburgh: Churchill Livingstone.

Cowan S.T. (1993) *Cowan and Steel's Manual for the Identification of Medical Bacterial*, 3rd edn. (eds G. Barrow & R.K.A. Feltham). Cambridge: Cambridge University Press.

Davis B.D., Dulbecco R., Eisen H. & Ginsberg H.S. (1990) *Microbiology*, 4th edn. Philadelphia: J.B. Lippincott.

Dawes I.W. & Sutherland I.W. (1991) *Microbial Physiology*, 2nd edn. Oxford: Blackwell Scientific Publications.

Gould G.W. (1983) Mechanisms of resistance and dormancy. In: *The Bacterial Spore* (eds A. Hurst & G.W. Gould), vol. 2, pp. 173–209. London: Academic Press.

Gould G.W. (1985) Modification of resistance and dormancy. In: *Fundamental and Applied Aspects of Bacterial Spores* (eds G.J. Dring, D.J. Ellar & G.W. Gould), pp. 371–382. London: Academic Press.

Hugo W.B. (1972) *An Introduction to Microbiology*, 2nd edn. London: Heinemann Medical Books.

Logan N.A. (1994) *Bacterial Systematics*. Oxford: Blackwell Science.

Olds R.J. (1975) *A Colour Atlas of Microbiology*. London: Wolfe Publishing.

Oxoid Manual (1990) Compiled by Bridson, E.Y. 6th edn. Alton: Alphaprint.

Parker M.T. & Collier L.H. (eds) (1990) *Topley and Wilson's Principles of Bacteriology, Virology and Immunity*, 8th edn., vols 1–5. London: Edward Arnold.

Rose A.H. (1976) *Chemical Microbiology*, 3rd edn. London: Butterworths.

Russell A.D. (1982) *The Destruction of Bacterial Spores*. London: Academic Press.

Skerman V.B.D., McGowan V. & Sneath P.H.A. (1980) Approved list of bacterial names. *Int J Syst Bacteriol*, **30**, 225–240.

Stokes E.J. & Ridgway G.L. (1993) *Clinical Microbiology*, 7th edn. London: Edward Arnold.

Stryer L. (1995) *Biochemistry*, 5th edn. San Francisco: W.H. Freeman & Co.

The following references are included because, although of an advanced nature, they concern the interaction of drugs and bacteria.

Chopra I. (1988) Efflux of antibacterial agents from bacteria. *FEMS Symposium No. 44: Homeostatic Mechanisms of Microorganisms*, pp. 146–58. Bath: Bath University Press.

Costerton J.W., Cheng K.-J., Geesey G.G., Ladd T.I., Nickel J.C., Dasgupta M. & Marrie T.J. (1987) Bacterial biofilms in nature and disease. *Annu Rev Microbiol*, **41**, 435–464.

Hammond S.M., Lambert P.A. & Rycroft A.N. (1984) *The Bacterial Cell Surface*. London: Croom Helm.

Hinkle P.C. & McCarty R.E. (1976) How cells make ATP. *Sci Am*, **238**, 104–123.

Nikaido H. & Vaara T. (1986) Molecular basis of bacterial outer membrane permeability. *Microbiol Rev*, **49**, 1–32.

Russell A.D. & Chopra I. (1996) *Understanding Antibacterial Action and Resistance*, 2nd edn. Chichester: Ellis Horwood.

The references below refer to the subject matter in 5.6.

Microscopy, DEFT

Pettipher G.J., Mansell R., McKinnon C.H. & Cousins, C.M. (1980) Rapid membrane filtration—epifluorescent technique for direct inumeration of bacteria in raw milk. *Appl Environ Microbiol*, **39**, 423–429.

Denyer S.P. & Ward K.H. (1983) A rapid method for the detection of bacterial contaminants in intravenous fluids using membrane filtration and epifluorescent microscopy. *J Parental Sci Technol*, **37**, 156–158.

Flow cytometry

Shapiro H.M. (1990) Flow cytometry in laboratory microbiology: new directions. *Am Soc Microbiol News*, **56**, 584–586.

Microcalorimetry

Beezer A.E. (1980) *Biological Microcalorimetry*. London: Academic Press.

Impedance

Silley P. & Forsythe S. (1996) Impedance microbiology—a rapid change for microbiologists. *J Bacteriol* **80**, 233–243.

Bioluminescence

Stanley P.E., McCarthy B.J. & Smither R. (eds) (1989) *ATP Luminescence: Rapid Methods in Microbiology*. Society of Applied Bacteriology Technical Series No. 26. Oxford: Blackwell Scientific Publications.

Stewart G.S.A.B., Loessner M.J. & Scherer S. (1996) The bacterial lux gene bioluminescent biosensor revisited. *Am Soc Microbiol News*, **62**, 297–301.

General reference

Stannard C.J., Petit S.B. & Skinner F.A. (1989) *Rapid Microbiological Methods for Foods, Beverages and Pharmaceuticals*. Society of Applied Bacteriology Technical Series No. 25. Oxford: Blackwell Scientific Publications.

2 Yeasts and moulds

1 Introduction

2 *Saccharomyces cerevisiae*
2.1 The life cycle
2.2 Metabolism and physiology
2.3 Cell wall

3 *Candida albicans*
3.1 Pharmaceutical and clinical significance
3.2 Alternative morphologies

4 *Cryptococcus neoformans*

5 *Neurospora crassa*

6 *Penicillium* and *Aspergillus*

7 *Epidermophyton, Microsporum* and *Trichophyton*

8 References

1 Introduction

Yeasts and moulds are members of the fungi. Yeasts are characterized as being essentially unicellular, whereas moulds are composed of filaments which *en masse* frequently appear fuzzy or powdery. The familar budding yeast *Saccharomyces cerevisiae*, also known as Baker's or Brewer's yeast, is usually thought of as the typical yeast. The green mould *Penicillium digitatum,* a frequent spoiler of fruits such as apples or oranges, and the bread mould *Neurospora crassa* will also be well-known to many. These latter two organisms are properly considered as typical moulds. As is usually the case, however, life is not completely straightforward for there are a considerable number of so-called 'dimorphic fungi' which can alternate between yeast-like and filamentous forms. One such organisms is *Candida albicans.* To make matters more complicated, it has been rediscovered that the would-be typical yeast *S. cerevisiae* can also form filaments under a variety of different conditions (Gimeno *et al.* 1992). All of these fungi have pharmaceutical and medical significance. The precise nature of this significance is different in each case. For example, *S. cerevisiae* is generally regarded as a totally safe organism suitable for use in human food and drink; the reason for its importance is because it is by far the best understood eukaryotic organism on the planet. In contrast, *Cryptococcus neoformans* has a variety of ways by which it can evade defence mechanisms of the immune system, but is relatively little studied. In between these two extremes are many yeasts and moulds, which are omnipresent in the environment, in or on our foods, or a part of the normal flora of humans, but all of which can opportunistically contaminate pharmaceutical preparations or cause post-operative disease. All fungi pose a threat to immunocompromised individuals. This knowledge should be weighed against a background of a general lack of suitable antifungal agents (see Chapter 5). The approach of this chapter will be to first describe *S. cerevisiae* in considerable detail because so much is known about it. Then, other yeasts and moulds will be considered in turn, pointing out (where appropriate) significant differences from *S. cerevisiae* or from each other.

2 *Saccharomyces cerevisiae*

Saccharomyces cerevisiae has a predominant place in the realms of cell biology and molecular biology where it has become accepted as the universal model eukaryote. The main reason for this is its genetic tractability. Traditionally, for reasons associated with its importance to the food and drink industry, a great deal was known about the biochemistry and physiology of this yeast. Later, with the advent of yeast genetics, a vast range of well-characterized mutants became available. In turn, because *S. cerevisiae* can be transformed and is readily amenable to genetic manipulation, this permitted the isolation and characterization of many yeast genes. Ultimately, in mid 1996 the nucleotide sequence of the entire genome of the organism was reported. This achievement is still only a far-off dream for molecular biologists studying most other eukaryotic organisms. Nevertheless, it is possible to identify genes from other organisms by means of genetic complementation in *S. cerevisiae*. Explained briefly, only one piece of DNA from another organism will be able to substitute for a mutation in a known gene in *S. cerevisiae*—this is a segment of DNA which carries the homologous gene (i.e. codes for the same function) in the other organism. The availability of well-defined mutants in *S. cerevisiae* combined with the facility of genetic manipulation and this yeast's short generation time, make this a very rapid way to identify heterologous (i.e. belonging to *another* organism) genes. Many of the latest concepts in cell and molecular biology (e.g. concerning control of the cell cycle) have been developed and tested in this organism. Naturally then, since it is the prime model eukaryote, it is also the best understood fungus.

2.1 The life cycle

The life cycle of *S. cerevisiae* is shown in Fig. 2.1. It can exist both as a haploid (one copy of each chromosome per cell) or as a diploid (two copies of each chromosome per cell). Haploids exists as one of two sexes referred to as mating type **a** and mating type *α*. When two haploid cells come close together they cause each other to arrest in the G1 phase of the cell cycle. Each subsequently produces a special protuberance enabling growth towards the mating partner. These somewhat abnormal looking cells are termed 'schmoos'. A haploid will only mate with another haploid of the opposite mating type. This is achieved by the expression of specific oligopeptide mating pheromones (hormones with brings about behavioual change in cells of the opposite sex) and the possession of surface receptors only for the opposite pheromone (hence, mating type **a** strains produce only **a**-factor and have receptors for *α*-factor, whilst mating type *α* strains produce only *α*-factor and have receptors for **a**-factor). The resulting diploid, like the haploids from which it arose, is capable of repeated rounds of vegetative reproduction.

The vegetative cell cycle of *S. cerevisiae* has received extensive attention. There are many justifications for this. Firstly, the cell cycle in this organism has many convenient 'landmarks' (Hartwell 1974, 1978; Pringle 1978) which make it very easy to identify the exact point in the cell cycle at which a cell happens to be. Examples of these landmark events include bud emergence, the size of the bud, mitosis (nuclear division takes place through the neck between the 'mother' cell and the bud), and cell

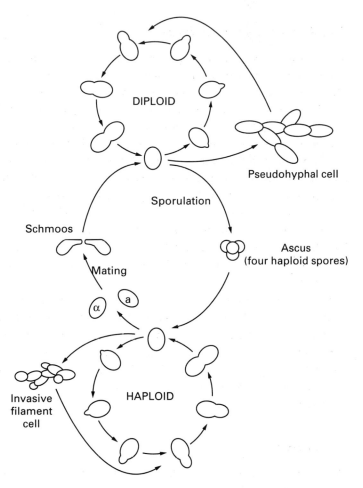

Fig. 2.1 The life cycle of *Saccharomyces cerevisiae*.

separation. Other markers of cell cycle progress are also apparent to the more experienced observer (Fig. 2.2). The reader will notice from Fig. 2.2 that the 'daughter' which is formed is smaller than the mother cell from which it arose. There is a size control which operates over initiation of a new cell cycle (Pringle & Hartwell 1981), and since the mother is larger than the minimum size necessary to pass this control, but the daughter is not, the consequence is that the mother cell can immediately start a new cell cycle, whereas the daughter must first grow for a period until it is large enough. Hence, mother and daughter do not proceed through the next cell cycle synchronously. The significant extent of morphological change throughout the cell cycle provides another reason for studying this yeast as the construction of defined morphology.

A third justification for studying the cell cycle of this yeast is that it affords a convenient system in which to study cell polarity. Together with asymmetric cell division (inherent in the *S. cerevisiae* cell cycle with the unequal sized mothers and daughters), the development of polarity is crucial in many aspects of development and differentiation. Furthermore, as explained in more detail later in this chapter, the correct

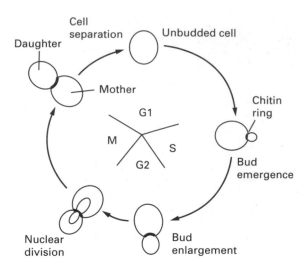

Fig. 2.2 'Landmark' events in the cell cycle of *Saccharomyces cerevisiae*. G1, S, G2 and M are the classical phases of the eukaryotic cell cycle.

development of polarity is an essential aspect in the life of most fungi. The development of polarity and the resulting asymmetric division can be considered as five constituent processes (Lew & Reed 1995) shown schematically in Fig. 2.3. These are:

1   the F-actin cytoskeleton;
2   the polarity of growth achieved by the way new cell wall material is arranged;
3   the location of 10-nm neck filaments;
4   formation of the cell 'cap';
5   the distribution of DNA and microtubules.

The construction of a yeast cell requires isotropic growth. Bud emergence is signalled by the accumulation of secretory vesicles, the rho protein Cdc42p and a cap of membrane-localized actin patches. Once the cap is established, subsequent bud emergence is accomplished entirely by polarized growth. Following bud emergence, the rings of 10-nm filaments remain at the mother/bud neck, whereas the proteins in the cap concentrate at the tip of the bud where secretion takes place. Later, there is a critical switch back to isotropic growth which brings about swelling of the bud. Most of the proteins of the cap appear to disperse simultaneously with the apical/isotropic switch. At cytokinesis, secretion is redirected to the neck and the proteins of the cap redistribute to this region. Mutants have been isolated which distinguish between the separate components and processes. In turn, the genes which the mutations have identified have all been characterized.

The pattern of budding in haploids differs from that in diploids (Friefelder 1960). Haploids grown in rich medium bud in an axial pattern, i.e. each new bud site is placed adjacent to the previous one. In the same rich nutrient conditions diploids exhibit bipolar budding, in this case choosing new bud sites at either end of the cell (Fig. 2.4). Under a variety of other conditions, all presumably involving some form of nutrient limitation, diploids will form pseudohyphae and haploids will form invasive filaments. As alluded to earlier in this chapter, this represents a 'rediscovery' in the case of *S. cerevisiae* because it had been known for a long time and forms part of the basic taxonomy. Its significance had been ignored. This situation arose because the ability to form these structures had been crossed-out of the genetic background of many academic strains

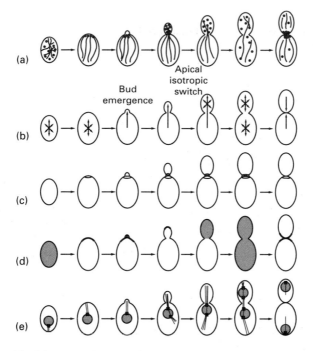

Fig. 2.3 The development of polarity and asymmetric division in *Saccharomyces cerevisiae*. The diagram is reproduced in a slightly simplified form from the work of Lew & Reed (1995) with the permission of *Current Opinion in Genetics and Development*. (a) The F-actin cytoskeleton: strands = actin cables; (●) cortical actin patches. (b) The polarity of growth is indicated by the direction of the arrows; (arrows in many directions signifies isotropic growth). (c) 10-nm filaments which are assembled to form a ring at the neck between mother and bud. (d) Construction of the 'cap' at the pre-bud site. Notice that the proteins of the cap become dispersed at the apical/isotropic switch, first over the whole surface of the bud, then more widely. Finally, secretion becomes refocussed at the neck in time for cytokinesis. (e) The status and distribution of the nucleus and microtubules of the spindle. Notice how the spindle pole body (■) plays an important part in orientation of the mitotic spindle.

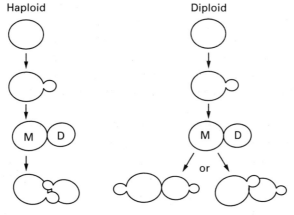

Fig. 2.4 The budding pattern in haploid and diploid *Saccharomyces cerevisiae*. The original cell which formed a bud is the mother (M). The daughter cell (D) is shown remaining attached as might be the case in colonies growing on the surface of agar.

around the world. Pseudohyphae are chains of regular-shaped, elongated cells in which unipolar budding predominates. The analogous situation in colonies of haploids growing on solid media is the formation of invasive filaments which are capable of penetrating the agar. The generally accepted view is that starvation of nitrogen is the signal for the switch from the yeast to a filamentous form (Kron *et al.* 1994), although it has also been shown that pseudohyphal growth is strictly oxygen-dependent (Wright *et al.* 1993) and that limitation of oxygen during continuous cultivation can result in the formation of pseudohyphae (Kuriyama & Slaughter 1995). In 1996 Dickinson showed that, dependent upon the concentration used, 'fusel' alcohols, i.e. *n*-amyl, isoamyl alcohol, etc., caused the formation of hyphal-like extensions or pseudohyphae in a wide number of different yeast species which were being cultured in rich liquid media where the cells would normally proliferate as yeasts rather than in any other form (Dickinson 1996). It seems reasonable to conclude that since fusel alcohols are produced when the yeasts are under various conditions of nutrient stress, the many situations which have been reported to induce pseudohyphal formation are triggered by fusel alcohols. As we have already noted, yeast-form proliferation is asymmetric and asynchronous; in contrast, as others have already observed (Kron & Gow 1995), pseudohyphal growth is symmetric and synchronous and, as will become apparent later in this chapter, hyphal growth is symmetric and asynchronous (Fig. 2.5).

The diplophase and haplophase are equally stable. Hence, in the presence of adequate nutrients, both are capable of repeated rounds of vegetative growth and mitosis. However, in the presence of a poorly utilized carbon source such as acetate, and usually in the absence of a nitrogen source, diploid strains switch to the alternative developmental pathway of meiosis and spore formation. This process of sporulation gives rise to structures termed 'asci'. Each single ascus contains four haploid ascospores (usually referred to simply as 'spores'). Sporulation in diploid strains of *S. cerevisiae* has been studied as a simple unicellular model of differentiation because it involves the co-ordination of a complex sequence of genetic, biochemical and morphological events (Fig. 2.6). The developmental switch occurs only in the G1 phase of the cell cycle, in normal (**a**/α) diploids which are respiratorily complete. Hence, it requires the co-ordination of signals about the environment, about the physiological and metabolic

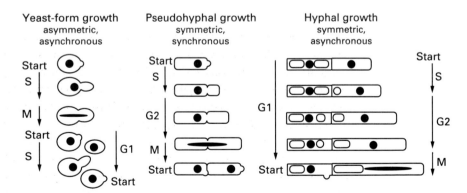

Fig. 2.5 Cell cycles resulting in yeast-form cells, pseudohyphae and hyphae. In many respects the cell cycle of pseudohyphal cells is similar to that of yeast-form cells, except that in pseudohyphae G2 is prolonged, thus larger daughter cells are produced which are identical in size to the mother cell. Hence, mother and daughter are both sufficiently large to start the next cell cycle and so bud synchronously. In hyphae the apical cell becomes progressively longer. The diagram is reproduced from the review of Kron & Gow (1995) with the permission of *Current Opinion in Cell Biology*.

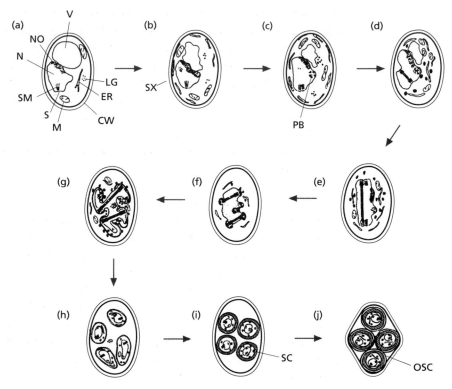

Fig. 2.6 The morphological events of sporulation in *Saccharomyces cerevisiae*. (a) starved cell: V, vacuole; LG, lipid granule; ER, endoplasmic reticulum; CW, cell wall; M, mitochondrion; S, spindle pole; SM, spindle microtubules; N, nucleus; NO, nucleolus. (b) Synaptonemal complex (SX) and development of polycomplex body (PB) along with division of spindle pole body in (c). (d) First meiotic division which is completed in (e). (f) Prepararation for meiosis II. (g) Enlargement of prospore wall, culminating in enclosure of separate haploid nuclei (h). (i) Spore coat (SC) materials produced and deposited, giving rise to the distinct outer spore coat (OSC) seen in the completed spores of the mature ascus (j). Reproduced from the review by Dickinson (1988) with permission from Blackwell Science Ltd.

status of the cell along with a way of monitoring the cell's ploidy and position in the cell cycle. It is attractive for study because it involves meiosis, a relatively rare event that occurs only in cells of specialized tissues in higher eukaryotes, and because it allows the study of developmentally regulated gene expression. Transfer to the sporulation pathway also involves a number of distinct metabolic switches (Dickinson 1988; Dickinson & Hewlins 1991). The whole process can be completed within 24 hours. The products of sporulation (haploid ascospores) have far greater resistance to heat, solvents, dehydration, etc. than vegetative cells. If returned to good nutrient conditions the spores will germinate and commence proliferation as free-living haploids. This whole sequence of events forms the basis of conventional genetics and laboratory strain construction in this yeast. Two haploids of opposite mating type each carrying particular mutations are placed in close proximity to each other on the surface of an agar medium. After mating and subsequent formation of the diploid, the cells can be replica plated to a different medium to allow selection for the diploid and against the parental haploids. ('Replica plating' involves making a replica of a group of cells which are growing on one type of medium onto one, or more, different media. This is done by pressing the agar surface of a Petri dish carrying cells onto a sheet of sterile velvet. Subsequently, other, uninoculated, Petri dishes can receive doses of these cells by being pressed onto the surface of the velvet). This is most simply arranged by ensuring that each parental haploid has different auxotrophic requirements, hence the resultant diploid will be able to grow on a minimal medium (due to complementation) whereas neither of the parents can. After 1–3 days growth, the diploid will then be replica plated again onto a sporulation medium. When the asci have formed, the individual spore progeny can be separately grown as individual clones (a clone is a group of cells which are genetically identical). This final step is accomplished by enzymatic digestion of the ascus wall followed by micromanipulation of the individual spores (a process known as 'dissection'). Due to the fact that meiotic recombination took place during sporulation, the spores will have different combinations of mutations to those present in the original parents. The precise combination of mutations in each spore can be determined by analysing the phenotypes.

2.2 Metabolism and physiology

Saccharomyces cerevisiae is normally described as a faculative anaerobe which means that it is able to proliferate under either anaerobic or aerobic conditions. It is able to utilize a wide range of mono-, di- and oligosaccharides, ethanol, acetate, glycerol, pyruvate and lactate. The favourite carbon source is glucose and the preferred mode of metabolism is fermentative using the Embden–Meyerhof pathway (EMP) resulting in the formation of ethanol. Many aspects of metabolism and physiology in this organism (not merely carbon metabolism) are subject to catabolite repression which in most cases means glucose repression. In the presence of glucose, synthesis of the enzymes necessary for disaccharide (sucrose and maltose) or galactose utilization and for growth on non-fermentable carbon sources (ethanol, acetate, glycerol, pyruvate and lactate) as well as mitochondrial development are repressed. As the repressing substrate (glucose) is consumed its concentration falls and the cells are said to become 'derepressed'; this occurs typically at glucose concentrations below 0.2%. In other words, induction of respiratory enzymes and components of the mitochondrial electron transport chain occurs. This metabolic switch takes place late in the exponential phase of a batch culture. As the cells pass through the deceleration phase and enter the stationary phase they will be fully derepressed and will start to consume the ethanol that was produced earlier. This requires the full participation of the tricarboxylic acid (TCA) and glyoxylate cycles for the complete oxidation of ethanol to carbon dioxide and water. Cells utilizing any of the non-fermentable carbon sources are also carrying out gluconeogenesis. The glucose-6-phosphate produced as a result of this gluconeogenesis is used both for the production of storage carbohydrate (trehalose) and for 'shuttling' around the hexose monophosphate pathway (HMP) for synthesis of ribose which is required for nucleotide (and hence ultimately nucleic acid) biosynthesis. The importance of the glycolytic pathway to *S. cerevisiae* cannot be overstated. This is underlined by the frequently quoted figure that the enzymes of glycolysis represent 30–65% (depending upon physiological conditions) of soluble protein (Fraenkel 1982). The storage material trehalose is produced in large quantities during sporulation (Dickinson *et al.* 1983). It confers to the spore the ability to withstand dehydration. A wide range of organisms in low water environments utilize trehalose for the same purpose including most insects and the remarkable drought-resisting resurrection plant *Selaginella lepidophylla* which can survive protracted desiccation until rains return (Leopold 1986). Trehalose does this by preventing phase transitions within membranes (Crowe *et al.* 1984). The compound is now added to a considerable number of laboratory products in order to extend their shelf-life and its use in pharmaceutical and medical materials including plasma, blood-based products, whole cells and tissues is under active investigation for the same reason.

Notwithstanding the foregoing, an important constraint on this otherwise metabolically flexible organism is the fact that proliferation under truly anaerobic conditions (something that is very difficult to achieve in the laboratory) is not possible without the provision of unsaturated fatty acid and sterol (Andreasen & Stier 1953, 1954). These are required for the assembly of membranes. Naturally, mutants defective in fatty acid or sterol biosynthesis have such requirements, but so do mutants with defects in porphoryin biosynthesis due to the involvement of haematin in the synthesis of both groups of compounds. Wild-type *S. cerevisiae* do not take up sterol under aerobic conditions. It is possible to supply a limited range of alternative sterols instead of the yeast's usual ergosterol. The ability of such an alternative sterol to support growth of anaerobic *S. cerevisiae* is a way of assessing the structural specificity of sterol requirement (Henry 1982). Some yeast sterol mutants were isolated as auxotrophs requiring ergosterol whilst others were obtained on the basis of resistance to the polyene antibiotic nystatin. Polyene antibiotics alter membrane permeability by interaction with specific membrane sterols (Cass *et al.* 1970; Norman *et al.* 1972; see Chapter 8) and seem not to inhibit lipid synthesis. Hence, mutants resistant to polyene antibiotics have been useful in identifying the effects of altered sterol composition on different membranes within the cell. This can be reflected in, for example, altered permeability to a specific molecule or ion.

2.3 Cell wall

The cell wall of *S. cerevisiae,* like that of other fungi, is very strong. Despite its great strength, one should remember that the cell wall is a dynamic structure (unlike a brick wall). There are three major components:

1   an internal glucan layer,
2   the external layer of mannoproteins;
3   chitin which occupies various specialized locations.

Cell wall composition varies according to physiological conditions and developmental status. For example, the wall of cells from stationary phase is much more resistant to degradation by β-glucanase than that from exponential phase cells (Necas 1971). The glucan of *S. cerevisiae* is mainly β(1–3)-linked glucoses with branching via β(1–6)-linked glucose units (Manners *et al.* 1973a, b). Most of the mannoproteins can only be released after enzymatic degradation of the glucan layer. There are long α(1–6)-mannose chains with α(1–2) and α(1–3) side chains *N*-linked to asparagine. There are also short mannose chains *O*-linked to serine or threonine (Van Rinsum *et al.* 1991). The carbohydrate chains of the mannoprotein layer are the main antigenic determinants when *S. cerevisiae* is injected into laboratory mammals. Chitin is a $\beta(1-4)$-linked polymer of *N*-acetylglucosamine. It confers enormous mechanical strength. In *S. cerevisiae* a ring of chitin is formed at the mother-bud junction (see Fig. 2.2). This ring persists after cell separation and is referred to as the 'bud scar'. Chitin is readily stained with the optical brightener Calcofluor White, and all of the bud scars on a cell can easily be visualized. Thus, it is possible to determine both the 'age' of a cell (by counting the number of bud scars) and the ploidy of the cell (by observing the pattern of bud scars, because, as explained earlier, haploids and diploids have different patterns of bud formation). Indeed, ageing research is also possible in this organism (Kennedy & Guarente 1996). In spore walls, the outermost layers contain a special polymer which is based upon dityrosine (Briza *et al.* 1990).

3 · *Candida albicans*

3.1 · Pharmaceutical and clinical significance

Candida albicans is a dimorphic organism which is part of the normal body flora of humans. For the majority of normal healthy individuals it will never cause any problems. However, in a number of settings it can cause severe disruption to lifestyle or even death. In the USA it is now the third most frequent cause of nosocomial (hospital acquired) infections. Post-operative infection arises typically where a patient has been in intensive care for weeks and has undergone several cycles of bacterial infections and high dose antibacterial therapy. In excess of 50% of deep-seated *Candida* infections are lethal. Persons suffering from AIDS, transplant patients and other immuno-compromised individuals are at even greater risk. The azole family of antifungal compounds (see Chapter 5) is frequently deployed but several of these block the metabolism of cyclosporins (which are administered for chronic immunosuppressive therapy) and thereby increase immunosupressivity. A possible alternative antifungal drug is amphotericin B, but this interacts with cyclosporins to give increased nephro-toxicity. Catheterized patients can become infected with *C. parapsilosis* which causes problems by virtue of its ability to form biofilm. In many apparently normal women, *C. albicans* causes vaginal thrush which can be so extreme as to incapacitate. Some denture-wearers and malnourished children can develop thrush in the mouth; in the case of the latter this can extend to large portions of the face.

It would be reasonable to imagine that the cell wall would be a focus for attacking this organism. In reality, whilst there have been studies of the biosynthesis of cell wall materials, the precise molecular organization within the cell walls is largely unknown. β-glucans and chitin form a skeleton for the mannoproteins which are found both at the outer surface and throughout the entire cell wall. By using wheat germ agglutinin it has been shown that chitin is concentrated in the cross-walls between mother and daughter cells, but is also distributed throughout the whole of the cell wall. It has not been possible to examine the distribution of glucans using plant lectins because there is no known lectin which reacts specifically with glucans. However, the use of a monoclonal antibody that reacts with $(1,6)$-β-glucan has enabled the linkages which connect $(1,6)$-β-glucan to mannoproteins and the distribution of $(1,6)$-β-glucan in the cell walls to be studied (Sanjuán *et al.* 1995). In *S. cerevisiae,* the synthesis of $(1,6)$-β-glucan begins early in the secretory pathway whereas in *C. albicans* it is apparently incorporated at a later stage. In both yeasts, (1,6)-β-glucan is located within an inner layer of the cell wall which can be rendered accessible with tunicamycin.

In the yeast form, *C. albicans* could be confused with *S. cerevisiae* upon simple microscopic inspection. However, major differences exist which would soon become apparent even to one not familiar with yeast taxonomy. *Candida albicans* is diploid and has no sexual cycle. This means that classical genetic methods like those described for *S. cerevisiae* are not possible with this organism. Attempts to isolate mutants by the use of mutagenic agents are almost bound to fail because of the improbability of producing mutations in both copies of a given gene and nowhere else in the genome. Naturally occurring mutants do, of course, exist. The more recent developments of molecular genetics are now being applied to *Candida,* but the reader should not conclude that this organism is understood to anything like the extent of *S. cerevisiae.* The isolation of *C. albicans* genes homologous to those in *S. cerevisiae* by means of complementation of *S. cerevisiae* mutants has been particularly useful as have techniques such as 'Ura blasting' in which first one copy of a given *Candida* gene is disrupted with the coding sequence of the *URA3* gene and then the second copy is treated likewise. This process can be applied sequentially to produce a strain with defined mutations in known genes (Gow *et al.* 1993).

3.2   Alternative morphologies

One spectacular difference between *S. cerevisiae* and *C. albicans* is the ability of the latter to switch to a hyphal pattern of proliferation (Gow 1994). A variety of different factors and conditions have been described which can elicit this switch. These include serum, neutral pH, certain temperature profiles, the addition of *N*-acetylglucosamine and many more (Odds 1988). In germ tube formation, a protuberance develops from the cell and thereafter growth remains highly polarized (Fig. 2.7). The cell which forms the tip of the developing germ tube remains polarized throughout the cell cycle. It must be emphasized that this is hyphal growth where cell division is symmetric, but in contrast to pseudohyphal development (where the next cell cycle is started synchronously), in this case growth is asynchronous with the result that the apical cell becomes progressively longer (see Fig. 2.5). It has not been shown that the virulence or pathogenicity of *C. albicans* are uniquely due to either the yeast or hyphal form. Nonetheless, the ability to be able to interconvert between the distinct morphologies must surely be to its advantage. The hyphal form is considered to be specialized for foraging (Kron & Gow 1995). Even if this is not the correct conclusion, it certainly conveys the ability to penetrate tissue, whilst the yeast form would seem to be more effective for dispersal, e.g. through the blood system. One of the justifications for studying morphological switching in *C. albicans* is that this may reveal a unique target for therapy or prophylaxis.

Another form of switching is well-known in *C. albicans.* This is the phenomenon of 'phenotypic switching' (Soll 1992) whereby colony morphologies vary dramatically (e.g. white, opaque, fuzzy, wrinkled.) These may seem trivial to the pharmacist or physician, but the variability extends far beyond the mere appearance of the colonies. It can encompass a vast array of biochemical alterations, antigenicities and drug

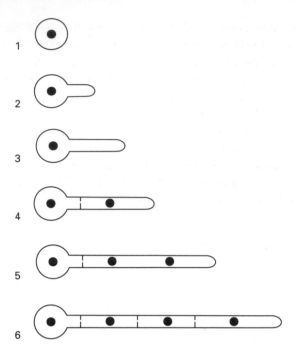

Fig. 2.7 Germ tube formation by *Candida albicans*. For simplicity the diagram merely illustrates the nuclear content of the parental yeast cell and the developing germ tube. In real life there is a complex rearrangement of cytoplasmic constituents which results in all parts except the apex becoming highly vacuolated.

sensitivities. Furthermore, it is documented that patients who have suffered from repeated vaginal candidosis have yielded the same strain which has presented an alternative phenotype on each occasion (Soll *et al.* 1989). Thus, this phenomenon seems to represent a mechanism which has evolved to enable *C. albicans* to escape destruction by the immune system. Phenotypic switching is so-called because it has been assumed that a mutational event could not be responsible due to the high frequencies (up to 10%)

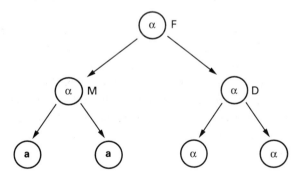

Fig. 2.8 Mating type switching in *Saccharomyces cerevisiae*. The founder cell (F) is a virgin (i.e. has not formed a bud previously), carries the *HO* gene and is mating type α. After the first cell cycle there will be the mother cell (M) and the daughter (D), both of which are mating type α. Mother cells which carry *HO* are able to switch mating type whilst in the G1 phase of the cell cycle. Assuming that M switches to mating type **a**, the progeny which result from M (a mother and a daughter) will thus both be mating type **a**. Daughters cannot switch mating type, hence D will produce two cells of mating type α. Note that two of the cells present at the four cell stage are mothers and hence capable of switching mating type before entering the next budding cycle.

observed. However, there clearly has to be a genetic basis to such variation. In *S. cerevisiae,* mating type switching can occur (Herskowitz *et al.* 1992) due to the presence of the *HO* gene. This gene confers on a haploid strain of either mating type the ability to switch to the opposite mating type. The opportunity to switch is only available to mother cells which are in the G1 phase of the cell cycle. Thus, it is quite easy to calculate that a single cell that was (say) mating type α could give rise after two complete cell cycles to a colony that comprised two cells of mating type **a** and two of mating type α (Fig. 2.8.) Hence, one could say that mating type switching in *S. cerevisiae* has a frequency of approximately 50% in appropriate strains, i.e. even higher than the frequency of phenotypic switching in *C. albicans.* The molecular basis of phenopic switching remains unclear at the time of writing.

4   *Cryptococcus neoformans*

Cryptococcus neoformans is an encapsulated yeast which causes cryptococcosis, a subacute or chronic infection of the central nervous system. In extreme cases, tissue damage can also occur in the skin, bones and internal organs. Cryptococcal meningitis is very frequent in AIDS patients. Despite this, it is not a newly discovered organism and its pathogenic capabilities have been known for many years. For example, in 1955 it was known that *Cr. neoformans* was the causative agent in 10% of all fatal human mycoses in the USA (Emmons 1955). It does not form a pseudomycelium, neither does it develop hyphae. Surely this yeast provides adequate proof that neither is necessary to be pathogenic to any warm-blooded animal! The yeast cells are almost spherical and in conditions of high osmolarity they produce a much reduced capsule, such that the overall size is less than $5\,\mu$m in diameter. This renders them small enough to remain as dust in the atmosphere and be inhaled. This is reckoned to be the route of all infections. The yeast is inhaled and carried to the alveoli of the lungs. When in the warm, moist alveoli, the yeast cells regenerate their thick capsules with the consequent release of polysaccharides and glycoproteins into the host's bloodstream, both of which serve as virulence factors (Murphy 1996). The capsule products cause neutrophils to lose their surface L-selectin, which is required for leukocytes to attach to endothelial cells before moving from the blood system to the tissues. Since the leukocytes are not sent to the site of infection in the tissue, the yeast escapes. The immune system is further confused by yeast cell products in the bloodstream due to the induction of suppressor T lymphocytes which attenuate immune responses. It is believed that the release of melanin from the yeast also helps it to evade the immune system. Melanin is thought to act as an antioxidant which thereby protects cryptococci from oxidative killing. With such an armoury of virulence, the reader will appreciate why rapid identification of this organism is so important.

5   *Neurospora crassa*

Neurospora crassa is a filamentous pink mould. It became famous to scientists due to the work of Beadle and Tatum in the 1940s when they developed the 'one gene—one enzyme' hypothesis. Its life cycle is shown in Fig. 2.9. Unfortunately, the full force of fungal nomenclature comes into play when considering this organism. Aerial hyphae

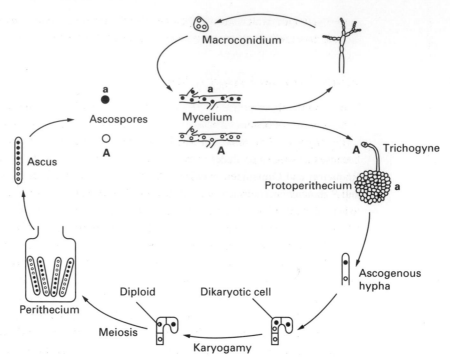

Fig. 2.9 The life cycle of *Neurospora crassa*. The figure illustrates both the asexual cycle via macroconidia and the sexual cycle. In the case of the latter, the diagram represents the interaction between a male of mating type **A** and a female of mating type **a**. The trichogyne grows towards the male. There is fusion, one male nucleus enters and pairs with a female nucleus. Rounds of synchronous nuclear divisions result in dikaryotic (i.e. containing two nuclei) cells. Karyogamy produces a true diploid which immediately undergoes meiosis and ascosporogenesis. The cycle is completed by germination of the individual ascospores to found fresh mycelia.

from the heterokaryotic (i.e. containing many separate nuclei) vegetative mycelium produce either macroconidia or microconidia. The macroconidia contain several nuclei and re-establish vegetative mycelium when they germinate. Each microconidium is uninucleate; their role in the life cycle is to fuse with the trichogyne (a specialized hypha of opposite mating type.) The trichogyne is carried on the protoperithecium, which, as its name suggests, is the precursor to the perithecium (fruiting body). Inside the perithecium, nuclear fusion takes place, followed by meiosis and further differentiation to produce an ascus containing eight ascospores. When the ascospores germinate, they produce haploid mycelia which can form heterokaryons by means of hyphal fusions with mycelia of the opposite mating type.

It is instructive to consider the similarities and differences in the life cycle of *S. cerevisiae* and *N. crassa*. Disregarding the obvious difference that the former is a yeast whilst the latter is a mould, it should be noted that both fungi have a vegetative haplophase. The diplophase of *S. cerevisiae* can proliferate, whereas in *N. crassa* the diploid rapidly undergoes meiosis and ascospore formation. Both organisms can exist in one of two mating types, each of which is controlled by a single genetic locus. *Neurospora crassa* has truly male and female thalli (singular, thallus, is the vegetative body of a fungus) which are morphologically distinct. *Neurospora crassa* is an obligate aerobe, hence, elimination of oxygen will prevent its growth.

6 *Penicillium* and *Aspergillus*

The scientifically informed layperson is aware that *Penicillium* species are associated with a number of beneficial products. These include the important antibiotic penicillin (originally from *P. notatum*, but which soon came to be prepared from *P. chrysogenum* because this species produces more: see Chapters 5 and 7), and the ripening of Stilton, Roquefort and Camembert cheeses with strains of *P. roquefortii* (blue vein cheeses) and *P. camembertii* (surface-ripened cheeses). However, many more would be surprised to learn that today's commercial penicillin-producing strains all derive from an organism which was originally isolated from a rotting Canteloupe melon. This fact emphasizes the real ecological place of such moulds where, of course, decomposition of fruits and vegetables is an essential part of the recycling of materials in the biosphere. Life could not continue on our planet in the absence of decomposer organisms.

A less desirable characteristic of many moulds is the production of mycotoxins. One group of mycotoxins, the aflatoxins, which are derived from decaketides, are a particular cause for concern. Aflatoxin B_1 is carcinogenic in animals and mammalian cell lines in tissue culture. It has been linked to specific mutations in the human tumour suppressor gene *p53* thus causing primary hepatocellular carcinoma. Hence, contamination by aflatoxins of food, feed, and medical, veterinary, pharmaceutical and laboratory preparations has serious health and economic consequences. *Aspergillus parasiticus* and *A. flavus* are notorious as producers of aflatoxins. As with other species of *Aspergillus,* they are very widespread in the environment and, aided by their rapid growth on a variety of substrates, they are commonly found as contaminants of all sorts of materials. Members of the genus can give rise to a group of diseases known collectively as aspergilloses. These includes allergies, toxicoses, tissue invasion and local colonization. *Aspergillus fumigatus* is the most common cause of aspergillosis. Not all members of the genus are wholly bad. *Aspergillus oryzae* has been used for centuries in the production of soy sauce. Although this is of little consequence in the West, the underlying technology became the foundation of the Japanese amino acid and nucleotide business which have worldwide economic importance.

It appears that the various strains of *Penicillium* used in cheese production do not produce any such toxins. Presumably this is an example of selection acting on the early human cheese-makers: the folk who produced cheese which contained mycotoxins ate their own cheese and died. Hence, they did not hand on their skills and strains of mould to subsequent generations! Microbiological contamination by wild moulds always carries the possibility of chemical contamination with their toxins, so we should not think of *Penicillium* species as being of universal benefit to humankind. Indeed, direct infections by *Penicillium* species have been reported to various parts of the human body including the cornea, ear, respiratory tract, urinary tract and heart (following the surgical insertion of artificial valves: Kwon-Chung & Bennett 1992).

Penicillium has no sexual cycle. The organisms merely produce conidia (asexually produced spores) which are readily dispersed by slight draughts (Fig. 2.10). New growth can commence after landing on a suitable substrate. The brush-like appearance is typical

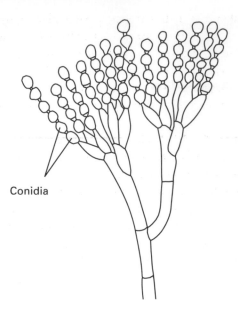

Fig. 2.10 A typical *Penicillium.*

Conidia

(Fig. 2.10). The organism *Penicillium marneffei* is said to be thermally dimorphic: at 25–30°C it produces colonies like any other of the genus. At 35–37°C it is yeast-like (Larone 1995). It is endemic in South-East Asia and is reported as causing deep-seated infections in both immunocompromised and normal individuals who have visited those parts. The wider significance of this to fungal biology and especially to the taxonomy of *Penicillium* species remains to be established, but the importance to human health is already clear.

7   *Epidermophyton, Microsporum* **and** *Trichophyton*

All three of these are dermatophytes, i.e. filamentous fungi which can utilize keratin for their nutrition. Keratin is the chief protein in skin, hair and nail. Hence, all of these organisms are responsible for superficial mycoses in mammals. It is often stated that dermatophytes are the only fungi to have evolved which rely upon infection for their own survival. This mistaken belief results from a view which is too human-centred and neglects, for example, the presence of symbiotic fungi in the stomachs of ruminants.

The genus *Microsporum* contains several interesting species including *M. audouinii,* which, in years gone by, caused epidemics of 'ringworm' in children, but rarely in adults: *M. ferrugineum* appears to fulfil this role today; *M. canis* which infects children, cats and dogs, but not adults—it is said that the children acquire the infection from the animals; *M. gypseum* affects mainly lower animals; *M. gallinae* infects poultry and humans; *M. nanum* can be common in pigs, but is rare in humans. The appearance of a tinea ('ringworm') is the host's reaction to the proteolytic (protein degrading) enzymes secreted by the fungus. In highly sensitized or hyper-allergic individuals this can be very pronounced.

Epidermophyton floccosum infects the skin and nails but not the hair, whereas different species of the genus *Trichophyton* display both geographical and anatomical variations. For example, *T. rubrum* is currently the most common dermatophyte of humans: it infects skin and nails but almost never hairy parts of the body; *T. mentagrophytes*, which is frequently the cause of athlete's foot, can infect all parts of the human body; the aptly-named *T. tonsurans* is the major causative agent of scalp ringworm in the USA whereas *T. megninii* is hardly ever found in the Western world. These varied distributions presumably reflect a complex matrix of variables including climate, nutrition, age, physiological status, the proximity of animals and other aspects of human lifestyle.

Certain identification of each individual dermatophyte requires great skill especially in the case of *Microsporum* where there is considerable morphological similarity between the species: hyphae are septate with numerous macroconidia which are thick-walled and rough in most cases. Microconidia are usually present. *Epidermophyton* is broadly similar except that microconidia are not formed. Distinguishing individual species of *Trichophyton* from each other is less problematical, although an unwary observer might confuse *T. mentagrophytes* with *T. rubrum*. Generally, in *Trichophyton* species, macroconidia are rare, thin-walled and smooth; there are numerous microconidia. Clearly, although these organisms only cause superficial infections, a rapid, genetic-based identification system would be a boon.

8   References

Andreasen A.A. & Stier J.B. (1953) Anaerobic nutrition of *Saccharomyces cerevisiae*. I. Ergosterol requirement for growth in a defined medium. *J Cell Comp Physiol*, **41**, 23–36.

Andreasen A.A. & Stier J.B. (1954) Anaerobic nutrition of *Saccharomyces cerevisiae*. II. Unsaturated fatty acid requirement for growth in a defined medium. *J Cell Comp Physiol*, **43**, 271–281.

Briza P., Ellinger A., Winkler G. & Breitenbach M. (1990) Characterization of a D, L-dityrosine-containing macromolecule from yeast ascospore walls. *J Biol Chem*, **265**, 15118–15123.

Cass A., Finklestein A. & Krespi V. (1970) The ion permeability induced in thin lipid membranes by the polyene antibiotics nystatin and amphotericin B. *J Gen Physiol*, **56**, 100–124.

Crowe J.H., Crowe L.M. & Chapman D. (1984) Preservation of membranes in anydrobiotic organisms: the role of trehalose. *Science*, **223**, 701–703.

Dickinson J.R. (1988) The metabolism of sporulation in yeast. *Microbiol Sci*, **5**, 121–123.

Dickinson J.R. (1996) 'Fusel' alcohols induce hyphal-like extensions and pseudohyphal formation in yeasts. *Microbiology*, **142**, 1391–1397.

Dickinson J.R. & Hewlins M.J.E. (1991) ^{13}C NMR analysis of a developmental pathway mutation in *Saccharomyces cerevisiae reveals* a cell derepressed for succinate dehydrogenase. *J Gen Microbiol*, **137**, 1033–1037.

Dickinson J.R., Dawes I.W., Boyd A.S.F. & Baxter R.L. (1983) ^{13}C NMR studies of acetate metabolism during sporulation of *Saccharomyces cerevisiae*. *Proc Nat Acad Sci USA*, **80**, 5847–5851.

Emmons C.W. (1955) Saprophytic sources of *Cryptococcus neoformans* associated with the pigeon. *Am J Hygiene*, **62**, 227–232.

Fraenkel D.G. (1982) Carbohydrate metabolism. In: *The Molecular Biology of the Yeast Saccharomyces, vol. 2. Metabolism and Biosynthesis* (eds J.N. Strathern, E.W. Jones & J.R. Broach), pp. 1–37. Cold Spring Harbor, NY: Cold Spring Harbor Laboratory.

Friefelder D.M. (1960) Bud formation in *Saccharomyces cerevisiae*. *J Bacteriol*, **80**, 567–568.

Gimeno C.J., Ljungdahl P.O., Styles C.A. & Fink G.R. (1992) Unipolar cell divisions in the yeast *S. cerevisiae* lead to filamentous growth: regulation by starvation and *RAS*. *Cell*, **68**, 1077–1090.

Gow N.A.R. (1994) Growth and guidance of the fungal hypha. *Microbiology*, **140**, 3139–3205.

Gow N.A.R., Swoboda R.K., Bertram G., Gooday G.W. & Brown A.J.P. (1993) Key genes in the regulation of dimorphism of *Candida albicans*. In: *Dimorphic Fungi* (eds H. Vanden Bossche, F.C. Odds & D. Kerridge), pp. 61–71. New York: Plenum Press.

Hartwell L.H. (1974) *Saccharomyces cerevisiae* cell cycle. *Bacteriol Rev*, **38**, 164–198.

Hartwell L.H. (1978) Cell division from a genetic perspective. *J Cell Biol*, **77**, 627–637.

Henry S.A. (1982) Membrane lipids of yeast: biochemical and genetic studies. In: *The Molecular Biology of the Yeast Saccharomyces, vol. 2. Metabolism and Biosynthesis* (eds J.N. Strathern, E.W. Jones & J.R. Broach), pp. 101–158. Cold Spring Harbor, NY: Cold Spring Harbor Laboratory.

Herskowitz I., Rine J. & Strathern J.N. (1992) Mating-type determination and mating-type inter-conversion in *Saccharomyces cerevisiae*. In: *The Molecular and Cellular Biology of the Yeast Saccharomyces cerevisiae. vol. 2, Gene Expression* (eds E.W. Jones, J.R. Pringle & J.R. Broach), pp. 583–656. Cold Spring Harbor, NY: Cold Spring Harbor Laboratory.

Kennedy B.K. & Guarente L. (1996) Genetic analysis of aging in *Saccharomyces cerevisiae*. *Trends Genet*, **12**, 355–359.

Kron S.J. & Gow N.A.R. (1995) Budding yeast morphogenesis: signalling, cytoskeleton and cell cycle. *Curr Opin Cell Biol*, **7**, 845–855.

Kron S.J., Styles C.A. & Fink G.R. (1994) Symmetric cell division in pseudohyphae of the yeast *Saccharomyces cerevisiae. Mol Biol Cell*, **5**, 1003–1022.

Kuriyama H. & Slaughter J.C. (1995) Control of cell morphology of the yeast *Saccharomyces cerevisiae* by nutrient limitation in continuous culture. *Lett Appl Microbiol*, **20**, 37–40.

Kwon-Chung K.J. & Bennett J.E. (1992) *Medical Mycology*. Philadelphia: Lea & Febiger.

Larone D.H. (1995) *Medically Important Fungi: A Guide to Identification*, 3rd edn. Washington: American Society for Microbiology.

Lew D.J. & Reed S.I. (1995) Cell cycle control of morphogenesis in budding yeast. *Curr Opin Genet Dev*, **5**, 17–23.

Leopold A.C. (1986) *Membranes, Metabolism and Dry Organisms*. Ithaca: Cornell University Press.

Manners D.J., Masson A.J. & Patterson J.C. (1973a) The structure of a β-(1-3)-D-glucan from yeast cell walls. *Biochem J*, **135**, 19–30.

Manners D.J., Masson A.J., Patterson J.C., Bjorndal H. & Lindberg B. (1973b) The structure of a β-(1-6)-D-glucan from yeast cell walls. *Biochem J*, **135**, 31–36.

Murphy J.W. (1996) Slick ways *Cryptococcus neoformans* foils host defences. *Am Soc Microbiol News*, **62**, 77–80.

Necas O. (1971) Cell wall synthesis in yeast protoplasts. *Bacteriol Rev*, **35**, 149–170.

Norman A.W., Demel R.A., DeKruyff B., Geurts Van Kessel W.S.M. & Van Deenen L.L.M. (1972) Studies on the biological properties of polyene antibiotics: comparison of the other polyenes with filipin in their ability to interact specifically with sterol. *Biochim Biophys Acta*, **290**, 1–14.

Odds F.C. (1988) *Candida and Candidosis*. London: Ballière Tindall.

Pringle J.R. (1978) The use of conditional lethal cell cycle mutants for temporal and functional sequence mapping of cell cycle events. *J Cell Physiol*, **95**, 393–406.

Pringle J.R. & Hartwell L.H. (1981) The *Saccharomyces cerevisiae* cell cycle. In: *The Molecular Biology of the Yeast Saccharomyces, vol. 1. Life Cycle and Inheritance* (eds J.N. Strathern, E.W. Jones & J.R. Broach), pp. 97–142. Cold Spring Harbor, NY: Cold Spring Harbor Laboratory.

Soll D.R. (1992) High frequency switching in *Candida albicans. Clin Microbiol Rev*, **5**, 183–203.

Sanjuán R., Zueco J., Stock R., Font de Mora J. & Sentandreu R. (1995) Identification of glucan-mannoprotein complexes in the cell wall of *Candida albicans* using a monoclonal antibody that reacts with a (1,6)-β-glucan epitope. *Microbiology*, **141**, 1545–1551.

Soll D.R., Galask R., Isley S. *et al.* (1989) Switching of *Candida albicans* during recurrent episodes of recurrent vaginitis. *J Clin Microbiol*, **27**, 681–690.

Van Rinsum J., Klis F.M. & van den Ende H. (1991) Cell wall glucomannoproteins of *Saccharomyces cerevisiae mnn9. Yeast*, **7**, 717–726.

Wright R.M., Repine T. & Repine J.E. (1993) Reversible pseudohyphal growth in haploid *Saccharomyces cerevisiae* is an aerobic process. *Curr Genet*, **23**, 388–391.

3 Viruses

1	**Introduction**	7.1.1	Cell culture	
		7.1.2	The chick embryo	
2	**General properties of viruses**	7.1.3	Animal inoculation	
2.1	Size			
2.2	Nucleic acid content	**8**	**Multiplication of human viruses**	
2.3	Metabolic capabilities	8.1	Attachment	
		8.2	Penetration and uncoating	
3	**Structure of viruses**	8.3	Production of viral proteins and	
3.1	Helical symmetry		replication of viral nucleic acid	
3.2	Icosahedral symmetry	8.4	Assembly and release of progeny	
			viruses	
4	**The effect of chemical and physical**			
	agents on viruses	**9**	**The problems of viral chemotherapy**	
		9.1	Interferon	
5	**Virus–host-cell interactions**			
		10	**Tumour viruses**	
6	**Bacteriophages**			
6.1	The lytic growth cycle	**11**	**The human immunodeficiency virus**	
6.2	Lysogeny			
6.3	Epidemiological uses	**12**	**Prions**	
7	**Human viruses**	**13**	**Further reading**	
7.1	Cultivation of human viruses			

1 Introduction

Following the demonstration by Koch and his colleagues that anthrax, tuberculosis and diphtheria were caused by bacteria, it was thought that similar organisms would, in time, be shown to be responsible for all infectious diseases. It gradually became obvious, however, that for a number of important diseases no such bacterial cause could be established. Infectious material from a case of rabies, for example, could be passed through special filters which held back all particles of bacterial size, and the resulting bacteria-free filtrate still proved to be capable of inducing rabies when inoculated into a susceptible animal. The term virus had, up until this time, been used quite indiscriminately to describe any agent capable of producing disease, so these filter-passing agents were originally called filterable viruses. With the passage of time the description 'filterable' has been dropped and the name virus has come to refer specifically to what are now known to be a distinctive group of microorganisms different in structure and method of replication from all others.

2 General properties of viruses

All forms of life—animal, plant and even bacterial—are susceptible to infection by viruses. Three main properties distinguish viruses from their various host cells: size, nucleic acid content and metabolic capabilities.

2.1 Size

Whereas a bacterial cell like a staphylococcus might be 1000 nm in diameter, the largest of the human pathogenic viruses, the poxviruses, measure only 250 nm along their longest axis, and the smallest, the poliovirus, is only 28 nm in diameter. They are mostly, therefore, beyond the limit of resolution of the light microscope and have to be visualized with the electron microscope.

2.2 Nucleic acid content

Viruses contain only a single type of nucleic acid, either DNA or RNA.

2.3 Metabolic capabilities

Virus particles have no metabolic machinery of their own. They cannot synthesize their own protein and nucleic acid from inanimate laboratory media and thus fail to grow on even nutritious media. They are obligatory intracellular parasites, only growing within other living cells whose energy and protein-producing systems they redirect for the purpose of manufacturing new viral components. The production of new virus particles generally results in death of the host cell and as the particles spread from cell to cell (e.g. within a tissue), disease can become apparent in the host.

3 Structure of viruses

In essence, virus particles are composed of a core of genetic material, either DNA or RNA, surrounded by a coat of protein. The function of the coat is to protect the viral genes from inactivation by adverse environmental factors, such as tissue nuclease enzymes which would otherwise digest a naked viral chromosome during its passage from cell to cell within a host. In a number of viruses the coat also plays an important part in the attachment of the virus to receptors on susceptible cells, and in many bacterial viruses the coat is further modified to facilitate the insertion of the viral genome through the tough structural barrier of the bacterial cell wall. The morphology of a variety of viruses is illustrated in Fig. 3.1.

The viral protein coat, or *capsid,* is composed of a large number of subunits, the *capsomeres.* This subunit structure is a fundamental property and is important from a number of aspects.

1 It leads to considerable economy of genetic information. This can be illustrated by considering some of the smaller viruses, which might, for example, have as a genome a single strand of RNA composed of about 3000 nucleotides and a protein coat with an overall composition of some 20000 amino acid units. Assuming that one amino acid is coded for by a triplet of nucleotides, such a coat in the form of a single large protein would require a gene some 60000 nucleotides in length. If, however, the viral coat comprised repeating units each composed of about 100 amino acids, only a section of

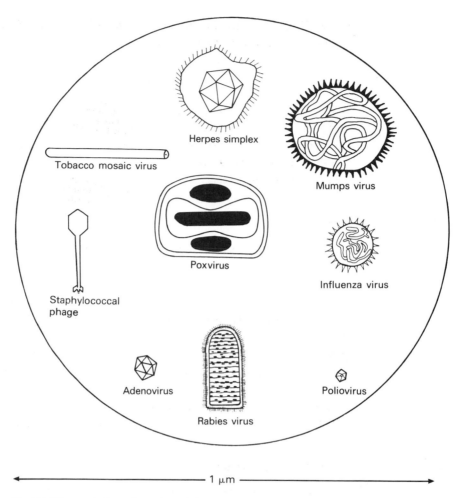

Fig. 3.1 The morphology of a variety of virus particles. The large circle indicates the relative size of a staphylococcus cell.

about 300 nucleotides long would be required to specify the capsid protein, leaving genetic capacity for other essential functions.

2 Such a subunit structure permits the construction of the virus particles by a process in which the subunits self-assemble into structures held together by non-covalent intermolecular forces as occurs in the process of crystallization. This eliminates the need for a sequence of enzyme-catalysed reactions for coat synthesis. It also provides an automatic quality-control system, as subunits which may have major structural defects fail to become incorporated into complete particles.

3 The subunit composition is such that the intracellular release of the viral genome from its coat involves only the dissociation of non-covalently bonded subunits, rather than the degradation of an integral protein sheath.

In addition to the protein coat, many animal virus particles are surrounded by a lipoprotein envelope which has generally been derived from the cytoplasmic membrane of their last host cell.

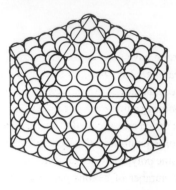

An icosahedral virus
particle composed of
252 capsomeres
240 being hexons and
12 being pentons

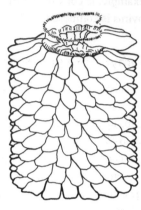

A helical virus partially
disrupted to show the
helical coil of viral
nucleic acid embedded
in the capsomeres

Fig. 3.2 Icosahedral and helical symmetry in viruses.

The geometry of the capsomeres results in their assembly into particles exhibiting one of two different architectural styles—helical or icosahedral symmetry (Fig. 3.2).

There is a third structural group comprising the poxviruses and many bacterial viruses, in which a number of major structural components can be identified and the overall geometry of the particles is complex.

3.1 Helical symmetry

Some virus particles have their protein subunits symmetrically packed in a helical array, forming hollow cylinders. The tobacco mosaic virus (TMV) is the classic example. X-ray diffraction data and electron micrographs have revealed that 16 subunits per turn of the helix project from a central axial hole that runs the length of the particle. The nucleic acid does not lie in this hole, but is embedded into ridges on the inside of each subunit and describes its own helix from one end of the particle to the other.

Helical symmetry was thought at one time to exist only in plant viruses. It is now known, however, to occur in a number of animal virus particles. The influenza and mumps viruses, for example, which were first seen in early electron micrographs as roughly spherical particles, have now been observed as enveloped particles; within the envelope, the capsids themselves are helically symmetrical and appear similar to the rods of TMV, except that they are more flexible and are wound like coils of rope in the centre of the particle.

3.2 Icosahedral symmetry

The viruses in this architectural group have their capsomeres arranged in the form of regular icosahedra, i.e. polygons having 12 vertices, 20 faces and 30 sides. At each of the 12 vertices or corners of these icosahedral particles is a capsomere, called a *penton,* which is surrounded by five neighbouring units. Each of the 20 triangular faces contains an identical number of capsomeres which are surrounded by six neighbours and called *hexons.* In plant and bacterial viruses exhibiting this type of symmetry, the hexons and pentons are composed of the same polypeptide chains; in animal viruses, however, they may be distinct proteins. The number of hexons per capsid varies considerably in different viruses. Adenovirus, for example, is constructed from 240 hexons and 12 pentons, while the much smaller poliovirus is composed of 20 hexons and 12 pentons.

4 The effect of chemical and physical agents on viruses

Heat is the most reliable method of virus disinfection. Most human pathogenic viruses are inactivated following exposure at 60°C for 30 minutes. The virus of serum hepatitis can, however, survive this temperature for up to 4 hours. Viruses are stable at low temperatures and are routinely stored at –40 to –70°C. Some viruses are rapidly inactivated by drying, others survive well in a desiccated state. Ultraviolet light inactivates viruses by damaging their nucleic acid and has been used to prepare viral vaccines. These facts must be taken into account in the storage and preparation of viral vaccines (Chapter 15).

Viruses that contain lipid are inactivated by organic solvents such as chloroform and ether. Those without lipid are resistant to these agents. This distinction has been used to classify viruses. Many of the chemical disinfectants used against bacteria, e.g. phenols, alcohols and quaternary ammonium compounds (Chapter 10), have minimal virucidal activity. The most generally active agents are chlorine, the hypochlorites, iodine, aldehydes and ethylene oxide.

5 Virus–host-cell interactions

The precise sequence of events resulting from the infection of a cell by a virus will vary with different virus–host systems, but they will be variations of four basic themes.
1   Multiplication of the virus and destruction of the host cell.
2   Elimination of the virus from the cell and the infection aborted without a recognizable effect on the cells occurring.
3   Survival of the infected cell unchanged, except that it now carries the virus in a latent state.
4   Survival of the infected cell in a dramatically altered or transformed state, e.g. transformation of a normal cell to one having the properties of a cancerous cell.

6 Bacteriophages

Bacteriophages, or as they are more simply termed, phages, are viruses that have bacteria as their host cells. The name was first given by D'Herelle to an agent which he found could produce lysis of the dysentery bacillus *Shigella shiga.* D'Herelle was convinced that he had stumbled across an agent with tremendous medical potential. His phage could destroy *Sh. shiga* in broth culture so why not in the dysenteric gut of humans? Similar agents were found before long which were active against the bacteria of many other diseases, including anthrax, scarlet fever, cholera and diphtheria, and attempts were made to use them to treat these diseases. It was a great disappointment, however, that phages so virulent in their antibacterial activity *in vitro* proved impotent *in vivo*. A possible exception was cholera, where some success seems to have been achieved, and cholera phages were apparently used by the medical corps of the German and Japanese armies during the Second World War to treat this disease. Since the development of antibiotics, however, phage therapy has been abandoned.

Interest in bacterial viruses did not cease with the demise of phage therapy. They proved to be very much easier to handle in the laboratory than other viruses and had conveniently rapid multiplication cycles. They have, therefore, been used extensively as the experimental models for elucidating the biochemical mechanisms of viral replication. A vast amount of information has been collected about them and many of the important advances in molecular biology, such as the discovery of messenger RNA (mRNA), the understanding of the genetic code and the way in which genes are controlled, have come from work on phage–bacterium systems.

It is probable that all species of bacteria are susceptible to phages. Any particular phage will exhibit a marked specificity in selecting host cells, attacking only organisms belonging to a single species. A *Staphylococcus aureus* phage, for example, will not infect *Staph. epidermidis* cells. In most cases, phages are in fact strain-specific, only being active on certain characteristic strains of a given species.

Most phages are tadpole-shaped structures with heads which function as containers for the nucleic acid and tails which are used to attach the virus to its host cell. There are, however, some simple icosahedral phages and others that are helically symmetrical cylinders. The dimensions of the phage heads vary from the large T-even group (Fig. 3.3) of *Escherichia coli* phages (60×90 nm) to the much smaller ones (30×30 nm) of certain *Bacillus* phages. The tails vary in length from 15 to 200 nm and can be quite

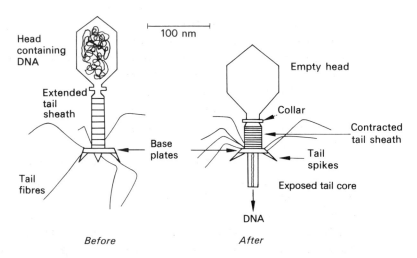

Fig. 3.3 T-even phage structure before and after tail contraction.

complex structures (Fig. 3.3). While the majority of phages have double-stranded DNA as their genetic material, some of the very small icosahedral and the helical phages have single-stranded DNA or RNA.

On the basis of the response they produce in their host cells, phages can be classified as *virulent* or *temperate*. Infection of a sensitive bacterium with a virulent phage results in the replication of the virus, lysis of the cell and release of new infectious progeny phage particles. Temperate phages can produce this lytic response, but they are also capable of a symbiotic response in which the invading viral genome does not take over the direction of cellular activity, the cell survives the infection and the viral nucleic acid becomes incorporated into the bacterial chromosome, where it is termed *prophage*. Cells carrying viral genes in this way are referred to as *lysogenic*.

6.1   The lytic growth cycle

The replication of virulent phage was initially studied using the T-even-numbered (T_2, T_4 and T_6) phages of *E. coli*. These phages adsorb, by their long tail fibres, on to specific receptors on the surface of the bacterial cell wall. The base plate of the tail sheath and its pins then lock the phage into position on the outside of the cell. At this stage, the tail sheath contracts towards the head, while the base plate remains in contact with the cell wall and, as a result, the hollow tail core is exposed and driven through to the cytoplasmic membrane (Fig. 3.3). Simultaneously, the DNA passes from the head, through the hollow tail core and is deposited on the outer surface of the cytoplasmic membrane, from where it finds its own way into the cytoplasm. The phage protein coat remains on the outside of the cell and plays no further part in the replication cycle.

Within the first few minutes after infection, transcription of part of the viral genome produces 'early' mRNA molecules, which are translated into a set of 'early' proteins. These serve to switch off host-cell macromolecular synthesis, degrade the host DNA and start to make components for viral DNA. Many of the early proteins duplicate enzymes already present in the host, concerned in the manufacture of nucleotides for cell DNA. However, the requirement for the production of 5-hydroxymethylcytosine-containing nucleotides, which replace the normal cytosine derivatives in T even phage DNA, means that some of the early enzymes are entirely new to the cell. With the build-up of its components, the viral DNA replicates and also starts to produce a batch of 'late' mRNA molecules, transcribed from genes which specify the proteins of the phage coat. These late messages are translated into the subunits of the capsid structures, which condense to form phage heads, tails and tail fibres, and then together with viral DNA are assembled into complete infectious particles. The enzyme digesting the cell wall, lysozyme, is also produced in the cell at this stage and it eventually brings about the lysis of the cell and liberation of about 100 progeny viruses, some 25 minutes after infection.

As other phage systems have been studied, it has become clear that the T-even model of virulent phage replication is atypical in a number of respects. The large T-even genomes, with their coding capacity for about 200 proteins, give these phages a relatively high degree of independence from their hosts. Although relying on the host energy and protein-synthesizing systems they are capable of specifying a battery of their own enzymes. Most other phages have considerably smaller genomes. They tend

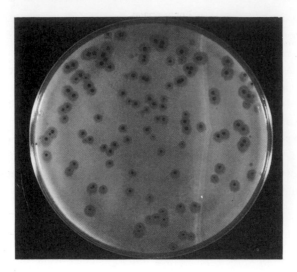

Fig. 3.4 Plaques formed by a phage on a plate seeded with *Bacillus subtilis.*

to disturb the host-cell metabolism to a much lesser extent than the T-even viruses, and also rely to a greater degree on pre-existing cell enzymes to produce components for their nucleic acid.

The lytic activity of the virulent phages can be demonstrated by mixing phage with about 10^7 sensitive indicator bacteria in 5 ml of molten nutrient agar. The mixture is then poured over the surface of a solid nutrient agar plate. On incubation, the phage particles will infect bacteria in their immediate neighbourhood, lysing them and producing a burst of progeny viruses. These particles then infect bacteria in the vicinity, producing a second generation of progeny and this sequence is repeated many times. In the meantime the uninfected bacteria produce a thick carpet or lawn of growth over the agar. As the lawn develops, clear holes or 'plaques' become obvious in it at each site of virus multiplication (Fig. 3.4). As each of these plaques is initiated by a single phage particle, they provide a means for titrating phage preparations.

6.2 **Lysogeny**

When a temperate phage is mixed with sensitive indicator bacteria and plated as described above, the reaction at each focus of infection is generally a combination of lytic and lysogenic responses. Some bacteria will be lysed and produce phage, others will survive as lysogenic cells, and the plaque becomes visible as a partial area of clearing in the bacterial lawn. It is possible to pick off cells from the central areas of these plaques and demonstrate that they carry prophage.

The phage lambda (λ) of *E. coli* is the temperate phage that has been most extensively studied. When any particular strain of *E. coli,* say K12, is infected with λ, the cells surviving the infection are designated *E. coli* K12(λ) to indicate that they are carrying the λ-prophage.

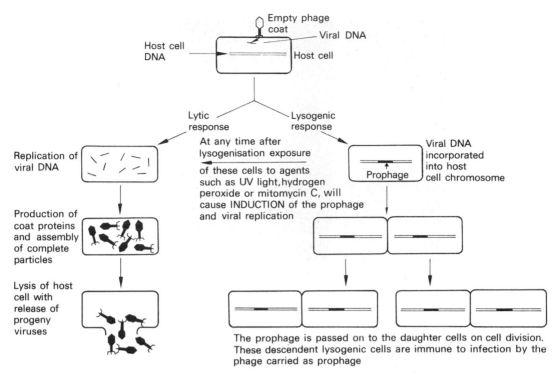

Fig. 3.5 Scheme to illustrate the lytic and lysogenic responses of bacteriophages.

The essential features of lysogenic cells and the phenomenon of lysogeny are listed below and summarized in Fig. 3.5.

1 Integration of the prophage into the bacterial chromosome ensures that, on cell division, each daughter cell will acquire the set of viral genes.

2 In a normally growing culture of lysogenic bacteria, the majority of bacteria manage to keep their prophages in a dormant state. In a very small minority of cells, however, the prophage genes express themselves. This results in the multiplication of the virus, lysis of the cells and liberation of infectious particles into the medium.

3 Exposure of lysogenic cultures to certain chemical and physical agents, e.g. hydrogen peroxide, mitomycin C and ultraviolet light, results in mass lysis and the production of high titres of phage. This process is called *induction.*

4 When a lysogenic cell is infected by the same type of phage as it carries as prophage, the infection is aborted, the activity of the invading viral genes being repressed by the same mechanism that normally keeps the prophage in a dormant state.

5 Lysogeny is generally a very stable state, but occasionally a cell will lose its prophage and these 'cured' cells are once more susceptible to infection by that particular phage type.

Lysogeny is an extremely common phenomenon and it seems that most natural isolates of bacteria carry one or more prophages, some strains of *Staph. aureus* have been shown to carry four or five different prophages.

The induction of a lysogenic culture to produce infectious phages, followed by lysogenization of a second strain of the bacterial species by these phages, results in the transmission of a prophage from the chromosome of one type of cell to that of another. On this migration, temperate bacteriophages can occasionally act as vectors for the transfer of bacterial genes between cells. This process is called *transduction* and it can be responsible for the transfer of such genetic factors as those that determine resistance to antibiotics (Chapter 9). In addition, certain phages have the innate ability to change the properties of their host cell. The classic example is the case of the β-phage of *Corynebacterium diphtheriae*. The acquisition of the β-prophage by non-toxin-producing strains of this species results in their conversion to diphtheria-toxin producers.

6.3	**Epidemiological uses**

Different strains of a number of bacterial species can be distinguished by their sensitivity to a collection of phages. Bacteria which can be typed in this way include *Staph. aureus* and *Salmonella typhi*. The particular strain of, say, *Staph. aureus* responsible for an outbreak of infection is characterized by the pattern of its sensitivity to a standard set of phages and then possible sources of infection are examined for the presence of that same phage type of *Staph. aureus*.

More recently, the fact that many of the chemical agents which cause the induction of prophage are carcinogenic has led to the use of lysogenic bacteria in screening tests for detecting potential carcinogens.

7	**Human viruses**

Viruses are, of course, important and common causes of disease in humans, particularly in children. Fortunately, most infections are not serious and, like the rhinovirus infections responsible for the common cold syndrome, are followed by the complete recovery of the patient. Many viral infections are in fact so mild that they are termed 'silent', to indicate that the virus replicates in the body without producing symptoms of disease. Occasionally, however, some of the viruses that are normally responsible for mild infections can produce serious disease. This pattern of pathogenicity is exemplified by the enterovirus group. Most enterovirus infections merely result in the symptomless replication of the virus in the cells lining the alimentary tract. Only in a small percentage of infections does the virus spread from this site via the bloodstream and the lymphatic system to other organs, producing a fever and possibly a skin rash in the host. On rare occasions enteroviruses like poliovirus can progress to the central nervous system where they may produce an aseptic meningitis or paralysis. There are a few virus diseases, such as rabies, which are invariably severe and have very high mortality rates.

Human viruses will cause disease in other animals. Some are capable of infecting only a few closely related primate species, others will infect a wide range of mammals. Under the conditions of natural infection viruses generally exhibit a considerable degree of tissue specificity. The influenza virus, for example, replicates only in the cells lining the upper respiratory tract.

Table 3.1 presents a summary of the properties of some of the more important human viruses.

Table 3.1 Important human viruses and their properties

Group	Virus	Characteristics	Clinical importance
DNA viruses			
Poxviruses	Variola Vaccinia	Large particles 200 × 250 nm: complex symmetry	Variola is the smallpox virus. It produces a systemic infection with a characteristic vesicular rash affecting the face, arms and legs, and has a high mortality rate. Vaccinia has been derived from the cowpox virus and is used to immunize against smallpox
Adenoviruses	Adenovirus	Icosahedral particles 80 nm in diameter	Commonly cause upper respiratory tract infections; tend to produce latent infections in tonsils and adenoids; will produce tumours on injection into hamsters, rats or mice
Herpesviruses	Herpes simplex virus (HSV1 and HSV2)	Enveloped, icosahedral particles 150 nm in diameter	HSV1 infects oral membranes in children, >80% are infected by adolescence. Following the primary infection the individual retains the HSV1 DNA in the trigeminal nerve ganglion for life and has a 50% chance of developing 'cold sores'. HSV2 is responsible for recurrent genital herpes
	Cytomegalovirus (CMV)	Enveloped, icosahedral particles 150 nm in diameter	CMV is generally acquired in childhood as a subclinical infection. About 50% of adults carry the virus in a dormant state in white blood cells. The virus can cause severe disease (pneumonia, hepatitis, encephalitis) in immunocompromised patients. Primary infections during pregnancy can induce serious congenital abnormalities in the fetus
	Epstein–Barr virus (EBV)	Enveloped, icosahedral particles 150 nm in diameter	Infections occur by salivary exchange. In young children they are commonly asymptomatic but the virus persists in a latent form in lymphocytes. Infection delayed until adolescence often results in glandular fever. In tropical Africa, a severe EBV infection early in life predisposes the child to malignant facial tumours (Burkitt's lymphoma)
Hepatitis viruses	Hepatitis B virus (HBV)	Spherical enveloped particle 42 nm in diameter enclosing an inner icosahedral 27-nm nucleocapsid	In areas such as South-East Asia and Africa, most children are infected by perinatal transmission. In the Western world the virus is spread through contact with contaminated blood or by sexual intercourse. There is strong evidence that chronic infections with HBV can progress to liver cancer

continued on p. 64

Table 3.1 *Continued*

Group	Virus	Characteristics	Clinical importance
Papovaviruses	Papilloma virus	Naked icosahedra 50 nm in diameter	Multiply only in epithelial cells of skin and mucous membranes causing warts. There is evidence that some types are associated with cervical carcinoma
RNA viruses Myxoviruses	Influenza virus	Enveloped particles, 100 nm in diameter with a helically symmetric capsid; haemagglutinin and neuraminidase spikes project from the envelope	These viruses are capable of extensive antigenic variation, producing new types against which the human population does not have effective immunity. These new antigenic types can cause pandemics of influenza. In natural infections the virus only multiplies in the cells lining the upper respiratory tract. The constitutional symptoms of influenza are probably brought about by absorption of toxic breakdown products from the dying cells on the respiratory epithelium
Paramyxoviruses	Mumps virus	Enveloped particles variable in size, 110–170 nm in diameter, with helical capsids	Infection in children produces characteristic swelling of parotid and submaxillary salivary glands. The disease can have neurological complications, e.g. meningitis, especially in adults
	Measles virus	Enveloped particles variable in size, 120–250 nm in diameter, helical capsids	Very common childhood fever, immunity is life-long and second attacks are very rare
Rhabdoviruses	Rabies virus	Bullet-shaped particles, 75–180 nm, enveloped, helical capsids	The virus has a very wide host range, infecting all mammals so far tested; dogs, cats and cattle are particularly susceptible. The incubation period of rabies is extremely varied, ranging from 6 days up to 1 year. The virus remains localized at the wound side of entry for a while before passing along nerve fibres to central nervous system, where it invariably produces a fatal encephalitis
Reoviruses	Rotavirus	An inner core is surrounded by two concentric icosahedral shells producing particles 70 nm in diameter	A very common cause of gastroenteritis in infants. It is spread through poor water supplies and when standards of general hygiene are low. In developing countries it is responsible for about a million deaths each year
Picornaviruses	Poliovirus	Naked icosahedral particles 28 nm in diameter	One of a group of enteroviruses common in the gut of humans. The primary site of multiplication is the lymphoid tissue of the alimentary tract. Only rarely do they cause systemic infections or serious neurological conditions like encephalitis or poliomyelitis

continued

Table 3.1 *Continued*

Group	Virus	Characteristics	Clinical importance
	Rhinoviruses	Naked icosahedra 30 nm in diameter	The common cold viruses; there are over 100 antigenically distinct types, hence the difficulty in preparing effective vaccines. The virus is shed copiously in watery nasal secretions
	Hepatitis A virus (HAV)	Naked icosahedra 27 nm in diameter	Responsible for 'infectious hepatitis' spread by the oro-faecal route especially in children. Also associated with sewage contamination of food or water supplies
Togaviruses	Rubella	Spherical particles 70 nm in diameter, a tightly adherent envelope surrounds an icosahedral capsid	Causes German measles in children. An infection contracted in the early stages of pregnancy can induce severe multiple congenital abnormalities, e.g. deafness, blindness, heart disease and mental retardation
Flaviviruses	Yellow fever virus	Spherical particles 40 nm in diameter with an inner core surrounded by an adherent lipid envelope	The virus is spread to humans by mosquito bites; the liver is the main target; necrosis of hepatocytes leads to jaundice and fever
	Hepatitis C virus (HCV)	Spherical particles 40 nm in diameter consisting of an inner core surrounded by an adherent lipid envelope	The virus is spread through blood transfusions and blood products. Induces a hepatitis which is usually milder than that caused by HBV
Filoviruses	Ebola virus	Long filamentous rods composed of a lipid envelope surrounding a helical nucleocapsid 1000 nm long, 80 nm in diameter	The virus is widespread amongst populations of monkeys. It can be spread to humans by contact with body fluids from the primates. The resulting haemorragic fever has a 90% case fatality rate
Retroviruses	Human T-cell leukaemia virus (HTLV-1)	Spherical enveloped virus 100 nm in diameter, icosahedral cores contain two copies of linear RNA molecules and reverse transcriptase	HTLV is spread inside infected lymphocytes in blood, semen or breast milk. Most infections remain asymptomatic but after an incubation period of 10–40 years in about 2% of cases, adult T-cell leukaemia can result
	Human immunodeficiency virus (HIV)	Differs from other retroviruses in that the core is cone-shaped rather than icosahedral	HIV is transmitted from person to person via blood or genital secretions. The principal target for the virus is the CD4+ T-lymphocyte cells. Depletion of these cells induces immunodeficiency

7.1   Cultivation of human viruses

The cultivation of viruses from material taken from lesions is an important step in the diagnosis of many viral diseases. Studies of the basic biology and multiplication processes of human viruses also require that they are grown in the laboratory under experimental conditions. Human pathogenic viruses can be propagated in three types of cell systems.

7.1.1   *Cell culture*

Cells from human or other primate sources are obtained from an intact tissue, e.g. human embryo kidney or monkey kidney. The cells are dispersed by digestion with trypsin and the resulting suspension of single cells is generally allowed to settle in a vessel containing a nutrient medium. The cells will metabolize and grow and after a few days of incubation at 37°C will form a continuous film or monolayer one cell thick. These cells are then capable of supporting viral replication. Cell cultures may be divided into three types according to their history.

1   Primary cell cultures, which are prepared directly from tissues.

2   Secondary cell cultures, which can be prepared by taking cells from some types of primary culture, usually those derived from embryonic tissue, dispersing them by treatment with trypsin and inoculating some into a fresh batch of medium. A limited number of subcultures can be performed with these sorts of cells, up to a maximum of about 50 before the cells degenerate.

3   There are now available a number of lines of cells, mainly originating from malignant tissue, which can be serially subcultured apparently indefinitely. These established cell lines are particularly convenient as they eliminate the requirement for fresh animal tissue for such sets or series of cultures. An example of these continuous cell lines are the famous HeLa cells, which were originally isolated from a cervical carcinoma of a woman called Henrietta Lacks, long since dead but whose cells have been used in laboratories all over the world to grow viruses.

Inoculation of cell cultures with virus-containing material produces characteristic changes in the cells. The replication of many types of viruses produces the cytopathic effect (CPE) in which cells degenerate. This effect is seen as the shrinkage or sometimes ballooning of cells and the disruption of the monolayer by death and detachment of the cells (Fig. 3.6). The replicating virus can then be identified by inoculating a series of cell cultures with mixtures of the virus and different known viral antisera. If the virus is the same as one of the types used to prepare the various antisera, then its activity will be neutralized by that particular antiserum and CPE will not be apparent in that tube. Alternatively viral antisera labelled with a fluorescent dye can be used to identify the virus in the cell culture.

7.1.2   *The chick embryo*

Fertile chicken eggs, 10–12 days old, have been used as a convenient cell system in which to grow a number of human pathogenic viruses. Figure 3.7 shows that viruses generally have preferences for particular tissues within the embryo. Influenza viruses,

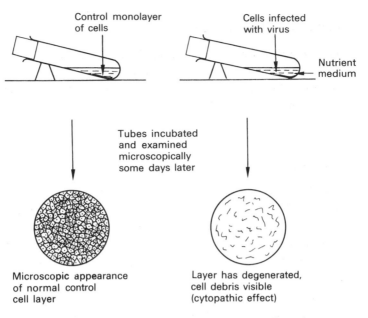

Tubes incubated and examined microscopically some days later

Control monolayer of cells

Cells infected with virus

Nutrient medium

Microscopic appearance of normal control cell layer

Layer has degenerated, cell debris visible (cytopathic effect)

Fig. 3.6 The cytopathic effect of a virus on a tissue culture cell monolayer.

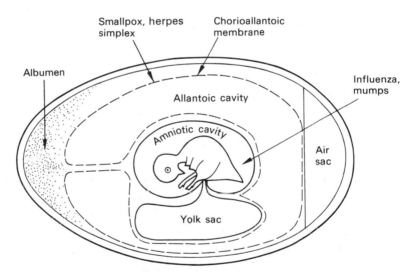

Smallpox, herpes simplex

Chorioallantoic membrane

Albumen

Influenza, mumps

Allantoic cavity

Amniotic cavity

Air sac

Yolk sac

Fig. 3.7 A chick embryo showing the inoculation routes for virus cultivation.

for example, can be grown in the cells of the membrane bounding the amniotic cavity, while smallpox virus will grow in the chorioallantoic membrane. The growth of smallpox virus in the embryo is recognized by the formation of characteristic pock marks on the membrane. Influenza virus replication is detected by exploiting the ability of these particles to cause erythrocytes to clump together. Fluid from the amniotic cavity of the infected embryo is titrated for its haemagglutinating activity.

Experimental animals such as mice and ferrets have to be used for the cultivation of some viruses. Growth of the virus is indicated by signs of disease or death of the inoculated animal.

8   Multiplication of human viruses

The long incubation times of many human virus diseases indicate that they replicate slowly in host cells. In tissue culture systems it has been shown that most human viruses take from 4 to 24 hours to complete a single replication cycle, contrasting with the 30 or so minutes for many bacterial viruses.

In general terms, four main stages can be recognized in the multiplication of human viruses. (i) attachment; (ii) penetration and uncoating (iii) production of viral proteins and replication of viral nucleic acid, (iv) assembly and release of progeny viruses.

8.1   Attachment

Specific proteins on the surface of virus particles, e.g. the haemagglutinins of influenza viruses (Fig. 3.8), mediate their adherence to glycoprotein receptors in the plasma membrane of host cells. Viruses make use of a variety of membrane glycoproteins as

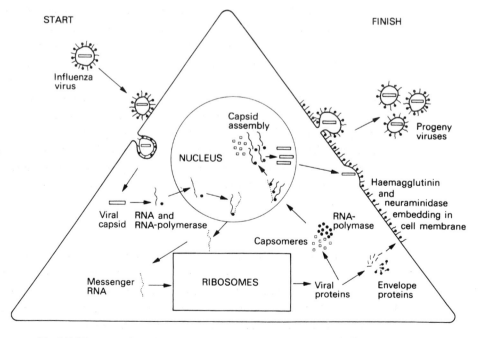

Fig. 3.8 Diagrammatic representation of the production and release of influenza virus particles from an infected cell.

their receptors. The primary functions of the cellular receptor molecules are not related to their role as viral attachment sites, some being membrane permeases or hormone receptors. Different viruses may use different receptors, e.g. different serotypes of human rhinoviruses use different receptors, in other cases unrelated viruses may share common receptors.

8.2 Penetration and uncoating

Viruses penetrate their host cells either by endocytosis or by fusion with the cell membrane. Macromolecules can be taken up into animal cells by attachment to membrane receptors and subsequent endocytosis. Many viruses use this essential cell function of receptor-mediated endocytosis to gain entry to their host cells. The virus-containing cytoplasmic vacuole fuses with endosomes and the resulting acidification generates conformational changes in the virus coat which can release the virus nucleocapsid into the cytosol. The membranes of some enveloped viruses fuse with the plasma membranes of their host cells and this releases the nucleocapsid directly into the cytoplasm. Some viruses then require only partial uncoating before transcription of their nucleic acid can begin, but in most cases the viral capsid completely disintegrates before viral functions start to be expressed. In some cases the nucleocapsid passes to the cell nucleus before uncoating occurs.

8.3 Production of viral proteins and replication of viral nucleic acid

During this phase most human viruses seem to bring host-cell macromolecular synthesis to a stop: the cell DNA, however, is generally not degraded. With the DNA-containing viruses, like adenovirus, the nucleic acid passes to the nucleus, where a host-cell RNA polymerase enzyme is used to transcribe part of the viral genome. These first messages are analogous to the 'early' messages of the T-even phages and are concerned in the production of enzymes for viral DNA synthesis. Viral DNA replication is then followed by formation of 'late' mRNA specifying capsid protein. The mRNA molecules are of course translated on the cytoplasmic ribosomes. The proteins produced are rapidly transported back to the nucleus, where capsid assembly takes place. An exception to this pattern of DNA virus replication is provided by the poxvirus, vaccinia. Within their complex structure these particles contain a DNA-dependent RNA polymerase enzyme, which is released during uncoating and proceeds to make mRNA molecules from the viral DNA. The whole of the replication of vaccinia takes place in the cell cytoplasm.

With some RNA viruses, e.g. poliovirus, the RNA strand from the particle can act directly as mRNA and is translated into viral proteins on the host-cell ribosomes. In many other RNA viruses, however (e.g. the influenza viruses), the RNA strands are negative-sense RNAs (antimessages) that have first to be transcribed to the complementary sequence by RNA-dependent RNA polymerases before they can function in protein synthesis. Since eukaryotic cells do not have these enzymes, the negative-sense RNA viruses must carry them in the virion.

Unlike eukaryotic cells which normally produce monocistronic mRNA, many viruses produce polycistronic messages. DNA viruses, which usually replicate in the cell nuclei, use nuclear RNA processing and splicing enzymes to cleave their polycistronic messages. Some RNA viruses such as human immunodeficiency virus (HIV) produce polycistronic messages which are translated into polyproteins. These then have to be cleaved by protease enzymes to produce functional proteins. Other RNA viruses (e.g. influenza) have segmented genomes in which each RNA molecule is a separate gene in its own nucleocapsid.

8.4 Assembly and release of progeny viruses

The non-enveloped human viruses all have icosahedral capsids. The structural proteins undergo a self-assembly process to form capsids into which the viral nucleic acid is packaged. Most non-enveloped viruses accumulate within the cytoplasm or nucleus and are only released when the cell lyses.

All enveloped human viruses acquire their phospholipid coating by budding through cellular membranes. The maturation and release of enveloped influenza particles is illustrated in Fig. 3.8. The capsid protein subunits are transported from the ribosomes to the nucleus, where they combine with new viral RNA molecules and are assembled into the helical capsids. The haemagglutinin and neuraminidase proteins that project from the envelope of the normal particles migrate to the cytoplasmic membrane where they displace the normal cell membrane proteins. The assembled nucleocapsids finally pass out from the nucleus, and as they impinge on the altered cytoplasmic membrane they cause it to bulge and bud off completed enveloped particles from the cell. Virus particles are released in this way over a period of hours before the cell eventually dies.

9 The problems of viral chemotherapy

Bacteria are vulnerable to the selective attack of chemotherapeutic agents because of the many metabolic and molecular differences between them and animal cells. The biology of virus replication, with its considerable dependence on host-cell energy-producing, protein-synthesizing and biosynthetic enzyme systems, severely limits the opportunities for selective attack. Another problem is that many virus diseases only become apparent after extensive viral multiplication and tissue damage has been done.

Recently, however, there have been a number of encouraging developments in the field of antiviral therapy. For example, acycloguanosine (acyclovir: see Chapter 5) has been shown to be non-toxic to host cells while specifically inhibiting the replication of herpes viruses. Successful clinical trials have led to the introduction of this drug for the treatment of a variety of herpetic conditions.

The control over human viral diseases is exercised by active immunization (Chapters 14 and 16) of the population, together with general hygiene and physical and chemical disinfection procedures.

9.1 Interferon

Although it is difficult to obtain drugs capable of interrupting viral replication, it had been known for many years that infection of a host with one virus could sometimes prevent infections with a second, quite unrelated virus. This phenomenon was called *interference* and in many cases it proved to be due to the production of a substance called *interferon.*

Interferons are low molecular weight proteins produced by virus-infected cells. They have no direct antiviral activity. They bind to the cell membranes and induce the synthesis of secondary proteins. If interferon-treated cells are then infected with a virus, although adsorption, penetration and uncoating can take place, the interferon-induced proteins inhibit viral nucleic acid and protein synthesis and the infection is aborted. Interferons have major roles to play in protecting the host against natural virus infections. They are produced more rapidly than antibodies and the outcome of many natural viral infections is probably determined by the relative early titres of interferon and virus, protection being most effective when the infecting dose of virus is low.

Potentially, interferon is an ideal antiviral agent in that it acts on many different viruses and is not toxic to host cells. However, the exploitation of this agent in the treatment of viral infections has been delayed by a number of factors. For example, it has proved to be species-specific and interferons raised in animal sources offered little protection to human cells. Human interferon is thus needed for the treatment of human infections and the production and purification of human interferon on a large scale has proved difficult. The insertion of human genes for interferon into *E. coli* has resolved the production problems (Chapter 24). Clinical trials have demonstrated that interferon prevents rhinovirus infection and has a beneficial effect in herpes, cytomegalovirus and hepatitis B virus infections.

Interferon does not only inhibit virus replication, it also has multiple effects on cell metabolism and slows down the growth and multiplication of treated cells. This is probably responsible for its widely reported antitumour effect. Encouraging results have been reported from clinical trials of interferon against several human tumours such as osteogenic sarcoma, myeloma, lymphoma and breast cancer.

10   Tumour viruses

Many viruses, both DNA and RNA containing, will cause cancer in animals. This so-called *oncogenic* activity of a virus can be demonstrated by the observation of tumour formation in inoculated experimental animals and by the ability of the virus to transform normal tissue culture cells into cells with malignant characteristics. These transformed cells are easily recognizable as they exhibit such properties as rapid growth and frequent mitosis, or loss of normal cell contact inhibition, so that they pile up on top of each other instead of remaining in a well-organized layer.

Studies on the transformation of tissue cultures with DNA-containing viruses have shown that, although complete virus particles cannot be found in the infected, transformed cells, viral DNA is present and is bound to the transformed cell DNA as *provirus,* analogous to the prophage of lysogenic bacteria.

RNA oncogenic viruses have an unusual enzyme, reverse transcriptase, which is capable of making DNA copies from an RNA template. Cells transformed by these retroviruses have been shown to possess DNA transcripts of the viral RNA. It appears that the transformation from normal to malignant is associated with the acquisition by the cell of viral DNA.

While human viruses like the adenoviruses can induce cancer in hamsters, rats and mice, the search for viruses causing human cancer is of course difficult because of the unacceptability of testing for oncogenic activity by infecting humans. In the last 10 years, however, it has been realized that viruses are a major cause of the disease in humans, being involved in the genesis of some 20% of human cancers worldwide. The characteristic features of the association between viruses and human cancers are that the incubation time between virus infection and development of the disease can be considerable, that less than 1% of infected individuals will develop the disease and that genetic and environmental cofactors are crucial for the progression to cancer. The Epstein–Barr virus (EBV), for example, is involved in the aetiology of Burkitt's lymphoma a malignant tumour of the jaw, found in African children. In fact this virus has a widespread distribution in the human population, being responsible for the condition of glandular fever which is common in young adults in Europe and America. The characteristic occurrence of Burkitt's lymphoma in hot humid areas of Africa where mosquitoes flourish has led to the hypothesis that infection with EBV has to be followed by malaria, which then induces immunosuppression and acts as the cofactor necessary for tumour formation.

The list of viruses involved in other human cancers includes hepatitis B, which is associated with hepatocellular carcinoma; human papilloma viruses with cervical, penile and some anal carcinomas; human T-cell lymphotropic virus type 1 associated with adult T-cell leukaemia/lymphoma syndrome; and HIV with Kaposi's sarcoma.

11   The human immunodeficiency virus

HIV is an enveloped particle with a cone-shaped nucleocapsid containing two copies of a positive sense single stranded RNA and the enzyme reverse transcriptase. The virus is transmitted from person to person by genital secretions and blood. From the original site of infection the virus is transported to lymph nodes where it replicates extensively in its target host cells, the CD4+ lymphocytes. After infection, most patients experience a brief glandular fever-like illness which is associated with a decline in the CD4+ cells and high titres of virus in the blood. The levels of virus in the blood then decline as the cellular and humoral immune responses are mounted. A long period of latency then follows which may last from 1 to perhaps 15 years or longer before any further clinical symptoms become apparent. In infected CD4+ cells the viral reverse transcriptase makes double stranded DNA copies of the HIV RNA and some of these become integrated into cellular chromosomes. These integrated proviruses may remain latent indefinitely. During this long asymptomatic phase only a small minority of CD4+ cells produce virus and only very low titres of HIV can be detected in the blood. As time goes by, however, there is a steady decline in the numbers of CD4+ cells in the blood and when the count falls below 200–400/µl the immune system becomes severely compromised. The consequent activation of other latent infections with organisms such cytomegalovirus or *Mycobacterium tuberculosis* and secondary infections with a variety of opportunistic pathogens such as *Pneumocystis carinii* will inevitably kill the AIDS patient.

Despite enormous research efforts, effective vaccines or chemotherapeutic agents against HIV have yet to be produced. There is no prospect that drugs will be able to eliminate the virus from the population of lymphocytes, the only hope is that compounds will be found that will achieve long-term suppression of viral replication and thus preserve the stock of CD4+ cells in infected individuals. It was hoped that inhibitors of reverse transcriptase such as azidothymidine (AZT) or dideoxyinosine (ddI) would act in this way; however, it is becoming increasing clear that these drugs do not consistently arrest the progress of the disease even when treatment is started in the asymptomatic phase.

In parts of the world (sub-Sahran African and southern and South-East Asia) the AIDS pandemic is out of control, with no effective chemotherapeutic agents and little prospect of a vaccine; the prognoses are bleak for the millions of HIV-infected individuals. Sexual intercourse is now the main mode of infection and if the pandemic is to be contained, sexually active individuals have to be persuaded to reduce the numbers of their sex partners and to practise safe sex using condoms.

12   Prions

The causative agents of the neurodegerative diseases of scrapie in sheep, bovine spongiform encephalopathy (BSE) and Creutzfeldt–Jakob disease (CJD) in humans used to be referred to as slow viruses. It is now clear, however, that they are caused by a distinct class of infectious agents termed *prions* (a word standing for 'proteinaceous infectious particle') that have unique and disturbing properties. These particles can be recovered from the brains of infected individuals as minute rod-like structures composed of oligomers of a 30-kDa polypeptide. They are devoid of nucleic acid and extremely resistant to heating and to ultraviolet irradiation. They also fail to produce an immune response in the host. Just how such proteins can replicate and be infectious has only recently become understood. It seems that a protein with the same amino acid sequence as the prion, but with a different conformation, is present in the membranes of normal neurones of the host. The evidence suggests that the prion form of the protein combines with the normal host cell form and alters its configuration to that of the prion. The newly formed prion can then in turn modify the folding of other normal protein molecules. In this way the prion protein is capable of autocatalytic replication. As the prions slowly accumulate in the brain, the neurones progressively vacuolate, holes eventually develop in the grey matter and the brain takes on a sponge-like appearance. The clinical symptoms take a long time to develop—up to 20 years in humans—but the disease has an inevitable progression to paralysis and death.

There has been great concern over the large-scale outbreak of BSE that occurred in the UK from 1988 as a result of feeding cattle with supplements prepared from sheep and cattle offal. Brain extracts from BSE cattle have transmitted the disease to mice, sheep, cattle, pigs and monkeys. Studies of 12 recent cases of atypical CJD in the UK have provided evidence that the bovine prions have infected humans through the consumption of contaminated beef.

13   Further reading

Dalgleish A.G. (1991) Viruses and cancer. *Br Med Bull*, **47**, 21–46.
Grady C. & Kelly G. (1996) HIV vaccine development. *Nursing Clin North Am*, **31**, 25–39.

Levie A.J. (1991) *Viruses.* Oxford: W.H. Freeman.

Norkin L.C. (1995) Virus receptors—implications for pathogenesis and the design of antiviral agents. *Clin Microbiol Rev*, **8**, 293–315.

Oxford J.S. (1995) Quo-vadis antiviral agents for herpes, influenza and HIV. *J Med Microbiol*, **43**, 1–3.

Pantaleo G. & Fauci A.S. (1996) Immunopathogenesis of HIV infection. *Ann Rev Microbiol*, **50**, 825–854.

Pauza C.D. & Streblow D.N. (1995) Therapeutic approaches to HIV infection based on virus structure and host-pathogen interaction. *Curr Topics Microbiol Immunol*, **202**, 117–132.

Prusiner S.B. (1996) Molecular biology and pathogenesis of prion disease. *Trends Biochem Sci*, **21**, 482–487.

White D.O. & Fenner F.J. (1994) *Medical Virology,* 4th edn. San Diego: Academic Press.

Whitley R.G. (1996) The past as a prelude to the future—history, status and future of antiviral drugs. *Ann Pharmacother*, **30**, 967–971.

4 Principles of microbial pathogenicity and epidemiology

1   Introduction

2   Portals of entry
2.1 Respiratory tract
2.2 Intestinal tract
2.3 Urinogenital tract
2.4 Conjunctiva

3   Consolidation
3.1 Resistance to host's defences
3.1.1 Modulation of the inflammatory
      response
3.1.2 Avoidance of phagocytosis
3.1.3 Survival following phagocytosis
3.1.4 Killing of phagocytes

4   Manifestation of disease
4.1 Non-invasive pathogens

4.2 Partially invasive pathogens
4.3 Invasive pathogens
4.3.1 Active spread
4.3.2 Passive spread

5   Damage to tissues
5.1 Direct damage
5.1.1 Specific effects
5.1.2 Non-specific effects
5.2 Indirect damage

6   Recovery from infection: exit of
     microorganisms

7   Epidemiology of infectious disease

8   Further reading

1   Introduction

The majority of microorganisms are free living and derive their nutrition from inert organic and inorganic materials. The association of such microorganisms with humans is generally harmonious, as the majority of those encountered are benign and, indeed, are often vital to balanced ecosystems. In spite of the ubiquity of microorganisms the tissues of healthy animals and plants are essentially microbe-free. This is achieved through provision of a number of non-specific defences to those tissues, and specific defences such as antibodies (see Chapters 14, 15) acquired after exposure to particular agents. Breach of these defences by microorganisms through the expression of virulence factors and adaptation to a pathogenic mode of life or following disease, accidental trauma, catheterization or implantation of medical devices may lead to the establishment of microbial infections.

The ability of bacteria and fungi to establish infections varies considerably. Some are rarely, if ever, isolated from infected tissues, whilst opportunist pathogens (e.g. *Pseudomonas aeruginosa*) can establish themselves only in compromised tissues. Only a few species of bacteria may be regarded as obligate pathogens, for which animals, plants or humans are the only reservoirs for their existence (e.g. *Neisseria gonorrhoeae*). Viruses (Chapter 3) on the other hand must parasitize host cells in order to replicate and are therefore inevitably associated with disease. Even amongst the viruses and obligate bacterial pathogens the degree of virulence varies, in that some are able to coexist with the host without causing the disease state (e.g. staphylococci), whilst others will always manifest disease. Organisms such as these invariably produce their effects, directly or indirectly, by actively growing on or in the host tissues.

Other groups of organisms may cause disease through ingestion by the victim of substances (toxins) produced during microbial growth on foods (e.g. *Clostridium botulinum,* botulism; *Bacillus cereus,* vomiting). The organisms themselves do not have to survive and grow in the victim in order for the effects of the toxin to be felt. Whether such organisms should be regarded as pathogenic is debatable, but they must be considered in any account of microbial pathogenicity.

The course of infection can be considered as a sequence of separate events (Fig. 4.1). In order for an infection to develop, pathogenic microorganisms must increase their number within the host more rapidly than the host can eliminate or kill them. Greater numbers of cells in the initial challenge to the host will increase the chances of successful colonization. The successful pathogen must therefore arrive at its 'portal of entry' to the body, or directly at the target tissue, in sufficient numbers as to allow establishment. The minimum number of infective organisms required to cause disease is called the 'minimum infective number' (MIN). MIN varies markedly between the various pathogens and is also affected by the general health and immune status of the individual host organisms, between individual hosts, and with the general state of health of the host. Growth and consolidation of the microorganisms at the portal of

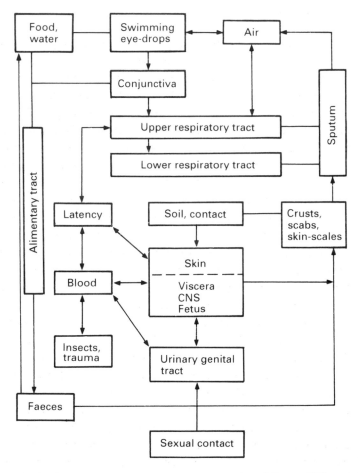

Fig. 4.1 Routes of infection and spread of transmission of disease. CNS, central nervous system.

entry commonly involves the formation of a microcolony (biofilm). Biofilms and microcolonies are collections of microorganisms that are attached to surfaces and enveloped within exopolymer matrices (glycocalyx) composed of polysaccharides, glycoproteins and/or proteins. Growth within the matrix not only protects the pathogens against phagocytosis and opsonization within the host but also modulates their micro-environment and reduces the effectiveness of some antibiotics. The high bacterial densities present within the biofilm communities also initiate the production of extracellular virulence factors such as toxins, proteases and siderophores (low molecular weight ligands responsible for the solubilization and transport of iron (III) in microbial cells) and may promote their acquisition of nutrients. Viruses are incapable of growing extracellularly and must therefore rapidly gain entry to the epithelial cells at their site of entry. Once internalized they are to a large extent, in the non-immune host, protected against the non-specific host defences. Following these initial consolidation events, the organisms may expand into surrounding tissues, and/or disperse via the circulatory systems to distant tissues to establish secondary sites of infection and consolidate further. Finally, the organism must exit the body, survive and/or immediately re-enter another susceptible host.

2   Portals of entry

The part of the body most widely exposed to microorganisms is the skin. Intact skin is usually impervious to microorganisms. Its surface contains relatively few nutrients and is of acid pH, which is unfavourable for microbial growth. The vast majority of organisms falling onto the skin surface will die, the remainder must compete for nutrients with the commensal microflora in order to grow. These commensals are highly adapted to growth on the skin and will normally prevent the establishment of adventitious contaminants. Infections of the skin itself, such as ringworm (*Trichophyton mentagrophytes*) rarely, if ever, involve penetration of the epidermis. Infections can, however, occur through the skin following trauma such as burns, cuts and abrasions and, in some instances, through insect or animal bites or the injection of contaminated medicines. In recent years extensive use of intravascular and extravascular medical devices and implants has led to an increase in the occurrence of hospital-acquired infection. Commonly these infections involve growth of skin commensals such as *Staphylococcus epidermidis* when associated with devices which penetrate the skin barrier. The organism grows as an adhesive biofilm upon the surfaces of the device, where infection arises either from contamination of the device during its implantation or by growth of the organism along it from the skin. In such instances the biofilm sheds bacterial cells to the body and gives rise to bacteraemias (the presence of bacteria in the blood). These readily respond to antibiotic treatment but the biofilm which is relatively recalcitrant towards even agressive antibiotic therapy, remains and acts as a continued focus of infection. In practice, such infected devices must be removed, and can be replaced only after successful chemotherapy of the bacteraemia.

The weak spots, or Achilles heels, of the body occur where the skin ends and mucous epithelial tissues begin (mouth, anus, eyes, ears, nose and urinogenital tract). These mucous membranes present a much more favourable environment for microbial growth than the skin, in that they are warm, moist and rich in nutrients. Such membranes, nevertheless, possess certain characteristics that allow them to resist infection. The majority, for example, possess their own highly adapted commensal microflora which must be displaced by any invading organisms. These resident flora vary greatly between different sites of the body but are usually common to particular host species. Each site can be additionally protected by physico-chemical barriers such as extreme acid pH in the stomach, the presence of freely circulating non-specific antibodies and/or opsonins, and/or by macrophages and phagocytes (see Chapter 14). All infections start from contact between these tissues and the potential pathogen. Contact may be direct, from an infected individual to a healthy one; or indirect, and involve inanimate vectors such as soil, food, drink, air and airborne particles being ingested, inhaled or entering wounds, or via infected bed-linen and clothing. Indirect contact may also involve animal vectors (carriers).

2.1   Respiratory tract

Air contains a large amount of suspended organic matter and, in enclosed occupied spaces, may hold up to 1000 microorganisms m^{-3}. Almost all of these airborne organisms are non-pathogenic bacteria and fungi of which the average person would inhale approximately 10 000 per day. The respiratory tract is protected against this assault by a mucociliary blanket which envelops the lower respiratory tract and nasal cavity. Particles becoming entrapped in this blanket of mucus are carried by ciliary action to the back of the throat and swallowed. The alveolar regions are, in addition, protected by a lining of macrophages. To be successful, a pathogen must avoid being trapped in the mucus and swallowed, and if deposited in the alveolar sacs must avoid engulfment by macrophages or resist subsequent digestion by them. The possession of surface adhesins, specific for epithelial receptors, aids attachment of the invading microorganism and avoidance of removal by the mucociliary blanket.

2.2   Intestinal tract

The intestinal tract must contend with whatever it is given in terms of food and drink. The lower gut is highly populated by commensal microorganisms ($10^{11} g^{-1}$ gut tissue). These organisms are often associated with the intestinal wall, either embedded in layers of protective mucus or attached directly to the epithelial cells. The pathogenicity of incoming bacteria and viruses depends upon their ability to survive passage through the stomach and duodenum and upon their capacity for attachment to, or penetration of, the gut wall in competition with the commensal flora, and in spite of the presence of secretory antibodies (Chapter 14).

2.3   Urinogenital tract

In healthy individuals, the bladder, ureters and urethra are sterile and sterile urine constantly flushes the urinary tract. Organisms invading the urinary tract must avoid being detached from the epithelial surfaces and washed out during urination. In the male, since the urethra is long (*ca.* 20 cm), bacteria must be introduced directly into the bladder, possibly through catheterization. In the female, the urethra is much shorter (*ca.* 5 cm) and is more readily traversed by microorganisms normally resident within the vaginal vault. Bladder infections are therefore much more common in the female. Spread of the infection from the bladder to the kidneys can easily occur through the reflux of urine into the ureter. As for the implantation of devices across the skin barrier (above), long-term catheterization of the bladder will promote the occurrence of bacterurias (the presence of bacteria in the urine) with all of the associated complications.

Lactic acid in the vagina gives it an acidic pH (5.0) which together with other products of metabolism inhibits colonization by most bacteria, except some lactobacilli, which constitute the commensal flora. Other types of bacteria are unable to establish themselves in the vagina unless they have become extremely specialized. These species of microorganism tend to be associated with venereal infections.

2.4 Conjunctiva

The conjunctiva is usually free of microorganisms and protected by the continuous flow of secretions from lachrymal and other glands, and by frequent mechanical cleansing of its surface by the eyelid periphery during blinking. Damage to the conjunctiva, caused through mechanical abrasion or reduction in tear flow, will increase microbial adhesion and allow colonization by opportunist pathogens. The likelihood of infection is thus promoted by the use of soft and hard contact lenses, physical damage, exposure to chemicals, or damage and infection of the eyelid border (blepharitis).

3 Consolidation

To be successful, a pathogen must be able to survive at its initial portal of entry, frequently in competition with the commensal flora and subject to the attention of macrophages and wandering white blood cells. Such survival invariably requires the organism to attach itself firmly to the epithelial surface. This attachment must be highly specific in order to displace the commensal microflora and subsequently governs the course of an infection. Attachment can be mediated through provision, on the bacterial surface, of adhesive substances, such as mucopeptide and mucopolysaccharide slime layers, fimbriae (Chapter 1), pili (Chapter 1) and agglutinins (Chapter 14). These are often highly specific in their binding characteristics, differentiating, for example, between the tips and bases of villi and the epithelial cells of the upper, mid and lower gut. Secretory antibodies which are directed against such adhesins block the initial attachment of the organism and confer resistance to infection.

The outcome of the encounter between the tissues and potential pathogens is governed by the ability of the microorganisms to multiply at a faster rate than they are removed from those tissues. Factors which influence this are the organisms's rate of growth, the initial number of organisms arriving at the site and their ability to resist the efforts of the host tissues at killing it. The definition of *virulence* for pathogenic microorganisms must therefore relate to the minimum number of cells required to initiate an infection. This will vary between individuals, but will invariably be lower in compromised hosts such as diabetics, cystic fibrotics and those suffering trauma such as malnutrition, chronic infection or physical damage.

Resistance to host's defences

Most bacterial infections confine themselves to the surface of epithelial tissue (e.g. *Bordetella pertussis, Corynebacterium diphtheriae, Vibrio cholerae)*. This is, to a large extent, a reflection of their inability to combat that host's deeper defences. Survival at these sites is largely due to firm attachment to the epithelial cells. Such organisms manifest disease through the production and release of toxins (see below).

Other groups of organisms regularly establish systemic infections (e.g. *Brucella abortus, Salmonella typhi, Streptococcus pyogenes)* after traversing the epithelial surfaces. This property is associated with their ability either to gain entry into susceptible cells and thereby enjoy protection from the body's defences, or to be phagocytosed by macrophages or polymorphs yet resist their lethal action and multiply within them. Other organisms are able to multiply and grow freely in the body's extracellular fluids. Microorganisms have evolved a number of different strategies which allow them to suppress the host's normal defences and thereby survive in the tissues. These are considered later.

3.1.1   *Modulation of the inflammatory response*

Growth of microorganisms releases cellular products into their surrounding medium, many of which cause non-specific inflammation associated with dilatation of blood vessels. This increases capillary flow and access of phagocytes to the infected site. Increased lymphatic flow from the inflamed tissues carries the organisms to lymph nodes where further antimicrobial and immune forces come into play (Chapter 14). Many of the substances released by microorganisms are chemotactic towards polymorphs which tend therefore to become concentrated at the site of infection. This is in addition to inflammation and white blood cell chemotaxis associated with antibody binding and complement fixation (Chapter 14). Many organisms have adapted mechanisms which allow them to overcome these initial defences. Thus, virulent strains of *Staphylococcus aureus* produce a mucopeptide (peptidoglycan), which suppresses early inflammatory oedema, and a related factor which suppresses the chemotaxis of polymorphs.

3.1.2   *Avoidance of phagocytosis*

Resistance to phagocytosis is sometimes associated with specific components of the cell wall and/or with the presence of capsules surrounding the cell wall. Classic examples of these are the M-proteins of the streptococci and the polysaccharide capsules of pneumococci. The acidic polysaccharide K-antigens of *Escherichia coli* and *Sal. typhi* behave similarly, in that (i) they can mediate attachment to the intestinal epithelial cells, and (ii) they render phagocytosis more difficult. Generally, possession of an extracellular capsule will reduce the likelihood of phagocytosis.

Microorganisms are more readily phagocytosed when coated with antibody (opsonized). This is due to the presence on the white blood cells of receptors for the Fc fragment of IgM and IgG (discussed in Chapter 14). Avoidance of opsonization will clearly enhance the chances of survival of a particular pathogen. A substance called protein A is released from actively growing strains of *Staph. aureus.* This acts by non-specific binding to IgG, at the Fc region (see also Chapter 14), at sites both close to and remote from the bacterial surface. This blocks the Fc region of bound antibody masking it from phagocytes. Protein A–IgG complexes will also bind complement, depleting it from the plasma and negating the associated chemotactic responses.

| 3.1.3 | *Survival following phagocytosis* |

Death following phagocytosis can be avoided if the microorganisms are not exposed to the intracellular processes (killing and digestion) within the phagocyte. This is possible if fusion of the lysosomes with phagocytic vacuoles can be prevented. Such a strategy is employed by virulent *Mycobacterium tuberculosis,* although the precise mechanism is unknown. Other bacteria seem able to grow within the vacuoles despite lysosomal fusion *(Listeria monocytogenes, Sal. typhi).* This can be attributed to cell wall components which prevent access of the lysosomal substances to the bacterial membranes (e.g. *Brucella abortus,* mycobacteria) or to the production of extracellular catalase which neutralizes the hydrogen peroxide liberated in the vacuole (e.g. staphylococci, streptococci).

If microorganisms are able to survive and grow within phagocytes then they will escape many of the other body defences and be distributed around the body.

| 3.1.4 | *Killing of phagocytes* |

An alternative strategy is for the microorganism to kill the phagocyte. This can be achieved by the production of leucocidins (e.g. staphylococci, streptococci) which promote the discharge of lysosomal substances into the cytoplasm of the phagocyte rather than into the vacuole, thus directing the phagocyte's lethal activity towards itself.

4 Manifestation of disease

Once established, the course of a bacterial infection can proceed in a number of ways. These can be related to the relative ability of the organism to penetrate and invade surrounding tissues and organs. The vast majority of pathogens, being unable to combat the defences of the deeper tissues, consolidate further on the epithelial surface. Others, which include a majority of viruses, penetrate the epithelial layers, but no further, and can be regarded as partially invasive. A small group of pathogens are fully invasive. These permeate the subepithelial tissues and are circulated around the body to initiate secondary sites of infection remote from the initial portal of entry.

Other groups of organisms may cause disease through ingestion by the victim of substances produced during microbial growth on foods. Such diseases may be regarded as intoxications rather than as infections and are considered further in section 5.1.1. Treatment in these cases is usually an alleviation of the harmful effects of the toxin rather than elimination of the pathogen from the body.

4.1 Non-invasive pathogens

Bordetella pertussis (the aetiological agent of whooping-cough) is probably the best described of these pathogens. This organism is inhaled and rapidly localizes on the mucociliary blanket of the lower respiratory tract. This localization is very selective and thought to involve agglutinins on the organisms' surface. Toxins, produced by the organism, inhibit ciliary movement of the epithelial surface and thereby prevent removal of the bacterial cells to the gut. A high molecular weight exotoxin is also produced during the growth of the organism which, being of limited diffusibility, pervades the subepithelial tissues to produce inflammation and necrosis. *C. diphtheriae* (the causal organism of diphtheria) behaves similarly, attaching itself to the epithelial cells of the respiratory tract. This organism produces a low molecular weight, diffusible toxin which enters the blood circulation and brings about a generalized toxaemia.

In the gut, many pathogens adhere to the gut wall and produce their toxic effect via toxins which pervade the surrounding gut wall or enter the systemic circulation. *Vibrio cholerae* and some enteropathic *E. coli* strains localize on the gut wall and produce toxins which increase vascular permeability. The end result is a hypersecretion of isotonic fluids into the gut lumen, acute diarrhoea and consequent dehydration which may be fatal in juveniles and the elderly. In all these instances, binding to epithelial cells is not essential but increases permeation of the toxin and prolongs the presence of the pathogen.

4.2 Partially invasive pathogens

Some bacteria and the majority of viruses are able to attach to the mucosal epithelia and then penetrate rapidly into the epithelial cells. These organisms multiply within the protective environment of the host cell, eventually killing it and inducing disease through erosion and ulceration of the mucosal epithelium. Typically, members of the genera *Shigella* and *Salmonella* utilize such mechanisms. These bacteria attach to the epithelial cells of the large and small intestines, respectively, and, following their entry into these cells by induced pinocytosis, multiply rapidly and penetrate laterally into adjacent epithelial cells. The mechanisms for such attachment and movement are unknown. Some species of salmonellae produce, in addition, exotoxins which induce diarrhoea (section 4.1). There are innumerable species and serotypes of *Salmonella*. These are primarily parasites of animals, but are important to humans in that they colonize farm animals such as pigs and poultry and ultimately infect such food. *Salmonella* food poisoning (salmonellosis), therefore, is commonly associated with inadequately cooked meats, eggs and also with cold meat products which have been incorrectly stored following contact with the uncooked product. Dependent upon the severity of the lesions induced in the gut wall by these pathogens, red blood cells and phagocytes pass into the gut lumen, along with plasma, and cause the classic 'bloody flux' of bacillary dysentery. Similar erosive lesions are produced by some enteropathic strains of *E. coli*.

Virus infections such as influenza and the 'common cold' (in reality 300–400 different strains of rhinovirus) infect epithelial cells of the respiratory tract and naso-pharynx, respectively. Release of the virus, after lysis of the host cells, is to the void rather than to subepithelial tissues. The epithelia is further infected resulting in general degeneration of the tracts. Such damage predisposes the respiratory tract to infection with opportunistic pathogens such as *Neisseria meningitidis* and *Haemophilus influenzae*.

4.3   **Invasive pathogens**

Invasive pathogens either aggressively invade the tissues surrounding the primary site of infection or are passively transported around the body in the blood, lymph, cerebrospinal fluid or pleural fluids. Some, especially aggressive organisms, do both, setting up a number of expansive secondary sites of infection in various organs.

4.3.1   *Active spread*

Active spread of microorganisms through normal subepithelial tissues is difficult in that the gel-like nature of the intracellular materials physically inhibits bacterial movement. Induced death and lysis of the tissue cells, in addition, produces a highly viscous fluid, partly due to undenatured DNA. Physical damage, such as wounds, rapidly seal with fibrin clots, thus reducing the effective routes of spread for opportunist pathogens. Organisms such as *Str. pyogenes*, *Cl. perfringens*, and to some extent the staphylococci, are able to establish themselves in tissues by virtue of their ability to produce a wide range of extracellular enzyme toxins. These are associated with killing of tissue cells, degradation of intracellular materials and mobilization of nutrients, and will be considered briefly.

1 *Haemolysins* are produced by most of the pathogenic staphylococci and streptococci. They have a lytic effect on red blood cells, releasing iron-containing nutrients.

2 *Fibrinolysins* are produced by both staphylococci (staphylokinase) and streptococci (streptokinase). These toxins dissolve fibrin clots, formed by the host around wounds and lesions to seal them, by indirect activation of plasminogen, thereby increasing the likelihood of organism spread. Streptokinase may be employed clinically in conjunction with streptodornase (Chapter 25) in the treatment of thrombosis.

3 *Collagenases* and *hyaluronidases* are produced by most of the aggressive invaders. These are able to dissolve collagen fibres and hyaluronic acids which function as intracellular cements. Their loss causes the tissues to break up and produce oedematous lesions.

4 *Phospholipases* are produced by organisms such as *Cl. perfringens* (α-toxin). These kill tissue cells by hydrolysing phospholipids present in cell membranes.

5 *Amylases, peptidases* and *deoxyribonuclease* mobilize many nutrients that are released from lysed cells. They also decrease the viscosity of fluids present at the lesion by depolymerization of their biopolymer substrates.

Organisms possessing the above toxins, particularly those also possessing leucocidins, are likely to cause expanding oedematous lesions at the primary site of infection. In the case of *Cl. perfringens,* a soil microorganism which has become adapted to a saprophytic mode of life, when it causes infection due to accidental contamination of deep wounds there ensues a process similar to that seen during the decomposition of a carcass. This organism is most likely to spread through tissues when blood circulation, and therefore oxygen tension, in the affected areas is minimal.

Abscesses formed by streptococci and staphylococci can be deep seated in soft tissues or associated with infected wounds or skin lesions. These become localized through the deposition of fibrin capsules around the infective site. Fibrin deposition is partly a response of the host tissues and partly a function of enzyme toxins such as coagulase. Phagocytic white blood cells can migrate into these abscesses in large numbers to produce significant quantities of pus; this might be digested by other phagocytes in the latter stages of the infection or discharged to the exterior or to the capillary and lymphatic network. In the latter case, blocked capillaries might serve as sites for secondary lesions. Toxins liberated from the microorganisms during their growth in such abscesses can freely diffuse to the rest of the body to set up a generalized toxaemia.

Particular strains of salmonellae (section 4.2) such as *Sal. typhi, Sal. paratyphi* and *Sal. typhimurium* are able not only to penetrate into intestinal epithelial cells and produce exotoxins but also to penetrate beyond into subepithelial tissues. These organisms therefore produce, in addition to the usual symptoms of salmonellosis, a characteristic systemic disease (typhoid and enteric fever). Following recovery from such infection the organism is commonly found associated with the gall bladder. In this state, the recovered person will excrete the organism and form a reservoir for the infection of others.

4.3.2   Passive spread

When invading microorganisms have crossed the epithelial barriers they will almost certainly be taken up, with lymph, in the lymphatic ducts and be delivered to the filtration and immune systems of the local lymph nodes. Sometimes this serves to spread infections further around the body. Eventually, spread may occur from local to regional lymph nodes and thence to the bloodstream. Direct entry to the bloodstream from the primary portal of entry is rare and will only occur when the organism damages the blood vessels or if it is injected directly into them. This might be the case following an insect bite or surgery. Bacteraemia such as this will often lead to secondary infections remote from the original portal of entry.

5   Damage to tissues

Damage caused to the host organism through infection can be direct and relate to the destructive presence, or to the production, of toxins by microorganisms in particular target organs; or it can be indirect and relate to interactions of the antigenic components of the pathogen with the host's immune system. Effects can therefore be closely related to, or remote from, the target organ.

Symptoms of the infection can in some instances be highly specific, relating to a single, precise pharmacological response to a particular toxin; or they might be non-specific and relate to the usual response of the body to particular types of trauma. Damage induced by infection will therefore be considered in these categories.

5.1   Direct damage

5.1.1   Specific effects

The consequences of infection to the host depend to a large extent upon the tissue or

organ involved. Soft tissue infections of skeletal muscle ɑ
than, for instance, infections of the heart muscle and centrɑ.
of the epithelial cells of small blood vessels can produce
tissues they supply. Cell and tissue damage is generally the rε.
by the microorganisms, usually concerning action at cell memι
are usually phagocytic cells and are generally killed (e.g. b.
Mycobacterium). Interference with membrane function, through th
such as phospholipase, cause the affected cells to leak. When lyso.   ɑnes
are affected, then lysosomal enzymes disperse into the cells and tissu   ɑsing them,
in turn, to autolyse. This is mediated through the vast battery of enzyme toxins available
to these organisms (section 4). If enough of these toxins are produced to enter the
circulation then a generalized toxaemia might result. During their growth, other
pathogens liberate toxins with precise pharmacological actions. Diseases mediated in
this manner include diphtheria, tetanus and scarlet fever.

In diphtheria, the organism *C. diphtheriae* confines itself to epithelial surfaces of
the nose and throat and produces a powerful toxin which affects the elongation factor
involved in protein biosynthesis. The heart and peripheral nerves are particularly affected
resulting in myocarditis (inflammation of the myocardium) and neuritis (inflammation
of a nerve). Little damage is produced at the infective site.

Tetanus occurs when *Cl. tetani*, ubiquitous in the soil and faeces, contaminates
wounds, especially deep puncture-type lesions. These might be minor traumas such as
a splinter, or major ones such as battle injury. At these sites, tissue necrosis and possibly
microbial growth reduce the oxygen tension to allow this anaerobe to multiply. Its
growth is accompanied by the production of a highly potent toxin which passes up
peripheral nerves and diffuses locally within the central nervous system. It acts like
strychnine by affecting normal function at the synapses. Since the motor nerves of the
brain stem are the shortest, the cranial nerves are the first affected, with twitches of the
eyes and spasms of the jaw (lockjaw).

A related organism, *Cl. botulinum*, produces a similar toxin which may contaminate
food if the organism has grown in it and conditions are favourable for anaerobic growth.
Meat pastes and pâtés are likely sources. This toxin interferes with acetylcholine release
at cholinergic synapses and also acts at neuromuscular junctions. Death from this toxin
eventually results from respiratory failure.

Many other organisms are capable of producing intoxication following their growth
on foods. Most common amongst these are the staphylococci and particular strains of
Bacillus such as *B. cereus*. Staphylococci such as *Staph. aureus* produce an enterotoxin
which acts upon the vomiting centres of the brain. Nausea and vomiting therefore
follow ingestion of contaminated foods, the delay between eating and vomiting varying
between 1 and 6 hours, depending on the amount of toxin ingested. *Bacillus cereus*
also produces an emetic toxin but its actions are delayed and vomiting can follow up to
20 hours after ingestion. The latter organism is often associated with rice products and
will propagate when the rice is cooked (spore activation) and subsequently reheated
after a period of storage.

Scarlet fever is produced following infection with certain strains of *Strep. pyogenes*.
These produce a potent toxin which causes an erythrogenic skin rash which accompanies
the more usual effects of a streptococcal infection.

If the infective agent damages an organ and affects its functioning, this can manifest itself as a series of secondary disease features. Thus, diabetes may result from an infection of the islets of Langerhans, paralysis or coma from infections of the central nervous system, and kidney malfunction from loss of tissue fluids and its associated hyper-glycaemia. In this respect virus infections almost inevitably result in the death and lysis of the host cells. This will result in some loss of function by the target organ. Similarly, exotoxins and endotoxins can also be implicated in non-specific symptoms, even when they have fairly well-defined pharmacological actions. Thus, a number of intestinal pathogens (e.g. *V. cholerae, E. coli*) produce potent exotoxins which affect vascular permeability. These generally act through adenyl cyclase, raising the intracellular levels of cyclic AMP (adenosine monophosphate). As a result of this the cells lose water and electrolytes to the surrounding medium, the gut lumen. A common consequence of these related, yet distinct, toxins is acute diarrhoea and haemoconcentration. Kidney malfunction might well follow and in severe cases lead to death. Symptomologically there is little difference between these conditions and food poisoning induced by ingestion of staphylococcal enterotoxin. The latter toxin is formed by the organisms during their growth on infected food substances and is absorbed actively from the gut. It acts, not at the epithelial cells of the gut, but at the vomiting centre of the central nervous system causing nausea, vomiting and diarrhoea within 6 hours.

Endotoxins form part of the cell envelopes of some bacterial species (see Chapter 1). They are shed into the surrounding medium during growth and following autolysis of the infecting organism. Endotoxins tend to be less toxic than exotoxins and less precise in their action. Classic endotoxins are the lipopolysaccharide/protein components of Gram-negative cells, i.e. *E. coli* and the salmonellae. Various toxic effects have been attributed to these endotoxins but their role in the establishment of the infection, if any, remains unclear. The most notable effect is their pyrogenicity (Chapters 1 and 18). This relates to release by the endotoxin of endogenous pyrogen from macrophages and phagocytes. Elevation of body temperature follows within 1–2 hours.

5.2   Indirect damage

Inflammatory materials are released from necrotic cells and directly from the infective agent. It is not always clear to what extent these can be related to actions by the host or by the pathogen. Inflammation causes swelling, pain and reddening of the tissues, and sometimes loss of function of the organs affected. These reactions may sometimes be the major sign and symptom of the disease.

Many microorganisms minimize the effects of the host's defence system against them by mimicking the antigenic structure of the host tissue. The eventual immunological response of the host to infection then leads to the autoimmune destruction of itself. Thus, infections with *Mycoplasma pneumoniae* can lead to production of antibody against normal Group O erythrocytes with concomitant haemolytic anaemia.

If antigen, released from the infective agent, is soluble then antigen–antibody complexes are produced. When antibody is present at a concentration equal to or greater than the antigen, such as in the case of an immune host, then these complexes precipitate and are removed by macrophages present in the lymph nodes. When antigen is present in excess the complexes, being small, continue to circulate in the blood and are eventually filtered off by the kidneys, becoming lodged in kidney glomeruli. A localized inflammatory response in the kidneys might then be initiated by the complement system (Chapter 14). Eventually the filtering function of the kidneys becomes impaired, producing symptoms of chronic glomerulonephritis.

6 Recovery from infection: exit of microorganisms

The primary requirement for recovery is that multiplication of the infective agent is brought under control, that it ceases to spread around the body and that the damaging consequences of its presence are arrested and repaired. Such control and recovery are brought about by the combined functioning of the phagocytic, immune and complement systems. A successful pathogen will not seriously debilitate its host; rather, the continued existence of the host must be ensured in order to maximize the dissemination of the pathogen within the host population. Ideally, the organism must persist within the host for the remainder of its lifespan and be constantly released to the environment. Whilst this is the case for a number of virus infections and for some bacterial ones, it is not common. Generally, recovery from infection is accompanied by complete destruction of the organism and restoration of a sterile tissue. Alternatively, the organism might return to a commensal relationship with the host on the epithelial and skin surface.

Where the infective agent is an obligate pathogen, a means must exist for it to infect other individuals before its eradication from the host organism. The route of exit is commonly related to the original portal of entry. Thus, pathogens of the intestinal tract are liberated in the faeces and might easily contaminate food and drinking water. Infective agents of the respiratory tract might be inhaled during coughing, sneezing or talking, survive in the associated water droplets and infect nearby individuals. Infective agents transmitted by insect and animal vectors may be spread through the same vectors, the insects/animals having been infected by the diseased host. For some 'fragile' organisms (e.g. *N. gonorrhoeae, Treponema pallidum*), direct contact transmission is the only means of transmission. In these cases, intimate contact between epithelial membranes, such as occurs during sexual contact, is required for transfer to occur. For opportunist pathogens, such as those associated with wound infections, transfer is less important because the pathogenic role is minor. Rather, the natural habitat of the organism serves as a constant reservoir for infection.

7 Epidemiology of infectious disease

Spread of a microbial disease through a population of individuals can be considered as vertical (transferred from one generation to another) or horizontal (transfer occurring within genetically unrelated groups). The latter can be divided into common-source outbreaks, relating to infection of a number of susceptible individuals from a single reservoir of the infective agent (i.e. infected foods), or propagated-source outbreaks, where each individual provides a new source for the infection of others.

Common-source outbreaks are characterized by a sharp onset of reported cases over the course of a single incubation period and relate to a common experience of the infected individuals. The number of cases will persist until the source of the infection is removed. If the source of the infection remains (i.e. a reservoir of insect vectors) then the disease becomes endemic to the exposed population with a constant rate of infection. Propagated-source outbreaks, on the other hand, show a gradual increase in reported cases over a number of incubation periods and eventually decline when the majority of susceptibles in the population have been affected. Factors contributing to propagated outbreaks of infectious disease are the infectivity of the agent (I), the population density (P) and the numbers of susceptible individuals in it (F). The likelihood of an epidemic is given by the product of these three factors (i.e. FIP). Changes in any one of them might initiate an outbreak of the disease in epidemic proportions. Thus, reported cases of particular diseases show periodicity, with outbreaks of epidemic proportion occurring only when FIP exceeds certain critical threshold values, related to the infectivity of the agent. Outbreaks of measles and chickenpox therefore tend to occur annually in the late summer amongst children attending school for the first time. This has the effect of concentrating all susceptible individuals in one, often confined, space at the same time. The proportion of susceptibles can be reduced through rigorous vaccination programmes (Chapter 16). Provided that the susceptible population does not exceed the threshold FIP value, then herd immunity against epidemic spread of the disease will be maintained.

Certain types of infectious agent (e.g. influenza virus) are able to combat herd immunity such as this through undergoing major antigenic changes. These render the majority of the population susceptible, and their occurrence is often accompanied by spread of the disease across the entire globe (pandemics).

8   Further reading

Bisno A.L. & Waidvogel F.A. (1994) *Infections Associated with Indwelling Medical Devices*, 2nd edn.
• Washington: American Society for Microbiology.
Mims C.A. (1991) *The Pathogenesis of Infectious Disease*, 4th edn. London: Academic Press.
Salyers A.A. & Drew D.D. (1994) *Bacterial Pathogenesis; a Molecular Approach.* Washington: American Society for Microbiology Press.
Smith H. (1990) Pathogenicity and the microbe *in vivo. J Gen Microbiol*, **136**, 377–393.

Part 2
Antimicrobial Agents

The theme of this section is antimicrobial agents; these are considered in three categories: first, antibiotics and *de novo* chemically synthesized chemotherapeutic agents; second, non-antibiotic antimicrobial compounds (disinfectants, antiseptics and preservatives); and third, immunological products. The subjects covered comprise the manufacture, evaluation and properties of antibiotics; the evaluation and properties of disinfectants, antiseptics and preservatives; the fundamentals of immunology; and the manufacture, quality control and clinical uses of immunological products. The mechanisms of action of antibiotics and non-antibiotic agents are also considered, together with an account of the ever-present problem of natural and acquired resistance. The principles involved in the clinical uses of antimicrobial drugs are discussed in Chapter 6.

Problems of recent years involving listeriosis, salmonellosis, giardiasis and Legionnaire's disease have received attention, as have the re-emergence of tuberculosis and the importance of methicillin-resistant *Staphylococcus aureus* (MRSA) and vancomycin-resistant enterococci (VRE).

Appropriate suggestions for additional reading are provided.

5 Types of antibiotics and synthetic antimicrobial agents

1	**Antibiotics**
1.1	Definition
1.2	Sources
2	**β-lactam antibiotics**
2.1	Penicillins and mecillinams
2.2	Cephalosporins
2.2.1	Structure–activity relationships
2.2.2	Pharmacokinetic properties
2.3	Clavams
2.4	1-oxacephems
2.5	1-carbapenems
2.5.1	Olivanic acids
2.5.2	Thienamycin and imipenem
2.6	1-carbacephems
2.7	Nocardicins
2.8	Monobactams
2.9	Penicillanic acid derivatives
2.10	Hypersensitivity
3	**Tetracycline group**
3.1	Tetracyclines
3.2	Glycylcyclines
4	**Rifamycins**
5	**Aminoglycoside-aminocyclitol antibiotics**
6	**Macrolides**
6.1	Older members
6.2	Newer members
7	**Polypeptide antibiotics**
8	**Glycopeptide antibiotics**

8.1	Vancomycin
8.2	Teicoplanin
9	**Miscellaneous antibacterial antibiotics**
9.1	Chloramphenicol
9.2	Fusidic acid
9.3	Lincomycins
9.4	Mupirocin (pseudomonic acid A)
10	**Antifungal antibiotics**
10.1	Griseofulvin
10.2	Polyenes
11	**Synthetic antimicrobial agents**
11.1	Sulphonamides
11.2	Diaminopyrimidine derivatives
11.3	Co-trimoxazole
11.4	Dapsone
11.5	Antitubercular drugs
11.6	Nitrofuran compounds
11.7	4-quinolone antibacterials
11.8	Imidazole derivatives
11.9	Flucytosine
11.10	Synthetic allylamines
11.11	Synthetic thiocarbamates
12	**Antiviral drugs**
12.1	Amantadines
12.2	Methisazone
12.3	Nucleoside analogues
12.4	Non-nucleoside compounds
12.5	Interferons
13	**Drug combinations**
14	**Further reading**

1 Antibiotics

1.1 Definition

An antibiotic was originally defined as a substance, produced by one microorganism, which inhibited the growth of other microorganisms. The advent of synthetic methods has, however, resulted in a modification of this definition and an antibiotic now refers to a substance produced by a microorganism, or to a similar substance (produced wholly or partly by chemical synthesis), which in low concentrations inhibits the growth of other microorganisms. Chloramphenicol was an early example. Antimicrobial agents such as sulphonamides (section 11.1) and the 4-quinolones (section 11.7), produced solely by synthetic means, are often referred to as antibiotics.

1.2 Sources

There are three major sources from which antibiotics are obtained.

1 Microorganisms. For example, bacitracin and polymyxin are obtained from some *Bacillus* species; streptomycin, tetracyclines, etc. from *Streptomyces* species; gentamicin from *Micromonospora purpurea;* griseofulvin and some penicillins and cephalosporins from certain genera *(Penicillium, Acremonium)* of the family Aspergillaceae; and monobactams from *Pseudomonas acidophila* and *Gluconobacter* species. Most antibiotics in current use have been produced from *Streptomyces* spp.

2 Synthesis. Chloramphenicol is now usually produced by a synthetic process.

3 Semisynthesis. This means that part of the molecule is produced by a fermentation process using the appropriate microorganism and the product is then further modified by a chemical process. Many penicillins and cephalosporins (section 2) are produced in this way.

2 β-lactam antibiotics

There are several different types of β-lactam antibiotics that are valuable, or potentially important, antibacterial compounds. These will be considered briefly.

2.1 Penicillins and mecillinams

The penicillins (general structure, Fig. 5.1A) may be considered as being of the following types.

1 Naturally occurring. For example, those produced by fermentation of moulds such as *Penicillium notatum* and *P. chrysogenum*. The most important examples are benzylpenicillin (penicillin G) and phenoxymethylpenicillin (penicillin V).

2 Semisynthetic. In 1959, scientists at Beecham Research Laboratories succeeded in isolating the penicillin 'nucleus', 6-aminopenicillanic acid (6-APA; Fig. 5.1A: R represents H). During the commercial production of benzylpenicillin, phenylacetic (phenylethanoic) acid ($C_6H_5.CH_2.COOH$) is added to the medium in which the *Penicillium* mould is growing (see Chapter 7). This substance is a precursor of the side

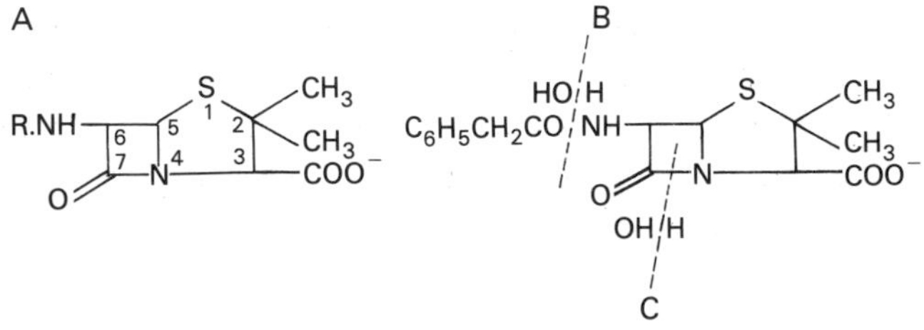

Fig. 5.1 A, General structure of penicillins; B, removal of side chain from benzylpenicillin; C, site of action of β-lactamases.

chain (R; see Fig. 5.2) in benzylpenicillin. Growth of the organism in the absence of phenylacetic acid led to the isolation of 6-APA; this has a different R_F value from benzylpenicillin which allowed it to be detected chromatographically.

A second method of producing 6-APA came with the discovery that certain microorganisms produce enzymes, penicillin amidases (acylases), which catalyse the removal of the side chain from benzylpenicillin (Fig. 5.1B).

Acylation of 6-APA with appropriate substances results in new penicillins being produced which differ only in the nature of the side chain (Table 5.1; Fig. 5.2). Some of these penicillins have considerable activity against Gram-negative as well as Gram-positive bacteria, and are thus broad-spectrum antibiotics. Pharmacokinetic properties may also be altered.

The sodium and potassium salts are very soluble in water but they are hydrolysed in solution, at a temperature-dependent rate, to the corresponding penicilloic acid (Fig. 5.3A; see also Fig. 9.3), which is not antibacterial. Penicilloic acid is produced at alkaline pH or (via penicillenic acid; Fig. 5.3B) at neutral pH, but at acid pH a molecular rearrangement occurs, giving penillic acid (Fig. 5.3C). Instability in acid medium logically precludes oral administration, since the antibiotic may be destroyed in the stomach; for example at pH 1.3 and 35°C methicillin has a half-life of only 2–3 minutes and is therefore not administered orally, whereas ampicillin, with a half-life of 600 minutes, is obviously suitable for oral use.

Benzylpenicillin is rapidly absorbed and rapidly excreted. However, certain sparingly soluble salts of benzylpenicillin (benzathine, benethamine and procaine) slowly release penicillin into the circulation over a period of time, thus giving a continuous high concentration in the blood. Simultaneous administration of benzylpenicillin (see Fortified Procaine Penicillin, BP) may be given initially.

Pro-drugs (e.g. carbenicillin esters, ampicillin esters; Fig. 5.2, Table 5.1) are hydrolysed by enzyme action after absorption from the gut mucosa to produce high blood levels of the active antibiotic, carbenicillin and ampicillin, respectively.

Several bacteria produce an enzyme, β-lactamase (penicillinase; see Chapter 9) which may inactivate a penicillin by opening the β-lactam ring, as in Fig. 5.1C. However, some penicillins (Table 5.1) are considerably more resistant to this enzyme than are others, and consequently may be extremely valuable in the treatment of infections caused by β-lactamase-producing bacteria. In general, the penicillins are active against Gram-positive bacteria; some members (e.g. ampicillin) are also effective against Gram-negative bacteria though not *Pseudomonas aeruginosa*, whereas others (e.g. carbenicillin) are active against this organism also. In particular, substituted ampicillins (piperacillin and the ureidopenicillins, azlocillin and mezlocillin) appear to combine the properties of ampicillin and carbenicillin. Temocillin is the first penicillin to be completely stable to hydrolysis by β-lactamases produced by Gram-negative bacteria.

The 6-β-amidinopenicillanic acids, mecillinam and its ester pivmecillinam, have unusual antibacterial properties, since they are active against Gram-negative but not Gram-positive organisms.

2.2   **Cephalosporins**

In the 1950s, a species of *Cephalosporium* (now known as *Acremonium:* see Chapter 7)

Drug	R	Drug	R	Drug	R

1 — $C_6H_5CH_2CO-$

2 — $C_6H_5OCH_2CO-$

3 — (with OCH_3, OCH_3 substituted ring)

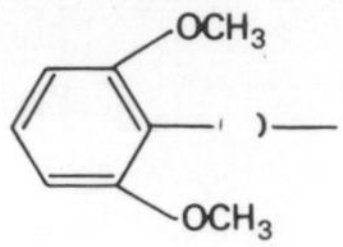

4 — (phenyl-isoxazole structure, $C=C-CO-$, N, O, CH_3)

5 — (2-Cl phenyl isoxazole structure, $C=C-CO-$, N, O, CH_3)

6 — (2-Cl, 6-F phenyl isoxazole structure, $C=C-CO-$, N, O, CH_3)

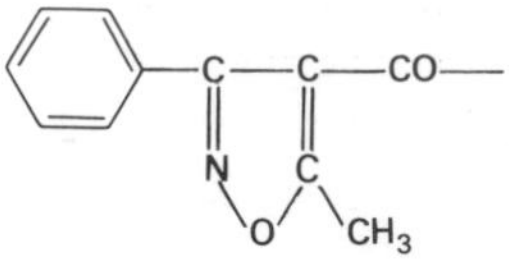

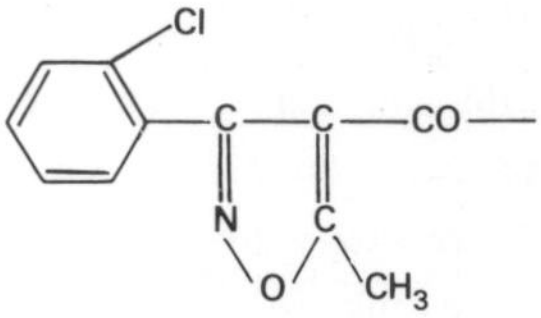

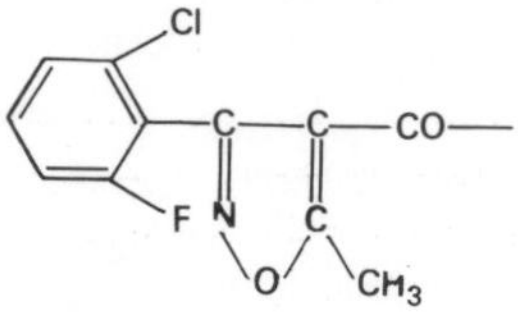

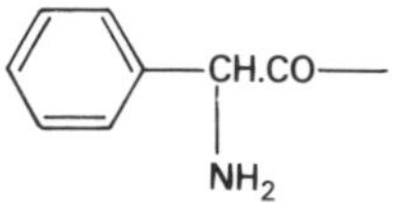

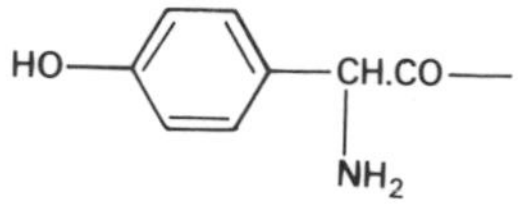

7 — phenyl $CH.CO-$, NH_2

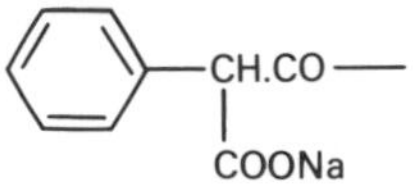

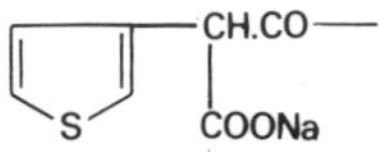

8 — HO-phenyl $CH.CO-$, NH_2

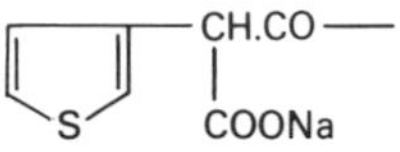

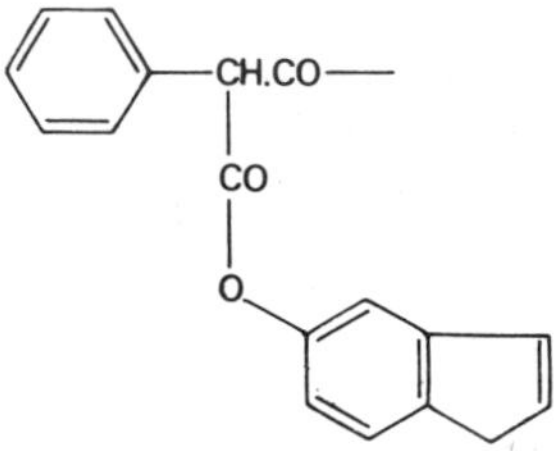

9 — phenyl $CH.CO-$, $COONa$

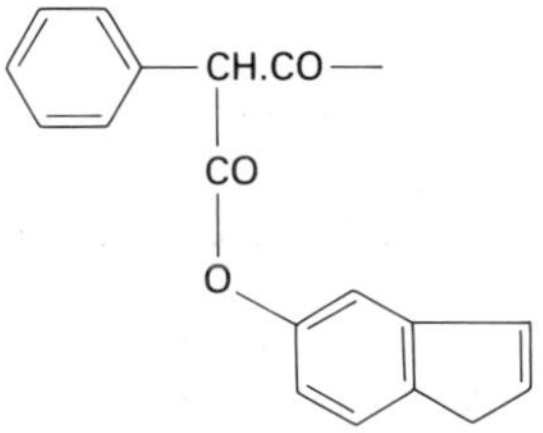

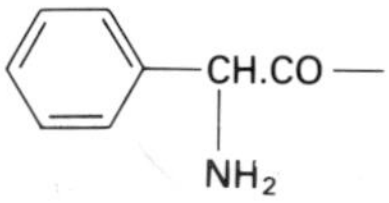

10 — thiophene $CH.CO-$, $COONa$

11 — thiophene $CH.CO-$, $COONa$

12 — phenyl $CH.CO-$, CO, O, (indanyl)

13 — phenyl $CH.CO-$, CO, O, (indanyl)

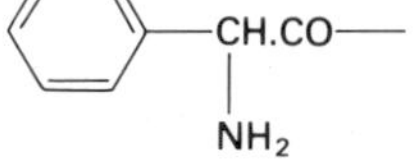

14 — phenyl $CH.CO-$, NH_2; At 3: $COOCH_2O.C.C(CH_3)_3$, O

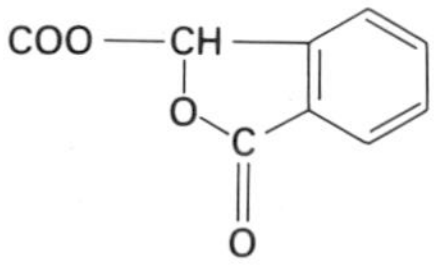

15 — phenyl $CH.CO-$, NH_2; At 3: $COO-CH$ (phthalidyl), $O-C$, O

16 — phenyl $CH.CO-$, NH_2; At 3: $COOCH_2CH_2O.COOC_2H_5$, $COOCH(CH_3)_3O.COOC_2H_5$

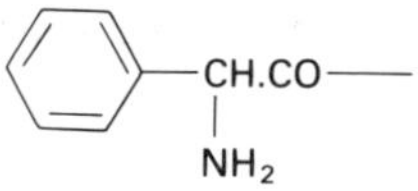

17 — phenyl $CH.CO-$, NH, CO, N (dioxopiperazine), O, O

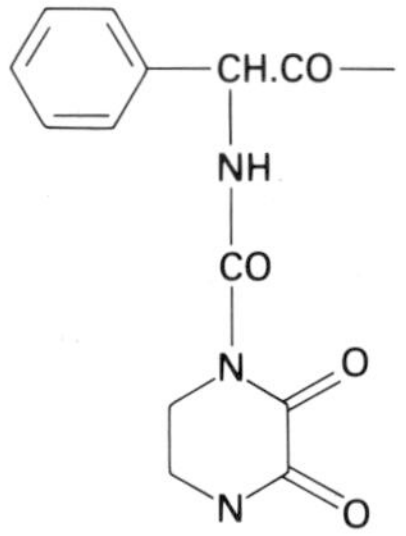

18 — phenyl $CH.CO-$, NH, CO, $N-NH$, O

19 — phenyl $CH.CO-$, NH, CO, N (imidazolidinone), O, $N-SO_2.CH_3$

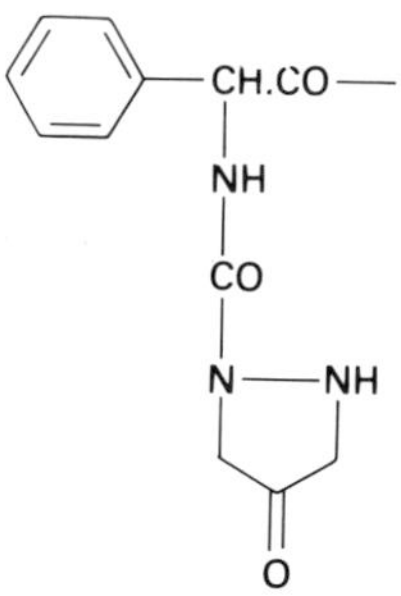

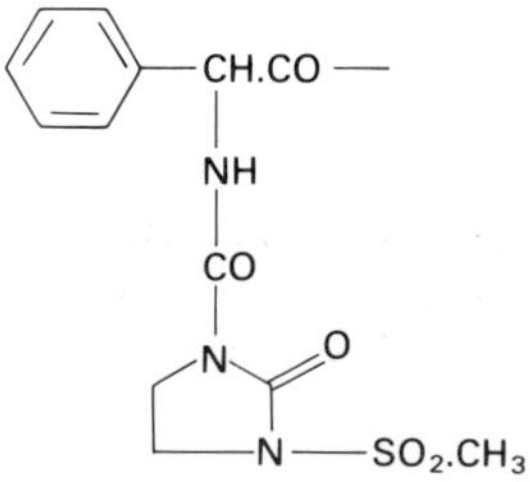

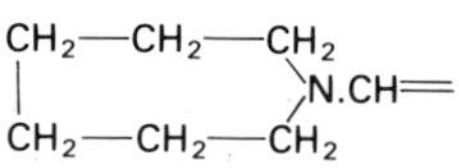

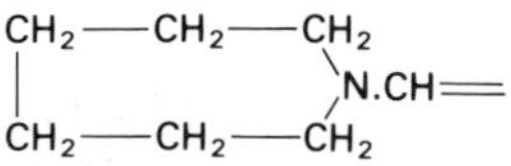

20 — $CH_2-CH_2-CH_2$ / $CH_2-CH_2-CH_2$ $N.CH=$

21 — $CH_2-CH_2-CH_2$ / $CH_2-CH_2-CH_2$ $N.CH=$; At 3: $COOCH_2O.C.C(CH_3)_3$, O

Table 5.1 The penicillins and mecillinams

Penicillin	Orally effective	Stability to β-lactamases from		Activity versus		Ester	Hydrolysed after absorption
		Staph. aureus	Gram −ve	Gram −ve*	Ps. aeruginosa		
1 Benzylpenicillin	−	−	−	−	−	−	−
2 Phenoxymethylpenicillin	+	−	−	−	−	−	−
3 Methicillin	−	+	+	−	−	−	−
4 Oxacillin	+	+	+	−	−	−	−
5 Cloxacillin	+	+	+	−	−	−	−
6 Flucloxacillin	+	+	+	−	−	−	−
7 Ampicillin	+	−	−	+	−	−	−
8 Amoxycillin	+	−	−	+	−	−	−
9 Carbenicillin	−	−	+	+	+	−	−
10 Ticarcillin	−	−	+	+	+	−	−
11 Temocillin	+	+	+	+	+	−	−
12 Carfecillin } Carbenicillin esters	+	−	+	+	+	+	+
13 Indanyl carbenicillin (carindacillin)	+	−	+	+	+	+	+
14 Pivampicillin } Ampicillin esters	+	−	−	+	−	+	+
15 Talampicillin	+	−	−	+	−	+	+
16 Bacampicillin	+	−	−	+	−	+	+
17 Piperacillin } Substituted ampicillins	−	−	−	+	+	−	−
18 Azlocillin	−	−	−	+	+	−	−
19 Mezlocillin	−	−	−	+	+	−	−
20 Mecillinam } 6-β-amidino-penicillins	−	NR	V	+	−	−	−
21 Pivmecillinam	+	NR	V	+	−	+	+

* Except *Ps. aeruginosa*. All penicillins show some degree of activity against Gram-negative cocci.

+, applicable. −, inapplicable. NR, not relevant: mecillinam and pivmecillinam have no effect on Gram-positive bacteria; V, variable.

Note: **1** Esters give high urinary levels. **2** Hydrolysis of these esters by enzyme action after absorption from the gut mucosa gives rapid and high blood levels. **3** For additional information on resistance to β-lactamase inactivation, see Chapter 9. **4** In general, all penicillins are active against Gram-positive bacteria, although this may depend on the resistance of the drug to β-lactamase (see column 3); thus, benzylpenicillin is highly active against strains of *Staphylococcus aureus* which do not produce β-lactamase, but is destroyed by β-lactamase-producing strains. **5** Temocillin (number 11) is less active against Gram-positive bacteria than ampicillin or the ureidopenicillins (substituted ampicillins).

isolated near a sewage outfall off the Sardinian coast was studied at Oxford and found to produce the following antibiotics.

1 An acidic antibiotic, cephalosporin P (subsequently found to have a steroid-like structure).

2 Another acidic antibiotic, cephalosporin N (later shown to be a penicillin, since its structure was based on 6-APA).

Fig. 5.2 (*Opposite*) Examples of the side chain R in various penicillins (the numbers 1–19 correspond to those in Table 5.1). Numbers 20 (mecillinam) and 21 (pivmecillinam) are 6-β-amidinopenicillanic acids (mecillinams). Number 11 (temocillin) has a methoxy (—OCH$_3$) group at position 6α: this confers high β-lactamase stability on the molecule.

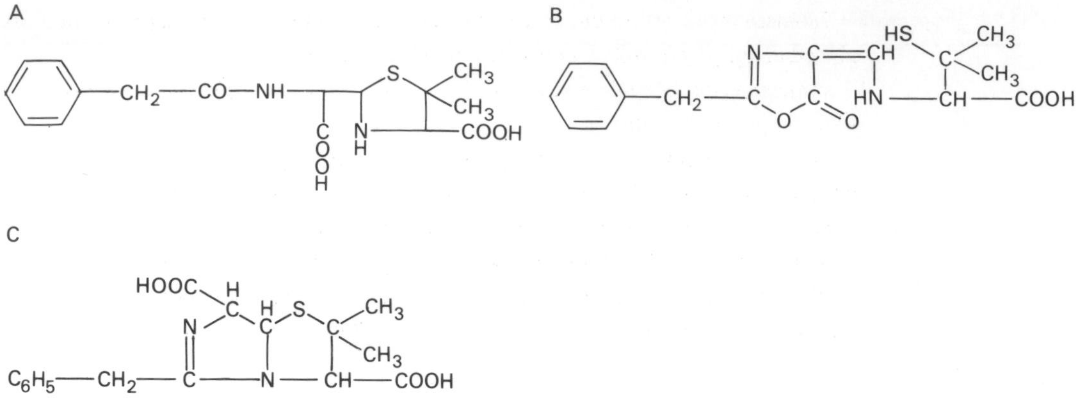

Fig. 5.3 Degradation products of benzylpenicillin in solution: A, penicilloic acid; B, penicillenic acid; C, penillic acid.

3 Cephalosporin C, obtained during the purification of cephalosporin N; this is a true cephalosporin, and from it has been obtained 7-aminocephalosporanic acid (7-ACA; Fig. 5.4), the starting point for new cephalosporins.

Cephalosporins consist of a six-membered dihydrothiazine ring fused to a β-lactam ring. Thus, the cephalosporins (Δ^3-cephalosporins) are structurally related to the penicillins (section 2.1). The position of the double bond in Δ^3-cephalosporins is important, since Δ^2-cephalosporins (double bond between 2 and 3) are not antibacterial irrespective of the composition of the side-chains.

2.2.1 Structure–activity relationships

The activity of cephalosporins (and other β-lactams) against Gram-positive bacteria depends on antibiotic affinity for penicillin-sensitive enzymes (PSEs) detected in practice as penicillin-binding proteins (PBPs). Resistance results from altered PBPs or, more commonly, from β-lactamases. Activity against Gram-negative bacteria depends upon penetration of β-lactams through the outer membrane, resistance to β-lactamases found in the periplasmic space and binding to PBPs. (For further information on mechanisms of action and bacterial resistance, see Chapters 8 and 9.) Modifications of the cephem nucleus (Fig. 5.4) at 7α, i.e. R^3, by addition of methoxy groups increase β-lactamase stability but decrease activity against Gram-positive bacteria because of reduced affinity for PBPs. Side-chains containing a 2-aminothiazolyl group at R^1, e.g. cefotaxime, ceftizoxime, ceftriaxone and ceftazidime, yield cephalosporins with enhanced affinity for PBPs of Gram-negative bacteria and streptococci. An iminomethoxy group ($—C{=}N.OCH_3$) in, for example, cefuroxime provides β-lactamase stability against common plasmid-mediated β-lactamases. A propylcarboxy group ($(CH_3)_2—C—COOH$) in, for example, ceftazidime increases β-lactamase resistance and also provides activity against *Ps. aeruginosa,* whilst at the same time reducing β-lactamase induction capabilities.

Further examples of the interplay of factors in antibacterial activity are demonstrated by the following findings.

1 7α-methoxy substitution of cefuroxine, cefamandole and cephapirin produces reduced activity against *E. coli* because of a lower affinity for PBPs;

2 similar substitution of cefoxitin produces enhanced activity against *E. coli* because of greater penetration through the outer membrane of the organism.

In cephalosporins susceptible to β-lactamases, opening of the β-lactam ring occurs with concomitant loss of the substituent at R^2 (except in cephalexin, where R^2 represents H; see Fig. 5.4). This is followed by fragmentation of the molecule. Provided that they are not inactivated by β-lactamases, the cephalosporins generally have a broad spectrum of activity, although there may be a wide variation. *Haemophilus influenzae*, for example, is particularly susceptible to cefuroxime; see also Table 5.2.

Pharmacokinetic properties

Pharmacokinetic properties of the cephalosporins depend to a considerable extent on their chemical nature, e.g. the substituent R^2. The 3-acetoxymethyl compounds such as cephalothin, cephapirin and cephacetrile are converted *in vivo* by esterases to the antibacterially less active 3-hydroxymethyl derivatives and are excreted partly as such. The rapid excretion means that such cephalosporins have a short half-life in the body. Replacement of the 3-acetoxymethyl group by a variety of groups has rendered other cephalosporins much less prone to esterase attack. For example, cephaloridine has an internally compensated betaine group at position 3 (R^2) and is metabolically stable.

Cephalosporins such as the 3-acetoxymethyl derivatives described above, cephaloridine and cefazolin are inactive when given orally. For good oral absorption, the 7-acyl group (R^1) must be based on phenylglycine and the amino group must remain unsubstituted. The R^2 substituent must be small, non-polar and stable; a methyl group is considered desirable but might decrease antibacterial activity. Earlier examples of oral cephalosporins are provided by cephalexin, cefaclor and cephradine (Table 5.2). Newer oral cephalosporins such as cefixime, cefpodoxime and ceftibuten show increased stability to β-lactamases produced by Gram-negative bacteria.

Like cefuroxime atexil (also given orally), cefpodoxime is an absorbable ester. During absorption, esterases remove the ester side-chain, liberating the active substance into the blood. Cefixime and ceftibuten are non-ester drugs characterized by activity against Gram-positive and Gram-negative bacteria, although *Ps. aeruginosa* is resistant.

Parenterally administered cephalosporins that are metabolically stable and that are resistant to many types of β-lactamases include cefuroxime, cefamandole, cefotaxime and cefoxitin, which has a 7α-methoxy group at R^2. Injectable cephalosporins with anti-pseudomonal activity include cefsulodin and cefoperazone.

Side-chains of the various cephalosporins, including those most recently developed, are presented in Fig. 5.4 and a summary of the properties of these antibiotics in Table 5.2.

Clavams

The clavams differ from penicillins (based on the penam structure) in two respects, namely the replacement of S in the penicillin thiazolidine ring (Fig. 5.1) with oxygen in the clavam oxazolidine ring (Fig. 5.5A) and the absence of the side-chain at position

6. Clavulanic acid, a naturally occurring clavam isolated from *Streptomyces clavuligerus,* has poor antibacterial activity but is a potent inhibitor of staphylococcal β-lactamase and of most types of β-lactamases produced by Gram-negative bacteria, especially those with a 'penicillinase' rather than a 'cephalosporinase' type of action.

A significant development in chemotherapy has been the introduction into clinical practice of a combination of clavulanic acid with a broad-spectrum, but β-lactamase-

Fig. 5.4 (*Above and opposite*) General structure of cephalosporins and examples of side-chains R^1 and R^2. (R^3 is —OCH$_3$ in cefoxitin and cefotetan and —H in other members.) Cephalosporins containing an ester group at position 3 are liable to attack by esterases *in vivo.*

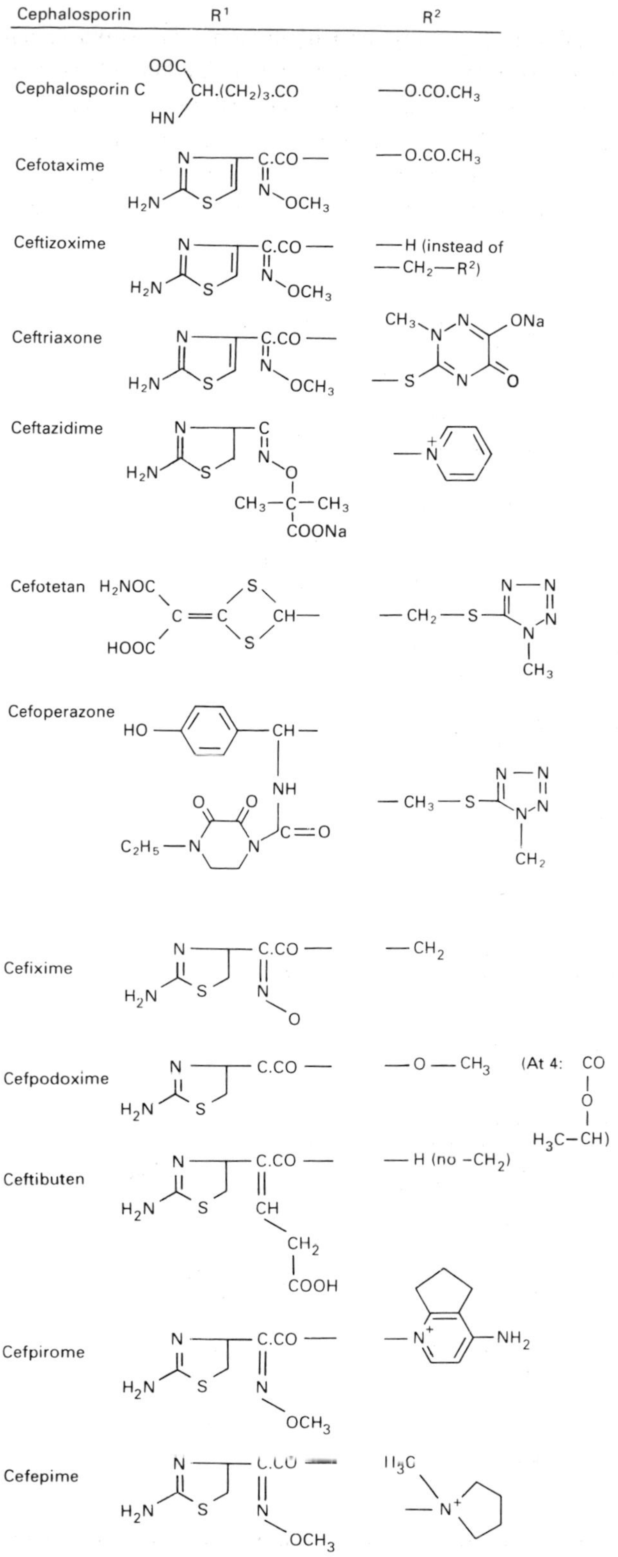

Cephalosporin	R^1	R^2
Cephalosporin C	^{OOC} CH.(CH$_2$)$_3$.CO, HN	—O.CO.CH$_3$
Cefotaxime	(aminothiazole) C.CO—, N—OCH$_3$, H$_2$N—S	—O.CO.CH$_3$
Ceftizoxime	(aminothiazole) C.CO—, N—OCH$_3$, H$_2$N—S	—H (instead of —CH$_2$—R^2)
Ceftriaxone	(aminothiazole) C.CO—, N—OCH$_3$, H$_2$N—S	CH$_3$–N–N, ONa, —S, N, O
Ceftazidime	(aminothiazole) C, N—O, H$_2$N—S, CH$_3$–C–CH$_3$, COONa	—N$^+$ (pyridinium)
Cefotetan	H$_2$NOC, C=C, CH—, HOOC, (dithietane S,S)	—CH$_2$—S, N—N tetrazole, N—N, CH$_3$
Cefoperazone	HO—⟨⟩—CH—, NH, C=O, O O, C$_2$H$_5$—N, N (piperazinedione)	—CH$_3$—S, N—N tetrazole, N—N, CH$_2$
Cefixime	(aminothiazole) C.CO—, N, O, H$_2$N—S	—CH$_2$
Cefpodoxime	(aminothiazole) C.CO—, H$_2$N—S	—O—CH$_3$ (At 4: CO, O, H$_3$C–CH)
Ceftibuten	(aminothiazole) C.CO—, CH, CH$_2$, COOH, H$_2$N—S	—H (no –CH$_2$)
Cefpirome	(aminothiazole) C.CO—, N—OCH$_3$, H$_2$N—S	—N$^+$ (cyclopenta-pyridine)—NH$_2$
Cefepime	(aminothiazole) C.CO—, N—OCH$_3$, H$_2$N—S	H$_3$C, —N$^+$ (pyrrolidine)

Fig. 5.4 *Continued.*

Table 5.2 The cephalosporins*

Group	Examples	Staphylococci†	Staphylococcal β-lactamase	Streptococci‡	Enterobacteria	Enterobacterial β-lactamases	Neisseria	Haemophilus	Ps. aeruginosa	Comment
		*Properties								
Oral cephalosporins	Cephalexin, cephradine, cefaclor, cefadroxil	++	++	+	V	V	+	(+)	R	
	Cefixime, ceftibuten	+	++	++	V	V	++	++	R	Newer oral cephalosporins
	Cefuroxime atexil	++	++	++	V	V	++	++	R	Absorbable ester
	Cefpodoxime	++	++	++	V	V	++	++	R	Absorbable ester
Injectable cephalosporins (β-lactamase-susceptible)	Cephaloridine, cephalothin, cephacetrile, cefazolin	++	+	+	V	V	+	(+)	R	
Injectable cephalosporins (improved β-lactamase stability)	Cefuroxime, cefoxitin, cefamandole	++	++	++	++	++	++	++	R	Cefoxitin shows activity against *Bacteroides fragilis*
Injectable cephalosporins (still higher β-lactamase stability)	Cefotaxime, ceftazidime, ceftizoxime, ceftriaxone (also the oxacephem, latamoxef, section 2.4)	++	++	+++	+++	+++	+++	+++	R (ceftazidime +++)	Latamoxef has high activity against *B. fragilis*
Injectable cephalosporins (anti-pseudomonal activity)	Cefoperazone Cefsulodin	++ (+)	++ ++	+ (+)	V	V	++	++ R	++ +++	
Injectable cephalosporins (other)	Cefotetan	(+)			+++	+++			R	Inhibits *B. fragilis*

* Early cephalosporins were spelt with 'ph', more recently with 'f'.

† Methicillin-resistant *Staph. aureus* (MRSA) strains are resistant to cephalosporins.

‡ Enterococci are resistant to cephalosporins.

+++, excellent; ++, good; +, fair; (+), poor; R, resistant; V, variable.

susceptible, penicillin, amoxycillin. The spectrum of activity has been extended to include *Ps. aeruginosa* by combining clavulanic acid with the β-lactamase-susceptible penicillin, ticarcillin.

2.4 1-oxacephems

In the 1-oxacephems, for example latamoxef (moxalactam, Fig. 5.5B), the sulphur

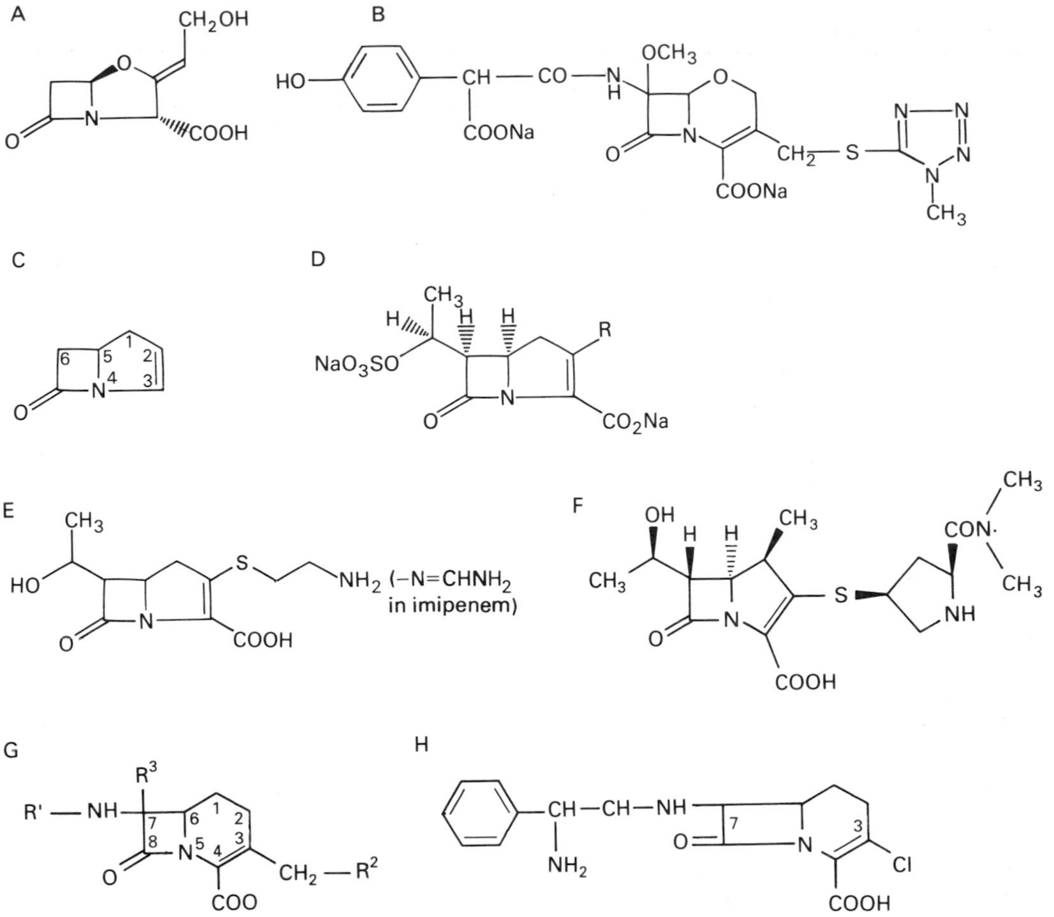

Fig. 5.5 A, clavulanic acid; B, latamoxef; C, 1-carbapenems; D, olivanic acid (general structure); E, thienamycin; F, meropenem; G, 1-carbacephems; H, loracarbef.

atom in the dihydrothiazine cephalosporin ring system is replaced by oxygen. This would tend to make the molecule chemically less stable and more susceptible to inactivation by β-lactamases. The introduction of the 7-α-methoxy group (as in cefoxitin, Fig. 5.4), however, stabilizes the molecule. Latamoxef is a broad-spectrum antibiotic with a high degree of stability to most types of β-lactamases, and is highly active against the anaerobe, *B. fragilis.*

2.5 1-carbapenems

The 1-carbapenems (Fig. 5.5C) comprise a new family of fused β-lactam antibiotics. They are analogues of penicillins or clavams, the sulphur (penicillins) or oxygen (calvams) atom being replaced by carbon. Examples are the olivanic acids (section 2.5.1) and thienamycin and imipenem (section 2.5.2).

2.5.1   *Olivanic acids*

The olivanic acids (general structure, Fig. 5.5D) are naturally-occurring β-lactam antibiotics which have, with some difficulty, been isolated from culture fluids of *Strep. olivaceus.* They are broad-spectrum antibiotics and are potent inhibitors of various types of β-lactamases.

2.5.2   *Thienamycin and imipenem*

Thienamycin (Fig. 5.5E) is a broad-spectrum β-lactam antibiotic with high β-lactamase resistance. Unfortunately, it is chemically unstable, although the *N*-formimidoyl derivative, imipenem, overcomes this defect. Imipenem (Fig. 5.5E) is stable to most β-lactamases but it readily hydrolysed by kidney dehydropeptidase and is administered with a dehydropeptidase inhibitor, cilastatin. Meropenem, which has yet to be marketed, is more stable than imipenem to this enzyme and may thus be administered without cilastatin. Its chemical structure is depicted in Fig. 5.5F.

2.6   **1-carbacephems**

In the 1-carbacephems (Fig. 5.5G), the sulphur in the six-membered dihydrothiazine ring of the cephalosporins (based on the cephem structure, see Fig. 5.4) is replaced by carbon. Loracarbef (Fig. 5.5H) is a new oral carbacephem which is highly active against Gram-positive bacteria, including staphylococci.

2.7   **Nocardicins**

The nocardicins (A to G) have been isolated from a strain of *Nocardia* and comprise a novel group of β-lactam antibiotics (Fig. 5.6A). Nocardicin A is the most active member, and possesses significant activity against Gram-negative but not Gram-positive bacteria.

2.8   **Monobactams**

The monobactams are monocyclic β-lactam antibiotics produced by various strains of bacteria. A novel nucleus, 3-aminomonobactamic acid (3-AMA, Fig. 5.6B), has been produced from naturally-occurring monobactams and from 6-APA. Several monobactams have been tested and one (aztreonam, Fig. 5.6C) has been shown to be highly active against most Gram-negative bacteria and to be stable to most types of β-lactamases. It is not destroyed by staphylococcal β-lactamases but is inactive against all strains of *Staph. aureus* tested. *Bacteroides fragilis,* a Gram-negative anaerobe, is resistant to aztreonam, probably by virtue of the β-lactamase it produces, and this conclusion is supported by the finding that a combination of the monobactam with clavulanic acid (section 2.3) is ineffective against this organism.

2.9   **Penicillanic acid derivatives**

Penicillanic acid derivatives are synthetically produced β-lactamase inhibitors.

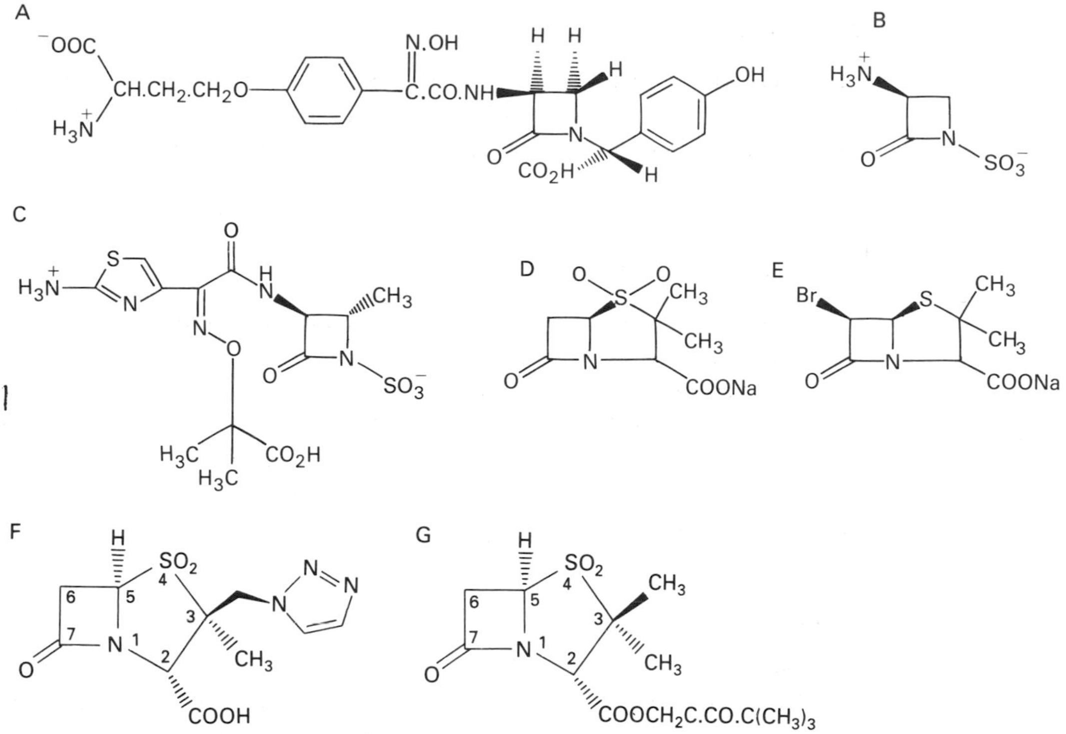

Fig. 5.6 A, Nocardicin A; B, 3-aminomonobactamic acid (3-AMA); C, aztreonam; D, penicillanic acid sulphone (sodium salt); E, β-bromopenicillanic acid (sodium salt); F, tazobactam; G, sulbactam.

Penicillanic acid sulphone (Fig. 5.6D) protects ampicillin from hydrolysis by staphylococcal β-lactamase and some, but not all, of the β-lactamases produced by Gram-negative bacteria, but is less potent than clavulanic acid. β-bromopenicillanic acid (Fig. 5.6E) inhibits some types of β-lactamases.

Tazobactam (Fig. 5.6F) is a penicillanic acid sulphone derivative marketed as a combination with piperacillin. Alone it has poor intrinsic antibacterial activity but is comparable to clavulanic acid in inhibiting β-lactamase activity.

Sulbactam (Fig. 5.6G) is a semisynthetic 6-desaminopenicillin sulphone structurally related to tazobactam. Not only is it an effective inhibitor of many β-lactamases but it is also active alone against certain Gram-negative bacteria. It is used in combination with ampicillin for clinical use.

2.10 Hypersensitivity

Some types of allergic reaction, for example immediate or delayed-type skin allergies, serum-sickness-like reactions and anaphylactic reactions, may occur in a proportion of patients given penicillin treatment. There is some, but not complete, cross-allergy with cephalosporins.

Contaminants of high molecular weight (considered to have arisen from mycelial residues from the fermentation process) may be responsible for the induction of allergy to penicillins; their removal leads to a marked reduction in the antigenicity of the penicillin. It has also been found, however, that varying amounts of a non-protein polymer (of unknown source) may also be present in penicillin and that this also may be antigenic.

The interaction of a non-enzymatic degradation product, D-benzylpenicillenic acid (formed by cleavage of the thiazolidine ring of benzylpenicillin in solution; see Fig. 5.3B), with sulphydryl or amino groups in tissue proteins, to form hapten–protein conjugates, is also of importance. In particular, the reaction between D-benzylpenicillenic acid and the ε-amino group of lysine (α,ε-diamino-n-caproic acid, $NH_2(CH_2)_4.CH(NH_2).COOH$) residues is to be noted, because these D-benzylpenicilloyl derivatives of tissue proteins function as complete penicillin antigens.

3   Tetracycline group

3.1   Tetracyclines

There are several clinically important tetracyclines, characterized by four cyclic rings (Fig. 5.7). They consist of a group of antibiotics obtained as by-products from the metabolism of various species of *Streptomyces,* although some members may now be thought of as being semisynthetic. Thus, tetracycline (by catalytic hydrogenation) and

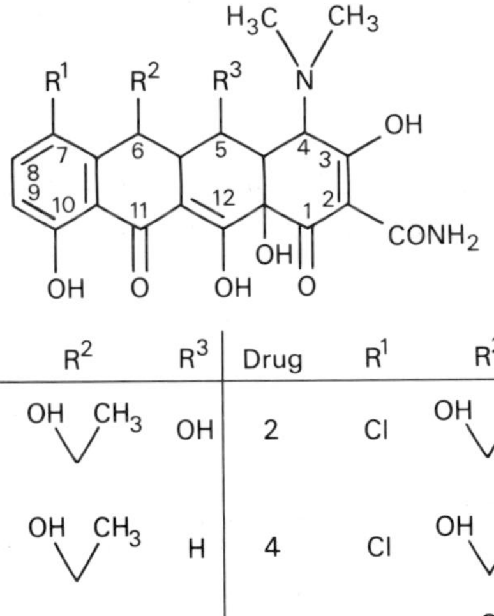

Drug	R^1	R^2	R^3	Drug	R^1	R^2	R^3
1	H	OH CH$_3$	OH	2	Cl	OH CH$_3$	H
3	H	OH CH$_3$	H	4	Cl	OH H	H
5	H	CH$_3$	OH	6	H	CH$_2$	OH
7	Cl	OH CH$_3$	H	8	CH$_3$ CH$_3$ N	H$_2$	H
		(At 2: CONHCH$_2$OH)		9	H	—	H

Fig. 5.7 Tetracycline antibiotics: 1, oxytetracycline; 2, chlortetracycline; 3, tetracycline; 4, demethylchlortetracycline; 5, doxycycline; 6, methacycline; 7, clomocycline; 8, minocycline; 9, thiacycline (a thiatetracycline with a sulphur atom at 6).

clomocycline are obtained from chlortetracycline, which is itself produced from *Strep. aureofaciens*. Methacycline is obtained from oxytetracycline (produced from *Strep. rimosus*) and hydrogenation of methacycline gives doxycycline. Demethyl-chlortetracycline is produced by a mutant strain of *Strep. aureofaciens*. Minocycline is a derivative of tetracycline.

The tetracyclines are broad-spectrum antibiotics, i.e. they have a wide range of activity against Gram-positive and Gram-negative bacteria. *Ps. aeruginosa* is less sensitive, but is generally susceptible to tetracycline concentrations obtainable in the bladder. Resistance to the tetracyclines (see also Chapter 9) develops relatively slowly, but there is cross-resistance, i.e. an organism resistant to one member is usually resistant to all other members of this group. However, tetracycline-resistant *Staph. aureus* strains may still be sensitive to minocycline. Suprainfection ('overgrowth') with naturally tetracycline-resistant organisms, for example *Candida albicans* and other yeasts, and filamentous fungi, affecting the mouth, upper respiratory tract or gastrointestinal tract, may occur as a result of the suppression of tetracycline-susceptible microorganisms.

Thiatetracyclines contain a sulphur atom at position 6 in the molecule. One derivative, thiacycline, is more active than minocycline against tetracycline-resistant bacteria. Despite toxicity problems affecting its possible clinical use, thiacycline could be the starting point in the development of a new range of important tetracycline-type antibiotics.

The tetracyclines are no longer used clinically to the same extent as they were in the past because of the increase in bacterial resistance.

3.2   **Glycylcyclines**

The glycylcyclines (Fig. 5.8) represent a new group of tetracycline analogues. They are novel tetracyclines substituted at the C-9 position with a dimethylglycylamido side-

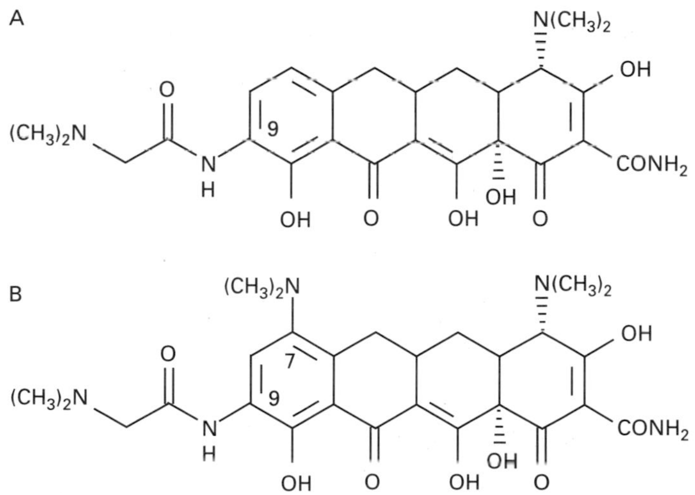

Fig. 5.8 Structures of two tetracycline analogues, which are members of the new glycylcycline group of antibiotics: A, *N,N*-dimethylglycylamido-6-demethyl-6-deoxytetracycline; B, *N,N*-dimethylglycylamidominocycline.

chain. They possess activity against bacteria that express resistance to the older tetracyclines by an efflux mechanism (Chapter 9).

4 Rifamycins

The rifamycins comprise a comparatively new antibiotic group and consist of rifamycins A to E. From rifamycin B are produced rifamide (rifamycin B diethylamide) and rifamycin SV, which is one of the most useful and least toxic of the rifamycins.

Rifampicin (Fig. 5.9), a bactericidal antibiotic, is active against Gram-positive bacteria (including *Mycobacterium tuberculosis*) and some Gram-negative bacteria (but not Enterobacteriaceae or pseudomonads). It has been found to have a greater bactericidal effect against *M. tuberculosis* than other antituberculosis drugs, is active orally, penetrates well into cerebrospinal fluid and is thus of use in the treatment of tuberculous meningitis (see also section 11.5).

Rifampicin possesses significant bactericidal activity at very low concentrations against staphylococci. Unfortunately, resistant mutants may arise very rapidly, both *in vitro* and *in vivo*. It has thus been recommended that rifampicin should be combined with another antibiotic, e.g. vancomycin, in the treatment of staphylococcal infections.

A newly introduced rifamycin is rifabutin. This may be used in the prophylaxis of *M. avium* complex infections in immunocompromised patients and in the treatment, with other drugs, of non-tuberculous mycobacterial infections.

5 Aminoglycoside–aminocyclitol antibiotics

Aminoglycoside antibiotics contain amino sugars in their structure. Deoxystreptamine-containing members are neomycin, framycetin, gentamicin, kanamycin, tobramycin, amikacin, netilmicin and sisomicin. Both streptomycin and dihydrostreptomycin contain streptidine, whereas the aminocyclitol spectinomycin has no amino sugar. Examples of chemical structures are provided in Fig. 5.10.

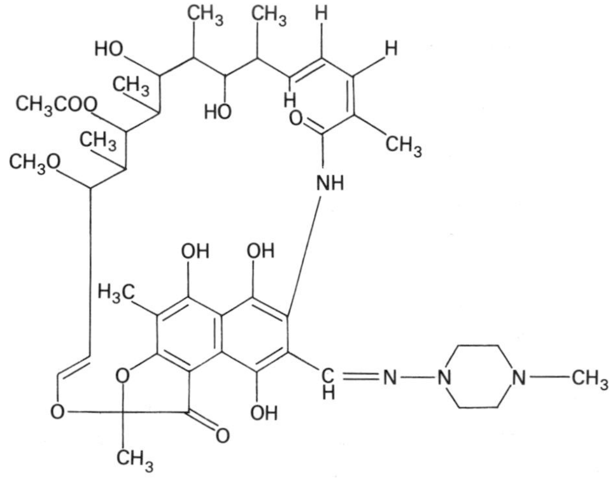

Fig. 5.9 Rifampicin.

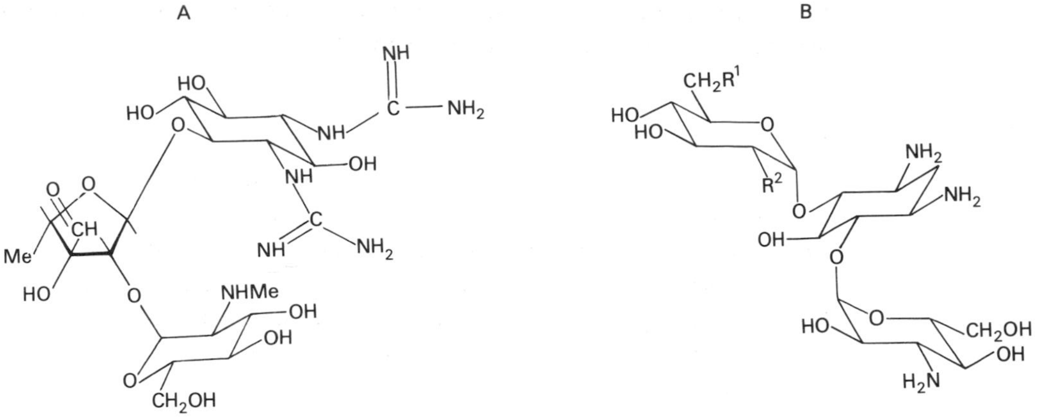

	R^1	R^2
Kanamycin A	NH_2	OH
Kanamycin B	NH_2	NH_2
Kanamycin C	OH	NH_2

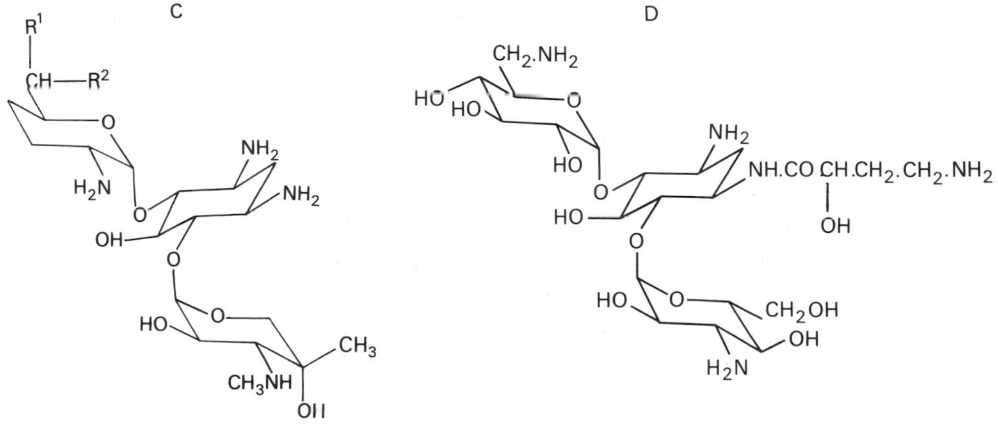

	R^1	R^2
Gentamicin C_{1a}	H	NH_2
Gentamicin C_1	CH_3	$NHCH_3$
Gentamicin C_2	CH_3	NH_2

Fig. 5.10 Some aminoglycoside antibiotics: A, streptomycin; B, kanamycins; C, gentamicins; D, amikacin.

Streptomycin was isolated by Waksman in 1944, and its activity against *M. tuberculosis* ensured its use as a primary drug in the treatment of tuberculosis. Unfortunately, its ototoxicity and the rapid development of resistance have tended to modify its usefulness, and although it still remains a front-line drug against tuberculosis it is usually used in combination with isoniazid and $p(4)$-aminosalicylic acid (section 11.5). Streptomycin also shows activity against other types of bacteria, for example against various Gram-negative bacteria and some strains of staphylococci. Dihydrostreptomycin has a similar antibacterial action but is more toxic.

Gentamicin (a mixture of three components, C_1, C_{1a} and C_2; Fig. 5.10C) is active against many strains of Gram-positive and Gram-negative bacteria, including some strains of *Ps. aeruginosa*. Its activity is greatly increased at pH values of about 8. It is often administered in conjunction with carbenicillin to delay the development of resistance. Gentamicin is the most important aminoglycoside antibiotic, is the aminoglycoside of choice in the UK and is widely used for treating serious infections. As with other members of this group, side-effects are dose related, dosage must be given with care, plasma levels should be monitored and treatment should not normally exceed 7 days.

Kanamycin (a complex of three antibiotics, A, B and C) is active in low concentrations against various Gram-positive (including penicillin-resistant staphylococci) and Gram-negative bacteria. It is a recognized second-line drug in the treatment of tuberculosis.

Paromomycin finds special use in the treatment of intestinal amoebiasis (it is amoebicidal against *Entamoeba histolytica*) and of acute bacillary dysentery.

Neomycin is poorly absorbed from the alimentary tract when given orally, and is usually used in the form of lotions and ointments for topical application against skin and eye infections. Framycetin consists of neomycin B with a small amount of neomycin C, and is usually employed locally.

A desirable property of newer aminoglycoside antibiotics is increased antibacterial activity against resistant strains, especially improved stability to aminoglycoside-modifying enzymes (Chapter 9). Alteration in the 3′ position of kanamycin B (Fig. 5.10B) to give 3′-deoxykanamycin B (tobramycin) changes the activity spectrum. Amikacin (Fig. 5.10D) has a substituted aminobutyryl in the amino group at position 1 in the 2-deoxystreptamine ring and this enhances its resistance to some, but not all, types of aminoglycoside-modifying enzymes, as it has fewer sites of modification. Netilmicin (*N*-ethylsisomicin) is a semisynthetic derivative of sisomicin but is less susceptible than sisomicin to some types of bacterial enzymes.

The most important of these antibiotics are amikacin, tobramycin, netilmicin and especially gentamicin.

6   Macrolides

6.1   Older members

The macrolide antibiotics are characterized by possessing molecular structures that contain large (12–16-membered) lactone rings linked through glycosidic bonds with amino sugars.

The most important members of this group are erythromycin (Fig. 5.11), oleandomycin, triacetyloleandomycin and spiramycin. Erythromycin is active against most Gram-positive bacteria, *Neisseria, H. influenzae* and *Legionella pneumophila,* but not against the Enterobacteriaceae; its activity is pH-dependent, increasing with pH up to about 8.5. Erythromycin estolate is more stable than the free base to the acid of gastric juice and is thus employed for oral use. The estolate produces higher and

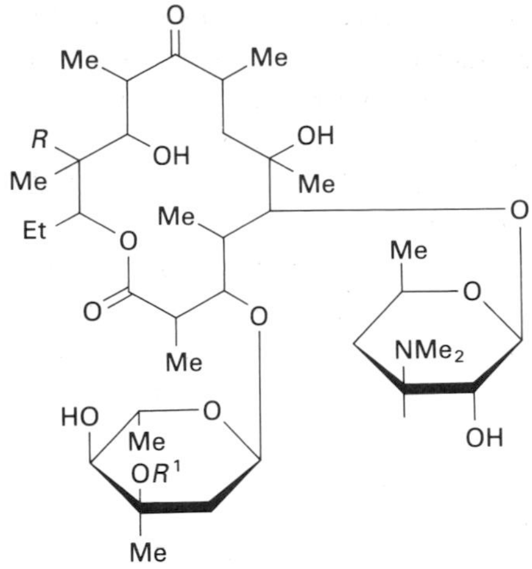

Erythromycin	R	R[1]
A	OH	Me
B	H	Me
C	OH	H

Fig. 5.11 Erythromycins: erythromycin is a mixture of macrolide antibiotics consisting largely of erythromycin A.

more prolonged blood levels and distributes into some tissues more efficiently than other dosage forms. *In vivo,* it hydrolyses to give the free base.

Staphylococcus aureus is less sensitive to erythromycin than are pneumococci or haemolytic streptococci, and there may be a rapid development of resistance, especially of staphylococci, *in vitro*. However, *in vivo* with successful short courses of treatment, resistance is not usually a serious clinical problem. On the other hand, resistance is likely to develop when the antibiotic is used for long periods.

Oleandomycin, its ester (triacetyloleandomycin) and spiramycin have a similar range of activity as erythromycin but are less active. Resistance develops only slowly in clinical practice. However, cross-resistance may occur between all four members of this group.

6.2 Newer members

The new macrolides are semisynthetic molecules that differ from the original compounds in the substitution pattern of the lactone ring system (Table 5.3, Figs 5.12 and 5.13).

Table 5.3 New macrolide derivatives of erythromycin

Lactone ring structure	Example	Derivative of erythromycin
14-membered	Erythromycin	–
	Roxithromycin	Methoxy-ethoxy-methyloxine
	Clarithromycin	Methyl
	Dirithromycin	Oxazine
15-membered	Azithromycin	Deoxo-aza-methyl-homo

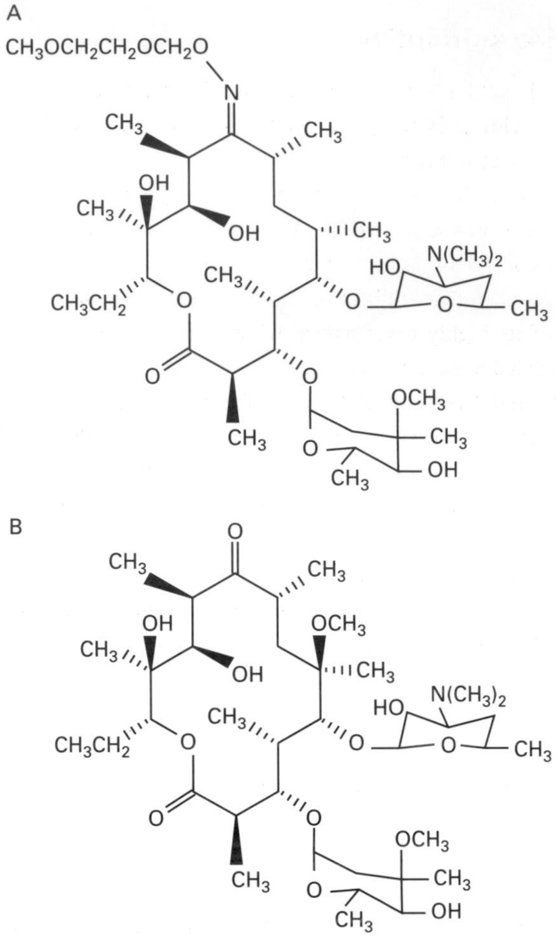

A

CH₃OCH₂CH₂OCH₂O

B

Fig. 5.12 Examples of newer 14-membered macrolides: A, roxithromycin; B, clarithromycin.

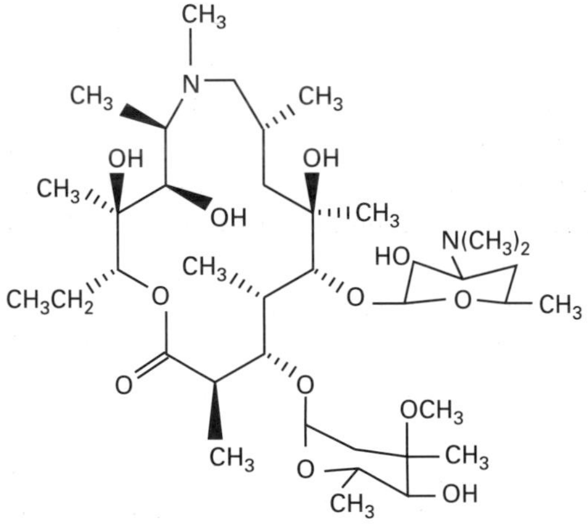

Fig. 5.13 Structure of azithromycin (15-membered macrolide).

Roxithromycin has similar *in vitro* activity to erythromycin but enters leucocytes and macrophages more rapidly with higher concentrations in the lysosomal component of the phagocytic cells. It is likely to become an important drug against *Legionella pneumophila*. Clarithromycin is also of potential value.

7   Polypeptide antibiotics

The polypeptide antibiotics comprise a rather diverse group. They include:

1 bacitracin, with activity against Gram-positive but not Gram-negative bacteria (except Gram-negative cocci);

2 the polymyxins, which are active against many types of Gram-negative bacteria (including *Ps. aeruginosa* but excluding cocci, *Serratia marcescens* and *Proteus* spp.) but not Gram-positive organisms; and

3 the two antitubercular antibiotics, capreomycin and viomycin.

Because of its highly toxic nature when administered parenterally, bacitracin is normally restricted to external usage.

The antibacterial activity of five members (A to E) of the polymyxin group is of a similar nature. However, they are all nephrotoxic although this effect is much reduced with polymyxins B and E (colistin). Colistin sulphomethate sodium is the form of colistin used for parenteral administration. Sulphomyxin sodium, a mixture of sulphomethylated polymyxin B and sodium bisulphite, has the action and uses of polymyxin B sulphate, but is less toxic.

Capreomycin and viomycin show activity against *M. tuberculosis* and may be regarded as being second-line antituberculosis drugs.

8   Glycopeptide antibiotics

Two important glycopeptide antibiotics are vancomycin and teicoplanin.

8.1   Vancomycin

Vancomycin is an antibiotic isolated from *Strep. orientalis* and has an empirical formula of $C_{66}H_{75}Cl_2N_9O_4$ (mol. wt 1448); it has a complex tricyclic glycopeptide structure. Modern chromatographically purified vancomycin gives rise to fewer side-effects than the antibiotic produced in the 1950s.

Vancomycin is active against most Gram-positive bacteria, including methicillin-resistant strains of *Staph. aureus* and *Staph. epidermidis*, *Enterococcus faecalis*, *Clostridium difficile* and Gram-negative cocci. Gram-negative bacilli, mycobacteria and fungi are not susceptible. Vancomycin-resistant enterococci are now posing a clinical problem in hospitals, however.

Vancomycin is bactericidal to most susceptible bacteria at concentrations near its minimum inhibitory concentration (MIC) and is an inhibitor of bacterial cell wall peptidoglycan synthesis, although at a site different from that of β-lactam antibiotics (Chapter 9).

Employed as the hydrochloride and administered by dilute intravenous injection, vancomycin is indicated in potentially life-threatening infections that cannot be treated with other effective, less toxic, antibiotics. Oral vancomycin is the drug of choice in the treatment of antibiotic-induced pseudomembranous colitis associated with the administration of antibiotics such as clindamycin and lincomycin (section 9.3).

8.2 Teicoplanin

Teicoplanin is a naturally occurring complex of five closely related tetracyclic molecules. Its mode of action and spectrum of activity are essentially similar to vancomycin, although it might be less active against some strains of coagulase-negative staphylococci. Teicoplanin can be administered by intramuscular injection.

9 Miscellaneous antibacterial antibiotics

Antibiotics described here (Fig. 5.14) are those which cannot logically be considered in any of the other groups above.

9.1 Chloramphenicol

Chloramphenicol (Fig. 5.14A) has a broad spectrum of activity, but exerts a bacteriostatic effect. It has antirickettsial activity and is inhibitory to the larger viruses. Unfortunately, aplastic anaemia, which is dose-related, may result from treatment in a proportion of patients. It should thus not be given for minor infections and its usage should be restricted to cases where no effective alternative exists, e.g. typhoid fever (see Chapter 6). Some bacteria (see Chapter 9) can produce an enzyme, chloramphenicol acetyltransferase, that acetylates the hydroxyl groups in the side-chain of the antibiotic to produce, initially, 3-acetoxychloramphenicol and, finally, 1,3-diacetoxychloramphenicol, which lacks antibacterial activity. The design of fluorinated derivatives of chloramphenicol that are not acetylated by this enzyme could be a significant finding.

The antibiotic is administered orally as the palmitate, which is tasteless; this is hydrolysed to chloramphenicol in the gastrointestinal tract. The highly water-soluble chloramphenicol sodium succinate is used in the parenteral formulation, and thus acts as a pro-drug.

9.2 Fusidic acid

Employed as a sodium salt, fusidic acid (Fig. 5.14B) is active against many types of Gram-positive bacteria, especially staphylococci, although streptococci are relatively resistant. It is employed in the treatment of staphylococcal infections, including strains resistant to other antibiotics. However, bacterial resistance may occur *in vitro* and *in vivo*.

9.3 Lincomycins

Lincomycin and clindamycin (Fig. 5.14C, D) are active against Gram-positive cocci, except *Enterococcus faecalis*. Gram-negative cocci tend to be less sensitive and enterobacteria are resistant. Cross-resistance of staphylococci may occur between lincomycins and erythromycin, but some erythromycin-resistant organisms may be sensitive to lincomycins.

9.4 Mupirocin (pseudomonic acid A)

Mupirocin (Fig. 5.14E) is the main fermentation product obtained from *Ps. fluorescens*.

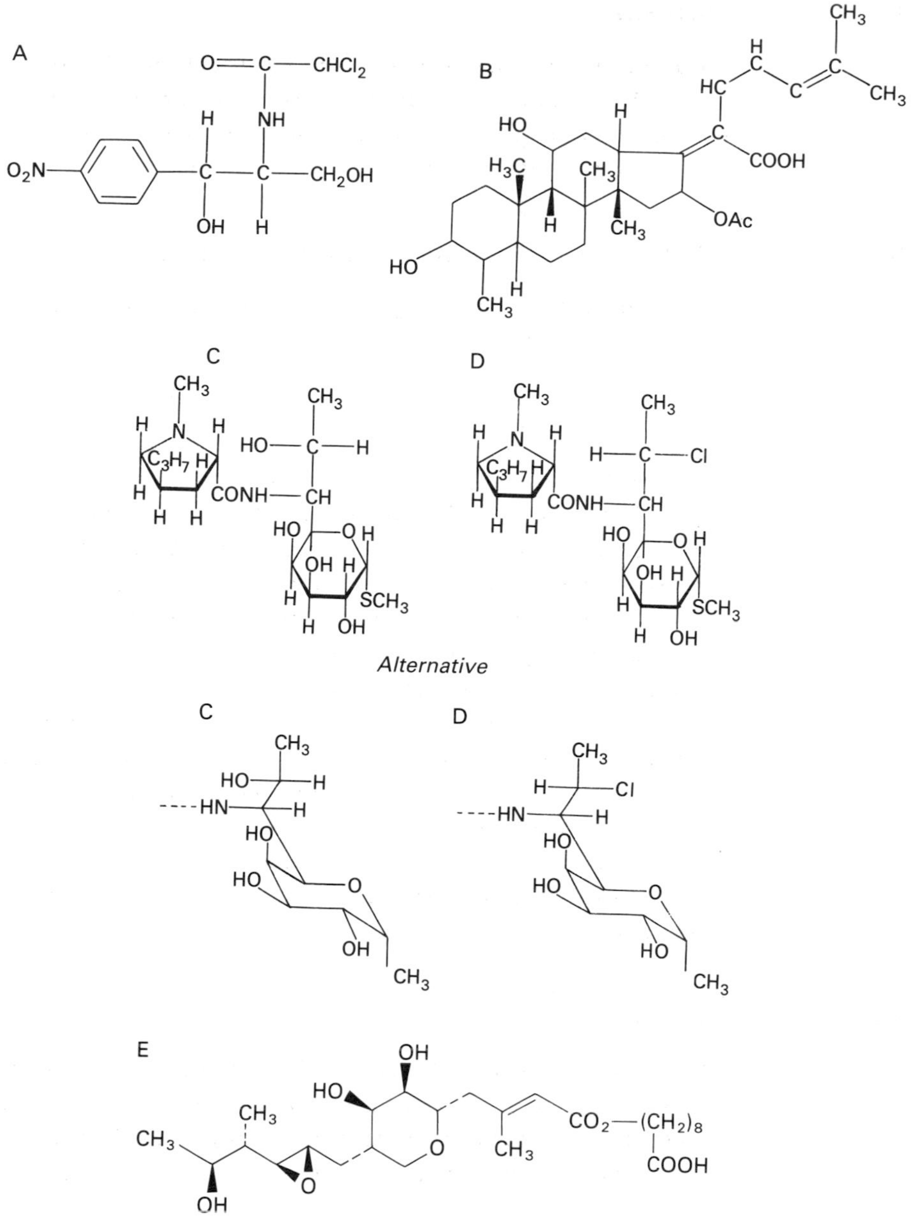

Fig. 5.14 Miscellaneous antibiotics: A, chloramphenicol; B, fusidic acid; C, lincomycin; D, clindamycin; E, mupirocin (pseudomonic acid A).

Other pseudomonic acids (B, C, D) are also produced. Mupirocin is active predominantly against staphylococci and most streptococci, but *Enterococcus faecalis* and Gram-negative bacilli are resistant. There is also evidence of plasmid-mediated mupirocin resistance in some clinical isolates of *Staph. aureus*.

Mupirocin is employed topically in eradicating nasal and skin carriage of staphylococci, including methicillin-resistant *Staph. aureus* colonization.

10   Antifungal antibiotics

In contrast to the wide range of antibacterial antibiotics, there are very few antifungal antibiotics that can be used systemically. Lack of toxicity is, as always, of paramount importance, but the differences in structure of, and some biosynthetic processes in, fungal cells (Chapter 2) mean that antibacterial antibiotics are usually inactive against fungi.

Fungal infections are normally less virulent in nature than are bacterial or viral ones but may, nevertheless, pose a problem in individuals with a depressed immune system, e.g. AIDS sufferers.

10.1   Griseofulvin

This is a metabolic by-product of *Penicillium griseofulvum*. Griseofulvin (Fig. 5.15A) was first isolated in 1939, but it was not until 1958 that its antifungal activity was discovered. It is active against the dermatophytic fungi, i.e. those such as *Trichophyton* causing ringworm. It is ineffective against *Candida albicans,* the causative agent of oral thrush and intestinal candidasis, and against bacteria, and there is thus no disturbance of the normal bacterial flora of the gut.

Griseofulvin is administered orally in the form of tablets. It is not totally absorbed when given orally, and one method of increasing absorption is to reduce the particle size of the drug. Griseofulvin is deposited in the deeper layers of the skin and in hair keratin, and is therefore employed in chemotherapy of fungal infections of these areas caused by susceptible organisms.

10.2   Polyenes

Polyene antibiotics are characterized by possessing a large ring containing a lactone group and a hydrophobic region consisting of a sequence of four to seven conjugated double bonds. The most important polyenes are nystatin and amphotericin B (Fig. 5.15B and C, respectively).

Nystatin has a specific action on *C. albicans* and is of no value in the treatment of any other type of infection. It is poorly absorbed from the gastrointestinal tract; even after very large doses, the blood level is insignificant. It is administered orally in the treatment of oral thrush and intestinal candidiasis infections.

Amphotericin B is particularly effective against systemic infections caused by *C. albicans* and *Cryptococcus neoformans.* It is poorly absorbed from the gastro-intestinal tract and is thus usually administered by intravenous injection under strict medical supervision. Amphotericin B methyl ester (Fig. 5.15C) is water-soluble, unlike amphotericin B itself, and can be administered intravenously as a solution. The two forms have equal antifungal activity but higher peak serum levels are obtained with the ester. Although the ester is claimed to be less toxic, neurological effects have been observed. An ascorbate salt has recently been described which is water-soluble, of similar activity and less toxic.

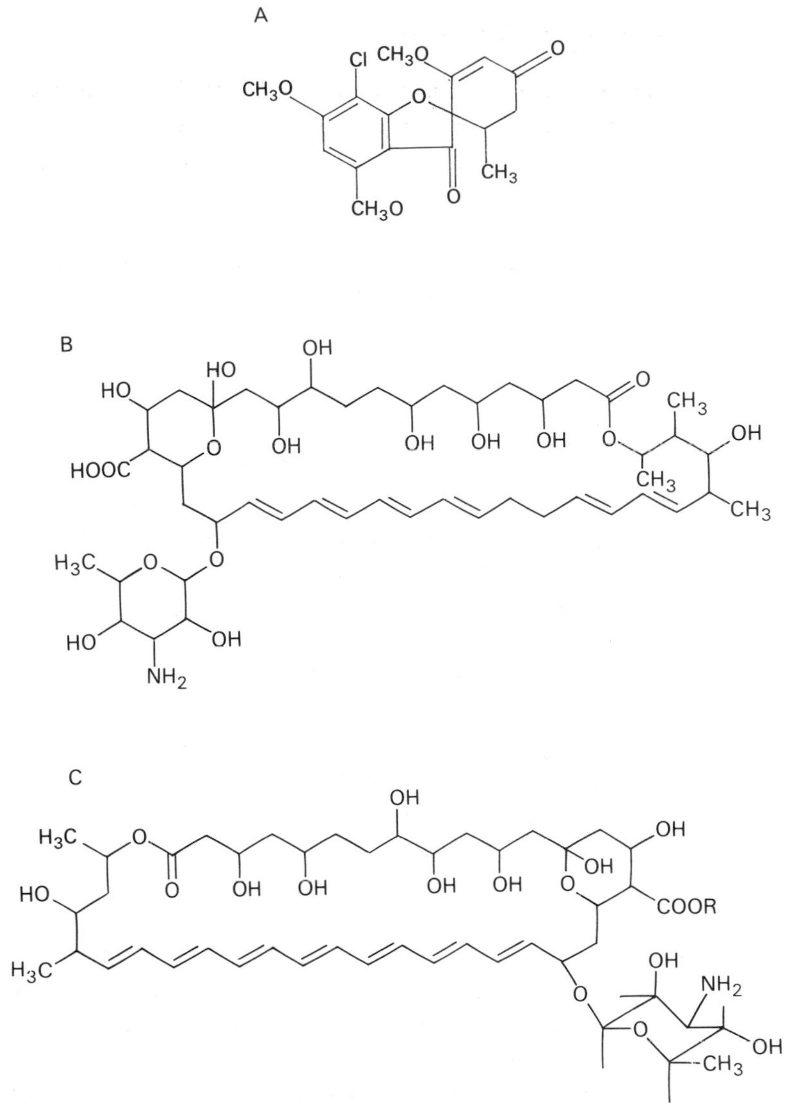

Fig. 5.15 Antifungal antibiotics: A, griseofulvin; B, nystatin; C, amphotericin (R = H) and its methyl ester (R = CH₃).

11   Synthetic antimicrobial agents

11.1   Sulphonamides

Sulphonamides were introduced by Domagk in 1935. It had been shown that a red azo dye, prontosil (Fig. 5.16B), had a curative effect on mice infected with β-haemolytic streptococci; it was subsequently found that *in vivo,* prontosil was converted into sulphanilamide. Chemical modifications of the nucleus of sulphanilamide (see Fig. 5.16A) gave compounds with higher antibacterial activity, although this was often accompanied by greater toxicity. In general, it may be stated that the sulphonamides

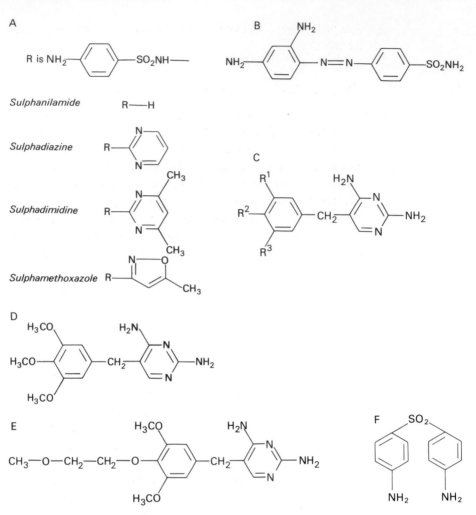

Fig. 5.16 A, some sulphonamides; B, prontosil rubrum; C, unsubstituted diaminobenzylpyrimidines; D, trimethoprim; E, tetroxoprim; F, dapsone.

have a broadly similar antibacterial activity but differ widely in pharmacological actions.

Bacteria which are almost always sensitive to the sulphonamides include *Strep. pneumoniae*, β-haemolytic streptococci, *Escherichia coli* and *Proteus mirabilis;* those almost always resistant include *Enterococcus faecalis, Ps. aeruginosa,* indole-positive *Proteus* and *Klebsiella;* whereas bacteria showing a marked variation in response include *Staph. aureus,* gonococci, *H. influenzae* and hospital strains of *E. coli* and *Pr. mirabilis.*

The sulphonamides show a considerable variation in the extent of their absorption into the bloodstream. Sulphadimidine and sulphadiazine are examples of rapidly absorbed ones, whereas succinylsulphathiazone and phthalylsulphathiazole are poorly absorbed and are excreted unchanged in the faeces.

From a clinical point of view, the sulphonamides are extremely useful for the treatment of uncomplicated urinary tract infection caused by *E. coli* in domiciliary practice. They have also been employed in treating meningococcal meningitis (a current problem is the number of sulphonamide-resistant meningococcal strains) and superficial eye infections.

11.2 Diaminopyrimidine derivatives

Small-molecule diaminopyrimidine derivatives were shown in 1948 to have an antifolate action. Subsequently, compounds were developed that were highly active against human cells (e.g. the use of methotrexate as an anticancer agent), protozoa (e.g. the use of pyrimethamine in malaria) or bacteria (e.g. trimethoprim: Fig. 5.16D). Unsubstituted diaminobenzylpyrimidines (Fig. 5.16C) bind poorly to bacterial dihydrofolate reductase (DHFR). The introduction of one, two or especially three methoxy groups (as in trimethoprim) produces a highly selective antibacterial agent. A recent antibacterial addition is tetroxoprim (2,4-diamino-5-(3′,5′-dimethoxy-4′-methoxyethoxybenzyl) pyrimidine; Fig. 5.16E) which retains methoxy groups at R^1 and R^3 and has a methoxyethoxy group at R^2. Trimethoprim and tetroxoprim have a broad spectrum of activity but resistance can arise from a non-susceptible target site, i.e. an altered DHFR (see Chapter 9).

11.3 Co-trimoxazole

Co-trimoxazole is a mixture of sulphamethoxazole (five parts) and trimethoprim (one part). The reason for using this combination is based upon the *in vitro* finding that there is a 'sequential blockade' of folic acid synthesis, in which the sulphonamide is a competitive inhibitor of dihydropteroate synthetase and trimethoprim inhibits DHFR (see Chapter 8, especially Fig. 8.5). The optimum ratio of the two components may not be achieved *in vivo* and arguments continue as to the clinical value of co-trimoxazole, with many advocating the use of trimethoprim alone. Co-trimoxazole is the agent of choice in treating pneumonias caused by *Pneumocystis carinii,* a yeast (although it had been classified as protozoa). *Pneumocystis carinii* is a common cause of pneumonia in patients receiving immunosuppressive therapy and in those suffering from AIDS.

11.4 Dapsone

Dapsone (diaminodiphenylsulphone; Fig. 5.16F) is used specifically in the treatment of leprosy. However, because resistance to dapsone is unfortunately now well known, it is recommended that dapsone be used in conjunction with rifampicin and clofazimine.

11.5 Antitubercular drugs

The three standard drugs used in the treatment of tuberculosis were streptomycin (considered above), *p*-aminosalicylic acid (PAS) and isoniazid (isonicotinylhydrazide, INH; synonym, isonicotinic acid hydrazine, INAH). The tubercle bacillus rapidly becomes resistant to streptomycin, and the role of PAS was mainly that of preventing this development of resistance. The current approach is to treat tuberculosis in two phases: an *initial* phase where a combination of three drugs is used to reduce the bacterial level as rapidly as possible, and a *continuation* phase in which a combination of two drugs is employed. Front-line drugs are isoniazid, rifampicin, streptomycin and ethambutol. Pyrazinamide, which has good meningeal penetration, and is thus particularly useful in tubercular meningitis, may be used in the initial phase to produce a highly bactericidal response.

Isoniazid has no significant effect against organisms other than mycobacteria. It is given orally. Cross-resistance between it, streptomycin and rifampicin has not been found to occur.

When bacterial resistance to these primary agents exists or develops, treatment with the secondary antitubercular drugs has to be considered. The latter group comprises capreomycin, cycloserine, some of the newer macrolides (azithromycin, clarithromycin), 4-quinolones (e.g. ciprofloxacin, ofloxacin) and prothionamide (no longer marketed in the UK). Prothionamide, pyrazinamide and ethionamide are, like isoniazid, derivatives of isonicotinic acid. The *British National Formulary* no longer lists ethionamide as being a suitable antitubercular drug. Chemical structures of the above, and of thiacetazone (not nowadays used because of its side-effects) are presented in Fig. 5.17.

There has, unfortunately, been a global resurgence of tuberculosis in recent years. Multiple drug-resistant *M. tuberculosis* (MDRTB) strains have been isolated in which resistance has been acquired to many drugs used in the treatment of this disease.

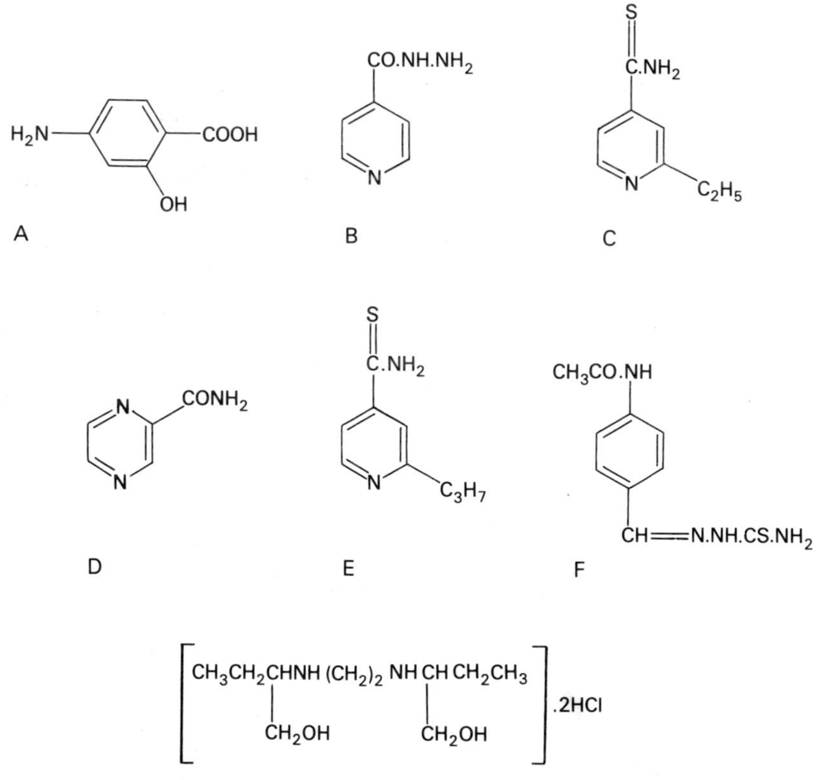

Fig. 5.17 Antitubercular compounds (see text also for details of antibiotics): A, PAS; B, isoniazid; C, ethionamide; D, pyrazinamide; E, prothionamide; F, thiacetazone; G, ethambutol.

Nitrofuran compounds

The nitrofuran group of drugs (Fig. 5.18) is based on the finding over 40 years ago that a nitro group in the 5 position of 2-substituted furans endowed these compounds with antibacterial activity. Many hundreds of such compounds have been synthesized, but only a few are in current therapeutic use. In the most important nitrofurans, an azomethine group, —CH=N—, is attached at C-2 and a nitro group at C-5. Less important nitrofurans have a vinyl group, —CH=CH—, at C-2.

Biological activity is lost if:

1   the nitro ring is reduced;
2   the —CH=N— linkage undergoes hydrolytic decomposition; or
3   the —CH=CH— linkage is oxidized.

The nitrofurans show antibacterial activity against a wide spectrum of micro-organisms, but furaltadone has now been withdrawn from use because of its toxicity. Furazolidone has a very high activity against most members of the Enterobacteriaceae, and has been used in the treatment of diarrhoea and gastrointestinal disturbances of bacterial origin. Nitrofurantoin is used in the treatment of urinary tract infections; anti-bacterial levels are not reached in the blood and the drug is concentrated in the urine. It is most active at acid pH. Nitrofurazone is used mainly as a topical agent in the treatment of burns and wounds and also in certain types of ear infections. The nitrofurans are believed to be mutagenic.

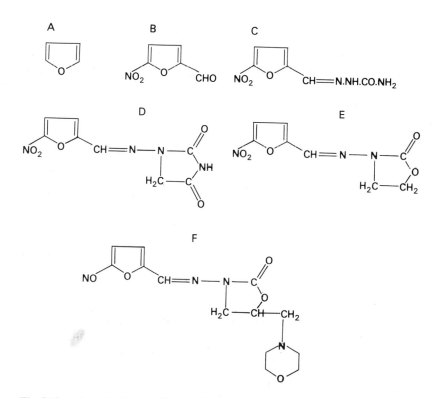

Fig. 5.18 A, furan; B, 5-nitrofurfural; C–F, nitrofuran drugs: respectively C, nitrofurazone, D, nitrofurantoin, E, furazolidone and F, furaltadone.

4-quinolone antibacterials

Over 10 000 quinolone antibacterial agents have now been synthesized. Nalidixic acid is regarded as the progenitor of the new quinolones. It has been used for several years as a clinically important drug in the treatment of urinary tract infections. Since its clinical introduction, other 4-quinolone antibacterials have been synthesized, some of which show considerably greater antibacterial potency. Furthermore, this means that many types of bacteria not susceptible to nalidixic acid therapy may be sensitive to the newer derivatives. The most important development was the introduction of a fluorine substituent at C-6, which led to a considerable increase in potency and spectrum of activity compared with nalidixic acid. These second-generation quinolones are known as fluoroquinolones, examples of which are ciprofloxacin and norfloxacin (Fig. 5.19).

Nalidixic acid is unusual in that it is active against several different types of Gram-negative bacteria, whereas Gram-positive organisms are resistant. However, the newer fluoroquinolone derivatives show superior activity against Enterobacteriacease and *Ps. aeruginosa,* and their spectrum also includes staphylococci but not streptococci. Extensive studies with norfloxacin have demonstrated that its broad spectrum, high urine concentration and oral administration make it a useful drug in the treatment of urinary infections. Ciprofloxacin may be used in the treatment of organisms resistant to other antibiotics; it can also be used in conjunction with a β-lactam or aminoglycoside antibiotic, e.g. when severe neutropenia is present.

The third and most recently developed generation of quinolones has maintained many of the properties of the second generation; examples are lomefloxacin, sparfloxacin (both difluorinated derivatives) and temafloxacin (a trifluorinated derivative). Lomefloxacin has a sufficiently long half-life to allow once-daily dosing, but adverse photosensitivity reactions are now being recognized. Sparfloxacin retains high activity against Gram-negative bacteria but has enhanced activity against Gram-positive cocci and anaerobes. Temafloxacin has, unfortunately, been withdrawn from clinical use because of unexpected severe haemolytic and nephrotoxic reactions.

Imidazole derivatives

The imidazoles comprise a large and diverse group of compounds with properties encompassing antibacterial (metronidazole), antiprotozoal (metronidazole), antifungal (clotrimazole, miconazole, ketoconazole, econazole) and anti-anthelmintic (mebendazole) activity: see Table 5.4. Metronidazole (Fig. 5.20A) inhibits the growth of pathogenic protozoa, very low concentrations being effective against the protozoa *Trichomonas vaginalis, Entamoeba histolytica* and *Giardia lamblia.* It is also used to treat bacterial vaginosis caused by *Gardnerella vaginalis.* Given orally, it cures 90–100% of sexually transmitted urogenital infections caused by *T. vaginalis.* It has also been found that metronidazole is effective against anaerobic bacteria, for example *B. fragilis,* and against facultative anaerobes grown under anaerobic, but not aerobic, conditions. Metronidazole is administered orally or in the form of suppositories.

Other imidazole derivatives include clotrimazole (Fig. 5.20B), miconazole (Fig. 5.20C) and econazole (Fig. 5.20D), all of which possess a broad antimycotic spectrum

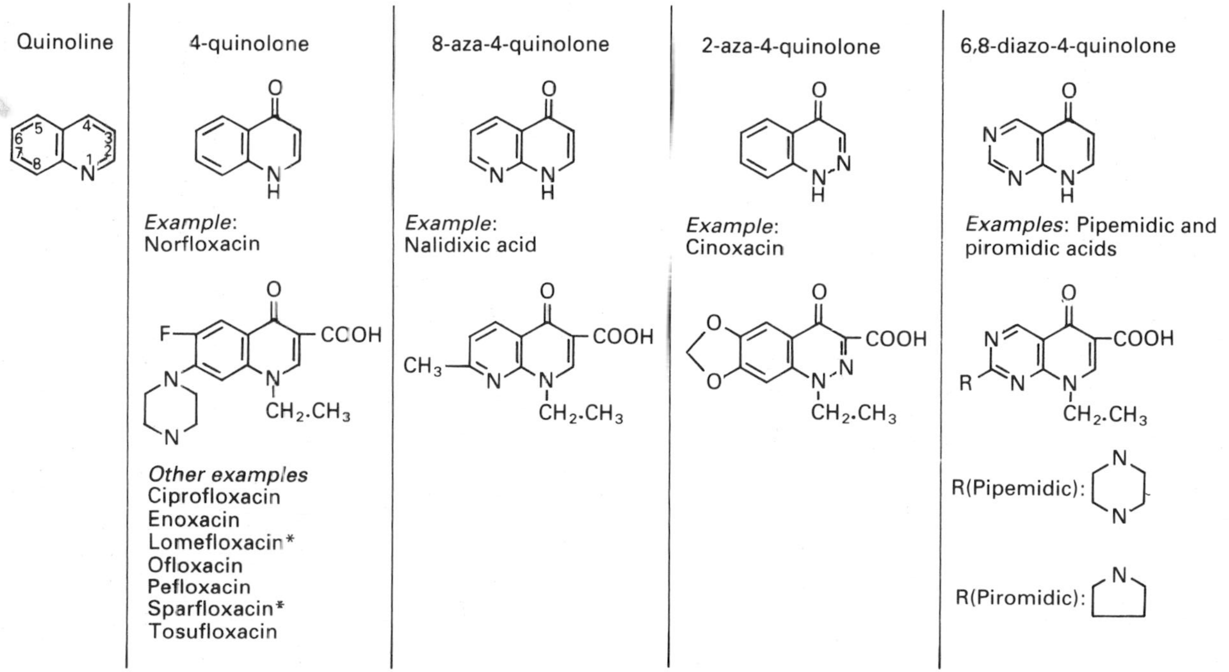

Fig. 5.19 Quinolone and antibacterial 4-quinolones. Note that the newer fluoroquine derivatives (e.g. norfloxacin, ciprofloxacin, ofloxacin) have a 6-fluoro and a 7-piperazino substituent. Drugs marked with an asterisk are difluorinated quinolones, with a second fluorine atom at C-8.

Table 5.4 Antimicrobial imidazoles

Antimicrobial or other activity	Examples
Antibacterial	Metronidazole, tinidazole: anaerobic bacteria only
Antiprotozoal	Metronidazole, tinidazole
Anthelmintic	Mebendazole
Antifungal	Clotrimazole, miconazole, econazole, ketoconazole
	Newer imidazoles: fluconazole, itraconazole

with some antibacterial activity and are used topically. Miconazole is used topically but can also be administered by intravenous or intrathecal injection in the treatment of severe systemic or meningeal fungal infections. Newer imidazoles are (a) ketoconazole (Fig. 5.20E) which is used orally for the treatment of systemic fungal infections (but not when there is central nervous system involvement or where the infection is life-threatening), (b) fluconazole (Fig. 5.20F), which is given orally or by intravenous infusion in the treatment of candidiasis and cryptococcal meningitis. Itraconazole is well absorbed when given orally after food.

11.9 Flucytosine

Flucytosine (5-fluorocytosine; Fig. 5.20G) is a narrow-spectrum antifungal agent with greatest activity against yeasts such as *Candida, Cryptococcus* and *Torulopsis.* Evidence has been presented which shows that, once inside the fungal cell, flucytosine is deaminated ot 5-fluorouracil (Fig. 5.20H). This is converted by the enzyme pyrophosphorylase to 5-fluorouridine monophosphate (FUMP), diphosphate (FUDP) and triphosphate (FUTP), which inhibits RNA synthesis; 5-fluorouracil itself has poor penetration into fungi. *Candida albicans* is known to convert FUMP to 5-fluorodeoxyuridine monophosphate (FdUMP), which inhibits DNA synthesis by virtue of its effect on thymidylate synthetase. Resistance can occur *in vivo* by reduced uptake into fungal cells of flucytosine or by decreased accumulation of FUTP and FdUMP.

11.10 Synthetic allylamines

Terbinafine (Fig. 5.17I), a member of the allylamine class of antimycotics, is an inhibitor of the enzyme squalene epoxidase in fungal ergosterol biosynthesis. Terbinafine is orally active, is fungicidal and is effective against a broad range of dermatophytes and yeasts. It can also be used topically as a cream.

11.11 Synthetic thiocarbamates

The synthetic thiocarbamates, of which tolnaftate (Fig. 5.20J) is an example, also inhibit squalene epoxidase. Tolnaftate inhibits this enzyme from *C. albicans*, but is inactive against whole cells, presumably because of its inability to penetrate the cell wall. Tolnaftate is used topically in the treatment or prophylaxis of tinea.

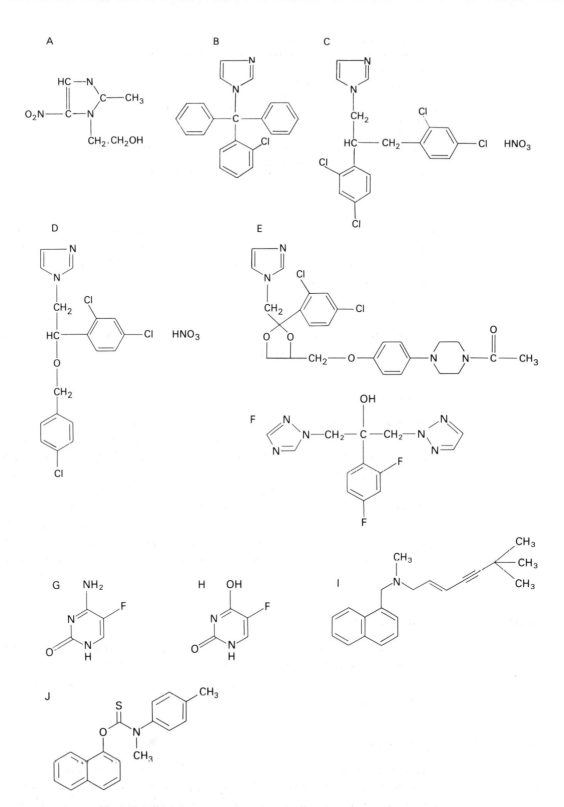

Fig. 5.20 Imidazoles (A–F): A, metronidazole; B, clotrimazole; C, miconazole; D, econazole; E, ketoconazole; F, fluconazole; G, flucytosine; H, 5-fluorouracil; I, terbinafine; J, tolnaftate.

12 Antiviral drugs

Several compounds are known that are inhibitory to mammalian viruses in tissue culture, but only a few can be used in the treatment of human viral infections. The main problem in designing and developing antiviral agents is the lack of selective toxicity that is normally possessed by most compounds. Viruses literally 'take over' the machinery of an infected human cell and thus an antiviral drug must be remarkably selectively toxic if it is to inhibit the viral particle without adversely affecting the human cell. Consequently, in comparison with antibacterial agents, very few inhibitors can be considered as being safe antiviral drugs, although the situation is improving. Possible sites of attack by antiviral agents include prevention of adsorption of a viral particle to the host cell, prevention of the intracellular penetration of the adsorbed virus, and inhibition of protein or nucleic synthesis.

Genetic information for viral reproduction resides in its nucleic acid (DNA or RNA: see Chapter 3). The viral particle (virion) does not possess enzymes necessary for its own replication; after entry into the host cell, the virus uses the enzymes already present or induces the formation of new ones. Viruses replicate by synthesis of their separate components followed by assembly.

Antiviral drugs are considered below with a summary in Table 5.5.

12.1 Amantadines

Amantadine hydrochloride (Fig. 5.21A) does not prevent adsorption but inhibits viral penetration. It has a very narrow spectrum and is used prophylactically against infection with influenza A virus; it has no prophylactic value with other types of influenza virus.

Table 5.5 Antiviral drugs and their clinical uses*

Group	Antiviral drug	Clinical uses
Nucleoside analogues	Idoxuridine	Skin including herpes labialis
	Ribavirin (tribavirin)	Severe respiratory syncytial virus bronchiolitis in infants and children
	Zidovudine	AIDS treatment
	Didanosine (DDI)	AIDS treatment
	Zalcitabine (DDC)	AIDS treatment
	Acyclovir (aciclovir) Famciclovir	Herpes simplex and varicella zoster
	Ganciclovir	Cytomegalovirus infections in immunocompromised patients only
Non-nucleoside analogues	Fascornet	Cytomegalovirus retinitis in patients with AIDS
	Amantadines	Prophylaxis: influenza A outbreak

* For further information, see the current issue of the *British National Formulary*.

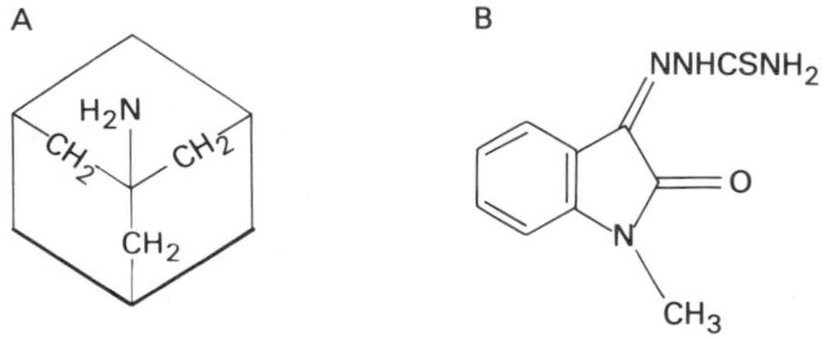

Fig. 5.21 A, Amantadine (used as the hydrochloride); B, methisazone.

12.2   **Methisazone**

Methisazone (Fig. 5.21B) inhibits DNA viruses (particularly vaccinia and variola) but not RNA viruses, and has been used in the prophylaxis of smallpox. It is now little used, especially as, according to the World Health Organization, smallpox has now been eradicated.

12.3   **Nucleoside analogues**

Various nucleoside analogues have been developed that inhibit nucleic acid synthesis. Idoxuridine (2′-deoxy-5-iodouridine; IUdR; Fig. 5.22C) is a thymidine analogue which inhibits the utilization of thymidine (Fig. 5.22A) in the rapid synthesis of DNA that normally occurs in herpes-infected cells. Unfortunately, because of its toxicity, idoxuridine is unsuitable for systemic use and it is restricted to topical treatment of herpes-infected eyes. Other nucleoside analogues include the following: cytarabine (cytosine arabinoside; Ara-C; Fig. 5.22D) which has antineoplastic and antiviral properties and which has been employed topically to treat herpes keratitis resistant to idoxuridine; adenosine arabinoside (Ara-A; vidarabine); and ribavirin (1-β-D-ribofuranosyl-1,2,4-triazole-3, carboxamide; Fig. 5.22E) which has a broad spectrum of activity, inhibiting both RNA and DNA viruses. Vidarabine, in particular, has a high degree of selectivity against viral DNA replication and is primarily active against herpesviruses and some poxviruses. It may be used systemically or topically. It is related structurally to guanosine (Fig. 5.22B).

Human immunodeficiency virus (HIV) is a retrovirus, i.e. its RNA is converted in human cells by the enzyme reverse transcriptase to DNA which is incorporated into the human genome and is responsible for producing new HIV particles. Zidovudine (azidothymidine, AZT; Fig. 5.22F) is a structural analogue of thymidine (Fig. 5.22A) and is used to treat AIDS patients. Zidovudine is converted in both infected and uninfected cells to the mono-, di- and eventually triphosphate derivatives. Zidovudine triphosphate, the active form, is a potent inhibitor of HIV replication, being mistaken for thymidine by reverse transcriptase. Premature chain termination of viral DNA ensues. However, AZT is relatively toxic because, as pointed out above, it is converted to the triphosphate by cellular enzymes and is thus also activated in uninfected cells.

2′3′-Dideoxycytidine (DDC, zalcitabine), a nucleoside analogue that also inhibits reverse transcriptase, is more active than zidovudine *in vitro,* and (unlike zidovudine) does not suppress erythropoiesis. DDC is not without toxicity, however, and a severe peripheral neurotoxicity, which is dose-related, has been reported. The chemical

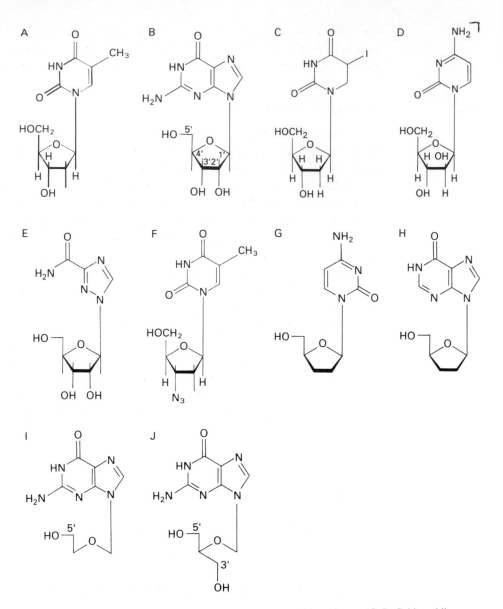

Fig. 5.22 Thymidine (A), guanosine (B) and some nucleoside analogues (C–J). C, idoxuridine; D, cytarabine; E, ribavirin; F, zidovudine (AZT); G, dideoxycytidine (DDC); H, dideoxyinosine (DDI); I, acyclovir; J, ganciclovir.

structures of DDC and of another analogue with similar properties, 2′3′-dideoxyinosine (DDI, didanosine), are presented in Fig. 5.22 (G, H, respectively).

Acyclovir (acycloguanosine, Fig. 5.22I) is a novel type of nucleoside analogue which becomes activated only in herpes-infected host cells by a herpes-specific enzyme, thymidine kinase. This enzyme initiates conversion of acyclovir initially to a monophosphate and then to the antiviral triphosphate which inhibits viral DNA polymerase. The host cell polymerase is not inhibited to the same extent, and the antiviral triphosphate is not produced in uninfected cells. Ganciclovir (Fig. 5.22J) is up to 100 times more active than acyclovir against human cytomegalovirus (CMV) but is also much more toxic; it is reserved for the treatment of severe CMV in immunocompromised patients. Famciclovir is similar, and valociclovir is a pro-drug ester of acyclovir.

12.4   Non-nucleoside compounds

Apart from the amantadines (section 12.1) and methisazone (section 12.2), various non-nucleoside drugs have shown antiviral activity. Two simple molecules with potent activity are phosphonoacetic acid (Fig. 5.23A) and sodium phosphonoformate (foscarnet, Fig. 5.23B). Phosphonoacetic acid has a high specificity for herpes simplex DNA synthesis, and has been shown to be non-mutagenic in experimental animals, but is highly toxic. Foscarnet inhibits herpes DNA polymerase and is non-toxic when applied to the skin and is a potentially useful agent in treating herpes simplex labialis (cold sores). It is used for cytomegalovirus retinitis in patients with AIDS in whom ganciclovir is inappropriate. Tetrahydroimidazobenzodiazepinone (TIBO) compounds have shown excellent activity *in vitro* against HIV reverse transcriptase in HIV type 1 (HIV-1) but not HIV-2 or other retroviruses.

Reverse transcriptase inhibitors prevent DNA from being produced in newly infected cells. They do not, however, prevent the reactivation of HIV from previously infected cells, the reason being that the enzyme is not involved in this process. Thus, agents that act at a later point in the replication cycle, possibly preventing reactivation, would be a major advance in the treatment of AIDs sufferers. The HIV protease inhibitors, which are currently receiving considerable attention, are believed to act in the manner depicted in Fig. 5.24.

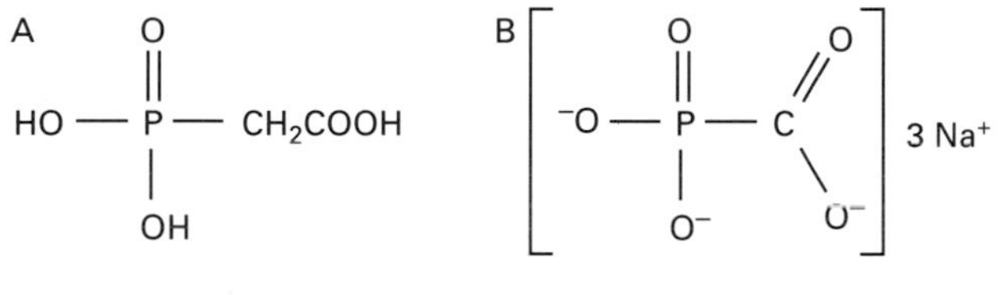

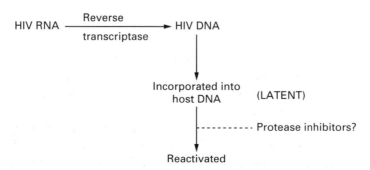

Fig. 5.23 A, phosphonoacetic acid; B, sodium phosphonoformate (foscarnet).

Fig. 5.24 Postulated mechanism of action of HIV protease inhibitors.

Interferons

Interferon is a low molecular weight protein, produced by virus-infected cells, that itself induces the formation of a second protein inhibiting the transcription of viral mRNA. Interferon is produced by the host cell in response to the virus particle, the viral nucleic and non-viral agents, including synthetic polynucleides such as polyinosinic acid : polycytidylic acid (poly I : C). There are two types of interferon.

Type I interferons. These are acid-stable and comprise two major classes, leucocyte interferon (Le-IFN, IFN-α) released by stimulated leucocytes, and fibroblast interferon (F-IFN, IFN-β) released by stimulated fibroblasts.

Type II interferons. These are acid-labile and are also known as 'immune' (IFN-γ) interferons because they are produced by T-lymphocytes (see Chapter 14) in the cellular immune system in response to specific antigens.

Type I interferons induce a virus-resistant state in human cells, whereas Type II are more active in inhibiting growth of tumour cells.

Disappointingly low yields of F-IFN and Le-IFN are achieved from eukaryotic cells. Recently, however, recombinant DNA technology has been employed to produce interferon in prokaryotic cells (bacteria). This aspect is considered in more detail in Chapter 24.

13   Drug combinations

A combination of two antibacterial agents may produce the following responses.

1   Synergism, where the joint effect is greater than the sum of the effects of each drug acting alone.

2   Additive effect, in which the combined effect is equal to the arithmetic sum of the effects of the two individual agents.

3   Antagonism (interference), in which there is a lesser effect of the mixture than that of the more potent drug action alone.

There are four possible justifications as to the use of antibacterial agents in combination.

1   The concept of clinical synergism, which may be extremely difficult to demonstrate convincingly. Even with trimethoprim plus sulphamethoxazole, where true synergism occurs *in vitro,* the optimum ratio of the two components may not always be present *in vivo,* i.e. at the site of infection in a particular tissue.

2   A wider spectrum of cover may be obtained, which may be (a) desirable as an emergency measure in life-threatening situations; or (b) of use in treating mixed infections.

3   The emergence of resistant organisms may be prevented. A classical example here occurs in combined antitubercular therapy (see earlier).

4   A possible reduction in dosage of a toxic drug may be achieved.

Indications for combined therapy are now considered to be much fewer than originally thought. There is also the problem of a chemical or physical incompatibility between two drugs. Examples where combinations have an important role to play in antibacterial chemotherapy were provided earlier (sections 2.3 and 2.9) in which a β-lactamase inhibitor and an appropriate β-lactamase-labile penicillin form a single pharmaceutical product. It must also be noted that a combination of two β-lactams does not necessarily produce a synergistic effect. Some antibiotics are excellent inducers of β-lactamase, and consequently a reduced response (antagonism) may be produced.

14   Further reading

Bean B. (1992) Antiviral therapy: current concepts and practices. *Clin Microbiol Rev*, **5**, 146–182.

Bowden K., Harris N.V. & Watson C.A. (1993) Structure–activity relationships of dihydrofolate reductase inhibitors. *J Chemother*, **5**, 377–388.

Bugg C.E., Carson W.M. & Montgomery J.A. (1993) Drugs by design. *Sci Am*, **269**, 92–98.

British National Formulary. London: British Medical Association & The Pharmaceutical Press. (The chapter on drugs used in the treatment of infections is a particularly useful section. New editions of the BNF appear at regular intervals.)

Brown A.G. (1981) New naturally occurring β lactam antibiotics and related compounds. *J Antimicrob Chemother*, **7**, 15–48.

Chopra I., Hawkey P.M. & Hinton M. (1992) Tetracyclines, molecular and clinical aspects. *J Antimicrob Chemother*, **29**, 245–277.

Greenwood D. (ed.) (1989) *Antimicrobial Chemotherapy*, 2nd end. London: Baillière Tindall.

Hamilton-Miller J.M.T. (1991) From foreign pharmacopoeias: 'new' antibiotics from old? *J Antimicrob Chemother*, **27**, 702–705.

Hooper D.C. & Wolfson J.S. (eds) (1993) *Quinolone Antimicrobial Agents*, 2nd edn. Washington: American Society for Microbiology.

Hunter P.A., Darby G.K. & Russell N.J. (eds) (1995) *Fifty Years of Antimicrobials: Past Perspectives and Future Trends*. 53rd Symposium of the Society for General Microbiology. Cambridge: Cambridge University Press

Kuntz I.D. (1992) Structure-based strategies for drug design and discovery. *Science*, **257**, 1079–1082.

Lambert H.P., O'Grady F., Greenwood D. & Finch R.G. (1992) *Antibiotic and Chemotherapy*, 7th edn. London & Edinburgh: Churchill Livingstone.

Neu H.C. (1985) Relation of structural properties of β-lactam antibiotics to antibacterial activity. *Am J Med*, **79** (Suppl. 2A), 2–13.

Power E.G.M. & Russell A.D. (1998) Design of antimicrobial chemotherapeutic agents. In: *Introduction to Principles of Drug Design* (ed. H.J. Smith), 3rd edn, Bristol: Wright.

Reeves D.S. & Howard A.J. (eds) (1991) New macrolides—the respiratory antibiotics for the 1990s. *J Hosp Infect*, **19** (Suppl. A).

Russell A.D. & Chopra I. (1996) *Understanding Antibacteral Action and Resistance,* 2nd edn. Chichester: Ellis Horwood.

Sammes P.G. (Ed.) *Topics in Antibiotic Chemistry*, vols 1–5. Chichester: Ellis Horwood.

Shanson D.C. (1989) *Microbiology in Clinical Practice*, 2nd edn. London: Wright.

Wolinski E. (1992) Antimycobacterial drugs. In: *Infections Diseases* (eds A. Gorbach, J.G. Bartlett & N.R. Blacklow), pp. 319–319. Philadelphia: W.B. Saunders.

Wood M.J. (1991) More macrolides. *Br Med J*, **303**, 594–595.

6 Clinical uses of antimicrobial drugs

1	**Introduction**	3.1.2	Lower respiratory tract infections
		3.2	Urinary tract infections
2	**Principles of use of antimicrobial drugs**	3.2.1	Pathogenesis
2.1	Susceptibility of infecting organisms	3.2.2	Drug therapy
2.2	Host factors	3.3	Gastrointestinal infections
2.3	Pharmacological factors	3.4	Skin and soft tissue infections
2.4	Drug resistance	3.5	Central nervous system infections
2.4.1	Multi-drug resistance		
2.5	Drug combinations	**4**	**Antibiotic policies**
2.6	Adverse reactions	4.1	Rationale
2.7	Superinfection	4.2	Types of antibiotic policies
2.8	Chemoprophylaxis	4.2.1	Free prescribing policy
		4.2.2	Restricted reporting
3	**Clinical use**	4.2.3	Restricted dispensing
3.1	Respiratory tract infections		
3.1.1	Upper respiratory tract infections	**5**	**Further reading**

1 Introduction

The worldwide use of antimicrobial drugs continues to rise; in 1995 these agents accounted for an expenditure of approximately £17 000 billion. In the UK antibiotic prescribing continues to rise. General practice use accounts for approximately 90% of all antibiotic prescribing and largely involves oral and topical agents. Hospital use accounts for the remaining 10% of antibiotic prescribing with a much heavier use of injectable agents. Although this chapter is concerned with the clinical use of antimicrobial drugs, it should be remembered that these agents are also extensively used in veterinary practice as well as in animal husbandry as growth promoters. In humans the therapeutic use of anti-infectives has revolutionized the management of most bacterial infections, many parasitic and fungal diseases and, with the availability of acyclovir and zidovudine (azidothymidine, AZT) (see Chapter 3 and 5), selected herpesvirus infections and human immunodeficiency virus (HIV) infection, respectively. Although originally used for the treatment of established bacterial infections, antibiotics have proved useful in the prevention of infection in various high-risk circumstances; this applies especially to patients undergoing various surgical procedures where perioperative antibiotics have significantly reduced postoperative infectious complications.

The advantages of effective antimicrobial chemotherapy are self-evident, but this has led to a significant problem in ensuring that they are always appropriately used. Surveys of antibiotic use have demonstrated that more than 50% of antibiotic prescribing can be inappropriate; this may reflect prescribing in situations where antibiotics are either ineffective, such as viral infections, or that the selected agent, its dose, route of administration or duration of use are inappropriate. Of particular concern is the prolonged use of antibiotics for surgical prophylaxis. Apart from being wasteful of health resources, prolonged use encourages superinfection by drug-resistant organisms and unnecessarily increases the risk of adverse drug reactions. Thus, it is essential that the clinical use of these agents be based on a clear understanding of the principles that have evolved to ensure safe, yet effective, prescribing.

Further information about the properties of antimicrobial agents described in this chapter can be found in Chapter 5.

2   Principles of use of antimicrobial drugs

2.1   Susceptibility of infecting organisms

Drug selection should be based on knowledge of its activity against infecting microorganisms. Selected organisms may be predictably susceptible to a particular agent, and laboratory testing is therefore rarely performed. For example, *Streptococcus pyogenes* is uniformly sensitive to penicillin. In contrast, the susceptibility of many Gram-negative enteric bacteria is less predictable and laboratory guidance is essential for safe prescribing. The susceptibility of common bacterial pathogens and widely prescribed antibiotics is summarized in Table 6.1. It can be seen that, although certain bacteria are susceptible *in vitro* to a particular agent, use of that drug may be inappropriate, either on pharmacological grounds or because other less toxic agents are preferred.

2.2   Host factors

In vitro susceptibility testing does not always predict clinical outcome. Host factors play an important part in determining outcome and this applies particularly to circulating and tissue phagocytic activity. Infections can progress rapidly in patients suffering from either an absolute or functional deficiency of phagocytic cells. This applies particularly to those suffering from various haematological malignancies, such as the acute leukaemias, where phagocyte function is impaired both by the disease and also by the use of potent cytotoxic drugs which destroy healthy, as well as malignant, white cells. Under these circumstances it is essential to select agents which are bactericidal, since bacteristatic drugs, such as the tetracyclines or sulphonamides, rely on host phagocytic activity to clear bacteria. Widely used bactericidal agents include the aminoglycosides, broad-spectrum penicillins, the cephalosporins and quinolones (see Chapter 5).

In some infections the pathogenic organisms are located intracellularly within phagocytic cells and, therefore, remain relatively protected from drugs which penetrate cells poorly, such as the penicillins and cephalosporins. In contrast, erythromycin, rifampicin and chloramphenicol readily penetrate phagocytic cells. Legionnaires' disease is an example of an intracellular infection and is treated with rifampicin and/or erythromycin.

2.3   Pharmacological factors

Clinical efficacy is also dependent on achieving satisfactory drug concentrations at the

Table 6.1 Sensitivity of selected bacteria to common antibacterial agents

	Staphylococcus aureus (pen. sensitive)	Staphylococcus aureus (pen. resistant)	Streptococcus pyogenes and Streptococcus pneumoniae	Enterococcus	Cl. perfringens	Neisseria gonorrhoeae	Neisseria meningitidis	Haemophilus influenzae	Escherichia coli	Klebsiella spp.	Proteus spp. (indole-negative)	Proteus spp. (indole-positive)	Serratia spp.	Salmonella spp.	Shigella spp.	Pseudomonas spp.	Bacteroides fragilis	Other Bacteroides spp.	Chlamydia spp.	Mycoplasma pneumoniae	Rickettsia spp.
Penicillin V/G	+	R	+	+	+	+*	+	±	R	R	R	R	R	R	R	R	R	+	R	R	R
Methicillin, flucloxacillin	+*	+*	+	R	(+)	(±)	(±)	R	R	R	R	R	R	R	R	R	R	(±)	R	R	R
Ampicillin, amoxycillin	+	R	+*	+	+	+*	+	±	±	R	+	R	R	±	±	R	R	+	R	R	R
Ticarcillin	(+)	R	(+)	+	+	(+)	(+)	(+)	±	±	+	±	±	(+)	(+)	+*	±	±	R	R	R
Cefazolin	+	+*	+	R	(±)	(+)	(+)	±	±	±	+	R	R	(+)	(+)	R	R	R	R	R	R
Cefamandole, cefuroxime	+	+	+	R	+	+	+	+	+	+	+	+	R	(+)	(+)	R	R	R	R	R	R
Cefoxitin	+	+	+	R	+	+	(+)	+	+	+	+	+	±	(+)	(+)	R	+	+	R	R	R
Cefotaxime, ceftriaxone	+	+	+	R	+	+	+	+	+	+	+	+	+	+	+	±	R/±	R/+	R	R	R
Ceftazidime	+	+	+	R	±	+	+	+	+	+	+	+	+	+	+	+	±	±	R	R	R
Erythromycin	+*	+	+	R	+*	+	(+)	±	R	R	R	R	R	R	R	R	R	±	+	+	R
Clindamycin	+*	+*	+	+	+*	R	R	R	R	R	R	R	R	R	R	R	+	+	R	R	R
Tetracyclines	+*	+*	±	+	+	+	+	+	+	±	±	±	R	(±)	(±)	R	±	±	+	+	+
Chloramphenicol	+	+	+	+	+	+	+	+*	+	+	+	+	+*	+*	+	R	+	+	+	+	+
Ciprofloxacin	±	±	+	±	R	+	+	+	+	+	+	+	+	+	+	(+)	R	R	+	+	+
Gentamicin, tobramycin, amikacin, netilmicin	+	+	R	R	R	R	R	+	+	+*	+	+	+*	(+)	(+)	+*	R	R	R	R	R
Sulphonamides	+	+	±	±	(±)	±	±	±	±	±	±	±	R	±	±	R	R	R	+	R	R
Trimethoprim–sulphamethoxazole	+	+	+	+	R	+	+	+	+	+	+	+	R	+	+	R	R	R	+	R	R

+, Sensitive; R, resistant; ±, some strains resistant; ( ), not appropriate therapy; *, rare strains resistant.

site of the infection; this is influenced by the standard pharmacological
absorption, distribution, metabolism and excretion. If an oral agent is s
gastrointestinal absorption should be satisfactory. However, it may be impair
factors such as the presence of food, drug interactions (including chelation), or impa
gastrointestinal function either as a result of surgical resection or malabsorptive states
Although effective, oral absorption may be inappropriate in patients who are vomiting
or have undergone recent surgery; under these circumstances a parenteral agent will be
required and has the advantage of providing rapidly effective drug concentrations.

Antibiotic selection also varies according to the anatomical site of infection. Lipid
solubility is of importance in relation to drug distribution. For example, the aminoglycosides are poorly lipid-soluble and although achieving therapeutic concentrations
within the extracellular fluid compartment, penetrate the cerebrospinal fluid (CSF)
poorly. Likewise the presence of inflammation may affect drug penetration into the
tissues. In the presence of meningeal inflammation, β-lactam agents achieve satisfactory
concentrations within the CSF, but as the inflammatory response subsides drug
concentrations fall. Hence it is essential to maintain sufficient dosaging throughout the
treatment of bacterial meningitis. Other agents such as chloramphenicol are little affected
by the presence or absence of meningeal inflammation.

Therapeutic drug concentrations within the bile duct and gall bladder are dependent
upon biliary excretion. In the presence of biliary disease, such as gallstones or chronic
inflammation, the drug concentration may fail to reach therapeutic levels. In contrast,
drugs which are excreted primarily via the liver or kidneys may require reduced dosaging
in the presence of impaired renal or hepatic function. The malfunction of excretory
organs may not only risk toxicity from drug accumulation, but will also reduce urinary
concentration of drugs excreted primarily by glomerular filtration. This applies to the
aminoglycosides and the urinary antiseptics, nalidixic acid and nitrofurantoin, where
therapeutic failure of urinary tract infections may complicate severe renal failure.

2.4   **Drug resistance**

Drug resistance may be a natural or an acquired characteristic of a microorganism.
This may result from impaired cell wall or cell envelope penetration, enzymatic
inactivation or altered binding sites. Acquired drug resistance may result from mutation,
adaptation or gene transfer. Spontaneous mutations occur at low frequency, as in the
case of *Mycobacterium tuberculosis* where a minority population of organisms is
resistant to isoniazid. In this situation the use of isoniazid alone will eventually result
in overgrowth by this subpopulation of resistant organisms.

A more recently recognized mechanism of drug resistance is that of efflux in which
the antibiotic is rapidly extruded from the cell by an energy-dependent mechanism.
This affects antibiotics such as the tetracyclines and macrolides.

Genetic resistance may be chromosomally or plasmid-mediated. Plasmid-mediated
resistance has been increasingly recognized among Gram-negative enteric pathogens.
By the process of conjugation (Chapter 9), resistance plasmids may be transferred
between bacteria of the same and different species and also different genera. Such
resistance can code for multiple antibiotic resistance. For example, the penicillins,
cephalosporins, chloramphenicol and the aminoglycosides are all subject to enzymatic

ctivation which may be plasmid-mediated. Knowledge of the local epidemiology of
tant pathogens within a hospital, and especially within high-dependency areas
as intensive care units, is invaluable in guiding appropriate drug selection.

...-drug resistance

In recent years multi-drug resistance has increased among certain pathogens. These include *Staph. aureus,* enterococci and *M. tuberculosis. Staphylococcus aureus* resistant to methicillin is known as methicillin-resistant *Staph. aureus* (MRSA). These strains are resistant to many antibiotics and have been responsible for major epidemics worldwide, usually in hospitals where they affect patients in high-dependency units such as intensive care units, burns units and cardiothoracic units. MRSA have the ability to colonize staff and patients and to spread readily among them. Several epidemic strains are currently circulating in the UK. The glycopeptides, vancomycin or teicoplanin, are the currently recommended agents for treating patients infected with these organisms.

Another serious resistance problem is that of drug-resistant enterococci. These include *Enterococcus faecalis* and, in particular, *E. faecium.* Resistance to the glycopeptides has again been a problem among patients in high-dependency units. Four different phenotypes are recognized (Van A, B, C and D). The Van A phenotype is resistant to both glycopeptides, while the others are sensitive to teicoplanin but demonstrate high (Van B) or intermediate (Van C) resistance to vancomycin; Van D resistance has only recently been described. Those fully resistant to the glycopeptides are increasing in frequency and causing great concern since they are essentially resistant to almost all antibiotics.

Tuberculosis is on the increase after decades in which the incidence has been steadily falling. Drug-resistant strains have emerged largely among inadequately treated or non-compliant patients. These include the homeless, alcoholic, intravenous drug abusing and immigrant populations. Resistance patterns vary but increasingly includes rifampicin and isoniazid. Furthermore, outbreaks of multi-drug-resistant tuberculosis have been increasingly reported from a number of hospital centres in the USA and more recently Europe, including the UK. These infections have occasionally spread to health care workers and is giving rise to considerable concern.

The underlying mechanisms of resistance are considered in Chapter 9.

2.5 Drug combinations

Antibiotics are generally used alone, but may on occasion be prescribed in combination. Combining two antibiotics may result in synergism, indifference or antagonism. In the case of synergism, microbial inhibition is achieved at concentrations below that for each agent alone and may prove advantageous in treating relatively insusceptible infections such as enterococcal endocarditis, where a combination of penicillin and gentamicin is synergistically active. Another advantage of synergistic combinations is that it may enable the use of toxic agents where dose reductions are possible. For example, meningitis caused by the fungus *Cryptococcus neoformans* responds to an abbreviated course of amphotericin B when it is combined with 5-flucytosine, thereby reducing the risk of toxicity from amphotericin B.

Combined drug use is occasionally recommended to prevent resistance emerging during treatment. For example, treatment may fail when fusidic acid is used alone to treat *Staph. aureus* infections, because resistant strains develop rapidly; this is prevented by combining fusidic acid with flucloxacillin. Likewise, tuberculosis is treated with a minimum of two agents, such as rifampicin and isoniazid; again drug resistance is prevented which may result if either agent is used alone.

The most common reason for using combined therapy is in the treatment of confirmed or suspected mixed infections where a single agent alone will fail to cover all pathogenic organisms. This is the case in serious abdominal sepsis where mixed aerobic and anaerobic infections are common and the use of metronidazole in combination with either an aminoglycoside or a broad-spectrum cephalosporin is essential. Finally, drugs are used in combination in patients who are seriously ill and in whom uncertainty exists concerning the microbiological nature of their infection. This initial 'blind therapy' frequently includes a broad-spectrum penicillin or cephalosporin in combination with an aminoglycoside. The regimen should be modified in the light of subsequent microbiological information.

| 2.6 | **Adverse reactions** |

Regrettably, all chemotherapeutic agents have the potential to produce adverse reactions with varying degrees of frequency and severity, and these include hypersensitivity reactions and toxic effects. These may be dose-related and predictable in a patient with a history of hypersensitivity or a previous toxic reaction to a drug or its chemical analogues. However, many adverse events are idiosyncratic and therefore unpredictable.

Hypersensitivity reactions range in severity from fatal anaphylaxis, in which there is widespread tissue oedema, airway obstruction and cardiovascular collapse, to minor and reversible hypersensitivity reactions such as skin eruptions and drug fever. Such reactions are more likely in those with a history of hypersensitivity to the drug, and are more frequent in patients with previous allergic diseases such as childhood eczema or asthma. It is important to question patients closely concerning hypersensitivity reactions before prescribing, since it precludes the use of all compounds within a class, such as the sulphonamides or tetracyclines, while cephalosporins should be used with caution in patients allergic to penicillin since these agents are structurally related. They should be avoided entirely in those who have had a previous severe hypersensitivity reaction to penicillin.

Drug toxicity is often dose-related and may affect a variety of organs or tissues. For example, the aminoglycosides are both nephrotoxic and ototoxic to varying degrees; therefore, dosaging should be individualized and the serum assayed, especially where renal function is abnormal, to avoid toxic effects and non-therapeutic drug concentrations. An example of dose-related toxicity is chloramphenicol-induced bone marrow suppression. Chloramphenicol interferes with the normal maturation of bone marrow stem cells and high concentrations may result in a steady fall in circulating red and white cells and also platelets. This effect is generally reversible with dose reduction or drug withdrawal. This dose-related toxic reaction of chloramphenicol should be contrasted with idiosyncratic bone marrow toxicity which is unrelated to dose and occurs at a much lower frequency of approximately 1 : 40 000 and is frequently irreversible, ending fatally. Toxic effects may also be genetically determined. For example, peripheral neuropathy may occur in those who are slow acetylators of isoniazid, while haemolysis occurs in those deficient in the red cell enzyme glucose-6-phosphate dehydrogenase, when treated with sulphonamides or primaquine.

<table>
<tr><td>2.7</td><td>

Superinfection

</td></tr>
</table>

2.7　　　**Superinfection**

Anti-infective drugs not only affect the invading organism undergoing treatment but also have an impact on the normal bacterial flora, especially of the skin and mucous membranes. This may result in microbial overgrowth of resistant organisms with subsequent superinfection. One example is the common occurrence of oral or vaginal candidiasis in patients treated with broad-spectrum agents such as ampicillin or tetracycline. A more serious example is the development of pseudo-membranous colitis from the overgrowth of toxin-producing strains of *Clostridium difficile* present in the bowel flora following the use of clindamycin and other broad-spectrum antibiotics. This condition is managed by drug withdrawal and oral vancomycin. Rarely, colectomy (excision of part or whole of the colon) may be necessary for severe cases.

2.8　　　**Chemoprophylaxis**

An increasingly important use of antimicrobial agents is that of infection prevention, especially in relationship to surgery. Infection remains one of the most important complications of many surgical procedures, and the recognition that peri-operative antibiotics are effective and safe in preventing this complication has proved a major advance in surgery. The principles that underly the chemoprophylactic use of anti-bacterials relate to the predictability of infection for a particular surgical procedure, both in terms of its occurrence, microbial aetiology and susceptibility to antibiotics. Therapeutic drug concentrations present at the operative site at the time of surgery rapidly reduce the number of potentially infectious organisms and prevents would sepsis. If prophylaxis is delayed to the post-operative period then efficacy is markedly impaired. It is important that chemoprophylaxis be limited to the peri-operative period, the first dose being administered approximately 1 hour before surgery for injectable agents and repeated for two to three repeat doses postoperatively. Prolonging chemoprophylaxis beyond this period is not cost-effective and increases the risk of adverse drug reactions and superinfection. One of the best examples of the efficacy of surgical prophylaxis is in the area of large-bowel surgery. Before the widespread use of chemoprophylaxis, postoperative infection rates for colectomy were often 30% or higher; these have now been reduced to around 5%.

Chemoprophylaxis has been extended to other surgical procedures where the risk of infection may be low but its occurrence has serious consequences. This is especially true for the implantation of prosthetic joint or heart valves. These are major surgical procedures and although infection may be infrequent its consequences are serious and on balance the use of chemoprophylaxis is cost-effective.

Examples of chemoprophylaxis in the non-surgical arena include the prevention of endocarditis with amoxycillin in patients with valvular heart disease undergoing dental surgery, and the prevention of secondary cases of meningococcal meningitis with rifampicin among household contacts of an index case.

3   Clinical use

The choice of antimicrobial chemotherapy is initially dependent upon the clinical diagnosis. Under some circumstances the clinical diagnosis implies a microbiological diagnosis which may dictate specific therapy. For example, typhoid fever is caused by *Salmonella typhi* which is generally sensitive to chloramphenicol, co-trimoxazole and ciproflaxin. However, for many infections, establishing a clinical diagnosis implies a range of possible microbiological causes and requires laboratory confirmation from samples collected, preferably before antibiotic therapy is begun. Laboratory isolation and susceptibility testing of the causative agent establish the diagnosis with certainty and make drug selection more rational. However, in many circumstances, especially in general practice, microbiological documentation of an infection is not possible. Hence knowledge of the usual microbiological cause of a particular infection and its susceptibility to antimicrobial agents is essential for effective drug prescribing. The following section explores a selection of the problems associated with antimicrobial drug prescribing for a range of clinical problems.

3.1   Respiratory tract infections

Infections of the respiratory tract are among the commonest of infections, and account for much consultation in general practice and a high percentage of acute hospital admissions. They are divided into infections of the upper respiratory tract, involving the ears, throat, nasal sinuses and the trachea, and the lower respiratory tract (LRT), where they affect the airways, lungs and pleura.

3.1.1   *Upper respiratory tract infections*

Acute pharyngitis presents a diagnostic and therapeutic dilemma. The majority of sore throats are caused by a variety of viruses; fewer than 20% are bacterial and hence potentially responsive to antibiotic therapy. However, antibiotics are widely prescribed and this reflects the difficulty in discriminating streptococcal from non-streptococcal infections clinically in the absence of microbiological documentation. Nonetheless, *Strep. pyogenes* is the most important bacterial pathogen and this responds to oral penicillin. However, up to 10 days' treatment is required for its eradication from the throat. This requirement causes problems with compliance since symptomatic improvement generally occurs within 2–3 days.

Although viral infections are important causes of both otitis media and sinusitis, they are generally self-limiting. Bacterial infections may complicate viral illnesses, and are also primary causes of ear and sinus infections. *Streptococcus pneumoniae* and *Haemophilus influenzae* are the commonest bacterial pathogens. Amoxycillin is widely prescribed for these infections since it is microbiologically active, penetrates the middle ear, and sinuses, is well tolerated and has proved effective.

Lower respiratory tract infections

Infections of the LRT include pneumonia, lung abscess, bronchitis, bronchiectasis and infective complications of cystic fibrosis. Each presents a specific diagnostic and therapeutic challenge which reflects the variety of pathogens involved and the frequent difficulties in establishing an accurate microbial diagnosis. The laboratory diagnosis of LRT infections is largely dependent upon culturing sputum. Unfortunately this may be contaminated with the normal bacterial flora of the upper respiratory tract during expectoration. In hospitalized patients, the empirical use of antibiotics before admission substantially diminishes the value of sputum culture and may result in overgrowth by non-pathogenic microbes, thus causing difficulty with the interpretation of sputum culture results. Alternative diagnostic samples include needle aspiration of sputum directly from the trachea or of fluid within the pleural cavity. Blood may also be cultured and serum examined for antibody responses or microbial antigens. In the community, few patients will have their LRT infection diagnosed microbiologically and the choice of antibiotic is based on clinical diagnosis.

Pneumonia. The range of pathogens causing acute pneumonia includes viruses, bacteria and, in the immunocompromised host, parasites and fungi. Table 6.2 summarizes these pathogens and indicates drugs appropriate for their treatment. Clinical assessment includes details of the evolution of the infection, any evidence of a recent viral infection, the age of the patient and risk factors such as corticosteroid therapy or pre-existing lung disease. The extent of the pneumonia, as assessed clinically or by X-ray, is also important.

Streptococcus pneumoniae remains the commonest cause of pneumonia and responds well to penicillin. In addition, a number of atypical infections may cause pneumonia and include *Mycoplasma pneumoniae*, *Legionella pneumophila*, psittacosis and occasionally Q fever. With psittacosis there may be a history of contact with parrots or budgerigars; while Legionnaires' disease has often been acquired during hotel holidays

Table 6.2 Microorganisms responsible for pneumonia and the therapeutic agent of choice

Pathogen	Drug(s) of choice
Streptococcus pneumoniae	Penicillin
Staphylococcus aureus	Flucloxacillin ± fusidic acid
Haemophilus influenzae	Amoxycillin or cefuroxime
Klebsiella pneumoniae	Cefotaxime ± gentamicin
Pseudomonas aeruginosa	Gentamicin ± azlocillin
Mycoplasma pneumoniae	Erythromycin or tetracycline
Legionella pneumophila	Erythromycin ± rifampicin
Chlamydia psittaci	Tetracycline
Mycobacterium tuberculosis	Rifampicin + isoniazid + ethambutol + pyrazinamide*
Herpes simplex, varicella/zoster	Acyclovir
Candida or *Aspergillus* spp.	Amphotericin B
Anaerobic bacteria	Penicillin or metronidazole

* Reduce to two drugs after 6–8 weeks.

in the Mediterranean area. The atypical pneumonias, unlike pneum
do not respond to penicillin. Legionnaires' disease is treated with e
the presence of severe pneumonia, rifampicin is added to the reg
infections are best treated with either erythromycin or tetracycli
drug is indicated for both psittacosis and Q fever.

Lung abscess. Destruction of lung tissue may lead to abscess formation and is a feature of aerobic Gram-negative bacillary and *Staph. aureus* infections. In addition, aspiration of oropharyngeal secretion can lead to chronic low-grade sepsis with abscess formation and the expectoration of foul-smelling sputum which characterizes anaerobic sepsis. The latter condition responds to high-dose penicillin, which is active against most of the normal oropharyngeal flora, while metronidazole may be appropriate for strictly anaerobic infections. In the case of aerobic Gram-negative bacillary sepsis, aminoglycosides, with or without a broad-spectrum cephalosporin, are the agents of choice. Acute staphylococcal pneumonia is an extremely serious infection and requires treatment with high-dose flucloxacillin alone or in combination with fusidic acid.

Cystic fibrosis. Cystic fibrosis is a multi-system, congenital abnormality which often affects the lungs and results in recurrent infections, initially with *Staph. aureus,* subsequently with *H. influenzae* and eventually leads on to recurrent *Ps. aeruginosa* infection. The latter organism is associated with copious quantities of purulent sputum which is extremely difficult to expectorate. *Pseudomonas aeruginosa* is a cofactor in the progressive lung damage which is eventually fatal in these patients. Repeated courses of antibiotics are prescribed and although they have improved the quality and longevity of life, infections caused by *Ps. aeruginosa* are difficult to treat and require repeated hospitalization and administration of parenteral antibiotics such as an aminoglycoside, either alone or in combination with an antipseudomonal penicillin. The dose of aminoglycosides tolerated by these patients is often higher than in normal individuals and is associated with larger volumes of distribution for these and other agents. Some benefit may also be obtained from inhaled aerosolized antibiotics. Unfortunately drug resistance may emerge and makes drug selection more dependent upon laboratory guidance.

3.2 Urinary tract infections

Urinary tract infection is a common problem in both community and hospital practice. Although occurring throughout life, infections are more common in pre-school girls and women during their childbearing years, although in the elderly the sex distribution is similar. Infection is predisposed by factors which impair urine flow. These include congenital abnormalities, reflux of urine from the bladder into the ureters, kidney stones and tumours and, in males, enlargement of the prostate gland. Bladder catheterization is an important cause of urinary tract infection in hospitalized patients.

3.2.1 *Pathogenesis*

In those with structural or drainage problems the risk exists of ascending infection to involve the kidney and occasionally the bloodstream. Although structural abnormalities may be absent in women of childbearing years, infection can become recurrent, symptomatic and extremely distressing. Of greater concern is the occurrence of infection in the pre-school child since normal maturation of the kidney may be impaired and result in progressive damage which presents as renal failure in later life.

From a therapeutic point of view, it is essential to confirm the presence of bacteriuria (a condition in which there are bacteria in the urine) since symptoms alone are not a reliable method of documenting infection. This applies particularly to bladder infection where the symptoms of burning micturition (dysuria) and frequency can be associated with a variety of non-bacteriuric conditions. Patients with symptomatic bacteriuria should always be treated. However, the necessity to treat asymptomatic bacteriuric patients varies with age and the presence or absence of underlying urinary tract abnormalities. In the pre-school child it is essential to treat all urinary tract infections and maintain the urine in a sterile state so that normal kidney maturation can proceed. Likewise in pregnancy there is a risk of infection ascending from the bladder to involve the kidney. This is a serious complication and may result in premature labour. Other indications for treating asymptomatic bacteriuria include the presence of underlying renal abnormalities such as stones which may be associated with repeated infections caused by *Proteus* spp.

3.2.2   *Drug therapy*

The antimicrobial treatment of urinary tract infection presents a number of interesting challenges. Drugs must be selected for their ability to achieve high urinary concentrations and, if the kidney is involved, adequate tissue concentrations. Safety in childhood or pregnancy is important since repeated or prolonged medication may be necessary. The choice of agent will be dictated by the microbial aetiology and susceptibility findings, since the latter can vary widely among Gram-negative enteric bacilli, especially in patients who are hospitalized. Table 6.3 shows the distribution of bacteria causing urinary tract infection in the community and in hospitalized patients. The greater tendency towards infections caused by *Klebsiella* spp. and *Ps. aeruginosa* should be noted since antibiotic sensitivity is more variable for these pathogens. Drug resistance has increased substantially in recent years and has reduced the value of formerly widely prescribed agents such as the sulphonamides and ampicillin.

Table 6.3 Urinary tract infection—distribution of pathogenic bacteria in the community and hospitalized patients

Organism	Community (%)	Hospital (%)
Escherichia coli	75	55
Proteus mirabilis	10	13
Kelbsiella or *Enterobacter spp.*	4	18
Enterococci	6	5
Staphylococcus epidermidis	5	4
Pseudomonas aeruginosa	–	5

Uncomplicated community-acquired urinary tract infection presents few problems with management. Drugs such as trimethoprim, co-trimoxazole, ciprofloxacin and ampicillin are widely used. Cure rates are high for ciprofloxacin and the trimethoprim-containing regimens, although drug resistance to ampicillin has increased. Treatment for 3 days is generally satisfactory and is usually accompanied by prompt control of symptoms, Single-dose therapy with amoxycillin 3 g or co-trimoxazole 1920 mg (4 tablets) has also been shown to be effective in selected individuals. Alternative agents include nitrofurantoin and nalidixic acid, although these are not as well tolerated.

It is important to demonstrate the cure of bacteriuria with a repeat urine sample collected 4–6 weeks after treatment, or sooner should symptoms fail to subside. Recurrent urinary tract infection is an indication for further investigation of the urinary tract to detect underlying pathology which may be surgically correctable. Under these circumstances it also is important to maintain the urine in a sterile state. This can be achieved with repeated courses of antibiotics, guided by laboratory sensitivity data. Alternatively, long-term chemoprophylaxis for periods of 6–12 months to control infection by either prevention or suppressions is widely used. Trimethoprim is the most commonly prescribed chemoprophylactic agent and is given as a single nightly dose. This achieves high urinary concentrations throughout the night and generally ensures a sterile urine. Nitrofurantoin is an alternative agent.

Infection of the kidney demands the use of agents which achieve adequate tissue as well as urinary concentrations. Since bacteraemia (a condition in which there are bacteria circulating in the blood) may complicate infection of the kidney, it is generally recommended that antibiotics be administered parenterally. Although ampicillin was formerly widely used, drug resistance is now common and agents such as cefotaxime or ciprofloxacin are often preferred, since the aminoglycosides, although highly effective and preferentially concentrated within the renal cortex, carry the risk of nephrotoxicity.

Infections of the prostate tend to be persistent, recurrent and difficult to treat. This is in part due to the more acid environment of the prostate gland which inhibits drug penetration by many of the antibiotics used to treat urinary tract infection. Agents which are basic in nature, such as erythromycin, achieve therapeutic concentrations within the gland but unfortunately are not active against the pathogens responsible for bacterial prostatitis. Trimethoprim, however, is a useful agent since it is preferentially concentrated within the prostate and active against many of the causative pathogens. It is important that treatment be prolonged for several weeks, since relapse is common.

3.3 Gastrointestinal infections

The gut is vulnerable to infection by viruses, bacteria, parasites and occasionally fungi. Virus infections are the most prevalent but are not susceptible to chemotherapeutic intervention. Bacterial infections are more readily recognized and raise questions concerning the role of antibiotic management. Parasitic infections of the gut are beyond the scope of this chapter.

Bacteria cause disease of the gut as a result of either mucosal invasion or toxin production or a combination of the two mechanisms as summarized in Table 6.4. Treatment is largely directed at replacing and maintaining an adequate intake of fluid and electrolytes. Antibiotics are generally not recommended for infective gastroenteritis,

Table 6.4 Bacterial gut infections—pathogenic mechanisms

Origin	Site of infection	Mechanism
Campylobacter jejuni	Small and large bowel	Invasion
Salmonella spp.	Small and large bowel	Invasion
Shigella spp.	Large bowel	Invasion ± toxin
Escherichia coli		
enteroinvasive	Large bowel	Invasion
enterotoxigenic	Small bowel	Toxin
Clostridium difficile	Large bowel	Toxin
Staphylococcus aureus	Small bowel	Toxin
Vibrio cholerae	Small bowel	Toxin
Clostridium perfringens	Small bowel	Toxin
Yersinia spp.	Small and large bowel	Invasion
Bacillus cereus	Small bowel	Invasion ± toxin
Vibrio parahaemolyticus	Small bowel	Invasion ± toxin

but deserve consideration where they have been demonstrated to abbreviate the acute disease or to prevent complications including prolonged gastrointestinal excretion of the pathogen where this poses a public health hazard.

It should be emphasized that most gut infections are self-limiting. However, attacks can be severe and may result in hospitalization. Antibiotics are used to treat severe *Campylobacter* and *Shigella* infections; erythromycin and co-trimoxazole, respectively, are the preferred agents. Such treatment abbreviates the disease and eliminates gut excretion in *Shigella* infection. However, in severe *Campylobacter* infection the data are currently equivocal, although the clinical impression favours the use of erythromycin for severe infections. The role of antibiotics for *Campylobacter* and *Shigella* infections should be contrasted with gastrointestinal salmonellosis, for which antibiotics are contraindicated since they do not abbreviate symptoms and are associated with more prolonged gut excretion and introduce the risk of adverse drug reactions. However, in severe salmonellosis, especially at extremes of age, systemic toxaemia and bloodstream infection can occur and under these circumstances treatment with either chloramphenicol or co-trimoxazole is appropriate.

Typhoid and paratyphoid fevers (known as enteric fevers), although acquired by ingestion of salmonellae, *Sal. typhi* and *Sal. paratyphi,* respectively, are largely systemic infections and antibiotic therapy is mandatory; ciprofloxacin is now the drug of choice although co-trimoxazole or chloramphenicol are satisfactory alternatives. Prolonged gut excretion of *Sal. typhi* is a well-known complication of typhoid fever and is a major public health hazard in developing countries. Treatment with ciprofloxacin or high-dose ampicillin can eliminate the gall-bladder excretion which is the major site of persistent infection in carriers. However, the presence of gallstones reduces the chance of cure.

Cholera is a serious infection causing epidemics throughout Asia. Although a toxin-mediated disease, largely controlled with replacement of fluid and electrolyte losses, tetracycline has proved effective in eliminating the causative vibrio from the bowel, thereby abbreviating the course of the illness and reducing the total fluid and electrolyte losses.

Traveller's diarrhoea may be caused by one of many gastrointest'
(Table 6.4). However, enterotoxigenic *Escherichia coli* is the most com
Whilst it is generally short-lived, traveller's diarrhoea can seriously m
abroad, be it for holiday or business purposes. Although not univers
use of short-course co-trimoxazole or quinolone such as norfloxacin can about
attack in patients with severe disease.

3.4 Skin and soft tissue infections

Infections of the skin and soft tissue commonly follow traumatic injury to the epithelium but occasionally may be blood-borne. Interruption of the integrity of the skin allows ingress of microorganisms to produce superficial, localized infections which on occasion may become more deep-seated and spread rapidly through tissues. Skin trauma complicates surgical incisions and accidents, including burns. Similarly, prolonged immobilization can result in pressure damage to skin from impaired blood flow. It is most commonly seen in patients who are unconscious.

Microbes responsible for skin infection often arise from the normal skin flora which includes *Staph. aureus*. In addition *Strep. pyogenes, Ps. aeruginosa* and anaerobic bacteria are other recognized pathogens. Viruses also affect the skin and mucosal surfaces, either as a result of generalized infection or localized disease as in the case of herpes simplex. The latter is amenable to antiviral therapy in selected patients, although for the majority of patients, virus infections of the skin are self-limiting.

Streptococcus pyogenes is responsible for a range of skin infections: impetigo is a superficial infection of the epidermis which is common in childhood and is highly contagious; cellulitis is a more deep-seated infection which spreads rapidly through the tissues to involve the lymphatics and occasionally the bloodstream; erysipelas is a rapidly spreading cellulitis commonly involving the face, which characteristically has a raised leading edge due to lymphatic involvement. Necrotizing fasciitis is a more serious, rapidly progressive infection of the skin and subcutaneous structures including the fascia and musculature. Despite early diagnosis and high-dose intravenous antibiotics, this condition is often life-threatening and may require extensive surgical debridement of devitalized tissue and even limb amputation to ensure survival. A fatal outcome is usually the result of profound toxaemia and bloodstream spread. Penicillin is the drug of choice for all these infections although in severe instances parenteral administration is appropriate. The use of topical agents, such as tetracycline, to treat impetigo may fail since drug resistance is now recognized.

Staphylococcus aureus is responsible for a variety of skin infections which require therapeutic approaches different from those of streptococcal infections. Staphylococcal cellulitis is indistinguishable clinically from streptococcal cellulitis and responds to cloxacillin or flucloxacillin, but generally fails to respond to penicillin owing to penicillinase (β-lactamase) production. *Staphylococcus aureus* is an important cause of superficial, localized skin sepsis which varies from small pustules to boils and occasionally to a more deeply invasive, suppurative skin abscess known as a carbuncle. Antibiotics are generally not indicated for these conditions. Pustules and boils settle with antiseptic soaps or creams and often discharge spontaneously, whereas carbuncles frequently require surgical drainage. *Staphylococcus aureus* may also cause postoperative wound infections, sometimes associated with retained suture material, and settles once the stitch is removed. Antibiotics are only appropriate in this situation if there is extensive accompanying soft tissue invasion.

Anaerobic bacteria are characteristically associated with foul-smelling wounds. They are found in association with surgical incisions following intra-abdominal procedures and pressure sores which are usually located over the buttocks and hips where they become infected with faecal flora. These infections are frequently mixed and include Gram-negative enteric bacilli which may mask the presence of underlying anaerobic bacteria. The principles of treating anaerobic soft tissue infection again emphasize the need for removal of all foreign and devitalized material. Antibiotics such as metronidazole or clindamycin should be considered where tissue invasion has occurred.

The treatment of infected burn wounds presents a number of peculiar facets. Burns are initially sterile, especially when they involve all layers of the skin. However, they rapidly become colonized with bacteria whose growth is supported by the protein-rich exudate. Staphylococci, *Strep. pyogenes* and, particularly, *Ps. aeruginosa* frequently colonize burns and may jeopardize survival of skin grafts and occasionally, and more seriously, result in bloodstream invasion. Treatment of invasive *Ps. aeruginosa* infections requires combined therapy with an aminoglycoside, such as gentamicin or tobramycin, and an antipseudomonal agent, such as azlocillin, ticarcillin or ceftazidime. This produces high therapeutic concentrations which generally act in a synergistic manner. The use of aminoglycosides in patients with serious burns requires careful monitoring of serum concentrations to ensure that they are therapeutic yet non-toxic, since renal function is often impaired in the days immediately following a serious burn. Excessive sodium loading may complicate the use of large doses of antipseudomonal penicillins such as carbenicillin and to a lesser extent ticarcillin.

3.5 Central nervous system infections

The brain, its surrounding covering of meninges and the spinal cord are subject to infection, which is generally blood-borne but may also complicate neurosurgery, penetrating injuries or direct spread from infection in the middle ear or nasal sinuses. Viral meningitis is the most common infection but is generally self-limiting. Occasionally destructive forms of encephalitis occur; an example is herpes simplex encephalitis. Bacterial infections include meningitis and brain abscess and carry a high risk of mortality, while, in those who recover, residual neurological damage or impairment of intellectual function may follow. This occurs despite the availability of antibiotics active against the responsible bacterial pathogens. Fungal infections of the brain, although rare, are increasing in frequency, particularly among immunocompromised patients who either have underlying malignant conditions or are on potent cytotoxic drugs.

The treatment of bacterial infections of the central nervous system highlights a number of important therapeutic considerations. Bacterial meningitis is caused by a variety of bacteria although their incidence varies with age. In the neonate, *E. coli* and group B streptococci account for the majority of infections, while in the preschool child *H. influenzae* is the commonest pathogen. *Neisseria meningitidis* has a peak incidence between 5 and 15 years of age, while pneumococcal meningitis is predominantly a disease of adults.

Penicillin is the drug of choice for the treatment of group B streptococcal, meningo-coccal and pneumococcal infections but, as discussed earlier, CSF concentrations of penicillin are significantly influenced by the intensity of the inflammatory response. To achieve therapeutic concentrations within the CSF, high dosages are required, and in the case of pneumococcal meningitis should be continued for 10–14 days.

Resistance of *H. influenzae* to ampicillin has increased in the past decade and varies geographically. Thus, it can no longer be prescribed with confidence as initial therapy, and cetotaxime or ceftriaxone are the preferred alternatives. However, once laboratory evidence for β-lactamase activity is excluded, ampicillin can be safely substituted.

Escherichia coli meningitis carries a mortality of greater than 40% and reflects both the virulence of this organism and the pharmacokinetic problems of achieving adequate CSF antibiotic levels. The broad-spectrum cephalosporins such as cefotaxime, ceftriaxone or ceftazidime have been shown to achieve satisfactory therapeutic levels and are the agents of choice to treat Gram-negative bacillary meningitis. Treatment again must be prolonged for periods ranging from 2 to 4 weeks.

Brain abscess presents a different therapeutic challenge. An abscess is locally destructive to the brain and causes further damage by increasing intracranial pressure. The infecting organisms are varied but those arising from middle ear or nasal sinus infection are often polymicrobial and include anaerobic bacteria, microaerophilic species and Gram-negative enteric bacilli. Less commonly, a pure *Staph. aureus* abscess may complicate blood-borne spread. Brain abscess is a neurosurgical emergency and requires drainage. However, antibiotics are an important adjunct to treatment. The polymicrobial nature of many infections demands prompt and careful laboratory examination to determine optimum therapy. Drugs are selected not only on their ability to penetrate the blood–brain barrier and enter the CSF but also on their ability to penetrate the brain substance. Metronidazole has proved a valuable alternative agent in such infections, although it is not active against microaerophilic streptococci which must be treated with high-dose benzylpenicillin. The two are often used in combination. Chloramphenicol is an alternative agent.

4   Antibiotic policies

4.1   Rationale

The plethora of available antimicrobial agents presents both an increasing problem of selection to the prescriber and difficulties to the diagnostic laboratory as to which agents should be tested for susceptibility. Differences in antimicrobial activity among related compounds are often of minor importance but can occasionally be of greater significance and may be a source of confusion to the non-specialist. This applies particularly to large classes of drugs, such as the penicillins and cephalosporins, where there has been an explosion in the availability of new agents in recent years. Guidance, in the form of an antibiotic policy, has a major role to play in providing the prescriber with a range of agents appropriate to his/her needs and should be supported by laboratory evidence of susceptibility to these agents.

In recent years, increased awareness of the cost of medical care has led to a major review of various aspects of health costs. The pharmacy budget has often attracted attention since, unlike many other hospital expenses, it is readily identifiable in terms of cost and prescriber. Thus, an antibiotic policy is also seen as a means whereby the economic burden of drug prescribing can be reduced or contained. There can be little argument with the recommendation that the cheaper of two compounds should be selected where agents are similar in terms of efficacy and adverse reactions. Likewise, generic substitution is also desirable provided there is bioequivalence. It has become increasingly impractical for pharmacists to stock all the formulations of every antibiotic currently available, and here again an antibiotic policy can produce significant savings by limiting the amount of stock held. A policy based on a restricted number of agents also enables price reduction on purchasing costs through competitive tendering. The above activities have had a major influence on containing or reducing drug costs, although these savings have often been lost as new and often expensive preparations become available, particularly in the field of biological and anticancer therapy.

Another argument in favour of an antibiotic policy is the occurrence of drug-resistant bacteria within an institution. The presence of sick patients and the opportunities for the spread of microorganisms can produce outbreaks of hospital infection. The excessive use of selected agents has been associated with the emergence of drug-resistant bacteria which have often caused serious problems within high-dependency areas, such as intensive care units or burns units where antibiotic use is often high. One oft-quoted example is the occurrence of a multiple-antibiotic resistant *K. aerogenes* within a neurosurgical intensive care unit in which the organism became resistant to all currently available antibiotics and was associated with the widespread use of ampicillin. By prohibiting the use of all antibiotics, and in particular ampicillin, the resistant organism rapidly disappeared and the problem was resolved.

In formulating an antibiotic policy, it is important that the susceptibility of microorganisms be monitored and reviewed at regular intervals. This applies not only to the hospital as a whole, but to specific high-dependency units in particular. Likewise general practitioner samples should also be monitored. This will provide accurate information on drug susceptibility to guide the prescriber as to the most effective agent.

4.2 Types of antibiotic policies

There are a number of different approaches to the organization of an antibiotic policy. These range from a deliberate absence of any restriction on prescribing to a strict policy whereby all anti-infective agents must have expert approval before they are administered. Restrictive policies vary according to whether they are mainly laboratory controlled, by employing restrictive reporting, or whether they are mainly pharmacy controlled, by restrictive dispensing. In many institutions it is common practice to combine the two approaches.

4.2.1 Free prescribing policy

The advocates of a free prescribing policy argue that strict antibiotic policies are both impractical and limit clinical freedom to prescribe. It is also argued that the greater the number of agents in use the less likely it is that drug resistance will emerge to any one agent or class of agents. However, few would support such an approach, which is generally an argument for mayhem.

4.2.2   *Restricted reporting*

Another approach that is widely practised in the UK is that of restricted reporting. The laboratory, largely for practical reasons, tests only a limited range of agents against bacterial isolates. The agents may be selected primarily by microbiological staff or following consultation with their clinical colleagues. The antibiotics tested will vary according to the site of infection, since drugs used to treat urinary tract infections often differ from those used to treat systemic disease.

There are specific problems regarding the testing of certain agents such as the cephalosporins where the many different preparations have varying activity against bacteria. The practice of testing a single agent to represent first generation, second generation or third generation compounds is questionable, and with the new compounds susceptibility should be tested specifically to that agent. By selecting a limited range of compounds for use, sensitivity testing becomes a practical consideration and allows the clinician to use such agents with greater confidence.

4.2.3   *Restricted dispensing*

As mentioned above, the most Draconian of all antibiotic policies is the absolute restriction of drug dispensing pending expert approval. The expert opinion may be provided by either a microbiologist or infectious disease specialist. Such a system can only be effective in large institutions where staff are available 24 hours a day. This approach is often cumbersome, generates hostility and does not necessarily create the best educational forum for learning effective antibiotic prescribing.

A more widely used approach is to divide agents into those approved for unrestricted use and those for restricted use. Agents on the unrestricted list are appropriate for the majority of common clinical situations. The restricted list may include agents where microbiological sensitivity information is essential, such as for vancomycin and certain aminoglycosides. In addition, agents which are used infrequently but for specific indications, such as parenteral amphotericin B, are also restricted in use. Other compounds which may be expensive and used for specific indications, such as broad-spectrum β-lactams in the treatment of *Ps. aeruginosa* infections, may also be justifiably included on the restricted list. Items omitted from the restricted or unrestricted list are generally not stocked, although they can be obtained at short notice as necessary.

Such a policy should have a mechanism whereby desirable new agents are added as they become available and is most appropriately decided at a therapeutics committee. Policing such a policy is best effected as a joint arrangement between senior pharmacists and microbiologists. This combined approach of both restricted reporting and restricted prescribing is extremely effective and provides a powerful educational tool for medical staff and students faced with learning the complexities of modern antibiotic prescribing.

5   Further reading

Finch R.G. (1996) Antibacterial chemotherapy: principles of use. *Medicine*, **24**, 24–26.

Greenwood D. (1995) *Antimicrobial Chemotherapy*, 3rd edn. Oxford: Oxford University Press.

Lambert H.P., O'Grady F., Greenwood D. & Finch R.G. (1996) *Antibiotic and Chemotherapy*, 7th edn. Edinburgh: Churchill Livingstone.

Mandell G.L., Douglas R.G. & Bennett J.E. (eds) (1995) *Principles and Practice of Infectious Diseases*, 4th edn. New York: John Wiley.

7 Manufacture of antibiotics

1   Introduction

2   Choice of examples

3   The production of benzylpenicillin
3.1   The organism
3.2   Inoculum preparation
3.3   The fermenter
3.3.1   Oxygen supply
3.3.2   Temperature control
3.3.3   Defoaming agents and instrumentation
3.3.4   Media additions
3.3.5   Transfer and sampling systems
3.4   Control of the fermentation

3.4.1   Batched medium
3.4.2   Fed nutrients
3.4.3   Stimulation by PAA
3.4.4   Termination
3.5   Extraction
3.5.1   Removal of cells
3.5.2   Isolation of benzylpenicillin
3.5.3   Treatment of crude extract

4   The production of penicillin V

5   The production of cephalosporin C

6   Further reading

1   Introduction

Industrial scale manufacture of the majority of antibiotics is fermentation-based. Strictly speaking, fermentations are biological processes occurring in the absence of air (oxygen). However, the term is now commonly applied to any large-scale cultivation of microorganisms, whether aerobic (with oxygen) or anaerobic (without oxygen).

Despite the ever-increasing use of complex instrumentation, the application of feedback control techniques and the use of computers, the science of antibiotic fermentation is still imperfectly developed. This technology is involved with a living cell population which is changing both quantitatively and qualitively throughout the production cycle: optimization is difficult, because no two ostensibly 'identical' batches are ever wholly alike. Dealing with the challenge of this variation is one of the attractions for those who practise in this field.

2   Choice of examples

The manufacture of benzylpenicillin (penicillin G, originally just 'penicillin') is chosen as a model for the antibiotic production process. It is the most renowned of antibiotics and is the first to have been manufactured in bulk. It is still universally prescribed and is also in demand as input material for semisynthetic antibiotics (Chapter 5). Developments associated with the penicillin fermentation process have been a significant factor in the development of modern biotechnology. It was a further 30 years, i.e. not until the 1970s, before there were significant new advances in industrial fermentations.

No single product can exemplify all the important features of antibiotic manufacture. Benzylpenicillin is a β-lactam. Brief accounts are given of the manufacture of two other β-lactams, penicillin V (phenoxymethylpenicillin) and cephalosporin C, to illustrate further key points.

However, important as the β-lactams are, they are but one of many families of antibiotics (Chapter 5). Furthermore, most industrial microorganisms used to make β-lactams are fungi; this is atypical of antibiotics as a whole where bacteria, particularly *Streptomyces* spp., predominate. Chapter 5 and some of the further reading at the end of this chapter provide the broad perspective, including information on those antibiotics made by total or partial chemical synthesis, against which this present account with its necessarily selective subject matter should be read.

All the examples are of 'batched' fermentations, i.e. of processes where sterile medium in a vessel is inoculated, the broth fermented for a defined period (usually hours or days), the tank emptied and the proceeds extracted ('downstream processing') to yield the antibiotic. During the fermentation, nutrients, antifoam agents and air are supplied, the pH is controlled and exhaust gases removed. After emptying the tank is turned around, that is cleaned and prepared for a new batch. In 'continuous' fermentations, sterile medium is added to the fermentation with a balancing withdrawal of broth for product extraction. This has a number of advantages providing the system can be run clean, i.e. without contamination. One is long fermentation runs of many weeks, hence greater productivity per vessel due to fewer turnrounds. In continuous culture the growth rate can be held at an optimum value for product fermentation. It is therefore suitable for products whose synthesis is proportional to cell density, but is not generally an economical process for antibiotic production where synthesis is not associated with growth and there are additional concerns about strain degeneration.

In this chapter there is little discussion of downstream processing operations after the fermentation stage, i.e. the recovery, purification, quality testing and sterile packaging of the products, even though these usually account for most of the total manufacturing costs. The limited discussion is because, beyond the basic principles, there is no simple model that can be used to illustrate downstream processing, no two processes are alike and different manufacturers are likely to employ different methods for the same product. The quality of the fermented material can markedly affect the efficiency of all the succeeding operations, for at the end of a typical fermentation, the antibiotic concentration will rarely exceed $20\,\mathrm{g}\,\mathrm{l}^{-1}$ and may be as low as $0.5\,\mathrm{g}\,\mathrm{l}^{-1}$.

Details of the manufacture of streptomycin and griseofulvin are to be found in previous editions of this book.

3   The production of benzylpenicillin

3.1   The organism

The original organism for the production of penicillin, *Penicillium notatum*, was isolated by Fleming in 1926 as a chance contaminant. In 1940, Florey and Chain produced purified penicillin and its tremendous curative potential became apparent. However, the liquid surface culture techniques necessary for the cultivation of this obligate aerobe were lengthy, labour-intensive and prone to contamination. The isolation of a higher-yielding organism, *P. chrysogenum*, from an infected Cantaloupe melon obtained in a market in Peoria, Illinois, USA, was the key advance. This organism could be grown in deep fermentations in sealed tanks under stirred and aerated conditions, in vessels as large as $250\,\mathrm{m}^3$.

From this one ancestral fungus each penicillin manufacturer has evolved a particular production strain by a series of mutagenic treatments, each followed by the selection of improved variants. These selected variants have proved capable of producing amounts of penicillin far greater than those produced by the 'wild' strain, especially when fermented on media under particular control conditions developed in parallel with the strains. These strain selection procedures have become a fundamental feature of industrial biotechnology.

Production strains are stored in a dormant form by any of the standard culture preservation techniques. Thus, a spore suspension may be mixed with a sterile, finely divided, inert support and desiccated. Alternatively, spore suspensions in appropriate media can be lyophilized or stored in a liquid culture biostat.

All laboratory operations are carried out in laminar flow cabinets in rooms in which filtered air is maintained at a slight positive pressure relative to their outer environment. Operators wear sterilized clothing and work aseptically. Antibiotic fermentations are, of strict necessity, pure culture aseptic processes, without contaminating organisms.

3.2   Inoculum preparation

The aim is to develop for the production stage fermenter a pure inoculum in sufficient volume and in the fast-growing (logarithmic) phase so that a high population density is soon obtained. Figure 7.1 shows a typical route by which the inoculum is produced. The time taken for each seed stage is measured in days and decreases as the sequence progresses. The final inoculum to the production stage is generally 1–10% of the total volume of the fementer. If the fermenter is under-inoculated there may be an extended lag before growth starts and the fermentation period will be prolonged. This is both uneconomic and may result in degenerative growth which affects performance, quality and hence also cost.

The inoculum stage media are designed to provide the organism with all the nutrients that it requires. Adequate oxygen is provided in the form of sterile air and the temperature is controlled at the desired level. Principal criteria for transfer to the next stage in the progression are freedom from contamination and growth to a pre-determined cell density.

Typical of fungi, the organism grows as branching filaments (hyphae) and by the time that the culture has progressed to the production stage it has a soup-like consistency.

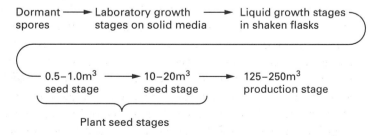

Fig. 7.1 Stages in the preparation of inoculum for the benzylpenicillin fermentation.

3.3   The fermenter

A typical fermenter is a closed, vertical, cylindrical, stainless steel vessel with convexly dished ends and of 25–250 m³ capacity. Its height is usually two to three times its diameter. Figure 7.2 shows such a vessel diagramatically, and Fig. 7.3 gives a view inside an actual vessel.

3.3.1   *Oxygen supply*

The penicillin fermentation needs oxygen, which is supplied as filter-sterilized air from a compressor. Oxygen is critical to aerobic processes and its supply is a crucial aspect of fementer design and batch control. As oxygen is poorly soluble in water, steps are taken to assist its passage into the liquid phase and from aqueous solution into the microorganism. In a conventional fermentation, air is introduced into the bottom of the vessel via a ring 'sparger' with multiple small holes rather than through a single large orifice. This breaks the air flow into smaller bubbles which have a greater surface area to volume ratio and hence greater oxygen transfer. These bubbles lose oxygen as they rise up the tank and, at the same time, carbon dioxide diffuses into them. The vessel is kept under a positive head pressure which promotes the dissolution of oxygen and in

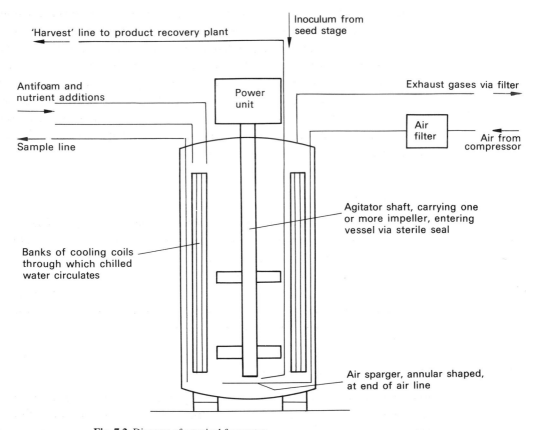

Fig. 7.2 Diagram of a typical fermenter.

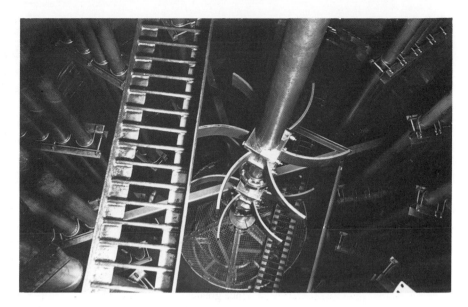

Fig. 7.3 View looking down into a 125 m³ stainless steel fermenter. (Courtesy of Glaxo Wellcome Operations.)

addition reduces the chances of contamination. The transfer of oxygen is further assisted by impellers mounted on a rotating vertical shaft driven by a powerful electric motor.

Baffles are also included to achieve the correct blend of shear and of bulk circulation from the power supplied, and generally to promote intimate contact of cells and nutrients. Aeration is a major expense as very large amounts of energy are consumed. The design, size and number of impellers relative to the fermenter design and type of microorganism form a science in their own right. There has been considerable research into novel, energetically more efficient methods of aeration, and the next generation of fermenters may include some that are radically different in design.

3.3.2 Temperature control

The production of benzylpenicillin is very sensitive to temperature. A lot of metabolic heat is generated and the fermentation temperature has to be reduced by controlled cooling. This heat transfer is achieved by circulating chilled water through banks of pipes inside the vessel (which also serve as baffles) or through external 'limpet' coils on the jacket of the vessel. These coils consist of continuous lengths of pipe welded in a shallow spiral round the vessel. This cooling water system is also used to cool batched medium sterilized in the vessel prior to its inoculation.

3.3.3 Defoaming agents and instrumentation

Microbial cultures may foam when they are subjected to vigorous mechanical stirring and aeration. If this foaming is not controlled, culture is lost by entrainment in the exhaust gases and so there are systems, often automatic, for detecting incipient foaming, for temporarily applying backpressure to contain the culture within the vessel and for the aseptic addition of defoaming agents.

Instrumentation is also fitted to provide a continuous display of important variables such as temperature and pH, the power used by the electric motor, airflow, dissolved oxygen and exhaust gas analysis. Manual or computer feedback control can be based either directly on the signals provided by the probes and sensors or on derived data calculated from those signals, such as the respiratory coefficient or the rate of change of pH. Mass spectronomical analysis of exhaust gases can provide valuable physiological information.

3.3.4 Media additions

Not all the nutrients required during fermentation are initially provided in the culture medium. Some are sterilized separately by batch or continuous sterilization and then added whilst the fermentation is in progress, usually via automatic systems that allow a preset programme of continuous or discrete aseptic additions.

3.3.5 Transfer and sampling systems

Aseptic systems are provided to transfer the inoculum to the vessel, to allow the taking of routine samples during fermentation, for early harvesting of aliquots when the vessel becomes full as a consequence of the media additions and to transfer the final contents to the extraction plant when fermentation is complete. Asepsis is assured by engineering design and by steam, which must reach all parts of the vessels and associated pipework. Any pockets of air or rough surfaces that steam does not penetrate could act as reservoirs for contaminating microorganisms.

Sampling is essential to monitor the amount of growth, the running levels of key nutrients and the penicillin concentration. It is necessary also to check that there has been no contamination by unwanted microorganisms.

3.4 Control of the fermentation

Should oxygen availability fall below a critical level, benzylpenicillin biosynthesis is greatly reduced although culture growth continues. Thus, if growth in the fermenter proceeds unchecked at the rate prevailing in the seed stages, the culture would become very dense and the available aeration would no longer be sufficient to maintain penicillin production. Accordingly, conditions are so adjusted that fast growth is achieved only until the cell population has reached the maximum density that the vessel can support. Further net growth is constrained by deliberately limiting the supply of a key nutrient (in practice, a sugar). The cells can then be stimulated to an 'overproduction' of benzylpenicillin while restricting the amount of growth and a stable, highly productive cell population can be sustained.

3.4.1 Batched medium

The medium initially placed in the fermenter is a complete one but designed only to support the desired amount of early growth. The principal nitrogen source is corn steep liquor (CSL), a by-product of the maize starch-producing industry. This material was originally found to be specifically useful for the penicillin fermentation, but it is recognized as valuable in many fungal antibiotic media. Apart from its primary purpose in supplying cheap and readily available nitrogen, CSL also contains a useful range of carbon compounds, such as acids and sugars, inorganic ions and growth factors—in short, it is virtually a complete growth medium in itself. However, like some of the fed nutrients, CSL is a complex nutrient, not chemically defined, derived from natural products and with significant batch-to-batch variation. It is therefore a source of variation and one of the reasons why no two fermentations are ever absolutely identical.

The medium contains subsidiary nitrogen sources and additional essential nutrients such as calcium (added in the form of chalk to counter the natural acidity of the CSL), magnesium, sulphate, phosphate, potassium and trace metals. The medium is sterilized with steam at 120°C either in the fermenter itself or in ancilliary plant, which may be worked continuously.

3.4.2   *Fed nutrients*

The sterile medium is stirred and aerated and its pH and temperature are set to the correct values on the process control monitors. It is then inoculated and the growth phase begins. The initial carbon source is sufficient in quantity to maintain early growth but not sufficient to provide the energy that penicillin production and maintenance of the cell population need during the rest of the fermentation. Carbon for these subsequent stages is 'fed' continuously in such a way as to limit net growth. Either sucrose or glucose is used, possibly as cheaper, impure forms, such as molasses or starch hydrolysate. As the concentration of residual sugar in the broth is too low to measure, the rate of feeding has to be learnt by experience and modified on the basis of systematic observation. An alternative way of attaining carbon limitation without the complication of a carefully monitored carbon feed rate is to supply all the carbohydrate at the outset as lactose. The rate-limiting hydrolysis of lactose to hexose is then relied upon to give a steady, slow feed of assimilable carbohydrate. Originally, all benzylpenicillin was manufactured using lactose in this way and some manufacturers still prefer this technique.

Calcium, magnesium, phosphate and trace metals added initially are usually sufficient to last throughout the fermentation, but the microorganisms need further supplies of nitrogen and sulphur to balance the carbon feed. Nitrogen is often supplied as ammonia gas. The word 'balance' is used quite deliberately; the whole system is a balanced one. Thus, the carbon and nitrogen feeds not only satisfy the organisms' requirements for these elements in the correct molar ratio, they also maintain an adequate reserve of ammonium ion and contribute to pH control, the carbon metabolism being acidogenic and balanced by the alkalinity of the ammonia. Sulphate is usually supplied in common with the sugar feed and, by obtaining the correct ratio, there is a balanced presentation of sulphate with an adequate pool of intermediates.

All feeds are sterilized before they are metered into the fermenter. Contaminants resistant to the antibiotic rarely find their way into the fermenter, but when they do, their effects are so damaging that prevention is of paramount importance. A resistant, β-lactamase-producing, fast-growing bacterial contaminant can destroy the penicillin already made, as well as consuming nutrients intended for the fungus, causing loss of pH control and interfering with the subsequent extraction process.

The growth phase passes rapidly into the antibiotic-production phase. The optimum pH and temperature for growth are not those for penicillin production and there may be changes in the control of these parameters. The only other event that marks the onset of the production phase is the addition of phenylacetic acid (PAA) by continuous feed.

<table>
<tr><td>3.4.3</td><td>Stimulation by PAA</td></tr>
</table>

Phenylacetic acid (PAA) supplies the side-chain of benzylpenicillin (see also Chapter 5); without PAA, the organisms synthesize only small quantities of this penicillin. Indeed, it was the chance presence of phenylacetyl compounds in CSL (formed from phenylalanine in the grain by the natural bacterial flora during processing) that caused it to be established in early experiments as the best of the cheap complex nitrogen sources and led to the use of PAA. Not only does PAA stimulate benzylpenicillin biosynthesis but it also suppresses the formation of other (unwanted) penicillins. High levels of PAA are, however, toxic to the organism and so it cannot be added indiscriminately. PAA is expensive. The feed provides an adequate standing level of PAA without approaching the toxic limit; the feed is reduced just before the end of the process so that the amount of unused (irrecoverable) precursor in the final culture is not excessive.

The building blocks for the biosynthesis of benzylpenicillin are three amino acids, α-aminoadipic acid, cysteine and valine, and PAA. The amino acids condense to a tripeptide, ring closure of which gives the penicillin ring structure with an α-aminoadipyl side-chain, isopenicillin N. The side-chain is then displayed by a phenylacetyl group from PAA to give benzylpenicillin.

α-Aminoadipic acid + Cysteine + Valine

↓

Tripeptide

↓

Isopenicillin N

PAA →   ↓   → α-Aminoadipic acid

Benzylpenicillin

There comes a time when sequential improvements in penicillin productivity obtained by standard strain improvement techniques (physical and chemical mutagenesis in conjunction with a variety of selection techniques that apply pressure for high-yielding variants) become subject to rate-limiting returns. At first, it is easy to double the 'titre' with each campaign; later in the genealogy even a 5% improvement would be regarded as excellent.

Recent developments by academic and industrial geneticists may well prove to have transformed this situation. Tremendous progress has been made since the mid-1980s both in the isolation and manipulation of the biosynthetic genes in this pathway and in the related routes to the cephalosporins (via the cephalosporin C-producing fungus *Acremonium chrysogenum*) and the cephamycins (via the cephamycin C-producing bacterium *Streptomyces clavuligerus*). Antibiotic manufacturers can now apply recombinant DNA technology to the industrial strains of filamentous micro-organisms used to produce β-lactams and there are exciting prospects of making genetic changes that will very significantly increase productivity. These are discussed further, later in this chapter. There is plenty of scope for improvement, because the best current industrial strains and processes convert little more than 10% of all elemental carbon into penicillin.

3.4.4   Termination

When to stop a fermentation is a very complex decision and several factors have to be taken into account. Quite often a manufacturer will find it appropriate to harvest shortly after the first signs of a faltering in the efficiency of conversion of the most costly raw material (the carbon source, e.g. glucose) into penicillin.

3.5   Extraction

3.5.1   Removal of cells

At harvest, the benzylpenicillin is in solution extracellularly, together with a range of other metabolites and medium constituents. The first step in downstream processing is to remove the cells by filtration or centrifugation. This stage is carried out under conditions that avoid contamination with β-lactamase-producing microorganisms which could lead to serious or total loss of product.

3.5.2   Isolation of benzylpenicillin

The next stage is to isolate the benzylpenicillin. Solvent extraction is the generally accepted process although other methods are available including ion-exchange chromatography and precipitation. In aqueous solution at pH 2–2.5 there is a high partition coefficient in favour of certain organic solvents such as amyl acetate, butyl acetate and methyl isobutyl ketone. The extraction has to be carried out quickly, as benzylpenicillin is very unstable at these low pH values. The penicillin is then extracted back into an aqueous buffer at pH 7.5, the partition coefficient now being strongly in favour of the aqueous phase. The solvent is recovered by distillation for re-use.

3.5.3   Treatment of crude extract

Benzylpenicillin is produced as various salts according to its intended use, whether as an input to semisynthetic β-lactam antibiotics manufacture or for clinical use in its own right.

The treatment of the crude penicillin extract varies according to the objective but involves formation of an appropriate salt, probably followed by treatment to remove pyrogens, and by sterilization. This last is usually achieved by filtration but pure metal salts of benzylpenicillin can be safely sterilized by dry heat if desired.

For parenteral use, the antibiotic is packed in sterile vials as a powder (reconstituted before use) or suspension. For oral use it is prepared in any of the standard presentations, such as film-coated tablets. Searching tests are carried out on an appreciable number of random samples of the finished product to ensure that it satisfies the stringent quality control requirements for potency, purity, freedom from pyrogens and sterility.

All stages of antibiotic manufacture from fermentation through to finished product are governed by the code of good manufacturing practice (GMP), of which quality control is one aspect. GMP requires that 'there should be a comprehensive system, so designed, documented, implemented and controlled, and so furnished with personnel, equipment and other resources as to provide assurance that products will consistently be of a quality appropriate to their intended use'.

4   The production of penicillin V

By the addition of different acyl donors to the medium, different penicillins can be biologically synthesized. For example, penicillin V is made by a similar process to benzylpenicillin, but with phenoxyacetic acid as the precursor instead of PAA. In the biosynthetic pathway, the α-aminoadipyl side-chain of isopenicillin N is replaced by a phenoxyacetyl group.

The microorganism is again *P. chrysogenum*. A manufacturer may use the same mutant strain to make both products or may have different mutants for the two penicillins. Parallel situations of a single organism producing more than one natural product occur with other types of antibiotics, for example strains of *Streptomyces aureofaciens* are used for both chlortetracycline and demethylchlortetracycline fermentations.

Like benzylpenicillin, penicillin V is still widely used in its own right but can also be used as a starting material for the manufacture of the semisynthetic penicillins, none of which can be made by direct fermentation.

5   The production of cephalosporin C

It is possible to convert penicillin V or benzylpenicillin to a cephalosporin by chemical ring expansion. The first-generation cephalosporin cephalexin, for example, can be made in this way. Most cephalosporins used in clinical practice, however, are semisynthetics produced from the fermentation product cephalosporin C.

The ancestral strain of *Acremonium chrysogenum* (at that time called *Cephalosporium acremonium*) was isolated on the Sardinian coast in 1945 following an observation that the local sewage outlet into the sea cleared at a quite remarkable rate. Advances were slow because the activity was associated with a number of different types of compound. Cephalosporin C was first isolated in 1952, but it was a further decade before clinically useful semisynthetic cephalosporins became available.

The biosynthetic route to cephalosporin C is identical to that of the penicillins as far as isopenicillin N (section 3.4.3). The further route to cephalosporin C is shown on p. 160. Note the branch into a third series of β-lactam drugs, the cephamycins (see Chapter 5).

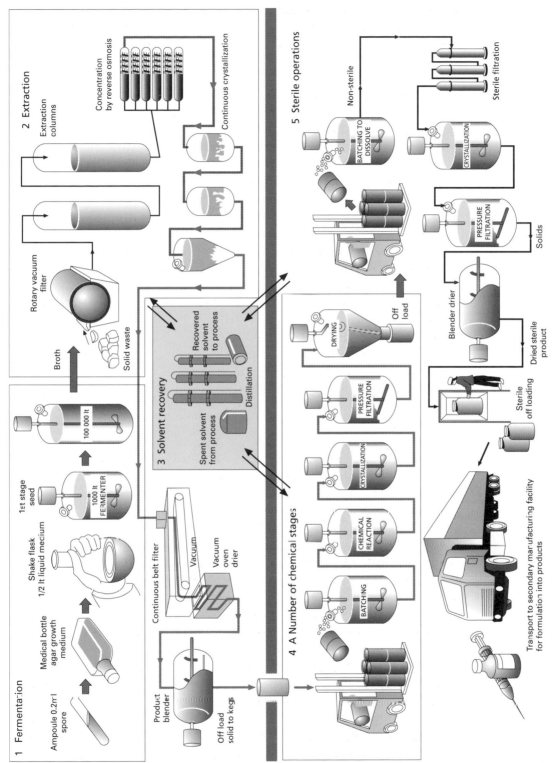

1 Fermentation

Ampoule 0.2ml spore

Medical bottle agar growth medium

Shake flask 1/2 lt liquid medium

1st stage seed

1000 lt FERMENTER

100 000 lt

2 Extraction

Extraction columns

Concentration by reverse osmosis

Continuous crystallization

Rotary vacuum filter

Broth

Solid waste

3 Solvent recovery

Recovered solvent to process

Spent solvent from process

Distillation

Continuous belt filter

Vacuum

Vacuum oven drier

Product blender

Off load solid to kegs

4 A Number of chemical stages

BATCHING

CHEMICAL REACTION

CRYSTALLIZATION

PRESSURE FILTRATION

DRYING

Off load

5 Sterile operations

Non-sterile

Sterile filtration

BATCHING TO DISSOLVE

CRYSTALLIZATION

PRESSURE FILTRATION

Solids

Blender drier

Dried sterile product

Sterile off loading

Transport to secondary manufacturing facility for formulation into products

Fig. 7.4 Typical production route for cephalosporins.

Isopenicillin N

↓

Penicillin N

↓

Desacetoxycephalosporin C

↓

Desacetylcephalosporin C → Cephamycin C (in certain *Streptomyces*)

↓

Cephalosporin C

The similarities in the routes to the three classes of antibiotics have facilitated progress in the understanding of the underlying molecular genetics. Most of the genes coding for the relevant enzymes have been isolated. Modern DNA techniques are being targetted at rate-limiting biosynthetic steps. Amplification of gene copy numbers, improving gene expression efficiencies, transferring genes to bacterial host organisms and manipulation of pathways of antibiotic synthesis all have potential in strain development. However, in the production of antibiotics, economic benefits from the application of recombinant DNA technology have thus far been limited.

Manufacturing processes for cephalosporin C and benzylpenicillin are broadly similar. In common with many other antibiotic fermentations, no specific precursor feed is necessary for cephalosporin C. There is sufficient acetyl group substrate for the terminal acetyltransferase reaction available from the organism's metabolic pool.

The product is extracted from the culture fluid by adsorption onto carbon or resins rather than by solvent. This illustrates an important general point that antibiotic manufacturing processes differ from one another much more in their product recovery stages than in their fermentation stages. Figure 7.4 illustrates a typical production route from inoculum to bulk antibiotic.

6   Further reading

Bu'Lock J.D., Nisbet L.J. & Winstanley D.J. (eds) (1983) *Bioactive Microbial Products,* vol. II, *Development and Production*. London: Academic Press.

Calam C.T. (1987) *Process Development in Antibiotic Fermentations*, Cambridge Studies in Biotechnology, 4 (eds Sir James Baddiley, N.H. Carey, J.F. Davidson, I.J. Higgins & W.G. Potter). Cambridge: Cambridge University Press.

Hugo W.B. & Mol H. (1972) Antibiotics and chemotherapeutic agents. In *Materials and Technology* (eds L.W. Codd, K. Dijkoff, J.H. Fearon, C.J. van Oss, H.G. Roeberson & E.G. Stanford). London: Longman & de Bussy.

Peberdy J.F. (ed.) (1987) *Penicillin and Acremonium*, Biotechnology Handbooks, 1 (Series eds T. Atkinson & R.F. Sherwood). New York: Plenum Press. (See, in particular, Chapters 2 and 5.)

Office for Official Publications of the European Community (1992) *The Rules Governing Medicinal Products in the European Community,* vol. IV, *Guide to Good Manufacturing Practice for the Manufacture of Medicinal Products*.

Queener S.W. (1990) Molecular biology of penicillin and cephalosporin biosynthesis. *Antimicrob Agents Chemother*, **34**, 943–948.

Rohm H.-J., Reed G., Pühler A. & Stadler P. (eds) (1993) *Biotechnology*, vol. III, Bioprocessing. New York: VCH.

Smith J.E. (1985) *Biotechnology Principles*. Aspects of Microbiology Series No. 11. Wokinham: Van Nostrand Reinhold.

Stowell J.D., Bailey P.J. & Winstanley D.J. (eds) (1986) *Bioactive Microbial Products*, vol. III, *Downstream Processing*. London: Academic Press.

Van Damme E.J. (1984) *Biotechnology of Industrial Antibiotics*. New York: Marcel Dekker.

Verrall M.S. (Ed) (1985) *Discovery and Isolation of Microbial Products*. Society of Chemical Industry Series in Biological Chemistry and Biotechnology. Chichester: Ellis Horwood.

A good source of articles on individual antibiotics, groups of antibiotics, fermentation plant and related topics is the series *Progress in Industrial Microbiology* edited originally by D.J.D. Hockenhull and published by Heywood Books, London. These articles normally carry extensive references to the original literature.

8 Mechanisms of action of antibiotics

1   Introduction

2   The bacterial cell wall
2.1   Peptidoglycan biosynthesis and its
      inhibition
2.1.1 D-Cycloserine
2.1.2 Glycopeptides—vancomycin and
       teicoplanin
2.1.3 β-Lactam antibiotics—penicillins,
       cephalosporins, carbapenems and
       monobactams
2.2   Mycolic acid and arabinogalactan
      synthesis in mycobacteria
2.2.1 Isoniazid
2.2.2 Ethambutol

3   Protein synthesis
3.1   Protein synthesis and selective
      inhibition
3.2   Aminoglycoside–aminocyclitol
      antibiotics
3.3   Tetracyclines
3.4   Chloramphenicol
3.5   Macrolides and azalides
3.6   Lincomycin and clindamycin
3.7   Fusidic acid
3.8   Mupirocin

4   Chromosome function and replication

4.1   The basis for selective inhibition
      of chromosome replication and
      function
4.1.1 Synthesis of precursors
4.1.2 Unwinding of the chromosome
4.1.3 Replication of DNA strands
4.1.4 Transcription
4.2   Quinolones
4.3   Nitroimidazoles (metronidazole) and
      nitrofurans (nitrofurantoin)
4.4   Rifampicin
4.5   5-Fluorocytosine

5   Folate antagonists
5.1   Folate metabolism in microbial and
      mammalian cells
5.2   Sulphonamides
5.3   DHFR inhibitors

6   The cytoplasmic membrane
6.1   Composition and susceptibility
      of membranes to selective
      disruption
6.2   Polymyxins
6.3   Polyenes
6.4   Imidazoles and triazoles
6.5   Naftidine

7   Further reading

1 Introduction

The antibiotics described in Chapter 5 are used to treat microbial infections caused by bacteria, fungi or protozoa. Most exert a highly selective toxic action upon their target microbial cells but have little or no toxicity towards mammalian cells. They can therefore be administered at concentrations sufficient to kill infecting organisms (or at least inhibit their growth) without damaging mammalian cells. By comparison, the disinfectants, antiseptics and preservatives described in Chapter 10 are too toxic for systemic treatment of infections. Study of the mechanism of action of the antibiotics reveals the basis of their selective toxicity. Table 8.1 lists the five broad target areas of action (cell wall, ribosome, chromosome, folate metabolism, cell membrane) with the major antibiotics which act upon them and a summary of the basis of selective action. Note that the majority of the antibiotics are used for treatment of bacterial infections; comparatively few agents are available for fungal or protozoal infections.

Table 8.1 Target sites for antimicrobial action

Target	Antibiotics†	Mechanism of action	Basis of selective toxicity
Bacterial cell wall	β-Lactams	Inhibit peptidoglycan synthesis	None in mammalian cells
	Glycopeptides	Inhibit peptidoglycan synthesis	None in mammalian cells
	Cycloserine	Inhibits peptidoglycan synthesis	None in mammalian cells
	Isoniazid*	Inhibits mycolic acid synthesis	None in mammalian cells
	Ethambutol*	Inhibits arabinogalactan synthesis	None in mammalian cells
Bacterial ribosome function	Aminoglycosides	Distort 30S ribosomal subunit	No action on 40S subunit
	Tetracyclines	Block 30S ribosomal subunit	Excluded by mammalian cells
	Chloramphenicol	Inhibits peptidyl transferase	No action on mammalian equivalent
	Macrolides, azalides	Block translocation	No action on mammalian equivalent
	Fusidic acid	Inhibits elongation factor	Excluded by mammalian cells
	Mupirocin	Inhibits isoleucyl-tRNA synthesis	No action on mammalian equivalent
Chromosome function	Quinolones	Inhibit DNA gyrase	No action on mammalian equivalent
	Metronidazole (also**)	DNA strand breakage	Requires anaerobic conditions not present in mammalian cells
	Nitrofurantoin	DNA strand breakage	No action on mammalian equivalent
	Rifampicin (also*)	Inhibits RNA polymerase	No action on mammalian equivalent
	5-Fluorocytosine***	Inhibits DNA synthesis	Converted to active form in fungi
Folate metabolism	Sulphonamides (also**)	Inhibit folate synthesis	Not present in mammalian cells
	Trimethoprim	Inhibits dihydrofolate reductase	Mammalian enzyme not inhibited
	Pyrimethamine**	Inhibits dihydrofolate reductase	Mammalian enzyme not inhibited
	Trimetrexate**/***	Inhibits dihydrofolate reductase	Toxicity overcome with leucovorin
Cytoplasmic membrane	Polymyxins	Disrupt bacterial membranes	Bind to LPS and phospholipids
	Polyenes***	Disrupt fungal membranes	Bind preferentially to ergosterol
	Imidazoles and triazoles***	Inhibit ergosterol synthesis	Pathway not in mammalian cells
	Naftidine***	Inhibits ergosterol synthesis	Pathway not in mammalian cells

† All antibacterial except: *antimycobacterial agent; **antiprotozoal agent; ***antifungal agent.
LPS, lipopolysaccharide.

The bacterial cell wall

2.1

Peptidoglycan biosynthesis and its inhibition

Peptidoglycan is a vital component of virtually all bacterial cell walls. It accounts for approximately 50% of the weight of Gram-positive bacterial walls, around 30% of mycobacterial cell walls and between 10 and 20% of the Gram-negative envelope. It is a macromolecule composed of sugar (glycan) chains which are crosslinked by short peptide bridges (Fig. 8.1).

One characteristic feature of peptidoglycan is the occurrence of D-amino acids, particularly D-alanine and D-glutamic acid. These D-stereoisomers of amino acids are not found in proteins. The precise nature of the peptide crosslinks varies among organisms but the essential structure is the same. The peptidoglycan polymer is responsible for both the shape of bacterial cells and their mechanical strength and integrity. If the synthesis of peptidoglycan is blocked selectively by antibiotic action

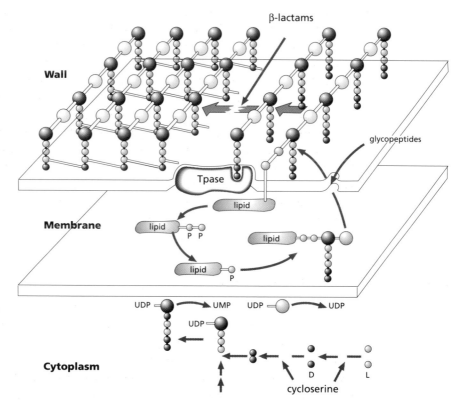

Fig. 8.1 Biosynthesis of peptidoglycan. The large circles represent *N*-acetylglucosamine or *N*-acetylmuramic acid; to the latter is linked initially a pentapeptide chain comprising L-alanine, D-glutamic acid and meso-diaminopimelic acid (small circles) terminating in two D-alanine residues (small, darker circles). The lipid molecule is undecaprenyl phosphate. In the initial (cytoplasm) stage where inhibition by the antibiotic D-cycloserine is shown, two molecules of L-alanine (small circles) are converted by an isomerase to the D-forms (small, darker circles), after which a ligase joins the two D-alanines together to produce a D-alanyl-D-alanine dipeptide.

the bacteria undergo a number of changes in shape and ultimately die following disruption (lysis) of the cells. Mammalian cells do not possess a cell wall and contain no other macromolecular structures resembling peptidoglycan. Consequently, antibiotics which interfere with peptidoglycan synthesis generally have excellent selective toxicity since the target is vital to the bacteria but absent from mammalian cells.

2.1.1   D-Cycloserine

There are three stages of peptidoglycan biosynthesis (Fig. 8.1). The first occurs in the cytoplasm where the precursors are synthesized. The formation and assembly of a D-alanyl-D-alanine dipeptide is the site of action of D-cycloserine. Two molecules of L-alanine are converted to the D-forms by an isomerase in the bacterial cytoplasm. A ligase then joins the two D-alanines together. Both of these enzymes are inhibited by binding cycloserine, which bears some structural similarities to D-alanine. Cycloserine binds covalently to the pyridoxal phosphate cofactor of the enzymes, effectively preventing them from forming D-alanyl-D-alanine. The D-alanyl-D-alanine dipeptide is then coupled to three other amino acids (in *Escherichia coli* these are L-alanine, D-glutamic acid and meso-diaminopimelic acid) which have been added sequentially to the sugar nucleotide, uridine diphosphate (UDP)-*N*-acetylmuramic acid. The sugar pentapeptide produced (*N*-acetylmuramylpentapeptide) is then transferred from the nucleotide to a hydrophobic lipid carrier molecule (undecaprenyl phosphate) which is located exclusively in the cytoplasmic membrane. The nucleotide uridine monophosphate (UMP) remains in the cytoplasm. Another sugar nucleotide precursor, UDP-*N*-acetylglucosamine is also produced in the cytoplasm and donates a molecule of *N*-acetylglucosamine to be coupled to the lipid carrier in the membrane forming a lipid pyrophosphate-linked disaccharide pentapeptide. This is the second stage of the biosynthetic pathway in which the disaccharide pentapeptide is transported across the membrane on the lipid carrier to be inserted into the cell wall at a growing point. The lipid carrier does not leave the cell membrane and is eventually recycled. It loses a single phosphate group whilst returning to the cytoplasmic face of the membrane to collect another disaccharide pentapeptide from the cytoplasm.

2.1.2   Glycopeptides—vancomycin and teicoplanin

It is in the third and final stage of the pathway that the glycopeptide antibiotics act. Here the disaccharide pentapeptide is first incorporated into the expanding cell wall linked to its lipid carrier. The growing glycan-peptide chain is transferred in turn to each molecule of lipid carrier as it brings its disaccharide pentapeptide precursor across the membrane. Each lipid carrier molecule thus acts in turn to hold the growing linear glycan strand before returning through the membrane to the cytoplasmic face. Incorporation of each disaccharide pentapeptide is catalysed by a transglycosylase and this step is effectively blocked by the glycopeptides. These antibiotics bind very tightly by hydrogen bonding to the terminal D-alanyl-D-alanine on each pentapeptide inhibiting extension of the linear glycan peptide in the cell wall. Vancomycin is thought to bind to the pentapeptides outside the cytoplasmic membrane. Possibly two vancomycin molecules form a back-to-back dimer which bridges between pentapeptides preventing further peptidoglycan assembly. Teicoplanin is a lipoglycopeptide which may act slightly differently by locating itself in the outer face of the cytoplasmic membrane and binding the pentapeptide as the precursors are transferred through the membrane.

β-Lactam antibiotics—penicillins, cephalosporins, carbapenems and monobactams

The β-lactam antibiotics block the final crosslinking stage of the pathway which occurs in the cell wall. Here the linear glycan strands are crosslinked via their peptide chains to the mature peptidoglycan in the cell wall. The crosslinking is catalysed by a group of enzymes called transpeptidases. These enzymes are located on the outer face of the cytoplasmic membrane. They first remove the terminal D-alanine residue from each pentapeptide on the linear glycan. This reaction involves breakage of the peptide between the two D-alanine residues on the linear glycan. The energy released is thought to be used in the formation of a new peptide bond between the remaining D-alanine on the glycan chain and an acceptor amino group on existing crosslinked peptidoglycan. In *Escherichia coli* this acceptor is the free amino group on *meso*-diaminopimelic acid (the third amino acid on each *N*-acetylmuramic acid). In other organisms, for example *Staphylococcus aureus*, it is the free amino group on lysine (replacing diaminopimelic acid) which acts as the acceptor. It should be noted that although there is considerable variation in the composition of the peptide crosslink among different species of bacteria, the essential transpeptidase mechanism is the same. Therefore virtually all bacteria can be inhibited by interference with this group of enzymes. The β-lactam antibiotics effectively inhibit the transpeptidases by acting as alternative substrates. They mimic the D-alanyl-D-alanine residues and react with the transpeptidases (Fig. 8.2).

The β-lactam bond is broken (instead of the equivalent peptide bond joining the alanine residues) but the remaining ring system in the β-lactam (a thiazolidine in penicillins) is not released (Fig. 8.3). Instead, the transpeptidase remains linked to the hydrolysed antibiotic with a half life of 10–15 minutes. Whilst bound to the β-lactam, the transpeptidase cannot participate in further rounds of peptidoglycan

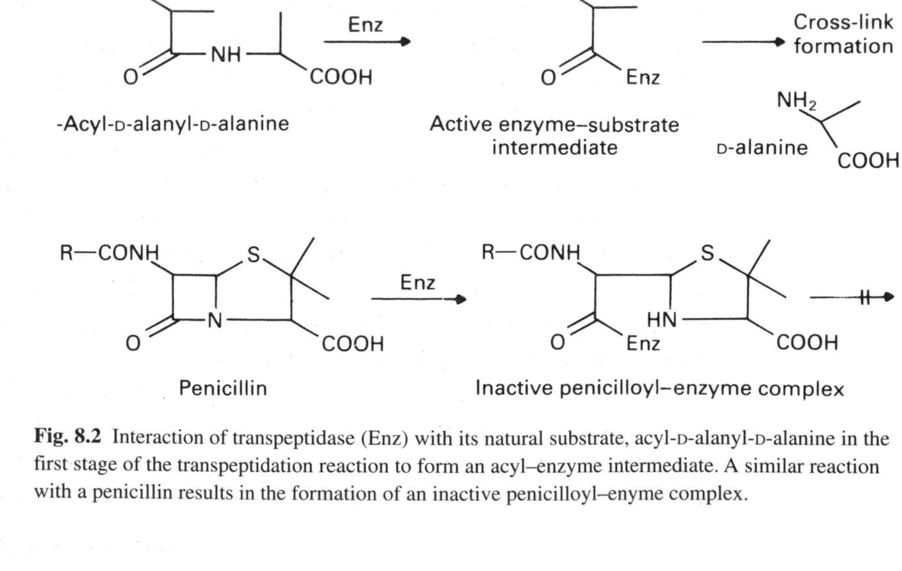

Fig. 8.2 Interaction of transpeptidase (Enz) with its natural substrate, acyl-D-alanyl-D-alanine in the first stage of the transpeptidation reaction to form an acyl–enzyme intermediate. A similar reaction with a penicillin results in the formation of an inactive penicilloyl–enyme complex.

A   B

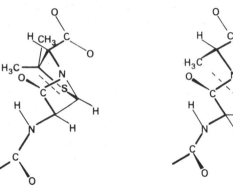

Fig. 8.3 A, comparison of the structure of the nucleus of the penicillin molecule with B, the D-alanyl-D-alanine end group of the precursor of bacterial peptidoglycan. The broken lines show the correspondence in position between the labile bond of penicillin and the bond broken during the transpeptidation reaction associated with the crosslinking in peptidoglycan.

crosslinking by reaction with its true substrate. All β-lactam antibiotics (penicillins, cephalosporins, carbapenems and monobactams) are thought to act in a similar way through interaction of their β-lactam ring with transpeptidases. However, there is considerable variation in the morphological effects of different β-lactams upon bacterial cells which is due to the existence of several types of transpeptidases. The transpeptidase enzymes are usually referred to as penicillin-binding proteins (PBPs) because they can be separated and studied after reaction with ^{14}C-labelled penicillin. This step is necessary because there are very few copies of each enzyme present in a cell. They are usually separated according to their size by electrophoresis and are numbered PBP1, PBP2, etc. starting from the highest molecular weight species. In Gram-negative bacteria the high molecular weight transpeptidases appear also to possess transglycosylase activity, i.e. they have a dual function in the final stages of peptidoglycan synthesis. Furthermore, the different transpeptidases have specialized functions in the cell; all crosslink peptidoglycan but some are involved with maintenance of cell integrity, some regulate cell shape and others produce new cross wall between elongating cells securing chromosome segregation prior to cell division.

Recognition of the existence of multiple transpeptidase targets and their relative sensitivity towards different β-lactams helps to explain the different morphological effects observed on treated bacteria. For example, benzylpenicillin (penicillin G), ampicillin and cephaloridine are particularly effective in causing rapid lysis of Gram-negative bacteria such as *E. coli*. These antibiotics act primarily upon PBP1B, the major transpeptidase of the organism. Other β-lactams have little activity against this PBP, for example mecillinam binds preferentially to PBP2 and it produces a pronounced change in the cells from a rod shape to an oval form. Many of the cephalosporins, for example cephalexin, cefotaxime and ceftazidime bind to PBP3 resulting in the formation of elongated, filamentous cells. The lower molecular weight PBPs, 4, 5 and 6, do not possess transpeptidase activity. These are carboxypeptidases which remove the terminal D-alanine from the pentapeptides on the linear glycans in the cell wall but do not catalyse the crosslinkage. Their role in the cells is to regulate the degree of crosslinking by denying the D-alanyl-D-alanine substrate to the transpeptidases but they are not essential for cell growth. Up to 90% of the amount of antibiotic reacting with the cells may be consumed in inhibiting the carboxypeptidases, with no lethal consequences to the cells.

Gram-positive bacteria also have multiple transpeptidases, but fewer than Gram-negatives. Shape changes are less evident than with Gram-negative rod-shaped organisms. Cell death follows lysis of the cells mediated by the action of endogenous autolytic enzymes (autolysins) present in the cell wall which are activated following β-lactam action. Autolytic enzymes able to hydrolyse peptidoglycan are present in most bacterial walls, they are needed to reshape the wall during growth and to aid cell separation during division. Their activity is regulated by binding to wall components such as the wall and membrane teichoic acids. When peptidoglycan assembly is disrupted through β-lactam action, some of the teichoic acids are released from the cells which are then susceptible to attack by their own autolysins.

2.2 Mycolic acid and arabinogalactan synthesis in mycobacteria

The cell walls of mycobacteria contain three structures: peptidoglycan, an arabino-galactan polysaccharide and long chain hydroxy fatty acids (mycolic acids) which are all covalently linked. Additional non-covalently attached lipid components found in the wall include glycolipids, various phospholipids and waxes. The lipid-rich nature of the mycobacterial wall is responsible for the characteristic acid-fastness on staining and serves as a penetration barrier to many antibiotics. Isoniazid and ethambutol have long been known as specific antimycobacterial agents but their mechanisms of action have only recently become more clearly understood.

2.2.1 Isoniazid

Mycolic acids are produced by a diversion of the normal fatty acid biosynthetic pathway in which short chain (16 carbon) and long chain (24 carbon) fatty acids are produced by addition of 7 or 11 malonate extension units from malonyl coenzyme A to acetyl coenzyme A. The long chain fatty acids are further extended and condensed to produce the 60–70 carbon β-hydroxymycolic acids. Isoniazid is thought to inhibit a desaturase (dehydrogenase) enzyme which inserts a double bond into the fatty acid chain at the 24 carbon stage of mycolic chain extension. Isoniazid itself is a prodrug which is activated inside mycobacteria by a catalase–peroxidase enzyme system called KatG. Unidentified reactive radicals then attack sensitive targets such as the C_{24}-desaturase involved in mycolic acid synthesis. *Mycobacterium tuberculosis* becomes resistant to isoniazid through loss of the activating KatG enzyme. Other targets involving metabolism of the nucleotide nicotinamide adenine dinucleotide (NAD) and DNA damage may also be involved in the killing mechanism.

2.2.2 Ethambutol

The antimicrobial action of ethambutol, like that of isoniazid, is specific for myco-bacteria, suggesting a target in the unique components of the mycobacterial cell wall. Cells treated with ethambutol accumulate an isoprenoid intermediate, decaprenyl-arabinose which is the source of arabinose in the arabinogalactan polymer. This suggests that ethambutol blocks assembly of the arabinogalactan through inhibition of an arabinosyl transferase enzyme.

3   Protein synthesis

3.1   Protein synthesis and selective inhibition

Figure 8.4 outlines the process of protein synthesis involving the ribosome, mRNA, a series of aminoacyl transfer RNA (tRNA) molecules (at least one for each amino acid)

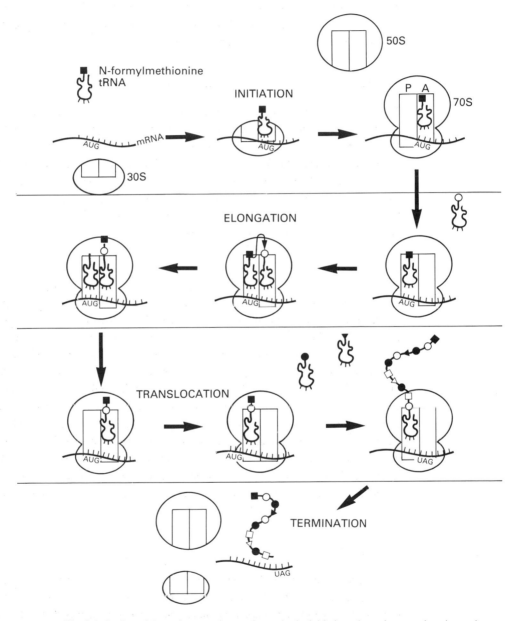

Fig. 8.4 Outline of the main events in protein synthesis; initiation, elongation, translocation and termination. AUG is an initiation codon on the mRNA; it codes for *N*-formylmethionine and initiates the formation of the 70S ribosome. UAG is a termination codon; it does not code for any amino acid and brings about termination of protein synthesis.

and accessory protein factors involved in initiation, elongation and termination. As the process is essentially the same in prokaryotic (bacterial) and eukaryotic cells (i.e. higher organisms and mammalian cells) it is surprising that there are so many selective agents which act in this area (see Table 8.1).

Bacterial ribosomes are smaller than their mammalian counterparts. They consist of one 30S and one 50S subunit (the S suffix denotes the size which is derived from the rate of sedimentation in an ultracentrifuge). The 30S subunit comprises a single strand of 16S rRNA and over 20 different proteins which are bound to it. The larger 50S subunit contains two single strands of rRNA (23S and 5S) together with over 30 different proteins. The subunits pack together to form an intact 70S ribosome. The equivalent subunits for mammalian ribosomes are 40S and 60S making an 80S ribosome. Some agents exploit subtle differences in structure between the bacterial and mammalian ribosomes. The macrolides, azalides and chloramphenicol act upon the 50S subunits in bacteria but not the 60S subunits of mammalian cells. By contrast, the tetracyclines derive their selective action through active uptake by microbial cells and exclusion from mammalian cells. They are equally active against both kinds of ribosomes by binding to the respective 30S and 40S subunits.

3.2   Aminoglycoside–aminocyclitol antibiotics

Most of the information on the mechanisms of action of aminoglycoside–aminocyclitol (AGAC) antibiotics comes from studies with streptomycin. One effect of the AGACs is to interfere with the initiation and assembly of the bacterial ribosome (Fig. 8.4). During assembly of the initiation complex, N-formylmethionyl-tRNA (fmet-tRNA) binds initially to the ribosome binding site on the untranslated 5′ end of the mRNA together with the 30S ribosomal subunit. Three protein initiation factors (designated IF_{1-3}) and a molecule of guanosine triphosphate (GTP) are involved in positioning the fmet-tRNA on the AUG start codon of mRNA. IF_1 and IF_3 are then released from the complex, GTP is hydrolysed to guanosine diphosphate (GDP) and released with IF_2 as the 50S subunit joins the 30S subunit and mRNA to form a functional ribosome. The fmet-tRNA occupies the peptidyl site (P site) leaving a vacant acceptor site (A site) to receive the next aminoacyl-tRNA specified by the next codon on the mRNA. Streptomycin binds tightly to one of the protein components of the 30S subunit. Binding of the antibiotic to the protein, which is the receptor for IF_3, prevents initiation and assembly of the ribosome.

Streptomycin binding to the 30S subunit also distorts the shape of the A site on the ribosome and interferes with the positioning and the aminoacyl-tRNA molecules during peptide chain elongation. Streptomycin therefore exerts two effects: inhibition of protein synthesis by freezing the initiation complex, and misreading of the codons through distortion of the 30S subunit. Simple blockage of protein synthesis would be bacteriostatic rather than bacteriocidal. Since streptomycin and the other AGACs exert a potent lethal action it seems that the formation of toxic, non-functional proteins through misreading of the codons on mRNA is a more likely mechanism of action. This can be demonstrated with cell-free translation systems in which isolated bacterial ribosomes are supplied with an artificial mRNA template such as polyU or polyC and all the other factors, including aminoacyl-tRNAs needed for protein synthesis.

In the absence of an AGAC the ribosomes will produce the artificial polypeptides, polyphenylalanine (as specified by the codon UUU) or polyproline (as specified by the codon CCC). However, when streptomycin is added, the ribosomes produce a mixture of polythreonine (codon ACU) and polyserine (codon UCU). The misreading of the codons does not appear to be random: U is read as A or C and C is read as A or U. If such misreading occurs in whole cells the accumulation of non-functional or toxic proteins would eventually prove fatal to the cells. There is some evidence that the bacterial cell membrane is damaged when the cells attempt to excrete the faulty proteins.

The effectiveness of the AGACs is enhanced by their active uptake by bacteria which proceeds in three phases. First, a rapid uptake occurs within a few seconds of contact which represents binding of the positively charged AGAC molecules to the negatively charged surface of the bacteria. This phase is referred to as the energy-independent phase (EIP) of uptake. In the case of Gram-negative bacteria the AGACs damage the outer membrane causing release of some lipopolysaccharide, phospholipid and proteins but this is not directly lethal to the cells. Second, there follows an energy-dependent phase of uptake (EDP I) lasting about 10 minutes, in which the AGAC is actively transported across the cytoplasmic membrane. A second energy-dependent phase (EDP II) which leads to further intracellular accumulation follows after some AGAC has bound to the ribosomes in the cytoplasm. Although the precise details of uptake by EDP I and EDP II are not clear, both require organisms to be growing aerobically. Anaerobes do not take up AGACs by EDP I or EDP II and are consequently resistant to their action.

3.3   Tetracyclines

This group of antibiotics is actively transported into bacterial cells, possibly as the magnesium complex, achieving a 50-fold concentration inside the cells. Mammalian cells do not take up the tetracyclines and it is this difference in uptake that determines the selective toxicity. Resistance to the tetracyclines is usually associated with failure of the active uptake system or with an active efflux pump which removes the drug from the cells before it can interfere with ribosome function. Protein synthesis by both bacterial and mammalian ribosomes is inhibited by the tetracyclines in cell-free systems. The action is upon the smaller subunit. Binding of just one molecule of tetracycline to the bacterial 30S subunit occurs at a site involving the 3′ end of the 16S rRNA, a number of associated ribosomal proteins and magnesium ions. The effect is to block the binding of aminoacyl-tRNA to the A site of the ribosome and halt protein synthesis. Tetracyclines are bacteriostatic rather than bacteriocidal, consequently they should not be used in combination with β-lactams, which require cells to be growing and dividing to exert their lethal action.

3.4   Chloramphenicol

Of the four possible optical isomers of chloramphenicol, only the D-*threo* form is active. This antibiotic selectively inhibits protein synthesis in bacterial ribosomes by binding to the 50S subunit in the region of the A site involving the 23S rRNA. The normal binding of the aminoacyl-tRNA in the A site is affected by chloramphenicol in such a way that the peptidyl transferase cannot form a new peptide bond with the growing peptide chain on the tRNA in the P site. Studies with aminoacyl-tRNA fragments containing truncated tRNA chains suggest that the shape of the region of tRNA closest to the amino acid is distorted by chloramphenicol. The altered orientation of this region of the aminoacyl-tRNA in the A site is sufficient to prevent peptide bond formation. Chloramphenicol has a broad spectrum of activity which covers Gram-positive and Gram-negative bacteria, mycoplasmas, rickettsia and chlamydia. It has the valuable property of penetrating into mammalian cells and is therefore the drug of choice for treatment of intracellular pathogens, including *Salmonella typhi*, the causative organism of typhoid. Although it does not inhibit 80S ribosomes, the 70S ribosomes of mammalian mitochondria are sensitive and therefore some inhibition occurs in rapidly growing mammalian cells with high mitochondrial activity.

3.5 Macrolides and azalides

Erythromycin is a member of the macrolide group of antibiotics; it selectively inhibits protein synthesis in a broad range of bacteria by binding to the 50S subunit. The site at which it binds is close to that of chloramphenicol and involves the 23S rRNA. Resistance to chloramphenicol and erythromycin can occur by methylation of different bases within the same region of the 23S rRNA. The sites are therefore not identical but binding of one antibiotic prevents binding of the other. Unlike chloramphenicol, erythromycin blocks translocation. This is the process by which the ribosome moves along the mRNA by one codon after the peptidyl transferase reaction has joined the peptide chain to the aminoacyl-tRNA in the A site. The peptidyl-tRNA is moved (translocated) to the P site, vacating the A site for the next aminoacyl-tRNA. Energy is derived by hydrolysis of GTP to GDP by an associated protein elongation factor, EF-G. By blocking the translocation process, erythromycin causes release of incomplete polypeptides from the ribosome. It is assumed that the azalides, such as azithromycin (Chapter 5), have a similar action to the macrolides. The azalides have improved intracellular penetration over the macrolides and are resistant to the metabolic conversion which reduces the serum half life of erythromycin.

3.6 Lincomycin and clindamycin

These agents bind selectively to a region of the 50S ribosomal subunit close to that of chloramphenicol and erythromycin. They block elongation of the peptide chain by inhibition of peptidyl transferase.

3.7 Fusidic acid

This steroidal antibiotic does not act upon the ribosome itself, but upon one of the associated elongation factors, EF-G. This factor supplies energy for translocation by hydrolysis of GTP to GDP. Another elongation factor, EF-Tu promotes binding of aminoacyl-tRNA molecules to the A site through binding and hydrolysis of GTP. Both EF-G and EF-Tu have overlapping binding sites on the ribosome. Fusidic acid binds the EF-G : GDP complex to the ribosome after one round of translocation has taken place.

This prevents further incorporation of aminoacyl-tRNA by blocking the binding of EF-Tu:GTP. Like the tetracyclines, fusidic acid owes its selective antimicrobial action to active uptake by bacteria and exclusion from mammalian cells. The equivalent elongation factor in mammalian cells, EF-2 is susceptible to fusidic acid in cell-free systems.

3.8 Mupirocin

The target of mupirocin is one of a group of enzymes which couple amino acids to their respective tRNAs for delivery to the ribosome and incorporation into protein. The particular enzyme inhibited by mupirocin is involved in producing isoleucyl-tRNA. The basis for the inhibition is a structural similarity between one end of the mupirocin molecule and isoleucine. Protein synthesis is halted when the ribosome encounters the isoleucine codon through depletion of the pool of isoleucyl-tRNA.

4 Chromosome function and replication

4.1 The basis for selective inhibition of chromosome replication and function

As with protein synthesis, the mechanisms of chromosome replication and function are essentially the same in prokaryotes and eukaryotes. There are, however, important differences in the detailed functioning and properties of the enzymes involved and these differences are exploited by a number of agents as the basis of selective inhibition. The microbial chromosome is large in comparison with the cell that contains it (approximately 1000 times the length of *E. coli*). During replication the circular double helix must be unwound to allow the DNA polymerase enzymes to synthesize new complementary strands. The shape of the chromosome is manipulated by the cell by the formation of regions of supercoiling. Positive supercoiling (coiling in the same sense as the turns of the double helix) makes the chromosome more compact. Negative supercoiling (generated by twisting the chromosome in the opposite sense to the helix) produces localized strand separation which is required both for replication and transcription. In a bacterium such as *E. coli*, four different topoisomerase enzymes are responsible for maintaining the shape of DNA during cell division. They act by cutting one or both of the DNA strands, they remove or generate supercoiling, then reseal the strands. Their activity is essential for the microbial cell to relieve the complex tangling of the chromosome (both knotting and chain link formation) which results from progression of the replication fork around the circular chromosome. Type I topoisomerases cut one strand of DNA and pass the other strand through the gap before resealing. Type II enzymes cut both strands and pass another double helical section of the DNA through the gap before resealing. In *E. coli* topoisomerase I and III are both type I enzymes whilst topoisomerases II and IV are type II enzymes. Topoisomerase II is also known as DNA gyrase and is the site of action of the quinolones.

The basic sequence of events for microbial chromosome replication is as follows.

4.1.1   *Synthesis of precursors*

Purines, pyrimidines and their nucleosides and nucleoside triphosphates are synthesized in the cytoplasm. At this stage the antifolate drugs (sulphonamides and dihydrofolate reductase inhibitors) act by blocking the production of thymine. The antifungal agent 5-fluorocytosine interferes with these early stages of DNA synthesis. Through conversion to 5-fluorouracil then to 5-fluorodeoxyuridylic acid (5-F-dUMP) it blocks thymidylic acid production through inhibition of the enzyme thymidylate synthetase. The antiviral nucleosides acycloguanosine (acyclovir) and iododeoxyuridine (idoxuridine) are converted to their respective nucleoside triphosphates in the cytoplasm of infected cells. They proceed to inhibit viral DNA replication either by inhibition of the DNA polymerase or by incorporation into DNA with subsequent termination of chain extension. Finally the anti-human immunodeficiency virus (HIV) drug azidothymidine (AZT) acts in an analogous manner, being converted to the corresponding triphosphate and inhibiting viral RNA synthesis by the HIV reverse transcriptase.

4.1.2 Unwinding of the chromosome

As described in section 4.1, the DNA double helix must unwind to allow access of the polymerase enzymes to produce two new strands of DNA. This is facilitated by DNA gyrase, the target of the quinolones. Some agents interfere with the unwinding of the chromosome by physical obstruction. These include the acridine dyes, of which the topical antiseptic proflavine is the most familiar, and the antimalarial acridine, mepacrine. They prevent strand separation by insertion (intercalation) between base pairs from each strand, but exhibit very poor selective toxicity.

4.1.3 Replication of DNA strands

The unwound DNA strands are kept unfolded during replication by binding a protein called Albert's protein. A series of enzymes produce new strands of DNA using each of the separated strands as templates. An RNA polymerase forms short primer strands of RNA on each template strand at specific initiator sites. DNA polymerase III then synthesizes and joins short DNA strands on to the RNA primers. These DNA strands are called Okasaki fragments. DNA polymerase I (which possesses nucleotidase activity) removes the RNA primers and replaces them with DNA strands. Finally a DNA ligase joins together the DNA strands producing two daughter chromosomes. The entire process is carefully regulated with proofreading stages to check that each nucleotide is correctly incorporated as specified by the template sequence. There are no therapeutic agents yet known which interfere directly with the DNA polymerases.

4.1.4 Transcription

The process of transcription, the copying of a single strand of mRNA sequence using one strand of the chromosome as a template, is carried out by RNA polymerase. This is a complex of four proteins (two α, one β and one β' subunits) which make up the core enzyme. Another small protein, the σ factor, joins the core enzyme, which binds to the promoter region of the DNA preceding the gene which is to be transcribed. The correct positioning and orientation of the polymerase is obtained by recognition of specific marker sites on the DNA at positions -10 and -35 nucleotide bases before the initiation site for transcription. The σ factor is responsible for recognition of the initiation signal for transcription and the core enzyme possesses the activity to join the nucleotides in the sequence specified by the gene. Mammalian genes possess an analogous RNA polymerase but there are sufficient differences in structure to permit selective inhibition of the microbial enzyme by the semisynthetic rifamycin antibiotic, rifampicin.

4.2 Quinolones

The quinolones selectively inhibit DNA gyrase (topoisomerase II), which is not found in mammalian cells. The gyrase, a tetramer comprising two A and two B subunits, is a highly versatile enzyme which is capable of catalysing a variety of changes in DNA topology. These include introduction of negative supercoiling and removal of positive supercoiling (relaxation), unknotting, and removal of linked structures (decatenation). Such activities ensure that the daughter chromosomes produced during replication can segregate in the cytoplasm prior to cell division. The gyrase binds to the chromosome at a point where two separate double stranded regions cross (this can be at a supercoiled region, a knotted or a linked (catenane) region). The A subunits cut both DNA strands on one chain with a 4 base pair stagger, the other chain is passed through the break which is then resealed. The B subunits derive energy for the reaction by hydrolysis of adenosine triphosphate (ATP). The precise details of the interaction are not clear but it appears that the quinolones bind to the A subunits at exposed single strand ends of the cut DNA chain. The gyrase is unable to reseal the DNA with the result that the chromosome in treated cells becomes fragmented. The number of fragments (approximately 100 per cell) is comparable to the number of supercoils in the chromosome. The action of the quinolones probably triggers secondary responses in the cells which are responsible for death. One notable morphological effect of quinolone treatment of Gram-negative rod-shaped organisms is the formation of filaments. Some of the quinolones may also act upon topoisomerase IV, which appears to be more important for chromosome segregation in staphylococci.

4.3 Nitroimidazoles (metronidazole) and nitrofurans (nitrofurantoin)

These agents also cause DNA strand breakage but by a direct chemical action rather than by inhibition of a topoisomerase. Metronidazole is active only against anaerobic organisms. The nitro group of metronidazole is converted to a nitronate radical by the low redox potential within cells. The activated metronidazole then attacks the DNA producing strand breakage. Nitrofurantoin is thought to act in a similar manner.

4.4 Rifampicin

The action of rifampicin is upon the β subunit of RNA polymerase. Binding of just one molecule of rifampicin inhibits the initiation stage of transcription in which the first nucleotide is incorporated in the RNA chain. Once started, transcription itself is not inhibited. It has been suggested that the structure of rifampicin resembles that of two adenosine nucleotides in RNA; this may form the basis of the binding of the antibiotic to the β subunit. One problem is the rapid development of resistance in organisms due to alterations in the amino acids comprising one particular region of the β subunit. These changes do not affect the activity of the polymerase but render it insensitive to rifampicin. The action of rifampicin is specific for the microbial RNA polymerase, the mammalian version being unaffected.

<table>
<tr><td>4.5</td><td>

5-Fluorocytosine

</td></tr>
</table>

This antifungal agent inhibits DNA synthesis at the early stages involving production of the nucleotide, thymidylic acid (dTMP). 5-Fluorocytosine (5-FC) is converted by a deaminase inside fungi to 5-fluorouracil then to the corresponding nucleoside phosphate, 5-fluorodeoxyuridylic acid (5-F-dUMP). This compound then acts as an inhibitor of thymidylate synthetase which normally produces dTMP from uridine monophosphate (dUMP) by addition of a methyl group (supplied by a folate cofactor, section 5.1) to the 5 position of the uracil ring. As this position is blocked by the fluoro group 5-F-dUMP acts as an inhibitor of the enzyme. 5-FC can be considered as a pro-drug, it has the value of being taken up by fungi as the pyrimidine base, whereas the active metabolite produced inside the cells would not be taken up because of its negative charge. Although 5-FC is an important antifungal agent in treatment of life-threatening infections, resistance can occur due to active efflux of the drug from the cells before it can inhibit DNA synthesis.

5   Folate antagonists

5.1   Folate metabolism in microbial and mammalian cells

Folic acid is an important cofactor in all living cells. In the reduced form, tetrahydrofolate (THF), it functions as a carrier of single carbon fragments which are used in the synthesis of adenine, guanine, thymine and methionine. One important folate-dependent enzyme is thymidylate synthetase, which produces dTMP by transfer of the methyl group from THF to dUMP. In this and other folate-dependent reactions THF is converted to dihydrofolic acid (DHF), which must be reduced back to THF before it can participate again as a carbon fragment carrier. The enzyme responsible for the reduction of DHF to THF is dihydrofolate reductase (DHFR; Fig. 8.5) which uses the nucleotide $NADPH_2$ as a cofactor. Bacteria, protozoa and mammalian cells all possess DHFR but there are sufficient differences in the enzyme structure for inhibitors such as trimethoprim and pyrimethamine to inhibit the bacterial and protozoal enzymes selectively without damaging the mammalian form. In the case of protozoa such as the *Plasmodium* species responsible for malaria, the DHFR is a double enzyme which also contains the thymidylate synthetase activity.

There is another fundamental difference between folate utilization in microbial and mammalian cells. Bacteria and protozoa are unable to take up exogenous folate and must synthesize it themselves. This is carried out in a series of reactions involving first the synthesis of dihydropteroic acid from one molecule each of pteridine and *p*-aminobenzoic acid (PABA). Glutamic acid is then added to form DHF which is reduced by DHFR to THF. Mammalian cells do not make their own DHF, instead they take it up from dietary nutrients and convert it to THF using DHFR.

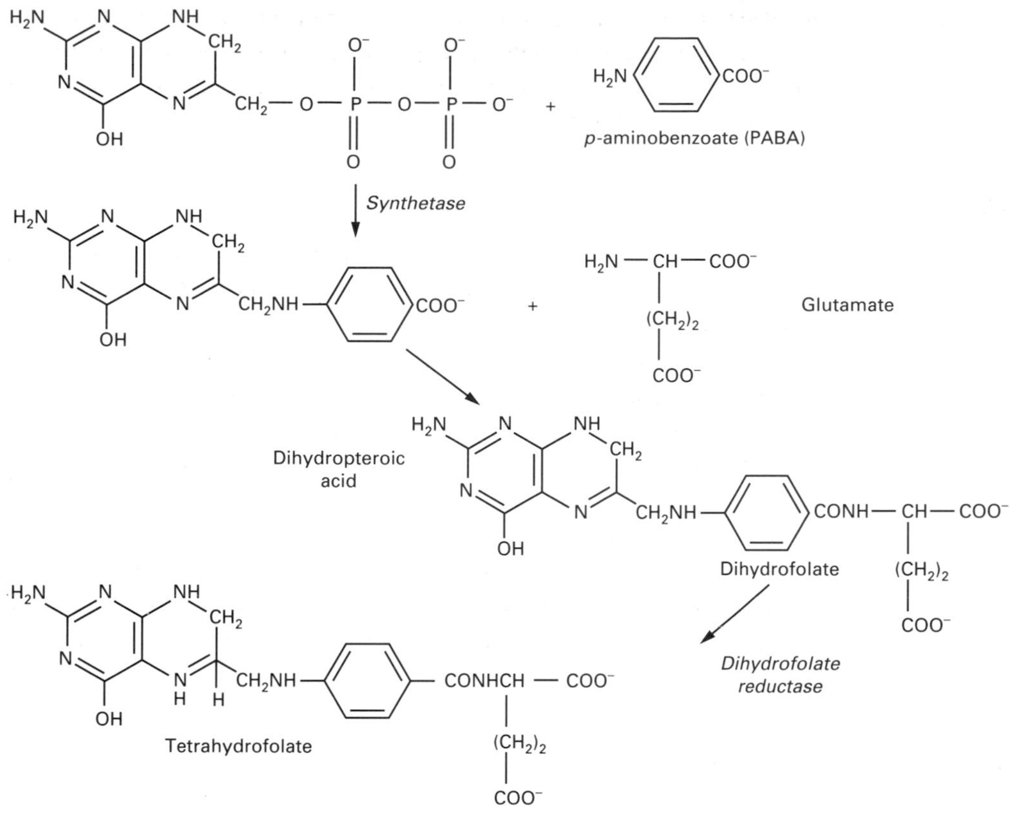

Fig. 8.5 Final steps in the biosynthesis of tetrahydrofolate by bacteria.

5.2   Sulphonamides

Sulphonamides are structural analogues of PABA. They competitively inhibit the incorporation of PABA into dihydropteroic acid and there is some evidence for their incorporation into false folate analogues which inhibit subsequent metabolism. The presence of excess PABA will reverse the inhibitory action of sulphonamides, as will thymine, adenine, guanine and methionine. However, these nutrients are not normally available at the site of infections for which the sulphonamides are used.

5.3   DHFR inhibitors

Trimethoprim is a selective inhibitor of bacterial DHFR. The bacterial enzyme is several thousand times more sensitive than the mammalian enzyme. Pyrimethamine, likewise, is a selective inhibitor of plasmodial DHFR. Both are structural analogues of the dihydropteroic acid portion of the DHF substrate. Crystal structures of the bacterial, plasmodial and mammalian DHFRs, each containing either bound substrate or the inhibitors have been determined by X-ray diffraction studies. These show how inhibitors fit tightly into the active site normally occupied by the DHF substrate, forming a pattern of strong hydrogen bonds with amino acid residues and water molecules lining the site. Another DHFR inhibitor is proguanil, a guanidine-containing pro-drug which is metabolized in the liver to cycloguanil, an active selective inhibitor of plasmodial DHFR. Methotrexate is a potent DHFR inhibitor which has an analogous structure to the whole DHF molecule, including the glutamate residue. It has no selectivity towards microbial DHFR and cannot therefore be used to treat infections; however, it is widely used as an anticancer agent. A derivative of methotrexate which is used for treatment of *Pneumocystis carinii* infections in acquired immunodeficiency syndrome (AIDS) patients is trimetrexate. Although it is very toxic to mammalian cells, simultaneous administration of leucovorin (formyl-THF or folinic acid) as an alternative source of folate which cannot be taken up by the organism protects host tissues. DHFR inhibitors can be used in combination with a sulphonamide to achieve a double interference with folate metabolism. Suitable combinations with matching pharmacokinetic properties are sulphamethoxazole and trimethoprim (the antibacterial, cotrimoxazole) and sulphadoxine and pyrimethamine (the antimalarial, fansidar).

6 The cytoplasmic membrane

6.1 Composition and susceptibility of membranes to selective disruption

The integrity of the cytoplasmic membrane is vital for the normal functioning of all cells. Bacterial membranes do not contain sterols and, in this respect differ from membranes of fungi and mammalian cells. Fungal membranes contain predominantly ergosterol as the sterol component whereas mammalian cells contain cholesterol. Gram-negative bacteria contain an additional outer membrane structure which provides a protective penetration barrier to potentially harmful substances, including many antibiotics. The outer membrane has an unusual asymmetric structure in which phospholipids occupy the inner face and the lipopolysaccharide (LPS) occupies the outer face. The outer membrane is attached to the peptidoglycan by proteins and lipoproteins. The stability of all membranes is maintained by a combination of non-covalent interactions between the constituents involving ionic, hydrophobic and hydrogen bonding. The balance of these interactions can be disturbed by the intrusion of molecules (membrane-active agents) which destroy the integrity of the membrane, thereby causing leakage of cytoplasmic contents or impairment of metabolic functions associated with the membrane. Most membrane-active agents which function in this way, e.g. the alcohols, quaternary ammonium compounds and bisbiguanides (considered in Chapter 10), have very poor selectivity. They cannot be used systemically because of their damaging effects upon mammalian cells; instead they are used as skin antiseptics, disinfectants and preservatives. A few agents can be used therapeutically: the polymyxins, which act principally upon the outer membrane of Gram-negative bacteria, and the antifungal polyenes, imidazoles naftidine.

6.2 Polymyxins

Polymyxin B and polymyxin E (colistin) are used in the treatment of serious Gram-negative bacterial infections, particularly those caused by *Pseudomonas aeruginosa*. They comprise a cyclic peptide containing positively charged groups linked by a tripeptide to a hydrophobic branched chain fatty acid. They bind tightly to negatively charged phosphate groups on LPS in the outer membrane of Gram-negative bacteria. The outer leaflet of the membrane structure is distorted, segments of which are released and the permeability barrier destroyed. The polymyxins can then penetrate to the cytoplasmic membrane where they disrupt membrane integrity, causing leakage of cytoplasmic components. Their detergent-like properties are a key feature of this membrane-damaging action which is similar to that of quaternary ammonium compounds. The high affinity of polymyxins for LPS is an advantage in treatment of *P. aeruginosa* lung infections where neutralization of the endotoxic action of LPS released from the organisms reduces inflammation.

6.3 Polyenes

Amphotericin B and nystatin are the most commonly used members of this group of antifungal agents. They derive their action from their strong affinity towards sterols, particularly ergosterol. The hydrophobic polyene region binds to the hydrophobic sterol ring system within fungal membranes. In so doing, the hydroxylated portion of the polyene is pulled into the membrane interior, destabilizing the structure and causing leakage of cytoplasmic constituents. It is possible that polyene molecules associate together in the membrane to form aqueous channels. The pattern of leakage is progressive, with small metal ions such as K^+ leaking first, followed by larger amino acids and nucleotides. The internal pH of the cells falls as K^+ ions are released, macromolecules are degraded and the cells are killed. The selective antifungal activity of the polyenes is poor, depending on the higher affinity for ergosterol than cholesterol. Kidney damage is a major problem when polyenes are used systemically to treat severe fungal infections. The problem can be reduced but not eliminated by administration of amphotericin as a lipid complex or liposome.

6.4 Imidazoles and triazoles

The azole antifungal drugs act by inhibiting the synthesis of the sterol components of the fungal membrane. They are inhibitors of one step in the complex pathway of ergosterol synthesis involving the removal of a methyl group from lanosterol. The 14α-demethylase enzyme responsible is dependent upon cytochrome P_{450}. The imidazoles and triazoles cause rapid defects in fungal membrane integrity due to reduced levels of ergosterol, with loss of cytoplasmic constituents leading to similar effects to the polyenes. The azoles are not entirely specific for fungal ergosterol synthesis and have some action upon mammalian steroid metabolism, for example they reduce testosterone synthesis.

6.5 Naftidine

This synthetic allylamine derivative inhibits the enzyme squalene epoxidase at an early stage in fungal sterol biosynthesis. Acting as a structural analogue of squalene, naftidine causes the accumulation of this unsaturated hydrocarbon, and a decrease in ergosterol in the fungal cell membrane.

7 Further reading

Arthur M., Reynolds P. & Courvalin P. (1996) Glycopeptide resistance in enterococci. *Trends Microbiol*, **4**, 401-407.

Barry C.E. & Mdluli K. (1996) Drug sensitivity and environmental adaptation of mycobacterial cell wall components. *Trends Microbiol*, **4**, 275–281.

Bentley P.H. & Ponsford R. (1993) *Recent Advances in the Chemistry of Antiinfective Agents*. London: Royal Society of Chemistry.

Brajtburg J., Powderly W.G., Kobayashi G.S. & Medoff G. (1990) Amphotericin B: current understanding of mechanism of action. *Antimicrob Agents Chemother*, **34**, 183–188.

Coulson C.J. (1994) *Molecular Mechanisms of Drug Action*. London: Taylor & Francis.

Franklin J.J. & Snow G.A. (1989) *Biochemistry of Antimicrobial Action*, 4th edn. London: Chapman & Hall.

Greenwood D. (1995) *Antimicrobial Chemotherapy*, 3rd edn. Oxford: Oxford University Press.

Hooper D.C. & Wolfson J.S. (1993) *Quinolone Antimicrobial Agents*. Washington: American Society for Microbiology.

Lancini G., Parenti F. & Hall G.G. (1995) *Antibiotics: a Multidisciplinary Approach*. New York: Plenum Press.

Nagarajan R. (1991) Antibacterial activities and modes of action of vancomycin and related glycopeptides. *Antimicrob Agents Chemother*, **35**, 605–609.

Russell A.D. & Chopra I. (1996) *Understanding Antibacterial Action and Resistance*, 2nd edn. New York: Ellis Horwood.

Sutcliffe J.A. & Georgopapadakou N.H. (1992) *Emerging Targets in Antibacterial and Antifungal Chemotherapy*. New York: Chapman & Hall.

Tipper D.J. (1988) *Antibiotic Inhibitors of Bacterial Cell Wall Biosynthesis*, 2nd edn. Oxford: Pergamon Press.

Williams R.A.D., Lambert P.A. & Singleton P. (1996) *Antimicrobial Drug Action*. Oxford: Bios.

9   Bacterial resistance to antibiotics

1	**Introduction**	3.2.5	Fusidic acid
		3.2.6	Mupirocin
2	**Intrinsic and acquired resistance**	3.3	Inhibitors of peptidoglycan synthesis
2.1	Genetic basis of acquired resistance	3.3.1	β-Lactams
2.1.1	Chromosomal mutations	3.3.2	Glycopeptides
2.1.2	Plasmids	3.3.3	Fosfomycin
2.1.3	Transposons	3.4	Membrane-active antibiotics
		3.4.1	Polymyxins
3	**Biochemical mechanisms of resistance**	3.5	Multidrug resistance pumps
3.1	Inhibitors of nucleic acid synthesis	3.6	Antibiotics with other resistance
3.1.1	Sulphonamides		mechanisms
3.1.2	Trimethoprim	3.6.1	Bacitracin
3.1.3	Quinolones	3.6.2	Antimycobacterial drugs
3.1.4	Rifampicin		
3.2	Inhibitors of protein synthesis	**4**	**The problem of antibiotic resistance**
3.2.1	Aminoglycoside–aminocyclitol group		
3.2.2	Tetracyclines	**5**	**Conclusions and comments**
3.2.3	Chloramphenicol		
3.2.4	Macrolide, lincosamide and	**6**	**References**
	streptogramin (MLS) antibiotics		

1   Introduction

Bacterial resistance to antibiotics has been recognized since the first drugs were introduced for clinical use. The sulphonamides were introduced in 1935 and approximately 10 years later 20% of clinical isolates of *Neisseria gonorrhoeae* had become resistant. Similar increases in sulphonamide resistance were found in streptococci, coliforms and other bacteria. Penicillin was first used in 1941, when less than 1% of *Staphylococcus aureus* strains were resistant to its action. By 1947, 38% of hospital strains had acquired resistance and currently over 90% of *Staph. aureus* isolates are resistant to penicillin. Increasing resistance to antibiotics is a consequence of selective pressure, but the actual incidence of resistance varies between different bacterial species. For example, ampicillin resistance in *Escherichia coli*, presumably under similar selective pressure as *Staph. aureus* with penicillin, has remained at a level of 30–40% for many years with a slow rate of increase. *Streptococcus pyogenes*, another major pathogen, has remained susceptible to penicillin since its introduction, with no reports of resistance in the scientific literature. Equally, it is well recognized that certain bacteria are unaffected by specific antibiotics. In other words, these bacteria have always been antibiotic-resistant.

2   Intrinsic and acquired resistance

Antibiotic resistance is classified into two broad types: intrinsic and acquired.
1   Intrinsic resistance. This suggests that inherent properties of the bacterium are

Table 9.1 Spectrum of activity of some antibacterial antibiotics*

Antibiotic	Gram-positive bacteria	Gram-negative bacteria
Penicillin	Streptococci, staphylococci, corynebacteria, clostridia, *Listeria*	Anaerobes
Fusidic acid	*Staph. aureus*	
Erythromycin	Streptococci, staphylococci, corynebacteria	*Legionella, Campylobacter*
Vancomycin	Streptococci, staphylococci, clostridia	
Aminoglycosides	*Staph. aureus* (gentamicin)	Coliforms, pseudomonads
Nalidixic acid†		Coliforms
Polymixins		Coliforms, pseudomonads
Metronidazole	Anaerobes only	Anaerobes only

* See also Chapters 5 and 6.
† Newer quinolones have a broad spectrum of activity against Gram-positive and Gram-negative bacteria. In general, Gram-negative bacteria tend to be more susceptible.

responsible for preventing antibiotic action (Godfrey & Bryan 1984). This type of resistance is also termed innate. There are many antibiotics active against Gram-positive bacteria which have no effect on Gram-negative bacteria and vice versa (Table 9.1). This intrinsic resistance is thought to be associated with the outer cell layers, such as the outer membrane, which are absent in Gram-positive cells. The Gram-negative cell envelope is effectively impermeable, preventing certain antibiotics from reaching their intracellular targets.

2   Acquired resistance. This occurs when bacteria which were previously susceptible become resistant, usually, but not always, after exposure to the antibiotic concerned. Intrinsic resistance is always chromosomally mediated, whereas acquired resistance may occur by mutations in the chromosome or by the acquisition of genes coding for resistance from an external source normally via a plasmid or transposon. Both types are clinically important and can result in treatment failure, although acquired resistance is more of a threat in the spread of antibiotic resistance (Russell & Chopra 1996).

2.1   Genetic basis of acquired resistance

Three genetic elements are responsible for acquired resistance: chromosomes, plasmids and transposons (Lewis 1989). Each of these will be considered in turn.

2.1.1   *Chromosomal mutations*

Resistance to certain antibiotics can arise as a consequence of mutations to chromosomal genes because of changes in the DNA sequence. Mutations can occur due to single base pair changes. Transitions involve the substitution of one purine (A or G) for another and therefore one pyrimidine (C or T) for another. Transversions involve a change from a pyrimidine to a purine and vice versa. Frameshift mutations occur when one or two bases are inserted into the DNA sequence, resulting in an altered reading frame and therefore an altered gene product.

More extensive changes in the DNA sequence (often referred to as macrolesions) can also occur. Deletions result in the loss of part of the DNA sequence. Insertions add extra base pairs to a gene. Transversions occur when a segment of the DNA is reversed and duplications occur when a segment of the DNA is repeated. Some of these changes also result in frameshifts.

The molecular basis of acquired chromosomal resistance for specific antibiotics is discussed later in this chapter.

2.1.2   *Plasmids*

The bacterial chromosome contains all the genes necessary for the growth and replication of cells. Many, if not most, bacteria also possess additional circular elements of DNA which are capable of replicating and transferring independently of the chromosome. These extrachromosomal genetic elements are known as plasmids and can code for a number of properties including antibiotic resistance. In a bacterial population under normal circumstances, it is not necessary for all cells within that population to harbour plasmids. This has the effect of avoiding the production of unnecessary gene products unless essential for the survival of the population. Assuming that a subset of the bacterial population maintains such plasmids, selective pressure following exposure to an antibiotic will ensure that plasmid-containing, and therefore resistant, cells and their progeny will survive the antibiotic challenge.

Plasmids have the ability to transfer within and between species and can therefore be acquired from other bacteria as well as a consequence of cell division. This property makes plasmid-acquired resistance much more threatening in terms of the spread of antibiotic resistance than resistance acquired due to chromosomal mutation. Plasmids also harbour transposons (section 2.1.3), which enhances their ability to transfer antibiotic resistance genes.

Plasmid transfer normally occurs by conjugation or transduction *in vivo*. Conjugation requires cell-to-cell contact and involves the transfer of DNA from a donor cell to a recipient cell. Plasmids which can mediate their own transfer are termed conjugative plasmids. Some plasmids which do not possess this property can nevertheless be transferred if they coexist with a conjugative plasmid. These are known as mobilizable plasmids. Both Gram-negative and Gram-positive bacteria have the ability to conjugate. Transduction is a process whereby DNA is transferred by bacteriophages, and plays an important role in the transfer of antibiotic resistance in Gram-positive bacteria such as *Staph. aureus, Strep. pyogenes* and the enterococci. Transduction is generally limited to organisms of the same species and therefore its role in the transfer of antibiotic resistance is less significant than conjugation.

A third mechanism of plasmid transfer is by transformation, which is the ability of certain microorganisms to acquire naked DNA from the environment. This is limited to certain bacteria, notably *Neisseria gonorrhoeae*, which is naturally competent to acquire DNA in this manner. *Neisseria gonorrhoeae* strains have the ability to recognize DNA from their own species, and are thus selective in their acquisition of naked DNA from the environment.

Transduction and transformation are generally limited to the same or related species and are therefore not effective as a means of antibiotic resistance transfer across species boundaries. However, our knowledge of transformation in nature is limited, and the significance of this mechanism of gene transfer is unknown.

2.1.3 Transposons

Transposons are mobile genetic elements capable of transferring or transposing independently from one DNA molecule to another. The DNA molecules may be chromosomes or plasmids. Transposons are normally flanked by short regions of almost identical DNA sequence known as repeats. These are termed direct repeats if they lie in the same direction relative to each other, or inverted repeats if they face in opposite directions. These repeats are thought to function as recognition sequences for enzymes involved in transposition (the ability of transposons to transfer and integrate into the recipient DNA molecule). The central region of the transposon often codes for antibiotic resistance genes. The ability of transposons to mobilize from one DNA molecule to another has led to them being referred to as jumping genes. Transposons do not require homologous regions of DNA in order to integrate into a DNA molecule unlike the normal recombination process in bacterial cells and are therefore a major cause of the transfer and spread of antibiotic resistance genes among different bacterial species. Furthermore, it is possible for bacteria to acquire a series of transposons coding for different antibiotic resistances by insertion in existing plasmids or the chromosome. Conjugative transposons which can mediate their own transfer have been described in the last 10 years. These make the transfer and spread of resistance genes more likely since they do not depend on insertion into conjugative plasmids for their mobilization. Known mechanisms of acquired resistance determined by chromosomes, plasmids or transposons are summarized in Table 9.2.

3   Biochemical mechanisms of resistance

Many different biochemical mechanisms of antibiotic resistance have been described,

Table 9.2 Genetic determinants of resistance

Chromosomally mediated resistance only	Plasmid-mediated resistance*	Transposons†
Methicillin	Aminoglycoside–	Single, e.g. ampicillin,
Quinolones	aminocyclitols	chloramphenicol, tetracycline
Rifampicin	β-Lactams	Multiple, e.g.
	Tetracyclines	ampicillin + streptomycin +
	Sulphonamides	sulphonamide
	Trimethoprim	
	Chloramphenicol	
	Erythromycin	
	Fusidic acid	

* Resistance may also be chromosomally mediated.
† Multiple resistance genes may be carried on a transposon.

though it is worth noting that more than one mechanism may be present at any one time in a resistant microorganism. This is particularly relevant in terms of the clinical efficacy of antibiotics. The acquisition of a single resistance mechanism may render a bacterium microbiologically resistant but therapeutically achievable levels of a drug may be sufficient to overcome such resistance. The acquisition of a second resistance mechanism may be necessary to achieve clinical resistance, i.e. the amount of antibiotic necessary to overcome the resistance mechanism is greater than can be achieved therapeutically.

Before considering specific mechanisms of resistance for particular classes of antibiotic it is worth considering potential mechanisms of resistance in bacterial cells. These are summarized in Fig. 9.1 and specific examples are listed in Table 9.3.

Gram-negative bacteria possess an outer membrane which can act as a barrier to the penetration of antibiotics. The main route of entry of hydrophilic molecules is via the porins, which form pores in the outer membrane. Qualitative or quantitative alterations in these porins can result in the decreased accumulation of antibiotic.

The cytoplasmic (cell) membrane of Gram-positive and Gram-negative bacteria can also act as an exclusion barrier. Alterations in membrane structure can reduce penetration or the presence of proteins functioning as efflux pumps can actively remove antibiotic molecules from the cytoplasm. Bacteria may produce enzymes which inactivate antibiotics, rendering them ineffective. These may destroy or alter the antibiotic molecule. Extracellular enzymes will be most effective in inactivating antibiotics since they will be kept away from their target sites. Gram-negative bacteria can also produce periplasmic enzymes which will act outside the cytoplasmic membrane.

These mechanisms of resistance rely on reducing or preventing access of antibiotic to their target sites, but other mechanisms of resistance involving the target sites themselves can be considered. Alterations in the target site which reduce the binding of

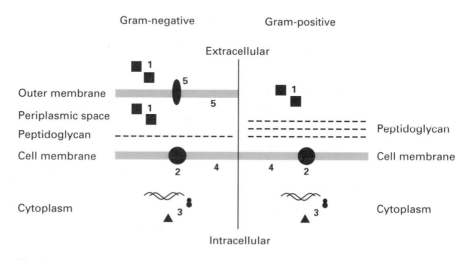

Fig. 9.1 Schematic representation of possible mechanisms of resistance in Gram-negative and Gram-positive bacteria. 1, antibiotic-inactivating enzymes; 2, antibiotic efflux proteins; 3, alteration or duplication of intracellular targets; 4, alteration of the cell membrane reducing antibiotic uptake; 5, alterations in porins or lipopolysaccharide reducing antibiotic uptake or binding.

Table 9.3 Mechanisms of antibiotic resistance

Expression of resistance	Example(s)	Comments
Enzymatic inactivation	Some β-lactam antibiotics	Hydrolysis of the β-lactam ring
	Chloramphenicol	Conversion to an inactive compound
Enzymatic trapping	Some β-lactam antibiotics	Penicillin-binding proteins
Enzymatic modification	Some aminoglycoside antibiotics	Alteration of the molecule by phosphorylation, adenylylation or acetylation
Bacterial impermeability*	Some β-lactam antibiotics	Mutational loss of porins
	Aminoglycoside antibiotics	Reduced ability of cells to take up drugs
	Tetracyclines, chloramphenicol, fusidic acid	Plasmid-mediated decreased drug accumulation
	Hydrophobic antibiotics: novobiocin, actinomycin D, erythromycin, rifampicin	Difficulty in entering Gram-negative cells
Antibiotic efflux	Tetracyclines	Energy-dependent efflux of accumulated drugs
Decreased affinity of target enzymes	β-Lactam antibiotics	Altered PBPs†
	Trimethoprim	Altered dihydroflolate reductase
	Sulphonamides	Altered dihydropteroate synthetase
Alteration in binding site	Streptomycin	Protein S12 component of 30S ribosomal subunit determines sensitivity or resistance
	Erythromycin	Ribosomes from resistant cells have lower affinity, resulting from enzymatic methylation of adenine in 23S rRNA
	Glycopeptides	Acquired ligase produces altered peptidoglycan precursors with lower affinity

* Depends on chemical nature of drug and on type of organism.
† Penicillin-binding proteins.

antibiotics, but allow the target to retain its normal function, are well known. An alternative is to bypass the antibiotic-sensitive step by duplicating the target site with an antibiotic-resistant version. A third related mechanism is to overproduce the target so that higher antibiotic concentrations are required to exert significant antibacterial action. In certain species, an enzyme or metabolic pathway may be absent, rendering the microorganism resistant to antibiotics effective against other bacterial species.

The following sections describe the biochemical mechanisms of resistance to different classes of antibiotics, with the antibiotics grouped according to their mechanism of action.

3.1   Inhibitors of nucleic acid synthesis

Antibiotics considered here can be divided into two mechanisms of action: those which inhibit nucleotide metabolism and those which inhibit enzymes involved in nucleic acid synthesis.

Sulphonamides

Chromosomal and plasmid-mediated resistance to the sulphonamides has been described (Huovinen *et al.* 1995).

Two mechanisms of chromosomal resistance have been identified. A mutation of dihydropteroate synthetase (DHPS) in *Strep. pneumoniae* produces an altered enzyme with reduced affinity for sulphonamides. Hyperproduction of *p*-aminobenzoic acid (PABA) overcomes the block imposed by inhibition of DHPS. The specific cause of PABA hyperproduction is unknown, though chromosomal mutation is the probable cause.

Duplication of DHPS, with the second version of the enzyme being resistant to the sulphonamides, is the cause of plasmid-acquired resistance. Two different enzymes have been identified, both with lowered affinity for the antibiotic.

Trimethoprim

Trimethoprim is a 2,4-diaminopyrimidine and all three genetic bases of resistance have been described (Huovinen *et al.* 1995).

Chromosomal mutations in *E. coli* result in overproduction of dihydrofolate reductase (DHFR). Higher concentrations of trimethoprim, which may not be therapeutically achievable, are therefore required to inhibit nucleotide metabolism. Other mutations lower the affinity of DHFR for trimethoprim. These two mechanisms of resistance may coexist in a single strain, effectively increasing the level of resistance to the antibiotic.

Plasmid- and transposon-mediated resistance is akin to that described for the sulphonamides, where the sensitive step is bypassed by duplication of the target with a resistant version. Many different resistant enzymes have been identified thus far.

Quinolones

The quinolones exert their action by binding to DNA gyrase (bacterial topoisomerase II) and inhibiting its functions. Acquired resistance to the quinolones arises due to chromosomal mutations in the genes coding for DNA gyrase (Hooper & Wolfson 1993). The most common mutations arise in the *gyrA* gene where a single base-pair change can be sufficient to cause resistance. Levels of resistance can be increased by the presence of multiple mutations with a region of the *gyr A* gene known as the quinolone resistance-determining region. The exact mechanism of resistance is unknown but is thought to involve a subtle conformational change in DNA gyrase which reduces binding of quinolones. Mutations in the *gyrB* gene have also been identified but these lead to lower levels of resistance. With certain *gyrB* mutations, bacteria become resistant to older quinolone analogues such as nalidixic acid, but become hypersusceptible to newer quinolones such as ciprofloxacin. Mutations in other bacterial topoisomerases have been identified in *Staph. aureus*. These are thought to be as important as DNA gyrase mutations in quinolone resistance in this microorganism.

Other chromosomal mutations resulting in quinolone resistance have been found to decrease permeability of the antimicrobial agent. *norB* mutants show a decrease in ompF porin. This is one of the major porins in Gram-negative bacteria. *norC* mutants have altered ompF and lipopolysaccharide, though the mutations are not in the *ompF* gene itself but appear to occur in a gene or genes whose products regulate OmpF. *norC* mutants are less susceptible to some quinolones such as ciprofloxacin but more susceptible to others.

Resistance to quinolones by efflux has been described in *Staph. aureus* and *Proteus mirabilis*. This gene has been designated *norA* in *Staph. aureus* and is homologous to membrane transport proteins coupled to the electromotive force. These proteins have the ability to remove small amounts of quinolone from cells normally and *norA* may have arisen as a result of mutations under selective pressure from quinolone use, resulting in a transport protein with increased affinity for these agents.

3.1.4   *Rifampicin*

Rifampicin is the semisynthetic derivative used widely in the UK. Resistance to rifampicin is primarily due to chromosomal mutations resulting in an altered RNA polymerase which is less well inhibited by the drug. The mutations tend to be clustered within short conserved regions of the β subunit gene of RNA polymerase. Similar mutations have been found in all bacterial species studied thus far.

3.2   Inhibitors of protein synthesis

Inhibition of protein synthesis is the antibacterial mechanism shared by most groups of antibiotics, though the exact action differs.

3.2.1   *Aminoglycoside–aminocyclitol group*

Three mechanisms of resistance to the aminoglycoside–aminocyclitol (AGAC) group of antibiotics are recognized (Shaw *et al.* 1993).

Alteration of the antibiotic molecule is plasmid- or transposon-encoded. Three classes of enzyme can alter the AGAC molecule. Aminoglycoside adenylyltransferases (AADs) use adenosine triphosphate (ATP) as a cofactor in modifying certain hydroxyl groups in the antibiotic molecule by adenylylating them (Fig. 9.2). Aminoglycoside phosphotransferases (APH) also use ATP to modify certain hydroxyl groups by phosphorylating them (Fig. 9.2). Aminoglycoside acetyltransferases (AACs) use acetyl CoA as a cofactor and acetylate susceptible amino groups on the molecule (Fig. 9.2). These three classes of enzyme have been further subdivided according to which site on the AGAC molecule is modified. For example, APH(6) phosphorylates the 6-hydroxyl group on the aminohexose group of streptomycin. Most AGAC antibiotics are susceptible to more than one modification reaction. Relatively small amounts of the antibiotic are modified, implying that resistance is determined by the relative rates of drug uptake and modification. A less efficient modifying enzyme will permit unmodified antibiotic to reach its ribosomal quantity. A more efficient enzyme, or greater quantities of the enzyme, will result in resistance.

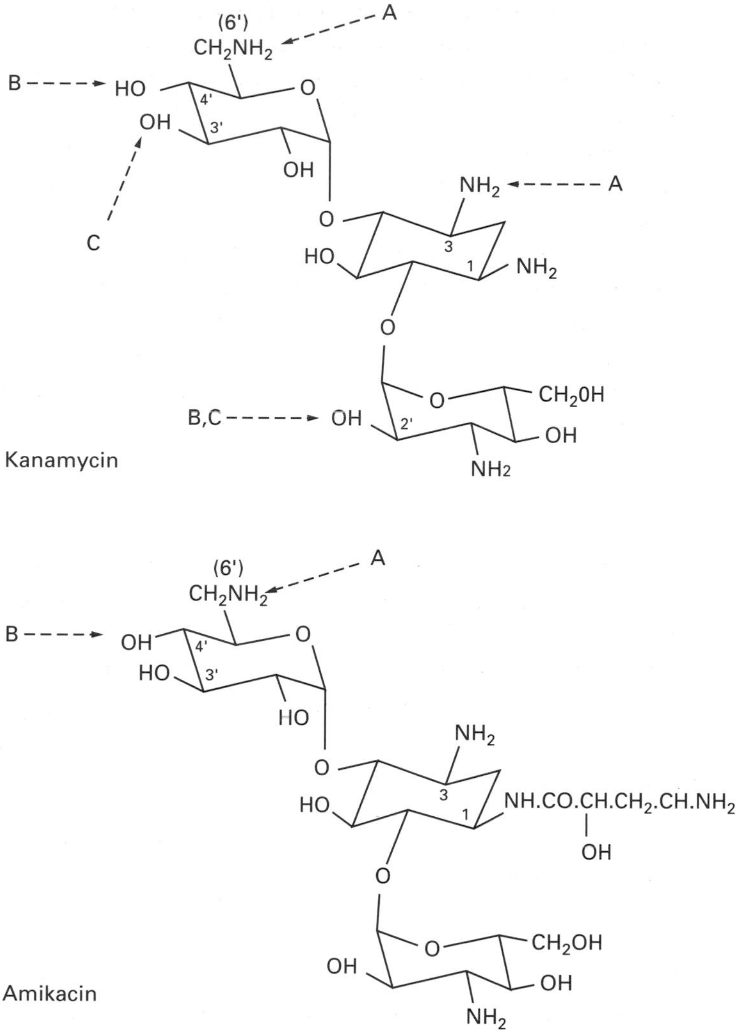

Fig. 9.2 Modification of AGACs (e.g. kanamycin and amikacin) by resistance enzymes. A, acetylation (AAC); B, adenylylation (AAD); C, phosphorylation (APH).

AGAC-modifying enzymes are active outside the cytoplasmic membrane, in the periplasmic space in Gram-negative bacteria and extracellularly in Gram-positives. Table 9.4 summarizes some of the enzymes involved in AGAC resistance and their spectrum of activity.

A second mechanism of resistance to the AGACs involves an alteration of the ribosomal target site. Mutations in the gene coding for ribosomal protein S12 (*rpsL* in *E. coli*) prevent the antibiotics from binding to their target. In mycobacteria, which possess only one ribosomal RNA operon, mutations in *rpoB*, coding for 16S rRNA, also inhibit binding of the drugs.

Acquired resistance due to decreased permeability by mutations affecting membrane transport have also been reported in other bacteria.

Table 9.4 Examples of aminoglycoside–aminocyclitol susceptibility to modifying enzymes

Aminoglycoside	Inactivation by
Streptomycin	APH(3″), APH(6), AAD(6), AAD(3″)(9)
Spectinomycin	AAD(3″)(9), AAD(9)
Gentamicin	APH(2″), AAD(2″), AAC(3), AAC(2′)
Kanamycin	APH(3′), APH(2″), AAD(2″), AAD(4′)(4″), AAC(6′)
Tobramycin	APH(2″), AAD(4′)(4″), AAD(2″), AAC(3), AAC(2′), AAC(6′)
Neomycin	APH(3′), AAD(4′)(4″), AAC(3), AAC(2′), AAC(6′)
Amikacin	AAD(4′)(4″), AAC(6′)

3.2.2 Tetracyclines

Three types of resistance mechanism have also been identified with this class of antibiotic (Chopra *et al.* 1992).

Plasmid- or transposon-encoded tetracycline efflux proteins have been described in a number of bacteria. These efflux proteins are thought to span the cytoplasmic membrane and are dependent on the proton-motive force for their action. It is thought that the efflux proteins bind tetracyclines and initiate proton transfer, although no functional domains have been identified. Eight distinct tetracycline efflux proteins have been identified thus far.

Plasmid- or transposon-encoded ribosomal protection factors are a second mechanism of resistance to the tetracyclines. These proteins are believed to alter the tetracycline binding site on the 30S ribosomal subunit, lowering the affinity for the drugs.

OmpF mutations in Gram-negative bacteria such as *E. coli* (see above) can result in low level resistance to the tetracyclines by reducing their uptake.

3.2.3 Chloramphenicol

Plasmid- or transposon-encoded chloramphenicol acetyltransferases (CATs) are responsible for resistance by inactivating the antibiotic. CATs convert chloramphenicol to an acetoxy derivative which fails to bind to the ribosomal target. Several CATs have been characterized and found to differ in properties such as electrophoretic mobility and catalytic activity.

Three other mechanisms of chloramphenicol resistance have been described. First, a transposon-encoded chloramphenicol efflux protein has been identified in *E. coli*. Second, some bacterial strains have been found to possess drug-resistant ribosomes, and third, low level resistance can arise by chromosomal mutations which reduce the amount of porins and therefore impair uptake. This last mechanism is essentially that described for the AGAC antibiotics.

Macrolide, lincosamide and streptogramin (MLS) antibiotics

These three classes of antibiotics are often grouped together because of their similar mode of action. They share a common mechanism of resistance, but there are some mechanisms specific to each group (Leclerq & Courvalin 1991).

Plasmid- or transposon-mediated resistance common to the MLS group is due to RNA methylase genes (*ermA, ermB* and *ermC*) which code for the methylation of an adenine residue in 23S rRNA. Methylation prevents the drugs from binding to the 50S ribosomal subunit and confers resistance to all MLS antibiotics.

A gene designated *msrA* has been identified in *Staph. aureus* which confers resistance to macrolides and streptogramins but not to lincosamides. Its function is unknown but the DNA sequence is homologous to genes coding for known efflux proteins.

Chromosomal mutations in *E. coli have* been identified as causing macrolide resistance. *eryA* alters protein L4 with a concomitant loss of binding to ribosomes. *eryB* alters protein L22 with a loss of macrolide binding, though the mutation is not in the structural gene for L22. *eryC* mutants are thought to alter the processing of rRNA and a 30S ribosomal subunit protein, though the precise mechanism of resistance is unclear. Macrolide resistance in mycobacteria is associated with point mutations in 23S rRNA. Plasmid-mediated inactivation of erythromycin (a 14-membered macrolide) is common in Gram-negative bacteria and has also been described in some Gram-positives. The lactone ring is hydrolysed by esterase in Gram-negatives, although no similar enzymes have been identified in Gram-positives. Erythromycin can also be phosphorylated, the altered molecule being rendered inactive. Plasmid-mediated resistance to the lincosamides is common in staphylococci. An enzyme nucleotidylates the antibiotics at a specific position rendering them inactive. Staphylococcal resistance to streptogramins is due to inactivation of the antibiotics by plasmid-encoded enzymes. Streptogramin A is inactivated by an acetyltransferase and streptogramin B by a hydrolase.

Fusidic acid

Gram-negative bacteria are intrinsically resistant to low levels of fusidic acid (a steroid) due to exclusion by the outer membrane. Nevertheless, acquired resistance does occur which has the effect of increasing the level of resistance to the antibiotic. Acquired resistance also occurs in Gram-positive bacteria normally susceptible to fusidic acid.

Plasmid-mediated resistance in Gram-positive bacteria is thought to involve decreased uptake of the drug, although the precise mechanism is unknown. Resistance to fusidic acid in Gram-negative bacteria is also poorly understood. A CAT-type enzyme has been identified in resistant strains but no modification or inactivation of the antibiotic has been observed. It is believed that the CAT forms a tight stoichiometric complex with the antibiotic, sequestering it and thus rendering it inactive (Davies 1994).

Chromosomal mutations have also been described which produce a modified translocation factor protein with lowered affinity for fusidic acid.

3.2.6   *Mupirocin*

Mupirocin is a topical antibiotic that inhibits isoleucyl tRNA synthetase with the subsequent inhibition of protein synthesis. Mupirocin has become a mainstay in the treatment of *Staph. aureus* infection and colonization during hospital outbreaks, and it is in this organism that acquired resistance has arisen (Gilbart *et al.* 1993).

High level mupirocin resistance, where strains can be up to 1000 times more resistant than susceptible strains, is due to the presence of an additional isoleucyl tRNA synthetase which is resistant to the antibiotic. Resistance is plasmid-encoded, but the resistant gene differs significantly from the normal susceptible version. The origins of high level mupirocin resistance are unclear but the low homology with existing genes would suggest that resistance is acquired from microorganisms other than *Staph. aureus*. High level mupirocin resistance is an example of duplication of the target site, the new version being resistant to the antibiotic. Low level mupirocin resistance results in strains approximately 50 times more resistant to the antibiotic than susceptible strains. No extra copies of the isoleucyl tRNA synthetase gene are found, indicating that resistance has been acquired by mutations in the normal chromosomal gene. Presumably, mupirocin has less affinity for the altered isoleucyl tRNA synthetase.

3.3   **Inhibitors of peptidoglycan synthesis**

3.3.1   *β-Lactams*

Acquired resistance to *β*-lactam antibiotics can occur by three different mechanisms: inactivation of the antibiotic, alteration of the target site and reduced permeability (Sanders 1992; Georgopapadakou 1993).

β-Lactams are inactivated by enzymes called *β*-lactamases which hydrolyse the cyclic amide bond in the antibiotic molecule (Fig. 9.3). Penicillins are converted to penicilloic acid which is unable to bind to penicillin-binding proteins (PBPs: see Chapter 8). A similar reaction occurs with cephalosporins, except that the cephalosporoic acid derivative is unstable and tends to break up. A wide variety of *β*-lactamases with different structures and substrate profiles has been identified in recent years and classified according to the scheme in Table 9.5. Many *β*-lactamases are plasmid- or transposon-

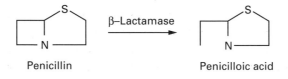

Penicillin   Penicilloic acid

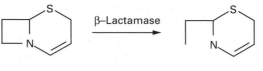

Cephalosporin   Cephalosporoic acid

Fig. 9.3 Hydrolysis of *β*-lactams. Cephalosporoic acid is unstable (see also Fig. 5.1 and sections 2.1 and 2.2 in Chapter 5).

Table 9.5 Examples of β-lactamases

Group of enzyme*	Preferred substrate	Inhibited by:		Representative enzymes
		Clavulanic acid	EDTA	
1	Cephalosporin	–	–	AmpC from Gram-negatives
2a	Penicillins	+	–	Penicillinases from Gram-positives
2b	Penicillins, cephalosporins	+	–	TEM-1†, TEM-2, SHV-1 from Gram negatives
2be	Penicillins, cephalosporins monobactams	+	–	TEM-3 to TEM-26
2br	Penicillins	+/–	–	TEM-30 to TEM-36
2c	Penicillins, carbenicillin	+	–	PSE-1, PSE-3, PSE-4
2d	Penicillins, cloxacillin	+/–	–	OXA-1 to OXA-11
2e	Cephalosporin	+	–	Inducible cephalosporinases from *Proteus vulgaris*
2f	Penicillins, cephalosporins, carbapenems	+	–	NMC-A from *Enterobacter cloacae*, Sme-I from *Serratia marcescens*
3	Most β-lactams, including carbapenems	–	+	L1 from *Xanthomonas maltophilia*, CcrA from *Bacteroides fragilis*
4	Penicillins	–	?	Penicillinase from *Pseudomonas cepacia*

* Based on Bush *et al.* (1995).
† Plasmid-encoded β-lactamases (TEM, PSE, OXA, SHV).

encoded but the Group 1 enzymes are mainly chromosomal. The origin of these is unclear but they may have diverged from existing PBPs. Transfer of these chromosomal enzymes by conjugation may be possible, but no evidence for this exists. Nevertheless, some reports indicate that these Group 1 genes may be mobilized into plasmids and then transferred to other bacteria. Some Group 1 enzymes are constitutive and expressed at low levels, but in other species these enzymes are inducible by β-lactams themselves. Mutations in regulatory genes can lead to constitutive high levels of expression. Such mutations are of clinical significance since they have led to the development of resistance to newer β-lactams previously thought to be resistant to β-lactamases.

It is worth noting that in Gram-negative organisms, β-lactamases are found in the periplasmic space where they inactivate β-lactams before the antibiotics can bind to their PBP targets on the cytoplasmic membrane. In Gram-positive organisms, however, β-lactamases are excreted extracellularly and therefore resistance is very much a characteristic of the population rather than individual β-lactamase-producing cells. If enough enzyme is synthesized, levels of β-lactam may be reduced sufficiently to permit growth of non-β-lactamase-producing strains.

A second mechanism of resistance involves alterations in PBPs which affect binding of β-lactams. These changes have been found to occur by multiple substitutions through recombination rather than point mutations. Acquired penicillin resistance in *Strep. pneumoniae* is because of such gene mosaics which code for an altered yet functional PBP with reduced affinity for penicillin. Sections of the susceptible PBP gene have been replaced by other DNA sequences, presumably via transformation.

Clinically, one of the most important examples of β-lactam resistance is that found in methicillin-resistant *Staph. aureus* (MRSA) strains. These are causing increasing concern in hospitals, especially because methicillin resistance is often accompanied by multiple resistance to unrelated antibiotics. Methicillin is resistant to β-lactamases and is a mainstay in the treatment of *Staph. aureus* since over 90% of hospital strains produce β-lactamase. Methicillin resistance is due to a novel PBP with low affinity for β-lactams. It is capable of functioning when all other PBPs have been inhibited and is sufficient to catalyse all the reactions necessary for cell growth. Resistance is mediated by the *mec* gene, whose origin is unknown. This is an example of resistance by duplication of an antibiotic target, the new version being resistant to the antibiotic.

A third resistance mechanism is akin to that described for the AGAC antibiotics and chloramphenicol, whereby changes in the outer membrane porins of Gram-negative bacteria reduce the penetration of β-lactams resulting in low levels of resistance.

3.3.2   *Glycopeptides*

Glycopeptide antibiotics interfere with peptidoglycan synthesis by binding to the D-alanyl-D-alanine terminus of peptidoglycan precursors. Resistance to glycopeptides was thought unlikely because the changes in integral structures and functions of the cell wall and the enzymes involved in its synthesis would render bacteria non-viable. As is often the case, bacteria have a nasty habit of surprising us!

Acquired resistance to the glycopeptides is transposon-mediated and has so far been largely confined to the enterococci. This has been a problem clinically because many of these strains have been resistant to all other antibiotics and were thus effectively untreatable. Fortunately, the enterococci are not particularly pathogenic and infections have been confined largely to seriously ill, long-term hospital patients. Two types of acquired glycopeptide resistance have been described (Woodford *et al.* 1995). The VanA phenotype is resistant to vancomycin and teicoplanin, whereas VanB is resistant

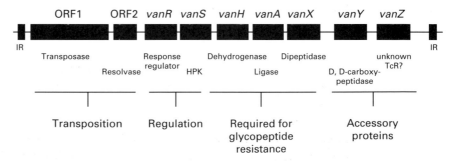

Fig. 9.4 Organization of glycopeptide-resistance genes in transposon Tn1546. IR, invested repeats; HPK, histidine protein kinase; TcR, low level teicoplanin resistance.

to vancomycin only. The VanA phenotype is conferred by a transposon which harbours nine genes coding for resistance (Fig. 9.4). The transposon is transferred by conjugative plasmids. VanA and VanH are essential for the expression or resistance, which is due to a modification of the peptidoglycan pathway to produce precursors with reduced affinity for glycopeptides. VanA is a ligase which catalyzes the synthesis of D-alanyl-D-lactate depsipeptide instead of D-alanyl-D-alanine. VanH is a dehydrogenase which catalyses the synthesis of D-lactate as the substrate for VanA. The glycopeptides have much reduced affinity for the depsipeptide. VanR and VanS are regulatory proteins which allow expression of the other resistance genes in the presence of glycopeptides. The VanX and VanY enzymes are responsible for removing D-alanyl-D-alanine dipeptides from precursors and peptidoglycan to increase levels of resistance. It should be noted that VanX is essential for resistance. The open reading frames (ORF1 and ORF2) code for transposition functions. The function of VanZ is unclear but is thought to have a role in the expression of high level teicoplanin resistance.

VanB-type has been less well-characterized but essentially operates in a similar manner to VanA. Both inducible and constitutive forms of resistance have been described, but the reasons for susceptibility to teicoplanin are unclear.

The origins of the glycopeptide-resistance genes are unknown and share little homology with genes found in intrinsically glycopeptide-resistant organisms.

3.3.3   *Fosfomycin*

Fosfomycin inhibits pyruvil transferase, which is an enzyme involved in peptidoglycan synthesis. Two mechanisms of acquired resistance have been described for fosfomycin (Davies 1994).

Plasmid- or transposon-mediated resistance occurs by inactivation of the antibiotic. Fosfomycin is combined with glutathione intracellularly to produce a compound lacking in antibacterial activity. The gene encoding the enzyme catalysing this reaction has been designated *for-r*.

A second mechanism of acquired resistance to fosfomycin involves chromosomal mutations in sugar phosphate uptake pathways which are responsible for transporting fosfomycin into the cell. The alterations decrease accumulation of the antibiotic to levels below those required for inhibition.

3.4   Membrane-active antibiotics

3.4.1   *Polymyxins*

Polymyxins are a group of antibiotics which disrupt bacterial cell membranes. Two mechanisms of acquired resistance to the polymyxins have been identified (Russell & Chopra 1996).

Acquired resistance to polymyxins in *E. coli* occurs because of chromosomal mutations which cause incorporation of aminoethanol and aminocarabinose in lipo-polysaccharide (LPS) in place of phosphate groups. The altered LPS has a decreased ionic charge which results in lowered binding of polymyxin and thus an increase in resistance to this group of antibiotics.

The mechanism of acquired resistance in *Pseudomonas aeruginosa* is different. Chromosomal mutations result in the increase of a specific outer membrane protein with a concomitant reduction in divalent cations. Polymyxins bind to the outer membrane at sites normally occupied by divalent cations, and therefore it is thought that a reduction in these sites will lead to decreased binding of the antibiotic with a consequent decreased susceptibility of the cell.

3.5   Multidrug resistance pumps

Some of the previous sections have described the acquisition of low-level resistance to various antibiotics by alterations in the cell membrane causing decreased uptake of the drugs. These have normally have characterized as changes in components such as porins which result in a decrease of penetration by antibiotics.

Acquired low-level resistance to many unrelated antibiotics by efflux has also increased in prominence in recent years (Cohen *et al.* 1993, George 1996). For example, MAR (multiple antibiotic resistance) mutants were first described in the early 1990s in *E. coli* and were resistant to low levels of chloramphenicol, tetracyclines, rifampicin, penicillins and quinolones, due to impaired uptake of the antibiotics. Increased active efflux of the drugs has been shown to be important in this type of resistance. These efflux pumps are normally regulated and inducible in response to external stimuli, and often mutations causing constitutive expression are responsible for the resistance phenotype. A number of multidrug resistance pumps (MDRs) have been identified and are widespread among bacteria. For example, seven distinct MDRs have been described in *E. coli* alone. The most common type belongs to a group of proteins involved in membrane translocation. This type of MDR is closely related to specific efflux proteins such as that responsible for tetracycline resistance. The origins of MDRs are unknown but a number of factors suggest that they may have arisen by mutations in specific drug efflux pumps causing a loss of specificity. These factors include the similarity of some MDRs to specific drug efflux pumps such as tetracycline, and the high incidence of apparently independent evolution of MDRs.

3.6   Antibiotics with other resistance mechanisms

3.6.1   *Bacitracin*

Acquired resistance to bacitracin has been observed in laboratory strains of *Staph. aureus*, but resistance has been unstable and no resistant mutants have yet been isolated *in vivo*. Gram-negative bacteria are intrinsically resistant to bacitracin, which inhibits the transfer of pentapeptide units to petidoglycan.

3.6.2   *Antimycobacterial drugs*

The advent of multidrug resistant strains of *Mycobacterium tuberculosis* (MDR-TB) has led to increased fears of untreatable infections by serious pathogens. Rifampicin, streptomycin and, occasionally, the quinolones are drugs used in the treatment of mycobacterial infections and resistance to those agents is as described previously. There are some drugs, important in the antimicrobial treatment of tuberculosis, where resistance has arisen in MDR-TB strains, but where the mechanisms are unclear. These drugs include isoniazid, pyrazinamide and ethambutol (Musser 1995).

There are two mechanisms of acquired resistance to isoniazid which have been proposed. The first suggests that mutations in the *katG* gene inhibit the metabolism of isoniazid into an active form which inhibits an essential protein, InhA, in mycobacteria. The mechanism of action of isoniazid remains theoretical and therefore the mechanism of resistance also must remain so. Nevertheless, genetic studies with laboratory strains would tend to support the above. Mutations in the gene *inhA* can also confer isoniazid resistance (and to the related drug ethionamide), presumably by reducing affinity of isoniazid metabolic by-products for InhA. However, clinical strains of *M. tuberculosis* resistant to isoniazid but with unknown mechanisms unrelated to *katG* or *inhA* have been isolated.

Pyrazinamide is a structural analogue of isoniazid and is converted to the active acid derivative intracellularly by a nicotinamidase. Pyrazinamide resistance has been linked to reduced levels of nicotinamidase but the genetic determinants of resistance have not been fully elucidated.

Mutations resulting in ethambutol resistance can arise spontaneously. The exact changes are unknown but may involve enzymes in carbohydrate synthesis pathways.

4 The problem of antibiotic resistance

Antibiotic resistance is becoming a cause for increasing concern and is the most common cause of treatment failure in bacterial infectious diseases (Tenover & Hughes 1996; Tenover & McGowan 1996). Furthermore, infections with antibiotic-resistant bacteria inevitably lead to the use of more expensive and often more toxic drugs, increased length of infection and subsequent hospital stay, and, of course, increased costs. It must be pointed out that at this time, the majority of infections, and particularly those caused by serious pathogens, remain susceptible to standard antibiotic treatment. However, this should not be taken as a signal to relax and ignore the increasing problems encountered in antimicrobial chemotherapy. The advent of MRSA must serve as a warning to be heeded. The ability of this important pathogen to spread within, and between, healthcare institutions is unparalleled, and the consequences to patients in terms of morbidity and mortality can be severe. The emergence of vancomycin-resistant enterococci (VRE) has caused great concern in the medical profession. Vancomycin (or teicoplanin) is often the only antibiotic effective against some MRSA strains. Acquisition of vancomycin resistance by MRSA would leave, for the first time since the introduction of antibiotics, a serious pathogen untreatable with any existing antibiotic. Transfer of vancomycin resistance from VRE to MRSA has already been demonstrated in the laboratory and it is possible the emergence of clinical strains of vancomycin-resistant MRSA will be encountered in the not-too-distant future. Some VRE strains are already resistant to all available antibiotics, but the relatively low virulence of the organism has meant that infections have been confined to seriously ill patients requiring lengthy hospitalization. Other multiply antibiotic-resistant bacteria also cause serious problems in hospitals. These tend to be Gram-negative bacteria, such as *E. coli* or *Klebsiella* spp., but the appearance of these microorganisms tends to be cyclical.

For example, gentamicin-resistant *Klebsiella* spp. caused problems in numerous UK hospitals during the 1980s, but their frequency has decreased in the 1990s, with resistance becoming more problematic in Gram-positive bacteria such as those mentioned above.

The problem is not confined to nosocomial bacteria. Certain community-acquired pathogens have become resistant to key antibiotics in the 1990s. MDR-TB has already been mentioned and the prospect of a resurgence of tuberculosis, especially in a drug-resistant form, is truly frightening. The severity of the infection is particularly acute in immunocompromised patients, such as those with human immunodeficiency virus (HIV). MDR-TB made headline news in the US and affluent European countries but the scale of the problem is several orders of magnitude greater in the developing world. The ease of long-distance travel means that these problems have to be considered globally and not in isolation.

Penicillin resistance in *Strep. pneumoniae* has also emerged in the 1990s. This microorganism is a community-acquired pathogen causing serious diseases such as pneumonia and meningitis. Penicillin is a mainstay in the treatment of infections caused by this bacterium and is often used empirically for urgent treatment when such cases are suspected. The delay in effective antimicrobial chemotherapy caused by infection with a penicillin-resistant strain can often be fatal. The resistance rate in the UK is relatively low, at around 6%, but this represents a significant increase since the 1980s. In some European countries, resistance rates are as much as 40%.

The ability of bacteria to disseminate and acquire antibiotic resistance genes is obviously a major cause of the spread of antibiotic resistance, but the factors involved in the maintenance and evolution of resistance genes must be considered. The single most important cause is selective pressure from the continuing use of antibiotics. Overuse and misuse undoubtedly exacerbate the problem. For example, resistance rates in the UK, which has relatively tight restrictions on the use of antibiotics, are considerably lower than those in countries with more lenient approaches. The preponderance of resistant organisms in healthcare institutions must be due to an environment where exposure to antibiotics is continuous, and therefore hospital-acquired strains would tend to be more resistant than community-acquired strains. The use of antibiotics in hospitals is difficult to control since a medical practitioner confronted with an infection will obviously treat the patient with the best tools at his or her disposal. Nevertheless, certain measures can be implemented to reduce the unnecessary or misguided use of antibiotics. These may include local antibiotic treatment policies, consultation with experts in antimicrobial chemotherapy such as microbiologists or infectious disease physicians, a local formulary with antibiotics restricted to those considered appropriate for the local situation, and effective infection control policies. Measures in the community might include restrictions of antibiotics to prescription-only status, which is the case in the UK, but often not enforced or regulated as tightly in other countries, and rational antibiotic prescribing by general practitioners. It is surprising how often antibiotics are prescribed inappropriately for viral infections such as the common cold or influenza.

The above addresses only part of the problem. The use of antibiotics is rife in areas such as animal husbandry, agriculture, aquaculture and even in the oil industry to prevent spoilage by contaminating microorganisms. A particularly pertinent example is the use of avoparcin in animal feed for many years. Avoparcin is related to the glycopeptides vancomycin and teicoplanin used for the treatment of infections in humans. There is mounting evidence to suggest that enterococci, which are commensals in the gut, have acquired resistance to avoparcin, and therefore cross-resistance to vancomycin and teicoplanin, in animals first due to constant exposure to the antibiotic. Transfer of resistance to human strains has resulted in the emergence of VRE. It seems that the similarities between avoparcin and the other two glycopeptides was not recognized initially because of their application in apparently unconnected areas. The prospect of legislating to avoid such occurrences appears daunting, but attempts must be made because the consequences may be disastrous.

5   Conclusions and comments

Bacterial resistance to antibiotics is often achieved by the constitutive possession or inducibility of drug-inactivating or -modifying enzymes. This problem can, at least to some extent, be overcome by designing new drugs that:

1 are unsusceptible to this enzyme attack; or

2 will inactivate the enzyme concerned thereby protecting susceptible antibiotics that, in the absence of the enzyme, would be highly active antibacterially.

Some degree of success has been achieved in both aspects, but the development of new antibiotics has concentrated on modifications to existing classes of drug rather than using completely novel compounds. The ability of bacteria to evolve mechanisms to surmount these derivatives should surprise us no longer, as the emergence of resistance to all known antibiotics has proved. The variety of resistance mechanisms and their ease of transfer is likely to overwhelm current attempts at producing 'new' antibiotics effective against resistant microorganisms. Rational design of novel antibiotics would require the elucidation of three-dimensional structures of essential bacterial enzymes with clues as to the important functional domains for potential targets.

Another problem concerns the lack of penetration of many drugs into Gram-negative bacteria. On the basis of current knowledge, it would seem logical that any design of new agents should at least consider the need for compounds that can penetrate the outer membrane of these cells even when there is a decrease in porins. In this context, the development of peptides with antibacterial activity is worthy of consideration. These are transported into cells via relatively non-specific permeases. One such example is alaphosphin which is rapidly accumulated by, and concentrated within, bacteria, where it is converted to L-1-aminoethylphosphonic acid which acts as an inhibitor of peptidoglycan synthesis. Alaphosphin belongs to a group of compounds, the phosphonopeptides, which are peptide mimics with C-terminal residues that simulate natural amino acids. Their mechanism of action results from transport into the bacterial cell followed by release of the alanine mimetic. These agents were considered as being an important concept in designing new antibacterially active compounds, but unfortunately these findings do not appear to have been followed by the development of any significant new drugs. There is, however, growing interest in other antibacterial peptides, many of which occur naturally in a wide range of eukaryotic organisms, but their full potential has yet to be established. Despite extensive research, the design of clinically effective antimetabolites seems to have been restricted largely to viruses, with little, if any, research into possible applications to bacteria.

At the present time we are faced with the real and frightening threat of a post-antibiotic era in years to come, where our existing antibiotic arsenal will become largely ineffective against bacterial infections.

6   References

Bush K., Jacoby G.A. & Medeiros A. (1995) A functional classification scheme for β-lactamases and its correlation with molecular structure. *Antimicrob Agents Chemother*, **39**, 1211–1233.

Chopra I., Hawkey P.M. & Hinton M. (1992) Tetracyclines, molecular and clinical aspects. *J Antimicrob Chemother*, **29**, 245–277.

Cohen S.P., Yan W. & Levy S.B. (1993) A multidrug resistance regulatory locus is widespread among enteric bacteria. *J Infect Dis*, **168**, 484–488.

Davies J. (1994) Inactivation of antibiotics and the dissemination of resistance genes. *Science*, **264**, 375–382.

George A.M. (1996) Multidrug resistance in enteric and other Gram-negative bacteria. *FEMS Microbiol Lett*, **139**, 1–10.

Georgopapadakou N.H. (1993) Penicillin-binding proteins and bacterial resistance to β-lactams. *Antimicrob Agents Chemother*, **37**, 2045–2053.

Gilbart J., Perry C.R. & Slocombe B. (1993) High-level mupirocin resistance in *Staphylococcus aureus*: evidence for two distinct isoleucyl-tRNA synthetases. *Antimicrob Agents Chemother*, **37**, 32–38.

Godfrey A.J. & Bryan L.E. (1984) Intrinsic resistance and whole cell factors contributing to antibiotic resistance. In: *Antimicrobial Drug Resistance* (ed. L.E. Bryan), pp. 113–145. New York: Academic Press.

Hooper D.C. & Wolfson J.S. (eds) (1993) *Quinolone Antimicrobial Agents*. Washington: American Society for Microbiology.

Huovinen P., Sundstrom L., Swedberg G. & Skold O. (1995) Trimethoprim and sulphonamide resistance. *Antimicrob Agents Chemother*, **39**, 279–289.

Leclerq R. & Courvalin P. (1991) Bacterial resistance to macrolide, lincosamide and streptogramin antibiotics by target modification. *Antimicrob Agents Chemother*, **35**, 1267–1272.

Lewis M.J. (1989) The genetics of resistance. In: *Antimicrobial Chemotherapy* (ed. D. Greenwood), 2nd edn, pp. 146–152. Oxford: Oxford University Press.

Musser J.M. (1995) Antimicrobial agent resistance in mycobacteria: molecular genetic insights. *Clin Microbiol Rev*, **8**, 496–514.

Power E.G.M. & Russell A.D. (1998) Design of antimicrobial chemotherapeutic agents. In *Introduction to Principles of Drug Design* (ed. H.J. Smith), 3rd edn, London: Gordon & Breach.

Russell A.D. & Chopra I. (eds) (1996) *Understanding Antibacterial Action and Resistance*. London: Ellis Horwood.

Sanders C.C. (1992) β-lactamases of Gram-negative bacteria: new challenges for new drugs. *Clin Infect Dis*, **14**, 1089–1099.

Shaw K.J., Rather P.N., Hare R.S. & Miller G.H. (1993) Molecular genetics of aminoglycoside resistance genes and familial relationships of the aminoglycoside-modifying enzymes. *Microbiol Rev*, **57**, 138–163.

Tenover F.C. & Hughes J.M. (1996) The challenges of emerging infectious diseases. Development and spread of multiplty resistant bacterial pathogens. *J Am Med Assoc*, **275**, 300–304.

Tenover F.C. & McGowan J.E., Jr. (1996) Reasons for the emergence of antibiotic resistance. *Am J Med Sci*, **311**, 9–16.

Woodford N., Johnson A.P., Morrison D. & Speller D.C. (1995) Current perspectives on glycopeptide resistance. *Clin Microbiol Rev*, **8**, 585–615.

10 Chemical disinfectants, antiseptics and preservatives

1   Introduction

2   Factors affecting choice of antimicrobial agent
2.1   Properties of the chemical agent
2.2   Microbiological challenge
2.2.1   Vegetative bacteria
2.2.2   *Mycobacterium tuberculosis*
2.2.3   Bacterial spores
2.2.4   Fungi
2.2.5   Viruses
2.2.6   Protozoa
2.2.7   Prions
2.3   Intended application
2.4   Environmental factors
2.5   Toxicity of the agent

3   Types of compound
3.1   Acids and esters
3.1.1   Benzoic acid
3.1.2   Sorbic acid
3.1.3   Sulphur dioxide, sulphites and metabisulphites
3.1.4   Esters of *p*-hydroxybenzoic acid (parabens)
3.2   Alcohols
3.2.1   Alcohols used for disinfection and antisepsis
3.2.2   Alcohols as preservatives
3.3   Aldehydes
3.3.1   Glutaraldehyde
3.3.2   Formaldehyde

3.3.3   Formaldehyde-releasing agents
3.4   Biguanides
3.4.1   Chlorhexidine and alexidine
3.4.2   Polyhexamethylene biguanides
3.5   Halogens
3.5.1   Chlorine
3.5.2   Hypochlorites
3.5.3   Organic chlorine compounds
3.5.4   Chloroform
3.5.5   Iodine
3.5.6   Iodophors
3.6   Heavy metals
3.6.1   Mercurials
3.7   Hydrogen peroxide and peroxygen compounds
3.8   Phenols
3.8.1   Phenol (carbolic acid)
3.8.2   Tar acids
3.8.3   Non-coal tar phenols (chloroxylenol and chlorocresol)
3.8.4   Bisphenols
3.9   Surface-active agents
3.9.1   Cationic surface-active agents
3.10   Other antimicrobials
3.10.1   Diamidines
3.10.2   Dyes
3.10.3   Quinoline derivatives
3.11   Antimicrobial combinations

4   Disinfection policies

5   Further reading

1   Introduction

Disinfectants, antiseptics and preservatives are chemicals which have the ability to destroy or inhibit the growth of microorganisms and which are used for this purpose.

Disinfectants. Disinfection is the process of removing microorganisms, including potentially pathogenic ones, from the surfaces of inanimate objects. The British Standards Institution further defines disinfection as not necessarily killing all microorganisms, but reducing them to a level acceptable for a defined purpose, for example a level which is harmful neither to health nor to the quality of perishable goods. Chemical disinfectants are capable of different levels of action. The term high level disinfection indicates destruction of all microorganisms but not necessarily bacterial spores; intermediate level disinfection indicates destruction of all vegetative bacteria including

Mycobacterium tuberculosis but may exclude some viruses and fungi and have little or no sporicidal activity; low level disinfection can destroy most vegetative bacteria, fungi and viruses, but this will not include spores and some of the more resistant microorganisms. Some high level disinfectants have good sporicidal activity and have been ascribed the name 'liquid chemical sterilant' or 'chemosterilant' to indicate that they can effect a complete kill of all microorganisms, as in sterilization.

Antiseptics. Antisepsis is defined as destruction or inhibition of microorganisms on living tissues having the effect of limiting or preventing the harmful results of infection. It is *not* a synomym for disinfection (British Standards Institution). The chemicals used are applied to skin and mucous membranes, therefore as well as having adequate antimicrobial activity, they must not be toxic or irritating for skin. Antiseptics are mostly used to reduce the microbial population on the skin prior to surgery or on the hands to help prevent spread of infection by this route. Antiseptics are often lower concentrations of the agents used for disinfection.

Preservatives. These are included in pharmaceutical preparations to prevent microbial spoilage of the product and to minimize the risk of the consumer acquiring an infection when the preparation is administered. Preservatives must be able to limit proliferation of microorganisms that may be introduced unavoidably during manufacture and use of non-sterile products such as oral and topical medications. In sterile products such as eye drops and multidose injections, preservatives should kill any microbial contaminants introduced inadvertently during use. It is essential that a preservative is not toxic in relation to the intended route of administration of the preserved preparation. Preservatives therefore tend to be employed at low concentrations and consequently levels of antimicrobial action also tend to be of a lower order than for disinfectants or antiseptics. This is illustrated by the requirements of the *British Pharmacopoeia* (1993) for preservative efficacy where a degree of bactericidal activity is necessary, although this should be obtained within a few hours or over several days of microbial challenge depending on the type of product to be preserved.

Other terms are considered in Chapter 11 (see section 1.1 and Fig. 11.1).

There are around 250 chemical entities that have been identified as active components of microbiocidal products in the European Union. The aim of this chapter is to introduce the range of chemicals in common use and to indicate their activities and applications.

2 Factors affecting choice of antimicrobial agent

Choice of the most appropriate antimicrobial compound for a particular purpose depends on:
1 properties of the chemical agent;
2 microbiological challenge;
3 intended application;
4 environmental factors;
5 toxicity of the agent.

2.1   Properties of the chemical agent

The process of killing or inhibiting the growth of microorganisms using an antimicrobial agent is basically that of a chemical reaction, and the rate and extent of this reaction will be influenced by the factors of concentration of chemical, temperature, pH and formulation. The influence of these factors on activity is discussed fully in Chapter 11 and is referred to in discussing the individual agents. Tissue toxicity influences whether a chemical can be used as an antiseptic or preservative and this unfortunately limits the range of chemicals for these applications or necessitates the use of lower concentrations of the chemical.

2.2   Microbiological challenge

The types of microorganism present and the levels of microbial contamination (the bioburden) both have a significant effect on the outcome of chemical treatment. If the bioburden is high, long exposure times or higher concentrations of antimicrobial may be required. Microorganisms vary in their sensitivity to the action of chemical agents. Some organisms, either because of their resistance to disinfection (for further discussion see Chapter 13) or because of their significance in cross-infection or nosocomial (hospital acquired) infections, merit attention.

The efficacy of an antimicrobial agent must be investigated by appropriate capacity, challenge and in-use tests to ensure that a standard is obtained which is appropriate to the intended use (Chapter 11). In practice, it is not usually possible to know which organisms are present on the articles being treated. Thus, it is necessary to categorize chemicals according to their antimicrobial capabilities and for the user to have an awareness of what level of antimicrobial action is required in a particular situation (Table 10.1).

Table 10.1 Levels of disinfection attainable

	Disinfection level		
	Low	Intermediate	High
Microorganisms killed	Most vegetative bacteria Some viruses Some fungi	Most vegetative bacteria including *M. tuberculosis* Most viruses including hepatitis B virus (HBV) Most fungi	All microorganisms unless extreme challenge or resistance exhibited
Microorganisms surviving	*M. tuberculosis* Bacterial spores HBV and prions as in Creutzfeldt–Jakob disease	Bacterial spores Prions	Extreme challenge of resistant bacterial spores Prions? (insufficient data)

2.2.1   Vegetative bacteria

At in-use concentrations, chemicals used for disinfection should be capable of killing most vegetative bacteria within a reasonable contact period. This includes 'problem' organisms such as *Listeria*, *Campylobacter*, *Legionella* and methicillin-resistant *Staphylococcus aureus* (MRSA). Antiseptics and preservatives are also expected to have a broad spectrum of antimicrobial activity but at the in-use concentrations, after exerting an initial biocidal effect, their main function may be biostatic. Gram-negative bacilli, which are the main causes of nosocomial infections, are often more resistant than Gram-positive species. *Pseudomonas aeruginosa*, an opportunistic pathogen (i.e. is pathogenic if the opportunity arises; see also Chapter 1), has gained a reputation as the most resistant of the Gram-negative organisms. However, problems mainly arise when a number of additional factors such as heavily soiled articles or diluted or degraded solutions are involved.

2.2.2   Mycobacterium tuberculosis

Mycobacterium tuberculosis (the tubercle bacillus) and other mycobacteria are resistant to many bactericides. Resistance is either (a) intrinsic, mainly due to reduced cellular permeability or (b) acquired, due to mutation or possibly the acquisition of plasmids, although this has yet to be shown: see also Chapter 13. Tuberculosis remains an important public health hazard, and indeed the annual number of tuberculosis cases is rising in many countries. The greatest risk of acquiring infection is from the undiagnosed patient. Equipment used for respiratory investigations can become contaminated with mycobacteria if the patient is a carrier of this organism. It is important to be able to disinfect the equipment to a safe level to prevent transmission of infection to other patients (Table 10.2). A synergistic mixture of alkyl polyguanides and alkyl quaternaries has recently been shown to be more effective than glutaraldehyde against *M. tuberculosis* and *M. avium-intracellulare* (see also section 3.11).

2.2.3   Bacterial spores

Bacterial spores are the most resistant of all microbial forms to chemical treatment. The majority of antimicrobial agents have no useful sporicidal action, with the exception of the aldehydes, halogens and peroxygen compounds. Such chemicals are sometimes used as an alternative to physical methods for sterilization of heat sensitive equipment. In these circumstances, correct usage of the agent is of paramount importance since safety margins are lower in comparison with physical methods of sterilization (Chapter 20).

The antibacterial activity of disinfectants and antiseptics is summarized in Table 10.2.

2.2.4   Fungi

The vegetative fungal form is often as sensitive as vegetative bacteria to antimicrobial agents. Fungal spores (conidia and chlamydospores; see Chapter 2) may be more

Table 10.2 Antibacterial activity of commonly used disinfectants and antiseptics

Class of compound	Activity against: Mycobacteria	Bacterial spores	General level* of antibacterial activity
Alcohols			
Ethanol/isopropyl	+	–	Intermediate
Aldehydes			
Glutaraldehyde	+	+	High
Formaldehyde	+	+	High
Biguanides			
Chlorhexidine	–	–	Intermediate
Halogens			
Hypochlorite/ chloramines	+	+	High
Iodine/iodophor	+	+	Intermediate, problems with *Ps. aeruginosa*
Peroxygens			
Peracetic acid	+	+	High
Hydrogen peroxide	+	–	Intermediate
Phenolics			
Clear soluble fluids	+	–	High
Chloroxylenol	–	–	Low
Bisphenols	–	–	Low, poor against *Ps. aeruginosa*
Quaternary ammonium compounds			
Benzalkonium	–	–	Intermediate
Cetrimide	–	–	Intermediate

* Activity will depend on concentration, time of contact, temperature, etc. (see Chapter 11) but these are activities expected if in-use concentrations were being employed.

resistant but this resistance is of much lesser magnitude than for bacterial spores. The ability to rapidly destroy pathogenic fungi such as the opportunistic yeast, *Candida albicans*, and filamentous fungi such as *Trichophyton mentagrophytes*, and spores of common spoilage moulds such as *Aspergillus niger*, is put to advantage in many applications of use. Many disinfectants have good activity against these fungi (Table 10.3).

2.2.5   *Viruses*

Susceptibility of viruses to antimicrobial agents can depend on whether the viruses possess a lipid envelope. Non-lipid viruses are frequently more resistant to disinfectants and it is also likely that such viruses cannot be readily categorized with respect to their sensitivities to antimicrobial agents. These viruses are responsible for many nosocomial infections, e.g. rotaviruses, picornaviruses and adenoviruses (see Chapter 3), and it may be necessary to select an antiseptic or disinfectant to suit specific circumstances. Certain viruses, such as Ebola and Marburg which cause haemorrhagic fevers, are highly infectious and their safe destruction by disinfectants is of paramount importance.

Table 10.3 Antifungal activity of disinfectants and antiseptics (adapted from Scott *et al.* 1986)

Antimicrobial agent	Time (min) to give >99.99% kill* of		
	Aspergillus niger	*Trichophyton mentagrophytes*	*Candida albicans*
Phenolic (0.36%)	<2	<2	<2
Chlorhexidine gluconate (0.02%, alcoholic)	<2	<2	<2
Iodine (1%, alcoholic)	<2	<2	<2
Povidone-iodine (10%, alcoholic and aqueous)	10	<2	<2
Hypochlorite (0.2%)	10	<2	5
Cetrimide (1%)	<2	20	<2
Chlorhexidine gluconate (0.05%) + cetrimide (0.5%)	20	>20	>2
Chlorhexidine gluconate (0.5%, aqueous)	20	>20	>2

* Initial viable counts were *ca.* 1×10^6.

There is much concern for the safety of personnel handling articles contaminated with pathogenic viruses such as hepatitis B virus (HBV) and human immunodeficiency virus (HIV) which causes acquired immune deficiency syndrome (AIDS). Some agents have been recommended for disinfection of HBV and HIV depending on the circumstances and level of contamination; these are listed in Table 10.4. Disinfectants must be able to treat rapidly and reliably accidental spills of blood, body fluids or secretions from HIV infected patients. Such spills may contain levels of HIV as high as 10^4 infectious units/ml. Recent evidence from the Medical Devices Agency evaluation of disinfectants against HIV indicated that few chemicals could destroy the virus in a

Table 10.4 Chemical disinfection of human immunodeficiency virus (HIV) and hepatitis B virus (HBV). Adapted from ACDP (1990) and Anon (1991)

Disinfecting agent	Application	Comment
Chlorine-releasing preparations, e.g. hypochlorite 10 000 ppm av. Cl_2, at least 30 min at room temperature	Spillage of HIV contaminated blood and body fluid	Use fresh solution Deteriorates on storage and may be adversely affected by organic matter
Hypochlorite 1000 ppm av. Cl_2	Minor contamination of inanimate surfaces	Corrosive to metals Bleaches fabrics
Aldehydes, e.g. glutaraldehyde 2% (w/v), 30 min at room temperature	Reserved for non-corrosive treatment of delicate items	Must be freshly activated Not recommended for surface decontamination due to vapour toxicity (see Table 10.5)
Alcohol 70% ethanol, at least 2 min for HIV but evaporation a problem	Limited application	Use alternative if possible as activity in presence of protein questionable

short time in the presence of high serum levels; only two of 13 products (glutaraldehyde and dichloroisocyanurate) were effective under the most stringent test conditions.

The virucidal activity of chemicals is difficult to determine in the laboratory. Tissue culture techniques are the most common methods for growing and estimating viruses; however, antimicrobial agents may also adversely affect the tissue culture: see also Chapter 11.

2.2.6 Protozoa

Acanthamoeba spp. can cause acanthamoeba keratitis with associated corneal scarring and loss of vision in soft contact lens wearers. The cysts of this protozoan, in particular, present a problem in respect of lens disinfection. The chlorine-generating systems in use are generally inadequate. Although polyhexamethylene biguanide shows promise as an acanthamoebacide, only hydrogen peroxide-based disinfection is considered completely reliable and consistent in producing an acanthomoebacidal effect.

2.2.7 Prions

Prions (small proteinaceous infectious particles, also known as unconventional slow viruses) are a unique class of infectious agent associated with causing spongiform encephalopathies such as bovine spongiform encephalopathy (BSE) in cattle and Creutzfeldt Jakob disease (CJD) in humans. There is considerable concern about the transmission of these agents from infected animals or patients. Risk of infectivity is highest in brain and spinal cord tissues. There are still many unknown factors regarding destruction of prions. It appears that they are resistant to most disinfectant procedures and that autoclaving or exposure to 1 N sodium hydroxide is required for decontamination. However, current advice is to destroy surgical instruments where procedures involve brain, spinal cord or eye in patients with confirmed or suspected CJD.

2.3 Intended application

The intended application of an antimicrobial agent, whether for preservation, antisepsis or disinfection, will influence its selection and also affect its performance. For example, in medicinal preparations the ingredients in the formulation may antagonize preservative activity. The risk to the patient will depend on whether the antimicrobial is in close contact with a break in the skin or mucous membranes or is introduced into a sterile area of the body.

In disinfection of instruments, the chemicals used must not adversely affect the instruments, e.g. cause corrosion of metals, affect clarity or integrity of lenses, or change texture of synthetic polymers. Many materials such as fabrics, rubber, plastics are capable of adsorbing certain disinfectants, e.g. quaternary ammonium compounds (QACs), are adsorbed by fabrics, while phenolics are adsorbed by rubber, the consequence of this being a reduction in concentration of active compound. A disinfectant can only exert its effect if it is in contact with the item being treated. Therefore access to all parts of an instrument or piece of equipment is essential. For small items, total immersion in the disinfectant must also be ensured.

2.4 Environmental factors

Organic matter can have a drastic effect on antimicrobial activity either by adsorption or chemical inactivation, thus reducing the concentration of active agent in solution or by acting as a barrier to the penetration of the disinfectant. Blood, body fluids, pus, milk, food residues or colloidal proteins, even present in small amounts, all reduce the effectiveness of antimicrobial agents to varying degrees and some are seriously affected. In their normal habitats, microorganisms have a tendency to adhere to surfaces and are thus less accessible to the chemical agent. Some organisms are specific to certain environments and their destruction will be of paramount importance in the selection of a suitable agent, e.g. *Legionella* in cooling towers and non-potable water supply systems, *Listeria* in the dairy and food industry and hepatitis in blood-contaminated articles.

Dried organic deposits may inhibit penetration of the chemical agent. Where possible, objects to be disinfected should be thoroughly cleaned. The presence of ions in water can also affect activity of antimicrobial agents, thus water for testing biocidal activity can be made artificially 'hard' by addition of ions.

These factors can have very significant effects on activity and are summarized in Table 10.5.

2.5 Toxicity of the agent

In choosing an antimicrobial agent for a particular application some consideration must be given to its toxicity. Increasing concern for health and safety is reflected in the Control of Substances Hazardous to Health (COSHH) Regulations which specify the precautions required in handling toxic or potentially toxic agents. In respect of disinfectant use these regulations affect, particularly, the use of phenolics, formaldehyde and glutaraldehyde. Toxic volatile substances, in general, should be kept in covered containers to reduce the level of exposure to irritant vapour and they should be used with an extractor facility. Limits governing the exposure of individuals to such substances are now listed, e.g. $0.7 \, \text{mg/m}^3$ (0.2 ppm) glutaraldehyde for both short- and long-term exposure. The aldehydes, glutaraldehyde less so than formaldehyde, may affect the eyes and skin (causing contact dermatitis), and may induce respiratory distress. Face protection and impermeable nitrile rubber gloves should be worn when using these agents. Table 10.5 lists the toxicity of many of the disinfectants in use and other concerns of toxicity are described for individual agents below.

Where the atmosphere of a workplace is likely to be contaminated, sampling and analysis of the atmosphere may need to be carried out on a periodic basis with a frequency determined by conditions.

3 Types of compound

The following section presents in alphabetical order by chemical grouping the agents most often employed for disinfection, antisepsis and preservation. This information is summarized in Table 10.6.

Table 10.5 Properties of commonly used disinfectants and antiseptics

Class of compound	Effect of organic matter	pH optimum	Toxicity and OES*	Other factors
Alcohols Ethanol	Slight		Avoid broken skin, eyes OES: 1000 ppm/1900 mg m^{-3}, 8 h only	Poor penetration, good cleansing properties
Aldehydes Glutaraldehyde	Slight	pH 8	Respiratory complaints and contact dermatitis reported Eyes, sensitivity OES: 0.2 ppm/0.7 mg m^{-3}, 10 min only	Non-corrosive, useful for heat sensitive instruments
Biguanides Chlorhexidine	Severe	pH 7–8	Avoid contact with eyes and mucous membranes Sensitivity may develop	Incompatible with soap and anionic detergents Inactivated by hard water, some materials and plastic
Chlorine compounds Hypochlorite	Severe	Acid/neutral pH	Irritation of skin, eyes and lungs OES: 1 ppm/3 mg m^{-3}, 10 min; 0.5 ppm/1.5 mg m^{-3}, 8 h	Corrosive to metals
Iodine preparations Iodophors	Severe	Acid pH	Eye irritation OES: 0.1 ppm/1 mg m^{-3}, 10 min only	May corrode metals
Phenolics Clear soluble fluids Black/white fluids Chloroxylenol	Slight Moderate/severe Severe	Acid pH	Protect skin and eyes Very irritant Sensitivity. May irritate skin OES: 10 ppm/38 mg m^{-3}, 10 min; 5 ppm/19 mg m^{-3}, 8 h	Adsorbed by rubber/plastic Greatly reduced by dilution Adsorbed by rubber/plastic
QACs Cetrimide and benzalkonium Chloride	Severe	Alkaline pH	Avoid contact with eyes	Incompatible with soap and anionic detergents Adsorbed by fabrics

* From the *Control of Substances Hazardous to Health (COSHH) Regulations* (1988).
OES, occupational exposure standard; QAC, quaternary ammonium compound.

Table 10.6 Examples of the main antimicrobial groups as antiseptics, disinfectants and preservatives

Antimicrobial agent	Antiseptic activity		Disinfectant Activity		Preservative activity	
	Concentration	Typical formulation/application	Concentration	Typical formulation/application	Concentration	Typical formulation/application
Acids and esters, e.g. benzoic acid, parabens					0.05–0.1% 0.25%	For oral and topical formulations
Alcohols, e.g. ethyl or isopropyl	50–90% in water	Skin prep.	50–90% in water	Clean surface prep., thermometers		
Aldehydes, e.g. glutaraldehyde	10%	Gel for warts	2.0%	Solution for instruments		
Biguanides, e.g. chlorhexidine† (gluconate, acetate etc)	0.02% 0.2% 0.5% (in 70% alcohol) 1.0% 4.0%	Bladder irrigation Mouthwash Skin prep. Dusting powder, cream dental gel Pre-op. scrub in surfactant	0.05% 0.5% (in 70% alcohol)	Storage of instruments, clean instrument disinfection (30 min) Emergency instrument disinfection (2 min)	0.0025% 0.01%	Solution for hard contact lenses Eye-drops
Chlorine, e.g. hypoclorite	≤0.5% avCl$_2$	Solution for skin and wounds	1–10%	Solution for surfaces and instruments		
Hydrogen peroxide	1.5% 3–6%	Stabilized cream Solution for wounds and ulcers, mouthwash	3.0%	Disinfection of soft contact lenses		

Compound				
Iodine compounds, e.g. free iodine, povidone-iodine	1.0%	Aqueous or alcoholic (70%) solution	10.0%	Aqueous or alc. solution
	1.0%	Mouthwash		
	2.5%	Dry powder spray		
	7.5%	Scalp and skin cleanser		
	10%	Pre-op. scrub, fabric dressing		
Phenolics, e.g. tar acids (clear soluble phenolics), non-coal tar (chloroxylenol), bisphenol (triclosan)	0.5%	Dusting powder	1–2%	Solution
	1.3%	Solution		
	2.0%	Skin cleanser		
QACs, e.g. cetyltrimethyl ammonium bromide (cetrimide)	0.1%	Solution for wounds and burns	0.1%	Storage or sterile instruments
	0.5%	Cream	1.0%	Instruments (1 h)
	1.0%	Skin solution	0.01%	Eye-drops

* Also used in combination with other agents e.g. chlorhexidine, iodine.

† Several forms available having $x\%$ chlorhexidine and $10x\%$ cetrimide.

QAC, quaternary ammonium compound.

3.1 Acids and esters

Antimicrobial activity, within a pharmaceutical context, is generally found only in the organic acids. These are weak acids and will therefore dissociate incompletely to give the three entities HA, H^+ and A^- in solution. As the undissociated form, HA, is the active antimicrobial agent, the ionization constant, K_a, is important and the pK_a of the acid must be considered especially in formulation of the agent.

3.1.1 Benzoic acid

This is an organic acid, C_6H_5COOH, which is included, alone or in combination with other preservatives, in many pharmaceuticals. Although the compound is often used as the sodium salt, the non-ionized acid is the active substance. A limitation on its use is imposed by the pH of the final product as the pK_a of benzoic acid is 4.2 at which pH 50% of the acid is ionized. It is advisable to limit use of the acid to preservation of pharmaceuticals having a maximum final pH of 5.0 and if possible less than 4.0. Concentrations of 0.05–0.1% are suitable for oral preparations. A disadvantage of the compound is the development of resistance by some organisms, involving in some cases metabolism of the acid resulting in complete loss of activity. Benzoic acid also has some use in combination with other agents, salicylic acid among others, in the treatment of superficial fungal infections.

3.1.2 Sorbic acid

This compound is a widely used preservative as the acid or its potassium salt. The pK_a is 4.8 and, as with benzoic acid, activity decreases with increasing pH and ionization. It is most effective at pH 4 or below. Pharmaceutical products such as gums, mucilages and syrups are usefully preserved with this agent.

3.1.3 Sulphur dioxide, sulphites and metabisulphites

Sulphur dioxide has extensive use as a preservative in the food and beverage industries. In a pharmaceutical context, sodium sulphite and metabisulphite or bisulphite have a dual role acting as preservatives and antioxidants.

3.1.4 Esters of p-hydroxybenzoic acid (parabens)

A series of alkyl esters (Fig. 10.1) of p(4)-hydroxybenzoic acid was originally prepared to overcome the marked pH-dependence on activity of the acids.

These parabens, the methyl, ethyl, propyl and butyl esters, are less readily ionized having pK_a values in the range 8–8.5 and exhibit good preservative activity even at pH

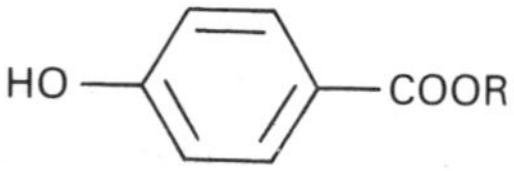

Fig. 10.1 p-Hydroxybenzoates (R is methyl, ethyl, propyl, butyl or benzyl).

levels of 7–8, although optimum activity is again displayed in acidic solutions. This broader pH range allows extensive and successful use of the parabens as pharmaceutical preservatives. The agents are active against a wide range of fungi but are less active against bacteria, especially the pseudomonads which may utilize the parabens as a carbon source. They are frequently used as preservatives of emulsions, creams and lotions where two phases exist. Combinations of esters are most successful for this type of product in that the more water-soluble methyl ester (0.25%) protects the aqueous phase whereas the propyl or butyl esters (0.02%) give protection to the oil phase. Such combinations are also considered to extend the range of activity. As inactivation of parabens occurs with non-ionic surfactants, due care should be taken in formulation of these.

3.2   Alcohols

3.2.1   *Alcohols used for disinfection and antisepsis*

The aliphatic alcohols, notably ethanol and isopropanol, which are used for disinfection and antisepsis, are bactericidal against vegetative forms, including *Mycobacterium* spp., but are not sporicidal. Alcohols have poor penetration of organic matter and their use is therefore restricted to clean conditions. They possess properties such as a cleansing action and volatility, are able to achieve a rapid and large reduction in skin flora and have been widely used for skin preparation prior to injection or other surgical procedures. However, the contact time of an alcohol-soaked swab with the skin prior to venepuncture is so brief that it is thought to be of doubtful value.

Ethanol (CH_3CH_2OH) is widely used as a disinfectant and antiseptic. The presence of water is essential for activity, hence 100% ethanol is ineffective. Concentrations between 60 and 95% are bactericidal but a 70% solution is usually employed for the disinfection of skin, clean instruments or surfaces. At higher concentrations, e.g. 90%, ethanol is also active against most viruses, including HIV. Ethanol is also a popular choice in pharmaceutical preparations and cosmetic products as a solvent and preservative.

Isopropyl alcohol (isopropanol, $CH_3CHOH.CH_3$) has slightly greater bactericidal activity than that of ethanol but is also about twice as toxic. It is less active against viruses, particularly non-enveloped viruses, and should be considered a limited-spectrum virucide. Used at concentrations of 60–70%, it is an acceptable alternative to ethanol for preoperative skin treatment and is also employed as a preservative for cosmetics.

3.2.2   *Alcohols as preservatives*

The aralkyl alcohols and more highly substituted aliphatic alcohols (Fig. 10.2) are used mostly as preservatives. These include:

1   Benzyl alcohol ($C_6H_5CH_2OH$). This has antibacterial and weak local anaesthetic properties and is used as an antimicrobial preservative at a concentration of 2%, although its use in cosmetics is restricted.

2   Chlorbutol (trichlorobutanol; trichloro-*t*-butanol; trichlorobutanol). Typical in-use concentration: 0.5%. It has been used as a preservative in injections and eyedrops. It is

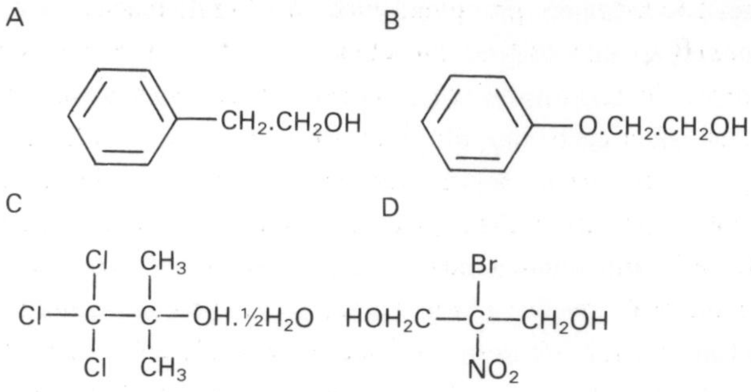

Fig. 10.2 Structural formulae of alcohols used in preserving and disinfection: A, 2-phenylethanol; B, 2-phenoxyethanol; C, chlorbutol (trichloro-*t*-butanol); D, Bronopol (2-bromo-2-nitropropan-1,3-diol).

unstable, decomposition occurring at acid pH during autoclaving, while alkaline solutions are unstable at room temperature.

3 Phenylethanol (phenylethyl alcohol; 2-phenylethanol). Typical in-use concentration: 0.25–0.5%. It is reported to have greater activity against Gram-negative organisms and is usually employed in conjunction with another agent.

4 Phenoxyethanol (2-phenoxyethanol). Typical in-use concentration: 1%. It is more active against *Ps. aeruginosa* than against other bacteria and is usually combined with other preservatives such as the hydroxybenzoates to broaden the spectrum of antimicrobial activity.

5 Bronopol (2-bromo-2-nitropropano-1,3-diol). Typical in-use concentration: 0.01–0.1%. It has a broad spectrum of antibacterial activity, including activity against *Pseudomonas* spp. The main limitation on the use of bronopol is that when exposed to light at alkaline pH, especially if accompanied by an increase in temperature, solutions decompose, turning yellow or brown. A number of decomposition products including formaldehyde are produced. In addition, nitrite ions may be produced and react with any secondary and tertiary amines present forming nitrosamines, which are potentially carcinogenic.

3.3 Aldehydes

A number of aldehydes possess antimicrobial properties, including sporicidal activity; however, only two, formaldehyde and glutaraldehyde, are used for disinfection. Both these aldehydes are highly effective biocides and their use as 'chemosterilants' reflect this.

3.3.1 *Glutaraldehyde*

Glutaraldehyde ($CHO(CH_2)_3CHO$) has a broad spectrum of antimicrobial activity and rapid rate of kill, most vegetative bacteria being killed within a minute of exposure, although bacterial spores may require 3 hours or more. The latter depends on the intrinsic resistance of spores which may vary widely. It has the further advantage of not being affected significantly by organic matter. The glutaraldehyde molecule possesses two aldehyde groupings which are highly reactive and their presence is an important component of biocidal activity. The monomeric molecule is in equilibrium with polymeric forms, and the physical conditions of temperature and pH have a significant effect on this equilibrium. At a pH of 8, biocidal activity is greatest but stability is poor due to polymerization. By contrast, acid solutions are stable but considerably less active, although as temperature is increased, there is a breakdown in the polymeric forms which exist in acid solutions and a concomitant increase in free active dialdehyde, resulting in better activity. In practice, glutaraldehyde is generally supplied as an acidic 2% aqueous solution, which is stable on prolonged storage. This is then 'activated' prior to use by addition of a suitable alkylating agent to bring the pH of the solution to its optimum for activity. The activated solution will have a limited shelf-life, in the order of 2 weeks, although more stable formulations are available. Glutaraldehyde is employed mainly for the cold, liquid chemical sterilization of medical and surgical materials that cannot be sterilized by other methods. Endoscopes, including for example, arthroscopes, laparoscopes, cystoscopes and bronchoscopes may be decontaminated by glutaraldehyde treatment. Contact times employed in practice for high level disinfection are often considerably less than the many hours recommended by manufacturers to achieve sterilization. The British Association of Urological Surgeons recommends that cystoscopes be routinely immersed for at least 10 minutes but that this should be increased to 1 hour if mycobacterial infection is known or suspected. Similarly, the British Thoracic Society recommends immersion of bronchoscopes for 20 minutes between immunocompetent patients one hour with immunocompromised patients to avoid opportunistic mycobacteria. Whilst *M. tuberculosis* is successfully eliminated from instruments after 1 hour with 2% glutaraldehyde, *M. avium-intracellulare* strains take much longer to inactivate as they are as much as 12 times more resistant to glutaraldehyde than *M. tuberculosis*. Gastroscopes from HIV-positive patients are required by the British Society of Gastroenterology to be immersed in 2% glutaraldehyde for 1 hour.

3.3.2 *Formaldehyde*

Formaldehyde (HCHO) can be used in either the liquid or gaseous state for disinfection purposes. In the vapour phase it has been used for decontamination of safety cabinets and rooms; however, recent trends have been to combine formaldehyde vapour with low temperature steam (LTSF) for the sterilization of heat-sensitive items (Chapter 20). Formaldehyde vapour is highly toxic and potentially carcinogenic if inhaled, thus its use must be carefully controlled. It is not very active at temperatures below 20°C and requires a relative humidity of at least 70%. The agent is not supplied as a gas but as either a solid polymer, paraformaldehyde, or a liquid, formalin, which is a 34–38% aqueous solution. The gas is liberated by heating or mixing the solid or liquid with potassium permanganate and water. Formalin, diluted 1:10 to give 4% formaldehyde, may be used for disinfecting surfaces. In general, however, solutions of either aqueous or alcoholic formaldehyde are too irritant for routine application to skin, while poor penetration and a tendency to polymerize on surfaces limit its use as a disinfectant.

Formaldehyde-releasing agents

Various formaldehyde condensates have been developed to reduce the irritancy associated with formaldehyde while maintaining activity and these are described as formaldehyde-releasing agents or masked-formaldehyde compounds.

Of these, noxythiolin (*N*-hydroxy-*N*-methylthiourea) has the greatest pharmaceutical use as an antimicrobial agent. The compound is supplied as a dry powder and on aqueous reconstitution slowly releases formaldehyde and *N*-methylthiourea. Antimicrobial activity is considered to be due to both the noxythiolin molecule and the released formaldehyde. Noxythiolin is used both topically and in accessible body cavities as an irrigation solution and in the treatment of peritonitis. The compound has extensive antibacterial and antifungal properties.

Polynoxylin (poly[methylenedi(hydroxymethyl)urea]) is a similar compound available in gel and lozenge formulations.

Taurolidine (bis-[1,1-dioxoperhydro-1,2,4-thiadiazinyl-4] methane) is a condensate of two molecules of the amino acid taurine and three molecules of formaldehyde. It is more stable than noxythiolin in solution and has similar uses. The activity of taurolidine is stated to be greater than that of formaldehyde.

3.4 Biguanides

3.4.1   *Chlorhexidine and alexidine*

Chlorhexidine is an antimicrobial agent first synthesized at Imperial Chemical Industries in 1954 in a research program to produce compounds related to the biguanide antimalarial, proguanil. Compounds containing the biguanide structure could be expected to have good antibacterial effect; thus, the major part of the proguanil structure is found in chlorhexidine. The chlorhexidine molecule, a bisbiguanide, is symmetric. A hexamethylene chain links two biguanide groups to each of which a *p*-chlorophenyl radical is bound (Fig. 10.3). A related compound is the bisbiguanide alexidine which has use as an oral antiseptic and antiplaque agent. Alexidine (Fig. 10.3A) differs from chlorhexidine (Fig. 10.3B) in that it possesses ethylhexyl end-groups.

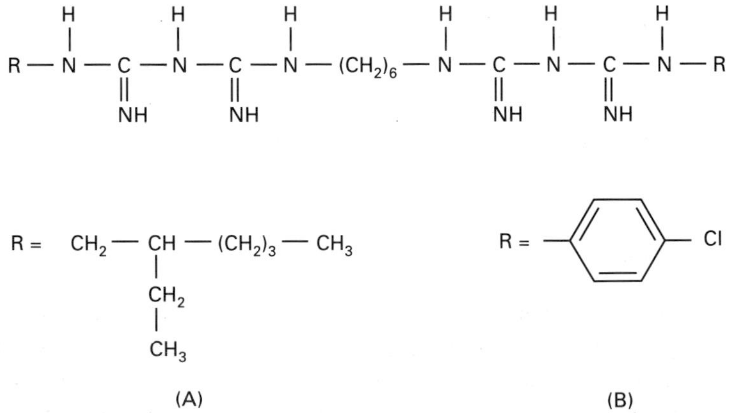

Fig. 10.3 Bisbiguanides: A, alexidine; B, chlorhexidine.

Chlorhexidine base is not readily soluble in water therefore the freely soluble salts, acetate, gluconate and hydrochloride, are used in formulation. Chlorhexidine exhibits the greatest antibacterial activity at pH 7–8 where it exists exclusively as a di-cation. The cationic nature of the compound results in activity being reduced by anionic compounds including soap and many anions due to the formation of insoluble salts. Anions to be wary of include bicarbonate, borate, carbonate, chloride, citrate and phosphate with due attention being paid to the presence of hard water. Deionized or distilled water should preferably be used for dilution purposes. Reduction in activity will also occur in the presence of blood, pus and other organic matter.

Chlorhexidine has widespread use, in particular as an antiseptic. It has significant antibacterial activity though Gram-negative bacteria are less sensitive than Gram-positive. A concentration of 1 : 2 000 000 prevents growth of, for example, *Staph. aureus* whereas a 1 : 50 000 dilution prevents growth of *Ps. aeruginosa*. Reports of pseudomonad contamination of aqueous chlorhexidine solutions have prompted the inclusion of small amounts of ethanol or isopropanol. Chlorhexidine is ineffective at ambient temperatures against bacterial spores and *M. tuberculosis*. A limited antifungal activity has been demonstrated which unfortunately restricts its use as a general preservative. Skin sensitivity has occasionally been reported, although, in general, chlorhexidine is well tolerated and non-toxic when applied to skin or mucous membranes and is an important preoperative antiseptic.

3.4.2   *Polyhexamethylene biguanides*

The antimicrobial activity of chlorhexidine, a bisbiguanide, exceeds that of monomeric biguanides. This has stimulated the development of polymeric biguanides containing repeating biguanide groups linked by hexamethylene chains. One such compound is a commercially available heterodisperse mixture of polyhexamethylene biguanides (PHMB, polyhexanide) having the general formula shown in Fig. 10.4, where n varies with a mean value of 5.5. The compound has a broad spectrum of activity against Gram-positive and Gram-negative bacteria and has low toxicity. PHMB is employed as an antimicrobial agent in various ophthalmic products.

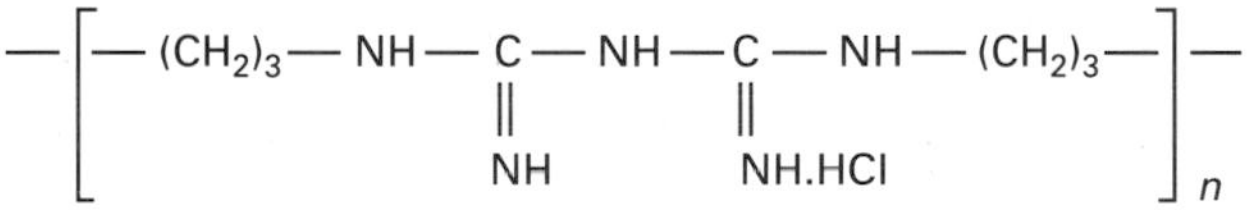

$$-\left[-(CH_2)_3 - NH - \underset{\underset{NH}{\|}}{C} - NH - \underset{\underset{NH.HCl}{\|}}{C} - NH - (CH_2)_3 - \right]_n -$$

Fig. 10.4 Polyhexamethylene biguanide (PHMB).

3.5   Halogens

Chlorine and iodine have been used extensively since their introduction as disinfecting agents in the early 19th century. Preparations containing these halogens such as Dakin's solution and tincture of iodine were early inclusions in many pharmacopoeiae and national formularies. More recent formulations of these elemens have improved activity, stability and ease of use.

Chlorine

A large number of antimicrobially active chlorine compounds are commercially available, one of the most important being liquid chlorine. This is supplied as an amber liquid by compressing and cooling gaseous chlorine. The terms liquid and gaseous chlorine refer to elemental chlorine whereas the word 'chlorine' is normally used to signify a mixture of OCl^-, Cl_2, $HOCl$ and other active chlorine compounds in aqueous solution. The potency of chlorine disinfectants is usually expressed in terms of parts per million (ppm) or percentage of available chlorine (avCl).

3.5.2   Hypochlorites

Hypochlorites are the oldest and remain the most useful of the chlorine disinfectants being readily available and inexpensive. They exhibit a rapid kill against a wide spectrum of microorganisms including fungi and viruses. High levels of available chlorine will enable eradication of acid-fast bacilli and bacterial spores. The compounds are compatible with most anionic and cationic surface-active agents and are relatively inexpensive to use. To their disadvantage they are corrosive, suffer inactivation by organic matter and can become unstable. Hypochlorites are available as powders or liquids, most frequently as the sodium or potassium salts of hypochlorous acid (HOCl). Sodium hypochlorite exists in solution as follows:

$$NaOCl + H_2O \rightleftharpoons HOCl + NaOH$$

Undissociated hypochlorous acid is a strong oxidizing agent and its potent antimicrobial activity is dependent on pH as shown:

$$HOCl \rightleftharpoons H^+ + OCl^-$$

At low pH the existence of HOCl is favoured over OCl^- (hypochlorite ion). The relative microbiocidal effectiveness of these forms is of the order of 100 : 1. By lowering the pH of hypochlorite solutions the antimicrobial activity increases to an optimum at about pH 5; however, this is concurrent with a decrease in stability of the solutions. This problem may be alleviated by addition of NaOH (see above equation) in order to maintain a high pH during storage for stability. The absence of buffer allows the pH to be lowered sufficiently for activity on dilution to use-strength. It is preferable to prepare use-dilutions of hypochlorite on a daily basis.

3.5.3   Organic chlorine compounds

A number of organic chlorine, or chloramine, compounds are now available for disinfection and antisepsis. These are the N-chloro ($=N$-Cl) derivatives of, for example, sulphonamides giving compounds such as chloramine-T and dichloramine-T and halazone (Fig. 10.5), which may be used for the disinfection of contaminated drinking water.

A second group of compounds, formed by N-chloro derivatization of heterocyclic compounds containing a nitrogen in the ring, includes the sodium and potassium salts of dichloroisocyanuric acid (e.g. NaDCC). These are available in granule or tablet

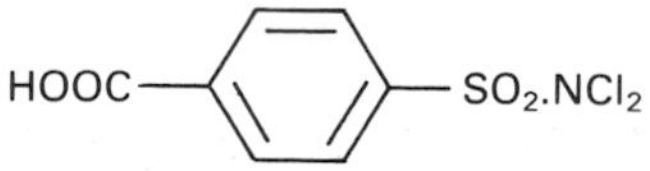

HOOC—⟨benzene ring⟩—SO$_2$.NCl$_2$

Fig. 10.5 Halazone.

form and, in contrast to hypochlorite, are very stable on storage, if protected from moisture. In water they will give a known chlorine concentration. The antimicrobial activity of the compounds is similar to that of the hypochlorites when acidic conditions of use are maintained. It is, however, important to note that where inadequate ventilation exists, care must be taken not to apply the compound to acidic fluids or large spills of urine in view of the toxic effects of chlorine production. The Health and Safety Executive (HSE) has set the occupational exposure standard (OES) short-term exposure limit at 1 ppm (see section 2.5 also).

3.5.4 Chloroform

Chloroform ($CHCl_3$) has a narrow spectrum of activity. It has been used extensively as a preservative in pharmaceuticals since the last century though recently has had limitations placed on its use. Marked reductions in concentration may occur through volatilization from products resulting in the possibility of microbial growth.

3.5.5 Iodine

Iodine has a wide spectrum of antimicrobial activity. Gram-negative and Gram-positive organisms, bacterial spores (on extended exposure), mycobacteria, fungi and viruses are all susceptible. The active agent is the elemental iodine molecule, I_2. As elemental iodine is only slightly soluble in water, iodide ions are required for aqueous solutions such as aqueous iodine solution, BP 1988 (Lugol's Solution) containing 5% iodine in 10% potassium iodide solution. Iodine (2.5%) may also be dissolved in ethanol (90%) and potassium iodide (2.5%) solution to give weak iodine solution, BP 1988 (Iodine Tincture).

The antimicrobial activity of iodine is less dependent than chlorine on temperature and pH, though alkaline pH should be avoided. Iodine is also less susceptible to inactivation by organic matter. Disadvantages in the use of iodine in skin antisepsis are staining of skin and fabrics coupled with possible sensitizing of skin and mucous membranes.

3.5.6 Iodophors

In the 1950s iodophors (*iodo* meaning iodine and *phor* meaning carrier) were developed to eliminate the side-effects of iodine while retaining its antimicrobial activity. These allowed slow release of iodine on demand from the complex formed. Essentially, four generic compounds may be used as the carrier molecule or complexing agent. These give polyoxymer iodophors (i.e. with propylene or ethyene oxide polymers), cationic (quaternary ammonium) surfactant iodophors, non-ionic (ethoxylated) surfactant iodophors and polyvinylpyrrolidone iodophors (PVP-I or povidone-iodine). The non-ionic or cationic surface-active agents act as solubilizers and carriers, combining detergency with antimicrobial activity. The former type of surfactant especially, produces a stable, efficient formulation the activity of which is further enhanced by the addition of phosphoric or citric acid to give a pH below 5 on use-dilution. The iodine is present in the form of micellar aggregates which disperse on dilution, especially below the critical micelle concentration (cmc) of the surfactant, to liberate free iodine.

When iodine and povidone are combined, a chemical reaction takes place forming a complex between the two entities. Some of the iodine becomes organically linked to povidone though the major portion of the complexed iodine is in the form of tri-iodide. Dilution of this iodophor results in a weakening of the iodine linkage to the carrier polymer with concomitant increases in elemental iodine in solution and antimicrobial activity.

The amount of free iodine the solution can generate is termed the 'available iodine'. This acts as a reservoir for active iodine releasing it when required and therefore largely avoiding the harmful side-effects of high iodine concentration. Consequently, when used for antisepsis, iodophors should be allowed to remain on the skin for 2 minutes to obtain full advantage of the sustained-release iodine.

Cadexomer-I_2 is an iodophor similar to povidone-iodine. It is a 2-hydroxymethylene crosslinked (1–4) α-D-glucan carboxymethyl ether containing iodine. The compound is used especially for its absorbent and antiseptic properties in the management of leg ulcers and pressure sores where it is applied in the form of microbeads containing 0.9% iodine.

3.6 Heavy metals

Mercury and silver have long been known to have antibacterial properties and preparations of these metals were among the earliest used antiseptics, but have been replaced by less toxic compounds. Other metals such as zinc, copper, aluminium and tin have weak antibacterial properties but are used in medicine for other functions, e.g. aluminium acetate and zinc sulphate are employed as astringents.

3.6.1 Mercurials

The organomercurial derivatives which are still in use in pharmacy are thiomersal and phenlymercuric nitrate or acetate (PMN or PMA) (Fig. 10.6).

Thiomersal is employed as a preservative for eye-drops and in lower concentration, 0.001–0.004%, as a preservative for contact lens solutions. The phenylmercuric salts (0.002%) are also used for preservation of eye-drops but long-term use has led to

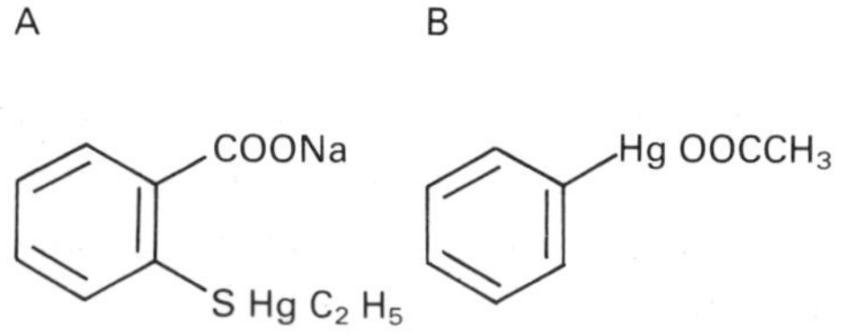

A   B

Fig. 10.6 Some organomercurials: A, thiomersal (sodium ethylmercurithiosalicylate); B, phenylmercuric acetate.

keratopathy and they are not recommended for prolonged use. Use of both mercurials has declined considerably due to risk of hypersensitivity and local irritation. They are absorbed from solution by rubber closures and plastic containers to a significant extent.

3.7 Hydrogen peroxide and peroxygen compounds

The germicidal properties of hydrogen peroxide (H_2O_2) have been known for more than a century, but use of low concentrations of unstable solutions did little for its reputation. However, stabilized solutions are now available and due to its unusual properties and antimicrobial activity, hydrogen peroxide has a valuable role for specific applications. It is used as an antiseptic for open wounds and ulcers where it provides additional cleansing due to its oxidation of organic debris. Its activity against the protozoa, *Acanthamoeba*, which can cause keratitis in contact lens wearers, has made it popular for disinfection of soft contact lenses. Concentrations of 3–6% are effective for general disinfection purposes. At high concentrations (up to 30%) and increased temperature hydrogen peroxide is sporicidal. Use has been made of this in vapour-phase hydrogen peroxide decontamination of laboratory equipment and enclosed spaces.

Peracetic acid (CH_3COOOH) is the peroxide of acetic acid and is a more potent biocide than hydrogen peroxide, with excellent rapid biocidal activity against bacteria, including mycobacteria, fungi, viruses and spores. It can be used in both the liquid and vapour phases and is active in the presence of organic matter. It is finding increasing use at concentrations of 0.2–0.35% as a chemosterilant of medical equipment. Its disadvantages are that it is corrosive to some metals. It is also highly irritant and must be used in an enclosed system.

Of the other peroxygen compounds with antimicrobial activity, potassium monoperoxysulphate is the main product marketed for disinfectant use. It is used for body fluid spillages and equipment contaminated with body fluids, but its activity against mycobacteria and some viruses is limited.

3.8 Phenols

Phenols (Fig. 10.7) are widely used as disinfectants and preservatives. The phenolics for disinfectant use have good antimicrobial activity and are rapidly bactericidal but generally are not sporicidal. Their activity is markedly diminished by dilution and is also reduced by organic matter. They are more active at acid pH. The main disadvantages of phenols are their caustic effect on skin and tissues and their systemic toxicity. The more highly substituted phenols are less toxic and can be used as preservatives and antiseptics; however, they are also less active than the simple phenolics, especially against Gram-negative organisms.

3.8.1 *Phenol (carbolic acid)*

Phenol no longer plays any significant role as an antibacterial agent. It is of historical interest, since it was introduced by Lister in 1867 as an antiseptic and has been used as a standard for comparison with other disinfectants, which are then given a phenol coefficient in tests such as the Rideal–Walker test.

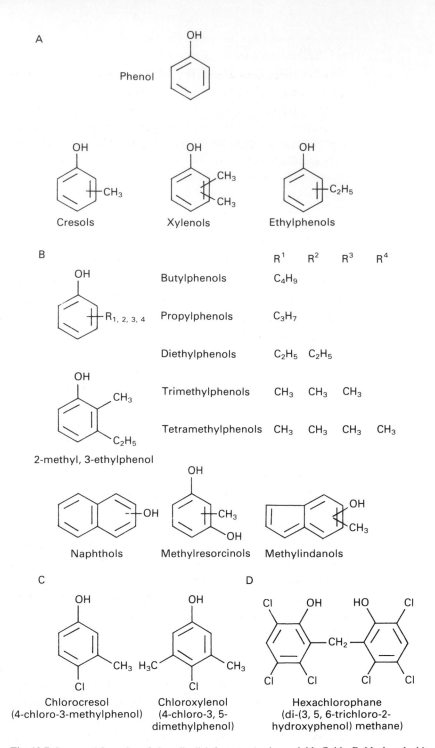

Fig. 10.7 Structural formulae of phenolic disinfectants: A, clear soluble fluids; B, black and white fluids; C, chlorinated phenols; D, bisphenols.

Tar acids

Many of the phenols which are used in household and other commercial disinfectant products are produced from the tar obtained by distillation of coal or more recently petroleum. They are known as the tar acids. These phenols are separated by fractional distillation according to their boiling point range into phenol, cresols, xylenols and high boiling point tar acids. As the boiling point increases the properties of the products alter as shown:

Phenols	Boiling point increases
Cresols	Bactericidal activity increases
Xylenols	Inactivation by organic matter increases
High boiling point	Water solubility decreases
Tar acids	Tissue toxicity decreases

The phenols from the higher boiling point fractions have greater antimicrobial activity but must be formulated so as to overcome their poor solubility. A range of solubilized and emulsified phenolic disinfectants are available including the *clear soluble fluids, black fluids* and *white fluids.*

Clear soluble fluids. Cresol is a mixture of *o-*, *m-* and *p-*methyl phenol (Fig. 10.7A). Because of its poor solubility, it is solubilized with a soap prepared from linseed oil and potassium hydroxide. It forms a clear solution on dilution. This preparation, known as Lysol (Cresol and Soap Solution BP 1968) has been widely used as a general purpose disinfectant but has largely been superseded by less irritant phenolics.

By using a higher boiling point fraction than cresols, consisting of xylenols and ethylphenols (Fig. 10.7A), a more active, less corrosive product which retains activity in the presence of organic matter, is obtained. It is also solubilized with a soap to give a clear soluble fluid. A variety of proprietary products for general disinfection purposes are available with these phenols as active ingredients. They possess rapid bactericidal activity, including mycobacteria, providing a major use for the terminal disinfection of rooms occupied by patients with open tuberculosis. Similarly, further use is made of these compounds for spills of faeces containing pathogens such as salmonellae and shigellae and for controlling outbreaks of methicillin-resistant *Staph. aureus* (MRSA).

Black fluids and white fluids. Black fluids and white fluids are prepared by solubilizing the high boiling point tar acids (Fig. 10.7B). Black fluids are homogenous solutions, which form an emulsion on dilution with water. White fluids are finely dispersed emulsions of tar acids, which on dilution with water produce more stable emulsions than do black fluids. Both types of fluid have good bactericidal activity. Preparations are very irritant and corrosive to the skin and are strong smelling; however, they are relatively inexpensive and are useful for household and general disinfection purposes. They must be used in adequate concentrations as activity is reduced by organic matter and is markedly affected by dilution.

Non-coal tar phenols (chloroxylenol and chlorocresol)

Many derivatives of phenol are now made by a synthetic process. Homologous series of substituted derivatives have been prepared and tested for antimicrobial activity. A combination of alkyl substitution and halogenation has produced useful derivatives including clorinated phenols which are constituents of a number of proprietary disinfectants. Two of the most widely used derivatives are *p*-chloro-*m*-cresol (4-chloro-3-methylphenol, chlorocresol, Fig. 10.7C) which is mostly employed as a preservative at a concentration of 0.1%, and *p*-chloro-*m*-xylenol (4-chloro-3,5-dimethylphenol, chloroxylenol, Fig. 10.7C) which is used for skin disinfection, although less than formerly. Chloroxylenol is sparingly soluble in water and must be solubilized, for example in a suitable soap solution in conjunction with terpineol or pine oil. Its antimicrobial capacity is weak and is reduced by the presence of organic matter.

3.8.4   *Bisphenols*

Bisphenols are composed of two phenolic groups connected by various linkages. Hydroxy halogenated derivatives, such as hexachlorophane (Fig. 10.7D) and triclosan, are the most active microbiologically, but are bacteriostatic at use-concentrations and have little antipseudomonal activity. The use of hexachlorophane is also limited by its serious toxicity. Both hexachlorophane and trichlosan have limited application in medicated soaps and washing creams.

3.9   Surface-active agents

Surface-active agents or surfactants are classified as anionic, cationic, non-ionic or ampholytic according to the ionization of the hydrophilic group in the molecule. A hydrophobic, water-repellent group is also present. Within the various classes a range of detergent and disinfectant activity is found. The anionic and non-ionic surface-active agents, for example, have strong detergent properties but exhibit little or no antimicrobial activity. They can, however, render certain bacterial species more sensitive to some antimicrobial agents, possibly by altering the permeability of the outer envelope. Ampholytic or amphoteric agents can ionize to give anionic, cationic and zwiterionic (positively and negatively charged ions in the same molecule) activity. Consequently, they display both the detergent properties of the anionic surface-active agents and the antimicrobial activity of the cationic agents. They are used quite extensively in Europe for pre-surgical hand scrubbing, medical instrument disinfection and floor disinfection in hospitals.

Of the four classes of surface-active agents, however, the cationic compounds arguably play the most important role in an antimicrobial context.

3.9.1   *Cationic surface-active agents*

The cationic agents used for their antimicrobial activity all fall within the group known as the quaternary ammonium compounds which are variously described as QACs, quats or onium ions. These are organically substituted ammonium compounds as shown in

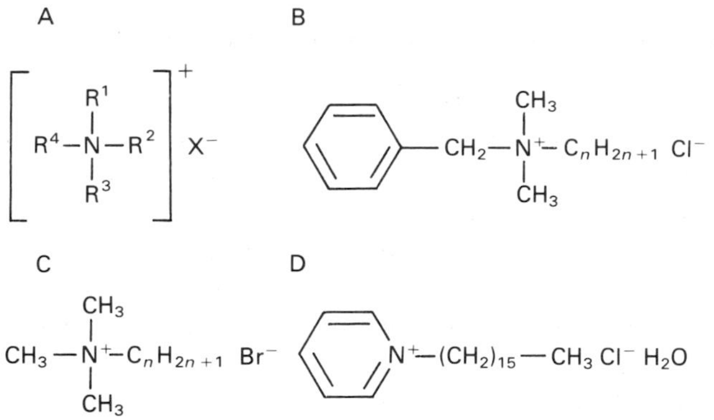

Fig. 10.8 Quaternary ammonium compounds (QACs): A, general structure of QACs; B, benzalkonium chloride ($n = 8 - 18$); C, cetrimide ($n = 12 - 14$ or 16); D, cetylpyridinium chloride.

Fig. 10.8A where the R substituents are alkyl or heterocyclic radicals to give compounds such as cetyltrimethylammonium bromide (cetrimide), cetylpyridinium chloride and benzalkonium chloride. Inspection of the structures of these compounds (Fig. 10.8B) indicates the requirement for good antimicrobial activity of having a chain length in the range C_8 to C_{18} in at least one of the R substituents. In the pyridinium compounds (Fig. 10.8C) three of the four covalent links may be satisfied by the nitrogen in a pyridine ring. Polymeric quaternary ammonium salts such as polyquaternium 1 are finding increasing use as preservatives.

The QACs are most effective against microorganisms at neutral or slightly alkaline pH and become virtually inactive below pH 3.5. Not surprisingly, anionic agents greatly reduce the activity of these cationic agents. Incompatibilities have also been recorded with non-ionic agents, possibly due to the formation of micelles. The presence of organic matter such as serum, faeces and milk will also seriously affect activity.

QACs exhibit greatest activity against Gram-positive bacteria with a lethal effect observed using concentrations as low as 1 : 200 000. Gram-negative bacteria are more resistant requiring a level of 1 : 30 000 or higher still if *Ps. aeruginosa* is present. Bacteriostasis is obtained at higher dilutions. A limited antifungal activity, more in the form of a static than a cidal effect, is exhibited. The QACs have not been shown to possess any useful sporicidal activity. This narrow spectrum of activity therefore limits the usefulness of the compounds. Since they are generally well tolerated and non-toxic when applied to skin and mucous membranes the compounds have considerable use in treatment of wounds and abrasions and they are used as preservatives in certain preparations. Benzalkonium chloride and cetrimide are employed extensively in surgery, urology and gynaecology as aqueous and alcoholic solutions and as creams. In many instances they are used in conjunction with a biguanide disinfectant such as chlorhexidine. The detergent properties of the QACs are also useful, especially in hospitals, for general environmental sanitation.

3.10   **Other antimicrobials**

The range of chemicals which can be shown to have antimicrobial properties is beyond the scope of this chapter. The agents included in this section have limited use or are of historic interest.

3.10.1   *Diamidines*

The activity of diamidines is reduced by acid pH and in the presence of blood and serum. Microorganisms may acquire resistance by serial subculture in the presence of increasing doses of the compounds. Propamidine and dibromopropamidine, as the isethionate salts, are the major diamidine derivatives employed as antimicrobial agents; propamidine in the form of eye-drops (0.1%) for amoebic infection and dibromopropamidine for topical treatment of minor infections.

3.10.2   *Dyes*

Crystal violet (Gentian violet), brilliant green and malachite green are triphenyl-methane dyes widely used to stain bacteria for microscopic examination. They also have bacteriostatic and fungistatic activity and have been applied topically for the treatment of infections. Staining of skin and clothes is a disadvantage of these agents. Due to concern about possible carcinogenicity, they are now rarely used.

The acridine dyes, including proflavine, acriflavine and aminacrine, have also been employed for skin disinfection and treatment of infected wounds or burns. They are slow-acting and mainly bacteriostatic in effect, with no useful fungicidal or sporicidal activity.

3.10.3   *Quinoline derivatives*

The quinoline derivatives of pharmaceutical interest are little used now. The antimicrobial activity of the derivatives is generally good against the Gram-positive bacteria though less so against Gram-negative species. The compound most frequently used in a pharmaceutical context is dequalinium chloride, a bisquaternary ammonium derivative of 4-aminoquinaldinium. As it is a cationic surface-active agent it is incompatible with anionic agents. It is formulated as a lozenge for the treatment of oropharyngeal infections.

3.11   Antimicrobial combinations

As is apparent from the above information, there is no ideal disinfectant, antiseptic or preservative. All chemical agents have their limitations either in terms of their antimicrobial activity, resistance to organic matter, stability, incompatibility, irritancy, toxicity or corrosivity. To overcome the limitations of an individual agent, formulations consisting of combinations of agents are available. For example, ethanol has been combined with chlorhexidine and iodine to produce more active preparations. The combination of chlorhexidine and cetrimide is also considered to improve activity. QACs and phenols have been combined with glutaraldehyde so that the same effect can be achieved with lower, less irritant concentrations of glutaraldehyde. Some combinations are considered to be synergistic, e.g. hydrogen peroxide and peroxy compounds.

4   Disinfection policies

The aim of a disinfection policy is to control the use of chemicals for disinfection and antisepsis and give guidelines on their use. The preceeding descriptions within this chapter of the activities, advantages and disadvantages of the many disinfectants available allow considerable scope for choice and inclusion of agents in a policy to be applied to such areas as industrial plant, walls, ceilings, floors, air, cleaning equipment and laundries and to the extensive range of equipment in contact with hospital patients.

The control of microorganisms is of prime importance in hospital and industrial environments. Where pharmaceutical products (either sterile or non-sterile) are manufactured, contamination of the product may lead to its deterioration and to infection in the user. In hospital there is the additional consideration of patient care, therefore protection from nosocomial (hospital-acquired) infection and prevention of cross-infection must also be covered. Hospitals generally have a disinfection policy, though the degree of adherence to, and implementation of, the policy content can vary. A specialized Infection Control Committee comprising the pharmacist, the consultant medical microbiologist and senior nurse responsible for infection control should formulate a suitable policy. This core team may usefully be expanded to include, for example, a physician, a surgeon, nurse teachers and nurses from several clinical areas, the sterile services manager and the domestic superintendent. Purchasing may also be represented. This expanded committee will meet regularly to help with the implementation of the policy and reassess its efficiency. Reference to Tables 10.2–10.4 indicates the susceptibility of various microorganisms to the range of agents available. Table 10.6 presents examples of the range of formulations and uses of the agents available.

Although scope exists for choice of disinfectant in many of the areas covered by a policy, in certain instances specific recommendations are made as to the type, concentration and usage of disinfectant in particular circumstances. For example, the Working Party of the British Society of Gastroenterology recommended aldehyde preparations as the first line antibacterial and antiviral disinfectant with a 4 minute soak of endoscopes sufficient for inactivation of hepatitis B virus and HIV. Similarly, the area of use of hypochlorite solutions will dictate the strength of solution (avCl) required. Where blood and body fluid spill occurs, a 1% avCl (10000 ppm) solution is required. Lower strengths, 0.1% and 0.125% avCl, are recommended for disinfection of general working surfaces and baby feeding bottles, respectively.

Categories of risk (to patients) may be assigned to equipment coming into contact with a patient, dictating the level of decontamination required and degree of concern. *High-risk* items have close contact with broken skin or mucous membrane or are those introduced into a sterile area of the body and should therefore be sterile. These include sterile instruments, gloves, catheters, syringes and needles. Liquid chemical disinfectants should only be used if heat or other methods of sterilization are unsuitable. *Intermediate-risk items* are in close contact with skin or mucous membranes and disinfection will normally be applied. Endoscopes, respiratory and anaesthetic equipment, wash bowls, bed-pans and similar items are included in this category. *Low-risk items* or areas include those detailed earlier such as walls, floors, etc., which are not in close contact with the patient. Cleaning is obviously important with disinfection being required, for example, in the event of contaminated spillage.

5   Further reading

Advisory Committee on Dangerous Pathogens (ACDP) (1990) *HIV—The Causative Agent of AIDS and Related Conditions*. Second revision of guidelines. London: Health and Safety Executive.

Anon (1991) *Decontamination of Equipment, Linen or other Surfaces Contaminated with Hepatitis B and/or Human Immunodeficiency Viruses*. Department of Health HC 33.

Anon (1988) Cleaning and disinfection of equipment for gastrointestinal flexible endoscopy: interim recommendations of a Working Party of the British Society of Gastroenterology. *Gut*, **29**, 1134–1151.

Ayliffe G.A.J., Coates D. & Hoffman P.N. (1993) *Chemical Disinfection in Hospitals*. London: PHLS.

British Medical Association (1989) *A Code of Practice for Sterilization of Instruments and Control of Cross Infection*. London: BMA (Board of Science and Education).

British Standards Institution (1986) *Terms Relating to Disinfectants*. BS 5283: 1986 Glossary. London: British Standards Institution.

Block S.S. (Ed) (1991) *Disinfection, Sterilization and Preservation*, 4th edn. Philadelphia: Lea & Febiger.

Coates D. & Hutchinson D.N. (1994) How to produce a hospital disinfection policy. *J Hosp Infect*, **26**, 57–68.

Control of Substances Hazardous to Health (COSHH) Regulations (1988). Statutary Instrument No. 1657.

Eggers H.J. (1990) Experiments on antiviral activity of hand disinfectants. Some theoretical and practical considerations. *Zentralblatt Bakt*, **273**, 36–51.

Health and Safety Executive (1991) Occupational Exposure Limits EH40/91. London: Health and Safety Executive.

Holton J., Nye P. & McDonald V. (1994) Efficacy of selected disinfectants against Mycobacteria and Cryptosporidia. *J Hosp Infect*, **27**, 105–115.

Russell A.D. (1990) Bacterial spores and chemical sporicidal agents. *Clin Microbiol Rev*, **3**, 99–119.

Russell A.D. (1996) Activity of biocides against mycobacteria. *J Appl Bacteriol Symp Suppl*, **81**, 87S–101S.

Russell A.D. & Chopra I. (1996) *Understanding Antibacterial Action and Resistance*, 2nd edn. Chichester: Ellis Horwood.

Russell A.D., Hugo W.B. & Ayliffe G.A.J. (ed.) (1998) *Principles and Practice of Disinfection, Preservation and Sterilization*, 3rd edn. Oxford: Blackwell Science.

Scott E.M., Gorman S.P. & McGrath S.J. (1986) An assessment of the fungicidal activity of antimicrobial agents used for hard-surface and skin disinfection. *J Clin Hosp Pharm*, **11**, 199–205.

Sterilization, Disinfection and Cleaning of Medical Equipment: Microbiology Advisory Committee (1993) Guidance on Decontamination from the Microbiology Advisory Committee to Department of Health Medical Devices Directorate. Part 1 Principles. London: HMSO.

van Bueren J., Salman H. & Cookson B.D. (1995) *The Efficacy of Thirteen Chemical Disinfectants against Human Immunodeficiency Virus (HIV)*. Medical Devices Agency Evaluation Report.

11 Evaluation of non-antibiotic antimicrobial agents

1	**Introduction**
1.1	Definition of terms
1.2	Dynamics of disinfection
2	**Factors affecting the disinfection process**
2.1	Effect of temperature
2.1.1	Practical meaning of the temperature coefficient
2.2	Effect of dilution
2.2.1	Practical meaning of the concentration exponent
2.3	Effect of pH
2.3.1	Rate of growth of the inoculum
2.3.2	Potency of the antibacterial agent
2.3.3	Effect on the cell surface
2.4	Effect of surface activity
2.5	Presence of interfering substances
2.6	Effect of inoculum size
3	**Evaluation of liquid disinfectants**
3.1	Suspension tests
3.1.1	Phenol coefficient tests
3.1.2	Capacity use-dilution test
3.2	Quantitative suspension tests
3.3	Mycobactericidal activity
3.4	Sporicidal activity
3.5	*In vivo* tests
3.5.1	Skin tests
3.5.2	Other *in vivo* tests
3.5.3	Toxicity tests
3.6	Estimation of bacteriostasis ✔
3.6.1	Serial dilution
3.6.2	Ditch-plate technique
3.6.3	Cup-plate technique
3.6.4	Solid dilution method
3.6.5	Gradient-plate technique
3.7	Tests for antifungal activity
3.7.1	Fungicidal activity
3.7.2	Fungistatic activity
3.7.3	Choice of test organism
3.8	Virucidal activity
3.8.1	Tissue culture or egg inoculation
3.8.2	Plaque assays
3.8.3	'Acceptable' animal model
3.8.4	Duck hepatitis B virus: a possible model of infectivity of human hepatitis B virus
3.8.5	Immune reaction
3.8.6	Virus morphology
3.8.7	Endogenous reverse transcriptase
3.8.8	Bacteriophage
4	**Semi-solid antibacterial preparations**
4.1	Tests for bacteriostatic activity
4.2	Tests for bactericidal activity
4.3	Tests on skin
4.4	General conclusions
5	**Solid disinfectants**
6	**Evaluation of air disinfectants**
6.1	Determination of viable airborne microorganisms
6.2	Experimental evaluation
7	**Preservatives**
7.1	Evaluation of preservatives
7.2	Preservative combinations
7.2.1	Synergy in preservative combinations
7.2.2	Evaluation of synergy
7.2.3	Rapid methods
8	**Appendix: British Standards**
9	**Further reading**

1   Introduction

1.1   Definition of terms

- *Bactericide*. An agency which kills bacteria.
- *Sporicide*. An agency which kills spores.
- *Bacteriostat*. An agency which prevents the reproduction and multiplication of bacteria.

- *Virucide (viricide)*. An agency which kills viruses.
- *Fungicide*. An agency which kills fungi.
- *Fungistat*. An agency which prevents fungal proliferation.

The foregoing terms are unequivocal and are the terms of choice in scientific writing; however, other terms are also in common use.

Disinfectant. This term implies a substance with bactericidal action. Clearly, if an environment is to be made free from the ability to reinfect, its bacterial population must be destroyed. A detailed description of the meaning of the terms 'disinfectant' and 'disinfection' is provided in Chapter 10.

Sanitizer. This term, sometimes used in the public health context, refers to an agent that reduces the number of bacterial contaminants to a safe level.

Antiseptic. This term means 'against sepsis' which in general means wound infection. A bacteriostatic agent may prevent sepsis developing in the body especially if the normal body defences against sepsis are operative. For further details, see Chapter 10.

Another common usage of the terms disinfectant and antiseptic is to use the former for preparations to be applied to inert surfaces and the latter to preparations for application to living tissues.

Many of the standard works include only the word 'disinfection' in their title yet deal with all classes of compounds and with a wide range of application. It is unrewarding to be too dogmatic about these terms; many substances can function in both capacities depending upon their concentration and time of contact. A more general term, *biocide*, is now widely used to denote a chemical agent that, literally, kills microorganisms.

It is doubtful if there is a difference other than degree between bacteriostatic and bactericidal action. The three situations, growth, bacteriostasis and killing, are represented graphically in Fig. 11.1. The question posed by this notion, to which often there is no precise answer, is: How long will a culture of bacteria remain viable when prevented from reproducing?

1.2   Dynamics of disinfection

Changes in the population of viable bacteria in an environment are determined by means of a viable count, and a plot of this count against time gives a dynamic picture of any pattern of change (see Fig. 11.1, curve A). The typical growth curve of a bacterial culture is constructed from data obtained in this way. The pattern of bacterial death in a lethal environment may be obtained by the same technique, when a death or mortality curve is obtained (Fig. 11.1, curve C).

Inspection of the death curves obtained from viable count data had early elicited the idea that because there was usually an approximate, and under some circumstances a quite excellent, linear relationship between the logarithm of the number of survivors and time, then the disinfection process was comparable to a unimolecular reaction. This implied that the rate of killing was a function of the amount of one of the participants in the reaction only, i.e. in the case of the disinfection process the number of viable cells. From this observation there followed the notion that the principles of first-order

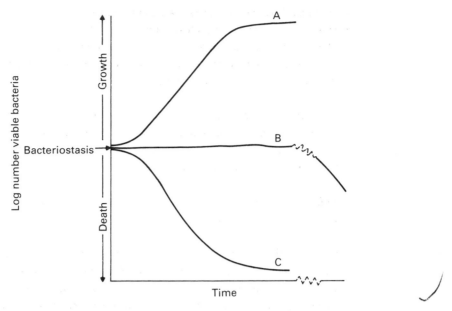

Fig. 11.1 The fate of a bacterial population when inoculated into: A, nutrient medium, normal growth curve. B, bacteriostatic environment. No change in viable population; after a prolonged time-interval the viable population will probably begin to fall. C, bactericidal environment. A sigmoid death curve is shown.

kinetics could be applied to the disinfection process and that a rate or velocity constant in an equation of the type shown below could be used as a measure of the efficiency of a disinfectant:

$$K = \frac{1}{t} \log \frac{N_0}{N}$$
(11.1)

where K is the rate or velocity constant, N_0 is the initial number of organisms, N is the final number of organisms, and t is the time for the viable count to fall from N_0 to N.

This may be understood more fully by reference to Fig. 11.2. Curve A shows the type of response which would be obtained if the lethal process followed precisely the pattern of a first-order reaction. Some experimental curves do, in fact, follow this pattern quite closely, hence the genesis of the original theory.

The more usual pattern found experimentally is that shown by B, which is called a sigmoid curve. Here the graph is indicative of a slow initial rate of kill, followed by a faster, approximately linear rate of kill where there is some adherence to first-order reaction kinetics; this is followed again by a slower rate of kill. This behaviour is compatible with the idea of a population of bacteria which contains a portion of susceptible members which die quite rapidly, an aliquot of average resistance, and a residue of more resistant members which die at a slower rate. When high concentrations of disinfectant are used, i.e. when the rate of death is rapid, a curve of the type shown by C is obtained; here the bacteria are dying more quickly than predicted by first-order kinetics and the rate 'constant' diminishes in value continuously during the disinfection process.

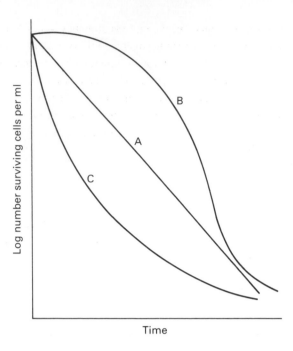

Fig. 11.2 Survivor/time curves for the disinfection process. A, obtained if the disinfection process obeyed the first-order kinetic law. B, sigmoid curve. This shows a slow initial rate of kill, a steady rate and finally a slower rate of kill. This is the form of curve most usually encountered. C, obtained if bacteria are dying more quickly than first-order kinetics would predict. The 'constant', K, diminishes in value continuously during the process.

The reason for this varied behaviour is not difficult to find. A population of bacteria does not possess the uniformity of properties inherent in pure chemical substances. This fact, together with the varied manner in which bactericides exert their effect and the complex nature of the bacterial cell, should provide adequate and satisfying reasons why the precise theories of reaction kinetics should have failed to explain the disinfection process.

The application of kinetic data is now being increasingly used in the evaluation of biocidal activity. As pointed out later (section 3.2), for example, data derived from viable counting procedures form the basis of modern suspension test methods.

The effects of temperature, pH and dilution on biocidal activity are of considerable significance and are dealt with in section 2.

2   Factors affecting the disinfection process

Apart from the obvious effect of concentration there are other important factors which affect the action of disinfectants.

2.1   Effect of temperature

In 1880, the bacteriologist Robert Koch had noted that anthrax spores were more rapidly killed by the same concentrations of phenol if the temperature was elevated. A former pharmacopoeial sterilization process 'heating with a bactericide' used an elevated temperature, 80–100°C, maintained for 30 minutes, to ensure that quite low concentrations of bactericides would sterilize parenteral injections and eye-drops.

The idea that disinfection could be treated as a first-order chemical reaction led to ideas equating the effect of heat on the process to the effect of heat on chemical reactions, invoking the Arrhenius equation. For reasons already given, attempts to fit equations derived from chemical reactions to the disinfection process are unrewarding, although as a generalization it is true that as the temperature is increased in arithmetical progression, the rate of disinfection (rate of kill) increases geometrically.

The effect of temperature on bactericidal activity may be expressed quantitatively by means of a temperature coefficient, either the temperature coefficient per degree rise in temperature, denoted by θ, or the coefficient per $10°$ rise, the Q_{10} value.

θ may be calculated from the equation

$$\theta^{(T_2-T2)} = \frac{t_1}{t_2} \tag{11.2}$$

where t_1 is the extinction time at $T_1°C$, and t_2 the extinction time at $T_2°C$ (i.e. $T_1 + 1°C$).

Q_{10} values may be calculated easily by determining the extinction time at two temperatures differing exactly by $10°C$. Then

$$Q_{10} = \frac{\text{Time to kill at } T°}{\text{Time to kill at } (T+10)°} \tag{11.3}$$

An overall picture of the whole process may be obtained by plotting rate of kill against temperature.

The value for Q_{10} of chemical and enzyme-catalysed reactions lies between 2 and 3. The Q_{10} values of disinfectants vary widely; thus, for phenol it is 4, for butanol 28, for ethanol 45, and for ethylene glycol monoethyl ether, nearly 300. These figures alone should suggest that pushing the analogy of disinfection and chemical reaction kinetics too far is unwarranted.

2.1.1 *Practical meaning of the temperature coefficient*

The value of Q_{10} for phenol is 4, which means that over the $10°C$ range used to determine the Q_{10} (actually 20–$30°C$) the activity will be increased by a factor of 4.

2.2 **Effect of dilution**

The effects of concentration or dilution of the active ingredient on the activity of a disinfectant are of paramount importance. Failure to be aware of these changes in activity is responsible for many misleading claims concerning the properties of a disinfectant.

It was realized at the end of the nineteenth century that there was an exponential relationship between potency and concentration. Thus, if the $\log_{10}$ of a death time, that is the time to kill a standard inoculum, is plotted against the $\log_{10}$ of the concentration, a straight line is usually obtained, the slope of which is the concentration exponent (η) (Fig. 11.3). Expressed as an equation,

$$\eta = \frac{(\text{Log death time at concentration } C_2) - (\log \text{death time at concentration } C_1)}{\text{Log } C_1 - C_2} \tag{11.4}$$

Thus, η may be obtained from experimental data either graphically or by substitution in the above equation. Some numerical values of η are given in Table 11.1.

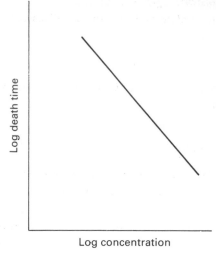

Fig. 11.3 Graphical determination of the concentration exponent, η, of a disinfectant.

Log death time (y-axis)

Log concentration (x-axis)

Table 11.1 Concentration exponents, η, for some disinfectant substances

Antimicrobial agent	η	Antimicrobial agent	η
Hydrogen peroxide	0.5	Parabens	2.5
Silver nitrate	0.9–1.0	Sorbic acid	2.6–3.2
Mercurials	0.03–3.0	Potassium laurate	2.3
Iodine	0.9	Benzyl alcohol	2.6–4.6
Crystal violet	0.9	Aliphatic alcohols	6.0–12.7
Chlorhexidine	2	Glycolmonophenyl ethers	5.8–6.4
Formaldehyde	1	Glycolmonoalkyl ethers	6.4–15.9
QACs	0.8–2.5	Phenolic agents	4–9.9
Acridines	0.7–1.9		
Formaldehyde donors	0.8–0.9		
Bronopol	0.7		
Polymeric biguanides	1.5–1.6		

QAC, quaternary ammonium compound.

2.2.1 *Practical meaning of the concentration exponent*

Mercuric chloride has a concentration exponent of 1; thus, the activity will be reduced by the power of 1 on dilution, and a threefold dilution means the disinfectant activity will be reduced by the value 3^1, or 3, that is to a third. Put another way the disinfection time will be three times as long. In the case of phenol, however, with a concentration exponent of 6, a threefold dilution will mean a decrease in activity of $3^6 = 729$, a figure 243 times the value for mercuric chloride. This explains why phenols may be rapidly inactivated by dilution and should sound a warning bell regarding claims for diluted phenol solutions based on data obtained at high concentrations.

2.3 Effect of pH

During the disinfection process a change of pH can, at one and the same time, affect:
1 the rate of growth of the inoculum;

2 the potency of the antibacterial agent itself;

3 the ability of the drug to combine with sites on the cell surface.

2.3.1 *Rate of growth of the inoculum*

In general, bacterial growth is optimal in the pH range 6–8; on either side of this bracket the rate of growth declines.

2.3.2 *Potency of the antibacterial agent*

If the agent is an acid or a base its degree of ionization will depend on the pH. If its acid dissociation constant, pK_a is known, the degree of ionization at any pH may be calculated or determined by reference to published tables.

It has been shown that in some compounds the active species is the non-ionized molecule while the ion is inactive (benzoic acid, phenols, nitrophenols, salicylic acid, acetic acid). Thus, conditions of pH which favour the formation of the ions of these compounds will also reduce their activity. The effect of pH on the ability of acetic acid and phenol to inhibit the growth of a mould is shown in Fig. 11.4.

In other cases the activity of the drug is due to the ionized molecule. For example, with the antibacterial acridine dyestuffs it is the cation which is the active agent and factors favouring ionization, all other things being equal, enhance their antibacterial activity (see Chapter 12).

Thus, at pH 7.3, 9-aminoacridine, which exists at this pH entirely as the cation, will inhibit the growth of *Streptococcus pyogenes* at a dilution of 1 : 160 000; the

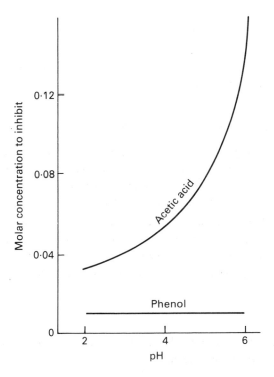

Fig. 11.4 The effect of pH on the concentration of phenol (pK_a 10) and of acetic acid (pK_a 4.7) to inhibit mould growth.

corresponding figure for 5-aminoacridine-3-carboxylic acid, which does not form cations at pH 7.3, is 1 : 5000.

Usually the antibacterial activity of cationic detergents such as cetrimide and the acridines increases with increase of pH (section 2.3.3).

2.3.3   *Effect on the cell surface*

Before an antibacterial agent can exert its effect on a cell it must combine with that cell. This process often follows the pattern of an adsorption isotherm. Clearly, factors which affect the state of the cell surface, as the pH of the cell's environment must do, must affect, to some extent, the adsorption process. An increase in the external pH renders the cell surface more negatively charged. Biocidal agents that are cationic in nature thus bind more strongly to the cell surface with a consequent increase in activity.

In most situations of practical disinfection, pH may not be a significant variable but it has long been recognized that phenols are less active in alkaline solution, an effect readily explained by the foregoing account.

2.4   **Effect of surface activity**

The possession of surface activity *per se* may be an important factor in the antibacterial action of a group of drugs, for example the cationic detergents. The addition of low concentrations of surface-active compounds may potentiate the biological effect of an antibacterial agent. Thus, phenols are often more active in the presence of soaps.

2.5   **Presence of interfering substances**

It has already been stated (section 2.3) that in most instances, before an antibacterial agent can act on a cell, it must first combine with it. It is not difficult to envisage the fact that the presence of other material, often referred to as organic matter, may reduce the effect of such an agent by adsorbing or inactivating it and thus reducing the amount available for combining with the cells it is desired to kill. Extraneous matter may be able to form a protective coat around the cell, thereby preventing the penetration of the active agent to its site of action. The possible influence, therefore, of other matter in the environment should not be overlooked.

2.6   **Effect of inoculum size**

This variable is often the one least controlled in the performance of tests upon disinfectants. Clearly, if it is postulated that disinfectant substances are first adsorbed on to a cell and thereafter kill it, the number of cells added to a given quantity of disinfectant may well be of significance. This is illustrated in Table 11.2.

In all experiments the inoculum size should be controlled and clearly stated in any account of the experiment.

Table 11.2 Effect of inoculum size on the minimum inhibitory concentration (MIC) of three antiseptics against *Staphylococcus aureus*

Antiseptic	MIC (μg ml^{-1}) vs. inoculum size		Increase (%)
	1×10^6	4×10^9	
Chlorocresol	225	350	55
Phenylethanol	3250	4750	65
Phenylmercuric acetate	3.5	5	70

3   Evaluation of liquid disinfectants

This evaluation may conveniently be classified into suspension tests (section 3.1) and counting methods, although the latter themselves use suspensions of microorganisms and hence are referred to here as quantitative suspension tests (section 3.2).

3.1   Suspension tests

These are essentially tests for sterility (Chapter 23) upon bacterial suspensions performed after treatment with the antibacterial agent for a prescribed time and under controlled conditions. They differ in the manner in which the experimental findings are calculated as well as in the details of experimental procedure.

They may be subdivided into phenol coefficient-type tests, of which there are many, quantitative suspension tests (which measure the rate at which test organisms are killed) and tests carried out at use-dilutions.

3.1.1   *Phenol coefficient tests*

The Rideal–Walker (RW) and Chick–Martin (CM) tests, long quoted, often in inappropriate circumstances, as standards for all disinfectants, were introduced at a time when typhoid fever was endemic. The tests were an attempt to standardize phenolic disinfectant claims or to kill the causal organism (*Salmonella typhi*) of typhoid fever. In the case of the CM test, account was taken of the presence of organic matter. During the first decade of the twentieth century, when the RW and CM tests were first described, it is true to say that these were valid tests. Phenols were the disinfectants almost invariably used, typhoid fever was still a present, although declining, menace to public health and it was utensils, rooms and surfaces at room temperature which were to be disinfected. The greatest single abuse of this type of test has been in the extrapolation of data to other situations and to disinfectants very different from phenol. Thus, it was not uncommon to find a preparation recommended for the treatment of wounds and declared able to kill staphylococci on the skin (at 37°C) in the presence of serum (organic matter), claimed as being six times as effective as pure phenol as judged by the RW test. If it is reiterated that the latter gives information about *Sal. typhi* at 17–18°C in an aqueous environment in the absence of organic matter, the extravagance of the extrapolation is plain. To use a phenol coefficient to evaluate non-phenolic disinfectants also contravened the fundamental concept of a biological assay, that is, that the standard and unknown should be of like mode of action. Not surprisingly, therefore, the RW and CM tests are falling into disuse, but full accounts will be found in the appropriate British Standards (BS 541: 1985 and BS 808: 1986). Both tests were fully described in the fourth edition (pp. 261–264) of the present book.

3.1.2   *Capacity use-dilution test*

The Kelsey–Sykes (KS) test. Having regard to the many disadvantages alleged against the RW and CM tests, attempts were made and published in the early 1960s to find improved test methods. The foundations for the new test were laid by Kelsey *et al.* in 1965, and with the collaboration of the late G. Sykes and of Isobel M. Maurer, the Kelsey–Sykes test was evolved. This test embodied several principles. Firstly, it was a capacity test. Here a bacterial inoculum was added to the disinfectant in three successive lots at 0, 1 and 5 minutes. This is the principle of a capacity test where the capacity or lack of capacity of the disinfectant to destroy successive additions of a bacterial culture is tested.

The total test is performed in separate repeats using four test organisms: *Staphylococcus aureus, Escherichia coli, Pseudomonas aeruginosa* and *Proteus vulgaris.* These were considered a more realistic choice than *Sal. typhi,* employed as the sole test organism in the RW and CM tests. The organisms, furthermore, are grown on a synthetic medium and survival is tested in a broth containing the non-ionic surface-active agent sorbitan mono-oleate (Tween 80). The disinfectant reaction is at 20°C and recovery of organisms at 32°C. Calibrated and dropping pipettes rather than loops are used for inoculation and other liquid manipulations, and disinfectants diluted at approximately the dilutions recommended for use are made in hard water. The test outlined above is carried out under clean and dirty conditions (compare RW, clean, and CM, dirty), the latter being simulated by dried yeast as in the CM test.

The disinfectant is assessed on its overall performance, namely its ability to kill microorganisms, as judged by subculture recovery or lack of it and not by comparison with phenol, i.e. a disinfectant would pass or fail according to its performance. A use-dilution concentration of a disinfectant must pass the test at three replications.

In summary, therefore, the KS suspension test differs from the RW and CM tests in that it is a capacity test, it reports the data as a pass or fail and not as a numerical cipher, i.e. not as a coefficient, and it uses a range of microorganisms. It combines an individual feature of the RW and CM tests in that it can report on disinfectant activity under both clean and dirty conditions.

This account highlights the main features of the test. It is described in detail by Kelsey and Maurer (1974).

Criticisms of the KS test. An extensive collaborative trial was carried out on the KS test and the conclusion (Cowen, 1978) was that the test was suitable for white and clear, soluble disinfectants providing due care was taken in interpreting the pass concentration. Further modification of the test is necessary before it can be applied to other disinfectants.

3.2	Quantitative suspension tests

There is no doubt that the maximum information concerning the fate of a bacterial population is obtained by performing viable counts at selected time intervals. Alternatively, the number of survivors expressed as the percentage remaining viable at the end of a given period of time may be determined by viable counts and this parameter is often used in assessing bactericidal activity.

Viable counting is a technique used in all branches of pure and applied bacteriology. Essentially, the method consists of dispersing the sample in a solid nutrient which is then incubated. Any developing colonies are counted and if the assumption is made that each countable colony arises from a single viable cell in the original sample and that each viable cell is capable of, eventually, producing a colony, the viable bacterial content of that sample is thus determined. Viable numbers are usually expressed as colony-forming units (cfu) per millilitre.

This type of test may be used to investigate bactericidal, sporicidal or fungicidal activity.

It will be recalled (section 1) that research on the time course of the disinfection process was carried out making extensive use of viable counts, and notions concerning the dynamics of the disinfection process were gathered by these means.

A far more useful parameter for practical disinfectant evaluation is to perform a viable count at the end of a chosen period and to determine the concentration of disinfectant to achieve a 99, 99.9, 99.99 or 99.999% kill. The use of a percentage kill calculated to three places of decimals may sound pedantic but these become significant when dealing with large populations. Thus, if 99.999% of a population of bacteria originally containing 1 000 000 cells are killed in a given time there are still 10 survivors. Expressed in another way, 90, 99, 99.9, 99.99 and 99.999% kills represent $\log_{10}$ reductions of 1, 2, 3, 4 and 5 respectively. This aspect provides the basis of a new European suspension test, currently being designed and still debated. The principle of this method is that a test bacterial suspension is exposed to a test disinfectant; after a specified time the numbers of cells remaining viable are compared with control (untreated) cells. A hypothetical example is provided in Table 11.3 together with an explanation of the calculation involved.

Tests should also be done in the presence of organic matter (e.g. albumin) and in hard water. It is important to remember when performing viable counts that care must be taken to ensure that, at the moment of sampling, the disinfection process is immediately arrested by the use of a suitable neutralizer or ensuring inactivation by dilution (Table 11.4). Membrane filtration is an alternative procedure, the principle of which is that treated cells are retained on the filter whilst the disinfectant forms the filtrate. After washing *in situ*, the membrane is transferred to the surface of a solid (agar) recovery medium and the colonies that develop on the membrane are counted.

A major source of error in performing viable counts results from clumping of the organism so that one colony on the final plate may arise, not from one organism, but perhaps from numbers which may be of the order of 100. Unfortunately, many antibacterial agents, by affecting the surface charge on the bacterial cell, actually promote clumping and steps must be taken to overcome this.

Table 11.3 Hypothetical example of a quantitative suspension test procedure (disinfectant used for 5 minutes at 20°C)

Subculture dilution	Control series (C)		Disinfectant series (D)	
	cfu	cfu ml^{-1}	cfu	cfu ml^{-1}
10^{-1}	TNTC*	—	88	8.8×10^2
10^{-2}	TNTC	—	8	8×10^2
10^{-3}	TNTC	—	0	—
10^{-4}	TNTC	—		
10^{-5}	110	1.1×10^7		
10^{-6}	11	1.1×10^7		

* TNTC, too numerous to count.

Microbicidal effect $(M_E) = \log N_C - \log N_D$
$$= \log 1.1 \times 10^7 - \log 8.8 \times 10^2$$
$$= 7.04 - 2.94$$
$$= 4.10 \text{ (after 5 minutes)}$$

where N_C and N_D represent the number of cfu ml^{-1} in the control and disinfectant series, respectively.

Table 11.4 Neutralizing agents for some antimicrobial agents*

Antimicrobial agent	Neutralizing agent
Benzoic acid and esters of p-hydroxybenzoic acid	Dilution or Tween 80
Bronopol	Cysteine hydrochloride
Chlorhexidine	Lubrol W and egg lecithin or Tween 80 and lecithin
Formaldehyde	Ammonium ions
Glutaraldehyde	Glycine
Halogens	Sodium thiosulphate
Hexachlorophane	Tween 80
Mercurials	Thioglycollic acid
Phenolic disinfectants	Dilution or Tween 80
QACs	Lubrol W and lecithin or Tween 80 and lecithin
Sulphonamides	p-Aminobenzoic acid

QAC, quaternary ammonium compound.
* This table should be read in conjunction with Table 23.3 in Chapter 23.

Quaternary ammonium compounds (QACs; Chapter 10) such as cetrimide, and also the bisbiguanide, chlorhexidine, are notoriously prone to promote clumping. A non-ionic surface-active agent of the type formed by condensing ethylene oxide with a long-chain fatty acid such as Cirrasol ALN-WF (ICI Ltd), formerly known as Lubrol W, together with lecithin, added to the diluting fluid has been used to overcome this effect.

A British Standard (BS 3286: 1960) dealt specifically with the laboratory evaluation of the biocidal activity of QACs. This has now been revised (BS 6471: 1984) and a specification (BS 6424: 1984) for QAC-based aromatic disinfectants introduced.

In certain instances it will be necessary to subject data obtained from viable counts to statistical analysis or, more sensibly, experiments should be designed so as to render them amenable to statistical treatment.

3.3 Mycobactericidal activity

Because of their hydrophobic nature, it is often difficult to prepare homogeneous suspensions of mycobacteria. Moreover, some, e.g. *Mycobacterium tuberculosis*, are slow-growing strains. It has been suggested that the non-pathogenic *M. terrae* can be used as an indicator organism for *M. tuberculosis*. Generally, the principle of testing methods is the same as for other non-sporing bacteria.

3.4 Sporicidal activity

Sporicidal activity can be determined against spores in liquid suspension or against spores dried on carriers. In principle, techniques are similar to those described for bactericidal tests. However, it should be realized that spores must germinate and outgrow before colony formation is observed. For this reason, incubation of recovery media should be continued for several days.

3.5 *In vivo* tests

Tests considered above have all been conducted in artificial or laboratory conditions. This may be satisfactory when disinfectants are required to act in non-living environments. However, many antibacterials are used on living tissue and on the skin, and so tests to evaluate them in these situations are called for.

3.5.1 *Skin tests*

The test organism may be placed on the skin, e.g. on the back of the hand, and the preparation to be evaluated placed on the same area. After a given time interval the area is swabbed with sterile cotton wool and the swab incubated in a suitable medium or washed in a suitable fluid, and viable counts are subsequently made.

One type of test measures the inhibition of respiration of bacterial cells on pieces of pig skin by the substance under test. Here, the factor of correlation between cell death and cessation of respiration should be borne in mind.

Hygienic hand disinfection. Hygienic hand disinfection is a term used to denote the killing and removal of transient microorganisms on the skin, i.e. those germs that literally 'come and go' and which do not therefore form part of the resident skin population. Essentially, hygienic hand disinfection is a measure to prevent the transmission of these organisms. It can be achieved in two ways.
1 Use of a hygienic hand rub, in which a suitable disinfectant or disinfectant–detergent is rubbed into dry hands for not more than 30 seconds. A suitable test method is to compare a product with a standard (70% ethanol or 60% isopropanol): the product must not be less effective than the standard.
2 Use of a hygienic hand wash, in which a suitable disinfectant or disinfectant-detergent is rubbed into wet or dry hands for not more than 30 seconds and then washing the hands in water. A suitable test method is to compare a product with a standard (soap and water): the product must be significantly more effective than the control.

Surgical hand disinfection. This term refers to the pre-operative disinfection of surgeons' hands, with the aim of preventing surgical wound infection. The most important criteria associated with surgical hand disinfection are:

1   a reduction of the resident skin flora to low levels;
2   a prolonged effect (lasting several hours);
3   minimal irritation to the skin.

The principle of tests evaluating the efficacy of surgical hand disinfectants is to sample the resident flora of the hands before and after surgical hand disinfection.

3.5.2   *Other in vivo tests*

Tests have been published for determining toxicity towards leucocytes. Evaluation on the infected chorioallantoic membrane of hens' eggs was suggested as being a useful method of testing potential wound disinfectants.

3.5.3   *Toxicity tests*

It is prudent to make an assessment of the systematic toxicity of a preparation to be used on wounds to guard against the possibility of general poisoning which may follow absorption of the medicament.

3.6   Estimation of bacteriostasis

Tests considered to date have, without exception, measured unequivocally the bactericidal effect. In some instances it is useful to know the minimum concentration which inhibits growth (reproduction) rather than those concentrations which achieve a rapid kill. The implications of the terms 'bactericide' and 'bacteriostat' were discussed earlier (see section 1.1, Fig. 11.1).

Methods which measure only growth inhibition (bacteriostasis) are given below.

3.6.1   *Serial dilution*

Graded doses of the test substance are incorporated into broth dispensed in McCartney boules and the bottles inoculated with the test organism and incubated. The point at which no growth occurs is taken as the bacteriostatic concentration (minimum inhibitory concentration, MIC). It is essential when performing these tests to determine the size of the inoculum as the position of the end-point varies considerably with inoculum size, which should always be defined in any description of result.

The test is carried out in practice by mixing the appropriate volume of the solution under test with double-strength broth and making it up to volume with water as illustrated in Table 11.5. If the volume of the inoculum is greater than 1–3 drops, this must be compensated for in planning a table of dilutions.

3.6.2   *Ditch-plate technique*

The test solution is placed in a ditch cut in nutrient agar contained in a Petri dish, or it

Table 11.5 Contents of containers for determining the MIC of phenol

	Final volume (ml) in container					
Double-strength broth	5	5	5	5	5	5
0.5% phenol solution	0	1	2	3	4	5
Sterile distilled water	5	4	3	2	1	0
Final conc. of phenol (% w/v)	0	0.05	0.1	0.15	0.2	0.25

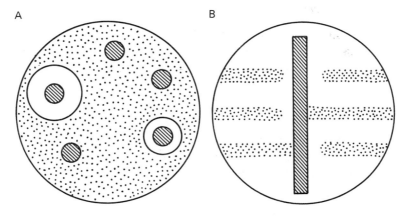

Fig. 11.5 Plates for the assessment of bacteriostatic effect of semi-solid preparations: A, cup-plate; B, ditch-plate.

may be mixed with a little agar before pouring into the ditch. The test organisms (as many as six may be tested) are streaked up to the ditch. The plate is then incubated. A typical result is shown in Fig. 11.5B. Organisms growing up to the ditch are considered resistant.

3.6.3 Cup-plate technique

The solution is placed in contact with agar, which is already inoculated with the test organism and after incubation zones of inhibition observed. The solution may be placed in a small cup sealed to the agar surface (a method used widely in antibiotic assays) in a well cut from the agar with a sterile cork-borer, or applied in the form of an impregnated disc of filter paper (Fig. 11.5A).

3.6.4 Solid dilution method

In this method the dilutions of the substance under test are made in agar instead of broth. The agar containing the substance under test is subsequently poured onto a Petri dish. It has the advantage that for any one concentration of the test substance, several organisms may be tested. Multipoint inoculators enable several organisms to be tested on one plate.

Gradient-plate technique

In this technique the concentration of a drug in an agar plate may (theoretically) be varied infinitely between zero and a given maximum. To perform the test, nutrient agar is melted, the solution under test added, and the mixture poured into a sterile Petri dish and allowed to set in the form of a wedge (Fig. 11.6A).

A second amount of agar is then poured onto the wedge and allowed to set with the Petri dish flat on the bench, giving the effect shown in Fig. 11.6B. The plates are incubated overnight to allow diffusion of the drug and to dry the surface. The test organisms must be streaked in a direction running from the highest to the lowest concentration. Up to six organisms may be tested in this way.

To calculate the result, the length of growth and the total length of the agar surface streaked is measured; then if total length of possible growth is x cm and total length of actual growth is y cm, the inhibitory concentration as determined by this method is:

$$\frac{c \times y}{x} \, \text{mg ml}^{-1}$$

where c is the final concentration, in μg or mg ml^{-1}, of the drug in the *total* volume of the medium. It should always be borne in mind that, in comparing results obtained on solid and in a liquid environment, the factor of drug diffusion may have a bearing on all results using solid environments.

3.7   **Tests for antifungal activity**

Fungi may be potential pathogens or occur as contaminants in pharmaceutical products. In performing tests on potential antifungal preparations the differing culture requirements of the fungi should be borne in mind, otherwise tests similar to those used for antibacterial activity may be employed.

Two typical media for growth of fungi are Sabouraud liquid medium and Czapek–Dox medium. Both these media may be solidified with agar if required.

A

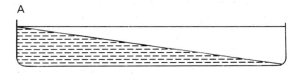

B

Maximum ———— Concentration gradient ———— Zero →

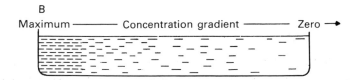

Fig. 11.6 Gradient-plate technique.

Fungicidal activity

Fungal spores or mycelium may be added to the solution under test. At selected time intervals, samples can be subcultured into suitable media and the presence or absence of growth noted after incubation. A quantitative assessment similar to that described for bactericidal activity (section 3.2, Table 11.3) can also be undertaken.

3.7.2   *Fungistatic activity*

Both the liquid and the solid dilution tests described above for bacteria (sections 3.6.1 and 3.6.4) may be used; suitable media must, of course, be employed.

3.7.3   *Choice of test organism*

For the evaluation of preparations to be used against pathogenic fungi, suitable cultures of these pathogens should be used. To test substances intended to inhibit general contaminants, cultures of common fungi obtained conveniently by exposing Petri dishes of solid media to the atmosphere may be used, or alternatively dust or soil may be used as a source of a mixed inoculum.

3.8   **Virucidal activity**

The testing of disinfectants for virucidal activity is not an easy matter. As pointed out earlier (Chapter 3), viruses are unable to grow in artificial culture media and thus some other system, usually employing living cells, must be considered. One such example is tissue culture, but not all virus types can propagate under such circumstances and so an alternative approach has to be adopted in specific instances. The principles of such methods are given below.

3.8.1   *Tissue culture or egg inoculation*

A standardized viral suspension is exposed, in the presence of yeast suspension, to appropriate dilutions of disinfectant in WHO hard water. At appropriate times, dilutions are made in inactivated horse serum and each dilution is inoculated into tissue cell culture or embryonated eggs (as appropriate for the test virus). The drop in infectivity of the treated virus is compared with that of the control (untreated) virus.

Since disinfectant itself might be toxic to the tissue culture or eggs, a toxicity test must also be carried out. Here, appropriate dilutions of disinfectant are mixed with inactivated horse serum and inoculated into tissue cells or eggs (as appropriate). These are examined daily for damage.

3.8.2   *Plaque assays*

Plaque assays, at present, apply to only a very limited number of viruses, e.g. poliovirus, herpes virus, human rotavirus. The principle of these assays is as follows: test virus is dried on to coverslips which are immersed in various concentrations of test disinfectant

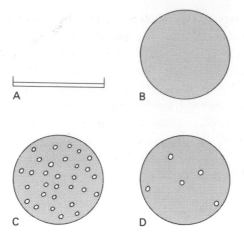

Fig. 11.7 A, diagrammatic representation of plaque assay for evaluating virucidal activity and B, monolayers of baby hamster kidney (BHK) cells; C, virus titre: *untreated* virus (o represents a plaque-forming unit, pfu, in BHK cells): D, virus titre: *disinfectant-treated* virus (before plating onto BHK, the disinfectant must be neutralized in an appropriate manner). Note the greatly reduced number of pfu in D, indicative of fewer uninactivated virus particles than in C.

for various time intervals and a plaque-counting method used to determine surviving viral particles. The plaques are similar to those described in Chapter 3, except that a host cell other than bacteria (Chapter 3) has to be employed.

For assaying herpes virus, monolayers of baby hamster kidney (BHK) cells are used. Virus titre is expressed as the number of plaque-forming units (pfu) per millilitre before and after exposure to a disinfectant, so that the virucidal efficacy of the test agent can be determined. A diagrammatic representation is given in Fig. 11.7.

3.8.3 *'Acceptable' animal model*

The hepatitis B virus (HBV) does not grow in tissue culture and an 'acceptable' animal model has been found to be the chimpanzee. This is observed for clinical infection after inoculation with treated and untreated virus, care being taken in the test series that residual disinfectant is removed by adequate means before inoculation into the animal.

This procedure is limited by the number of animals that can be used and by the strictures imposed by a humane approach. HBV has not yet been transmitted to non-primate animals.

3.8.4 *Duck hepatitis B virus: a possible model of infectivity of human hepatitis B virus*

Duck hepatitis B virus (DHBV) has been proposed as a possible model for the inactivation of human HBV by chemical disinfectants. The principle of the test method uses viral DNA polymerase (DNAP) as a target, total inhibition *in vitro* of DNAP by chemical disinfectants being predictive of inactivation of infectivity *in vivo*.

3.8.5 *Immune reaction*

Three types of particles are associated with HBV: small spherical particles, 22 nm in diameter; tubular particles, also having a diameter of 22 nm; and larger spherical particles (42 nm diameter) known as the Dane particles. The Dane particle alone has a typical virus structure and appears to be infectious but is the least common form. It consists of a complex, double-layered sphere with an electron-dense core. It contains partially double-stranded circular DNA and is regarded as the putative virion (for further information on virions see Chapter 3). The Dane particles contain three antigens: hepatitis B surface antigen (HBsAg) which is also present on 22-nm particles, hepatitis B core antigen (HBcAg) found in the inner core and hepatitis B e antigen (HBeAg) found in the core and responsible for infectivity.

The specific immunological detection of the HBV surface antigen (HBsAg) is considered as being presumptive evidence for the presence of viable HBV. The hypothesis, then, on which this method is based is that if the disinfectant can destroy the reactivity of the HBsAg, it can also destroy the infectivity of HBV. A problem with some disinfectants, e.g. formaldehyde and glutaraldehyde, is that their actions are essentially fixative in nature. The HBsAg immunological reaction is thus not destroyed at concentrations known to be high enough to kill the most resistant forms (bacterial spores) of microorganisms. Furthermore, concentrations of disinfectants necessary to inactivate HBsAg within a reasonable period of time are often comparatively high.

This type of procedure may thus suggest that an unnecessarily high disinfectant concentration (so-called overkill) may be employed in practice to achieve a virucidal effect.

3.8.6 Virus morphology

The serum from patients with clinical symptoms of hepatitis B commonly contain three distinct structures that possess HBsAg (section 3.8.5 above). The effects of different concentrations of various disinfectants on the structure of Dane particles have been studied, but it is unlikely that morphological changes can be related to virucidal activity.

3.8.7 Endogenous reverse transcriptase

The human immunodeficiency virus (HIV; lymphadenopathy-associated virus, LAV; human T-cell lymphotrophic virus type 3, HTLV III) is responsible for acquired immune deficiency syndrome (AIDS; see Chapter 3). Because of the hazard and difficulties of growing the virus outside humans, a different approach has to be examined for determining viral sensitivity to disinfectants.

Studies have demonstrated that one such method is to examine the effects of disinfectants on endogenous RNA-dependent DNA polymerase (i.e. reverse transcriptase) activity. In essence, HIV is an RNA virus; after it enters a cell the RNA is converted to DNA under the influence of reverse transcriptase. The virus induces a cytopathic effect on T lymphocytes, and in the assay reverse transcriptase activity is determined after exposure to different concentrations of various disinfectants. However, it has been suggested that monitoring residual viral reverse transcriptase activity is not a satisfactory alternative to tests whereby infectious HIV can be detected in systems employing fresh human peripheral blood mononuclear cells.

3.8.8 Bacteriophage

A model for evaluating virucidal agents has been described which employs bacteriophages as indicator organisms. Bacteriophages used include those infecting *Escherichia coli*, *Bacteroides fragilis* and *Pseudomonas aeruginosa*.

4   Semi-solid antibacterial preparations

The use of the term 'semi-solid' has been coined to embrace a group of pharmaceutical preparations known as pastes, ointments, creams and gels. The chief feature which distinguishes the first three is their viscosity or, to use a more descriptive word, their stiffness, which decreases in the order: paste, ointment, cream. They may consist of an intimate mixture of the active agent with either an oleaginous base or, alternatively, an emulsion with either water or an oleaginous substance as a continuous phase. Gels are preparations in which the base is usually a carbohydrate polymer (starch, pectin, methylcellulose, tragacanth, sterculia gum) and water, or more rarely having a base of protein origin, such as gelatin, with a suitable quantity of water. More recently polyethylene glycols and other organic polymers have been used.

When formulating antibacterial preparations it is imperative to realize that the properties of the base may seriously modify the antibacterial activity of the medicament. It is quite useless to formulate a well-proven antiseptic into an otherwise elegant pharmaceutical preparation without determining if the final formulation is, itself, an effective antibacterial agent.

4.1   Tests for bacteriostatic activity

The first official test was published by the Food, Drug and Insecticide Administration of the US Department of Agriculture, in which portions of the preparation were placed on the surface of nutrient agar inoculated with *Staph. aureus*. After incubation the zones of inhibition, if any, around the preparation were measured. This test was modified later by incorporating 10% of horse serum in the agar 'to simulate conditions in a wound' and a control consisting of unmedicated base was also used in each experiment. This test is known as the cup-plate test (see also section 3.6.3 and Fig. 11.5).

In addition to placing the test preparation onto sectors of seeded agar, it may be placed in a trough cut in uninoculated agar and test organisms streaked in parallel lines up to the edge of the trough. Failure to grow up to the edge is indicative of inhibition.

Thus, the cup-plate method is useful to test several preparations or varying formulations of the same preparation against one organism under identical conditions, and the ditch-plate method enables one preparation to be tested against several organisms (see Fig. 11.5A, B).

4.2   Tests for bactericidal activity

A number of tests have been described which imitate, at least in part, the principle of the phenol coefficient test for liquid disinfectants. A culture of the test organism is mixed intimately with the semi-solid preparation, and the mixture subcultured by means of a loop into a suitable broth designed to disperse the base and neutralize the antibacterial activity of the medicament.

Thus, the culture may be mixed and transferred to a hypodermic syringe surrounded by a constant-temperature jacket; at desired intervals, the mixture is subcultured by ejecting small volumes from the syringe nozzle into subculture medium.

A technique, devised by one of the authors (W.B.H.), was designed to test the preparation when spread on to an infected surface. The surface of a nutrient agar plate was inoculated evenly with the test organism and incubated to produce an even surface growth. The preparation under test was spread evenly upon this, and at selected time intervals a core of agar, cells and preparation were removed with a sterile cork-borer and the disc of agar and cell removed by means of a sterile needle and inoculated into recovery medium, which was then incubated. As much of the preparation is removed as is possible and care taken to ensure its dispersal in the medium. The organism should, if still viable, grow through the back of the agar disc to give growth in the subculture tube also.

4.3 Tests on skin

It is possible to also test semi-solid antibacterial preparations on the skin itself, as described for liquid disinfectants (section 3.5.1). A portion of the skin—the backs of the fingers between the joints is a useful spot—is treated with the test organism, the preparation is then applied and after a suitable interval the area is swabbed and the swab incubated in a suitable medium. Alternatively, the method employing pig skin, described in section 3.5.1, may well be adapted to the problem of testing semi-solid skin disinfectants.

4.4 General conclusions

It is suggested that, as a minimum routine for the final test of an alleged antibacterial semi-solid formulation, the following be used.
1 The cup-plate technique for bacteriostatic activity (section 3.6.3).
2 A test for bactericidal activity.
3 A skin test.

For routine assessment of test formulations during development work the cup-plate and ditch-plate methods are adequate.

5 Solid disinfectants

Solid disinfectants (disinfectant powders) usually consist of a disinfectant substance diluted by an inert powder. For example phenolic substances adsorbed onto kieselguhr form the basis of many disinfectant powders, while another widely used powder of respectable antiquity is hypochlorite powder. Disinfectant or antiseptic powders for use in medicine include substances such as acriflavine, or antifungal compounds such as zinc undecenoate or salicylic acid mixed with talc.

Solid disinfectants may be evaluated *in vitro* by applying them to suitable test organisms growing on solid medium. Discs may be cut from the agar and subcultured, observing the usual precautions.

To test their inhibitory power, the powders may be dusted onto the surface of seeded agar plates, using the inert diluent as a control and noting the extent of growth.

Disinfectant and sanitary powders are the subject of a British Standard (BS 1013:1946), now withdrawn, which describes a method of determining the RW coefficient of such powders. A weighed quantity was shaken with distilled water at 18°C for 30 minutes and this suspension was used in the test already described (section 3.1.1).

6   Evaluation of air disinfectants

One of the most potent routes for transmission of bacterial disease is via the air. Cross-infection in hospital wards, infection in operating theatres, the transmission of disease in closed spaces such as cinemas and other places of assembly, in the ward rooms and crew's quarters of ships and in submarines are all well known. Of equal importance is the provision of a bacteria-free environment for aseptic manipulations generally. Clearly, the disinfection of atmospheres is a worthwhile field of study and to this end much research has been done. It is equally clearly important to be able to evaluate preparations claimed to be air disinfectants.

Heretofore the milieu on or in which the disinfectant has been required to act has been either solid or liquid; now antibacterial action in the gas or vapour phase or in the form of aerosol (colloidal) interaction must be considered, and this presents the problem of determining the viable airborne population.

6.1   Determination of viable airborne microorganisms

The simplest way of assessing the viable microbial population of the air is to expose Petri dishes containing a solid nutrient medium to the air, followed by incubation; indeed this method was used in 1881 by Koch. Although this method does depend on the organisms or organism-bearing particles actually falling on the plate by gravity it is a method which is still used to assess the general cleanliness of air in pharmaceutical factories where aseptic operations are taking place, in food processing areas or in hospital wards. More positive data may be obtained, however, if a force other than gravity is used to collect airborne particles.

An early attempt at quantification consisted of placing a Petri dish containing a nutrient agar in a box beneath an inverted funnel, the stem of which passed out of the box into the atmosphere. By applying a partial vacuum to the box, air was drawn in through the stem of the funnel and impinged on the agar. The plate could be incubated directly and developing colonies counted. Provided the air drawn in was metered, a direct quantitative assessment of the viable airborne population could be made. This idea led logically to the development of the slit sampler illustrated in Fig. 11.8. The principle is similar to that described immediately above, but the Petri dish is placed on a turntable which can be revolved at varying speeds and the funnel is replaced by a cylinder in which the end nearest the nutrient medium is furnished with a slit ca. 2.5 mm wide. The arrangement is set so that the slit runs parallel to a radius of the dish but leaves a clear space around the circumference and at the centre of the plate. In operation,

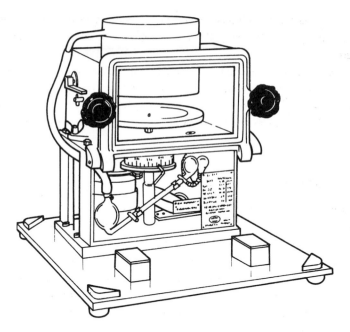

Fig. 11.8 Slit sampler (C.F. Casella & Co., Ltd).

a vacuum is applied to the chamber containing the turntable, air passes in through the slit and the nutrient medium revolves so that the airborne particles, if any, are trapped on the medium and spread in a sector over the medium.

6.2 Experimental evaluation

In brief, the experimental technique is to create a bacterial population in a close chamber, obtain a quantitative assessment of the viable airborne bacterial population by means of a suitable sampling device, submit the population to the disinfectant action, whether ultraviolet light, chemical vapour or aerosol, and then determine the airborne population at suitable intervals.

7 Preservatives

Preservatives may include disinfectant and antiseptic chemicals together with certain compounds used almost exclusively as preservatives. They are added to many industrial, including pharmaceutical, products which may, by their nature, support the growth of bacteria and moulds causing spoilage of the product and possibly infection of the user. In the field of pharmaceutical preservation, addition of an inhibitory substance to a multidose injection (Chapter 21) or the prevention of growth in aqueous suspensions of drugs intended for oral administration (Chapter 18) are prime examples.

Preservatives are widely employed in cosmetic preservation for lotions, creams and shampoos. Preservation is also an important aspect of formulation in emulsion paints and cutting fluids, i.e. fluids used to cool and lubricate lathe and drilling tools.

7.1 Evaluation of preservatives

Potential chemical preservatives may be evaluated in the first place by the methods outlined above, especially by determining MIC values (section 3.6) or by viable counts (section 3.2). The RW, CM and KS tests (sections 3.1.1 and 3.1.2) have no relevance in preservative evaluation. It will be recalled (section 2.5) that formula ingredients may reduce the efficiency of a preservative which has shown up well in conventional tests using culture media as the suspending fluid.

Emulsions, especially oil-in-water emulsions which, incidentally, figure widely in cosmetic products, are especially prone to failure because the preservative may partition into the oily phase of the emulsion while contaminants will flourish in the aqueous phase now deprived of preservative by partitioning (see Chapter 18 for further details).

The cardinal requirement, therefore, for preservative efficacy is the evaluation of the finally preserved preparation and this may be performed by means of a challenge test. In essence, the (hopefully) preserved product is deliberately inoculated (challenged) with suitable test organisms and incubated and examined to see if the inoculum has been able to grow or if its growth has been successfully suppressed. There has been extensive debate on challenge testing and the subject has been reviewed by Cowen and Steiger (1976).

The *British Pharmacopoeia* (1993) contains a test for efficacy of preservatives. In essence, the product is deliberately challenged separately by the fungus *Aspergillus niger*, the yeast *Candida albicans* and the bacteria *Ps. aeruginosa* and *Staph. aureus*. These organisms represent potential contaminants in the environment in which products are prepared, stored or used. Other organisms may be used in specified circumstances, e.g. the osmophilic yeast, *Zygosaccharomyces rouxii* for preparations with a high sucrose content, and *E. coli* for oral liquid preparations.

Different performance criteria are laid down for injectable and ophthalmic preparations, topical preparations and oral liquid preparations. Inhibition of the challenge organism is determined by viable counting techniques. The *British Pharmacopoeia* (1993) should be consulted for full details of the experimental procedures to be used.

The *United States Pharmacopeia* (1995, 23rd edn) also gives procedures for evaluating the efficacy of antimicrobial preservatives in pharmaceutical products.

7.2 Preservative combinations

The use of preservative combinations may be used to extend the range and spectrum of preservation. Thus, in the series of alkyl esters of 4-hydroxybenzoic (*p*-hydroxybenzoic) acid (parabens), water solubility decreases in the order: methyl, ethyl, propyl and butyl ester. By combining these products it is possible to achieve a situation where both the aqueous and oil phase of an emulsion are protected.

Combinations may also be used to extend the spectrum of a preservative system. Thus, the preservative Germall 115 has an essentially antibacterial activity and very low, if not zero, antifungal activity. By combining Germall 115 with parabens, which possess antifungal activity, a broader spectrum (antibacterial/antifungal) preservative system is obtained.

Synergy in preservative combinations

Very occasionally a combination of antimicrobial agents exhibits synergy. Synergy is measured against a single microorganism and is exhibited when a combination of two compounds exerts a greater inhibitory effect than could be expected from a simple additive effect of the two compounds in the mixture.

7.2.2

Evaluation of synergy

Synergy may be evaluated and displayed by preparing mixtures of the two compounds being investigated and determining their growth inhibitory power by means of an MIC determination (section 3.6.1).

The results may be plotted in the form of a graph (called an isobologram) and an example is given in Fig. 11.9. This graph may be interpreted as follows: 50×10^{-2} mg% and 35 mg% of phenylmercuric acetate and chlorocresol, respectively, used alone, inhibits the growth of *Staph. aureus*. In combination, 20×10^{-2} mg% of phenylmercuric acetate and 5 mg% of chlorocresol inhibit the growth of this organism. Thus, growth

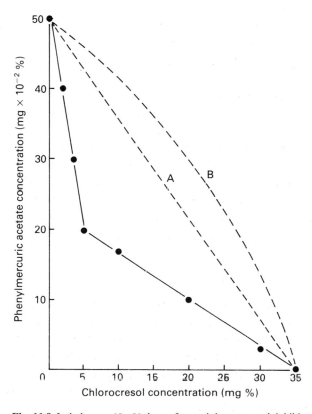

Fig. 11.9 Isobologram (●—●) drawn from minimum growth inhibitory concentrations (MIC values) of chlorocresol and phenylmercuric acetate used alone and in combination against *Staph. aureus*, showing synergy. A, result if combination was merely additive; B, result if combination was antagonistic.

Evaluation of non-antibiotic antimicrobial agents 253

inhibition is obtained with a lower total quantity of preservative. If the combinations were merely additive, the isobologram plot would follow the course of the dashed line (A), and if antagonistic the dashed curve (B).

Synergy has been discussed in depth by Denyer *et al.* (1985) and Hodges & Hanlon (1991).

7.2.3   *Rapid methods*

In many cases, especially in the food industry, it would be very useful if the performance of a biocide or the extent of contamination of product, apparatus and working surfaces could be deduced sooner than that provided by a method which depends on visible microbial growth (12–24 hours). Many methods have been devised to secure a more rapid result and have been designated rapid tests. They have recently been reviewed by Denyer (1990).

Two such methods will be mentioned here.

1 *Epifluorescence* depends on the fact that certain dyes, acridine orange being widely used, will stain cellular material. When examined in fluorescent light any living cells present will fluoresce green or greenish yellow, whereas dead cells will appear orange to red. The methods will be found in the literature under direct epifluorescent microscopy (DEM) and direct epifluorescent filter technique (DEFT). In DEM, material suspected of being contaminated or a sample in which living bacteria are sought are examined directly; in DEFT the sample being examined is filtered and the residue on the filter examined as above.

2 *Bioluminescence.* In another method, luminous bacteria, or bacteria not normally luminous but which have been manipulated genetically to become luminous, are used. Their death under chemical stress or presence in hygiene studies are assessed in a sensitive light meter. A variant of this method depends on the fact that bacterial adenosine triphosphatase (ATPase), present in bacteria, will catalyse the normal biological light-producing reaction to give detectable light in a sensitive meter.

This is a very brief summary but is included as readers may come across these methods or a reference to rapid methods in their general reading or work experience.

8   Appendix: British Standards

British Standards relating to disinfectants (date in brackets at end of an entry means that the Standard was confirmed on that date without further revision).

(1986) *'Specification for black and white disinfectants'.* BS 2462: 1986 [1991].

(1986) *'Glossary of terms relating to disinfectants'.* BS 5283: 1986 [1991].

(1976) *'Aromatic disinfectant fluids'.* BS 5197: 1976 [1991].

(1984) *'Method for determination of the antimicrobial activity of QAC disinfectant formulations'.* BS 6471: 1984 [1994].

(1990) *'Specification for QAC based aromatic disinfectant fluids'.* BS 6424: 1984 [1990].

(1985) *'Method for determination of the Rideal–Walker coefficient of disinfectants'.* BS 541: 1985 [1991].

(1986) *'Method for assessing the efficacy of disinfectants by the modified Chick–Martin test'.* BS 808: 1986 [1991].

9 Further reading

Akers M.J. & Taylor C.J. (1990) Official methods of preservative evaluation and testing. In: *Guide to Microbiological Control in Pharmaceuticals* (eds S.P. Denyer & R.M. Baird), pp. 292–303. Chichester: Ellis Horwood.

Cowen R.A. (1978) Kelsey–Sykes capacity test: a critical review. *Pharm J*, **220**, 202–204.

Cowen R.A. & Steiger B. (1976) Antimicrobial activity—a critical review of test methods of preservative efficiency. *J Soc Cosmet Chem*, **27**, 467–481.

Croshaw B. (1981) Disinfectant testing—with particular reference to the Rideal–Walker and Kelsey–Sykes tests. In: *Disinfectants: Their Use and Evaluation of Effectiveness* (eds C.H. Collins, M.C. Allwood, S.F. Bloomfield & A. Fox), pp. 1–15. London: Academic Press.

Denyer S.P. (1990) Monitoring microbiological quality: application of rapid microbiological methods to pharmaceuticals. In: *Guide to Microbiological Control in Pharmaceuticals* (eds S.P. Denyer & R.M. Baird), pp. 146–156. Chichester: Ellis Horwood.

Denyer S.P. & Hugo W.B. (eds) (1991) *Mechanisms of Action of Chemical Biocides*. Society for Applied Bacteriology Technical Series No. 27. Oxford: Blackwell Scientific Publications.

Denyer S.P., Hugo W.B. & Harding V.D. (1985) Synergy in preservative combinations. *Int J Pharm*, **25**, 245–253.

Hodges N.A. & Hanlon G.W. (1991) Detection and measurement of combined biocide action. In: *Mechanisms of Action of Chemical Biocides* (eds S.P. Denyer & W.B. Hugo), Society for Applied Bacteriology Technical Series No. 27, pp. 297–310. Oxford: Blackwell Scientific Publications.

Jones M.V., Bellamy K., Alcock R. & Hudson R. (1991) The use of bacteriophage MS2 as a model system to evaluate virucidal hand disinfectants. *J Hosp Infect*, **17**, 270–285.

Kelsey J.C. & Maurer I.M. (1974) An improved Kelsey–Sykes test for disinfectants. *Pharm J*, **207**, 528–530.

Leak R.E. & Leech R. (1988) Challenge tests and their predictive stability. In: *Microbial Quality Assurance in Pharmaceuticals, Cosmetics and Toiletries* (eds S.F. Bloomfield, R. Baird, R.E. Leak & R. Leach), pp. 129–146. Chichester: Ellis Horwood.

Maillard J.Y., Beggs T.S., Day M.J., Hudson R.A. & Russell A.D. (1993). Effect of biocides on *Pseudomonas aeruginosa* phage F116. *Lett Appl Microb*, **17**, 167–170.

Orth D.S. (1990) Preservative evaluation and testing: the linear regression method. In: *Guide to Microbiological Control in Pharmaceuticals* (eds S.P. Denyer & R.M. Baird), pp. 304–312. Chichester: Ellis Horwood.

Pinto R.M., Abad F.X., Roca R.M., Riera J.M. & Bosch A. (1991) The use of *Bacteroides fragilis* phages as indicators of the efficiency of virucidal products. *FEMS Microb Lett*, **82**, 61–66.

Resnick L., Veren K., Salahuddin S.Z., Tondreau S. & Markham P.D. (1986) Stability and inactivation of HTLV-III/LAV under clinical and laboratory environments. *J Am Med Assoc*, **255**, 1887–1891.

Reybrouck G. (1992) The evaluation of the antimicrobial activity of disinfectants. In: *Principles and Practice of Disinfection, Preservation and Sterilization* (eds A.D. Russell, W.B. Hugo & G.A.J. Ayliffe), 2nd edn, pp. 114–133. Oxford: Blackwell Scientific Publications.

Russell A.D. (1981) Neutralization procedures in the evaluation of bactericidal activity. In: *Disinfectants: Their Use and Evaluation of Effectiveness* (eds C.H. Collins, M.C. Allwood, S.F. Bloomfield & A. Fox), pp. 45–59. London: Academic Press.

Russell A.D. (1982) *The Destruction of Bacterial Spores*. London: Academic Press.

Russell A.D. & Chopra I. (1996) *Understanding Antibacterial Action and Resistance*. Chichester: Ellis Horwood.

Russell A.D., Hugo W.B. & Ayliffe G.A.J. (eds) (1998) *Principles and Practice of Disinfection, Preservation and Sterilization*, 3rd edn. Oxford: Blackwell Science.

Stannard C.J., Petitt S.B. & Skinner F.A. (eds) (1989) *Rapid Microbiological Methods for Foods, Beverages and Pharmaceuticals*. Society for Applied Bacteriology Technical Series No. 25. Oxford: Blackwell Scientific Publications.

Tyler R. & Ayliffe G.A.J. (1987) A surface test for virucidal activity of disinfectants: preliminary study with herpes virus. *J Hosp Infect*, **9**, 22–29.

12 Mode of action of non-antibiotic antibacterial agents

1   Cell wall

2   Cytoplasmic membrane
2.1   Action on membrane potentials
2.2   Action on membrane enzymes
2.2.1 Electron transport chain
2.2.2 Adenosine triphosphatase
2.2.3 Enzymes with thiol groups
2.3   Action on general membrane
       permeability
2.3.1 Permeabilization

3   Cytoplasm

3.1   General coagulation
3.2   Ribosomes
3.3   Nucleic acids
3.4   Thiol groups
3.5   Amino groups

**4   Highly reactive compounds: multitarget
       reactors**

5   Conclusions

6   Further reading

This group of drugs has often been classified as non-specific protoplasmic poisons and indeed such views are still expressed today. Such a broad generalization is, however, very far from the true position.

It is convenient to consider the modes of action in terms of the drugs' targets within the bacterial cell, and in the following pages various examples will be given. The targets to be considered are the cell wall, the cytoplasmic membrane and the cytoplasm. Much more detailed treatments of the subject will be found in the references at the end of this chapter. Experimental methods for determining the mode of action of an antimicrobial substance have recently been compiled (Denyer & Hugo, 1991).

1   Cell wall

This structure is the traditional target for a group of antibiotics which include the penicillins (Chapter 5), but a little-noticed report which appeared in 1948 showed that low concentrations of disinfectant substances caused cell wall lysis such that a normally turbid suspension of bacteria became clear. It was thought that these low concentrations of disinfectant cause enzymes whose normal role is to synthesize the cell wall to reverse their role in some way and effect its disruption or lysis.

In the original report, the disinfectants (at the following percentages: formalin, 0.12; phenol, 0.32; mercuric chloride, 0.0008; sodium hypochlorite, 0.005 and merthiolate, 0.0004) caused lysis of *Escherichia coli*, streptococci and staphylococci.

Glutaraldehyde also owes part of its mode of action to its ability to react with, and provide irreversible crosslinking in, the cell wall. As a result, other cell functions are impaired. This phenomenon is especially found in Gram-positive cells.

2   Cytoplasmic membrane

Actions on the cytoplasmic membrane may be divided into three categories.

1 Action on membrane potentials.

2 Action on membrane enzymes.

3 Action on general membrane permeability.

2.1 Action on membrane potentials

Recent work has shown that bacteria, in common with chloroplasts and mitochondria, are able, through the membrane-bound electron transport chain aerobically, or the membrane-bound adenosine triphosphate (ATP) anerobically, to maintain a gradient of electrical potential and pH such that the interior of the bacterial cell is negative and alkaline. This potential gradient and the electrical equivalent of the pH difference (1 pH unit $\equiv$ 58 mV at 37°C) give a potential difference across the membrane of 100–180 mV, with the inside negative. The membrane is impermeable to protons, whose extrusion creates the potential described.

These results may be expressed in the form of an equation, thus:

$$\Delta p = \Delta \psi - Z\Delta pH$$

where Δp is the protonmotive force, $\Delta \psi$ the membrane electrical potential and ΔpH the transmembrane pH gradient, i.e. the pH difference between the inside and outside of the cytoplasmic membrane. Z is a factor converting pH units to millivolts so that all the units of the equation are the same, i.e. millivolts. Z is temperature-dependent and at 37°C has a value of 62.

This potential, or protonmotive force as it is also called, in turn drives a number of energy-requiring functions which include the synthesis of ATP, the coupling of oxidative processes to phosphorylation, a metabolic sequence called oxidative phosphorylation and the transport and concentration in the cell of metabolites such as sugars and amino acids. This, in a few simple words, is the basis of the chemiosmotic theory linking metabolism to energy-requiring processes.

Certain chemical substances have been known for many years to uncouple oxidation from phosphorylation and to inhibit active transport, and for this reason they are named uncoupling agents. They are believed to act by rendering the membrane permeable to protons hence short-circuiting the potential gradient or protonmotive force.

Some examples of antibacterial agents which owe at least a part of their activity to this ability are tetrachlorosalicylanilide (TCS), tricarbanilide, trichlorocarbanilide (TCC), pentachlorophenol, di-(5-chloro-2-hydroxyphenyl) sulphide (fentichlor) and 2-phenoxyethanol.

2.2 Action on membrane enzymes

2.2.1 Electron transport chain

Hexachlorophane inhibits the electron transport chain in bacteria and thus will inhibit all metabolic activities in aerobic bacteria.

Adenosine triphosphatase

Chlorhexidine has been shown to inhibit the membrane ATPase and could thus inhibit anaerobic processes.

2.2.3   *Enzymes with thiol groups*

Mercuric chloride, other mercury-containing antibacterials and silver will inhibit enzymes in the membrane, and for that matter in the cytoplasm, which contain thiol, –SH, groups. A similar action is shown by 2-bromo-2-nitropropan-1,3-diol (bronopol) and *iso*-thiazolones. Under appropriate conditions the toxic action on cell thiol groups may be reversed by addition of an extrinsic thiol compound, for example cysteine or thioglycollic acid (see also Chapters 12 and 23).

2.3   Action on general membrane permeability

This lesion was recognized early as being one effect of many disinfectant substances. The membrane, as well as providing a dynamic link between metabolism and transport, serves to maintain the pool of metabolites within it.

Treatment of bacterial cells with appropriate concentrations of such substances as cetrimide, chlorhexidine, phenol and hexylresorcinol, causes a leakage of a group of characteristic chemical species. The potassium ion, being a small entity, is the first substance to appear when the cytoplasmic membrane is damaged. Amino acids, purines, pyrimidines and pentoses are examples of other substances which will leak from treated cells.

If the action of the drug is not prolonged or exerted in high concentration the damage may be reversible and leakage may only induce bacteriostasis.

2.3.1   *Permeabilization*

Drugs able to affect outer membrane integrity have also been exploited as potentiators of antimicrobial agents (biocides, i.e. redisinfectants, antiseptics and preservatives, and antibiotics) thereby helping these to penetrate the outer membrane of Gram-negative organisms and especially *Pseudomonas aeruginosa*.

Chelators, especially ethylenediamine tetra-acetic acid (EDTA), have been used as potentiators of the action of chloroxylenol. Vaara has extensively reviewed the subject of permeabilization and Ayres, Furr and Russell have described a rapid method of evaluating the permeabilization of *Ps. aeruginosa* (see Further Reading, Section 6).

3   Cytoplasm

Within the cytoplasm are a number of important subcellular particles which include the ribosome and oxy- and deoxyribonucleic acids. Enzymes other than those in the membrane are also present in the cytoplasm.

Many early studies measured overall enzyme inhibition in bacterial cultures and a search was made for a peculiarly sensitive enzyme which might be identified as a target, interference with which would cause death. No such enzyme has been found.

3.1 General coagulation

High concentrations of disinfectants, for example chlorhexidine, phenol or mercury salts, will coagulate the cytoplasm and in fact it was this kind of reaction which gave rise to the epithet 'general protoplasmic poison', already referred to, providing an uncritical and dismissive definition of the mode of action of disinfectants. There is little doubt, however, that the disinfectants in use in the 1930s had just this effect when applied at high concentrations.

3.2 Ribosomes

These organelles, the sites of protein synthesis, are well-established targets for antibiotic action.

Both hydrogen peroxide and p-chloromercuribenzoate will dissociate the ribosome into its two constituent parts but whether this is a secondary reaction of the two chemicals is difficult to assess. There is no real evidence that the ribosome is a prime target for disinfectant substances.

3.3 Nucleic acids

Acridine dyes used as antiseptics, i.e. proflavine and acriflavine, will react specifically with nucleic acids, by fitting into the double helical structure of this unique molecule. In so doing they interfere with its function and can thereby cause cell death.

3.4 Thiol groups

Mention has been made of thiol groups in the cytoplasmic membrane as targets for certain antibacterial compounds. Thiol groups also occur in the cytoplasm and these groups will also serve as targets.

Bronopol, *iso*-thiazolones, chlorine, chlorine-releasing agents, hypochlorites and iodine will oxidize or react with thiol groups.

3.5 Amino groups

Formaldehyde, sulphur dioxide and glutaraldehyde react with amino groups. If these groups are essential for metabolic activity, cell death will follow reactions of this nature. Chlorinated *iso*-thiazolones as well as acting on -SH groups, (Section 3.4), can react with -NH$_2$ groups.

4 Highly reactive compounds: multitarget reactors

There are one or two chemical sterilants in use whose chemical reactivity is so high

Table 12.1 Cellular-targets for non-antibiotic antibacterial drugs

No.	Target or reaction attacked	Acridine dyes	Alcohols	Anilides (TCS, TCC)	Bronopol	Chlorhexidine	Copper II salts	Ethylene oxide	Formaldehyde	Glutaraldehyde	Hexachlorophane	Hydrogen peroxide	Hypochlorites, chlorine releasers	Iodine	Mercury II salts, organic mercurials	Phenols	β-propiolactone	QACs	Silver salts	Sulphur dioxide, sulphites	Iso-thiazolones
1	Cell wall								+	+			+		+	+					
2	Cytoplasmic membrane		+													+					
2.1	Action on membrane potentials			+							+					+					
2.2	Action on membrane enzymes																				
2.2.1	Electron transport chain										+										
2.2.2	Adenosine triphosphatase						+														
2.2.3	Enzymes with thiol groups				+			+		+		+	+	+	+		+		+	+	+
2.3	Action on general membrane permeability		+	+		+										++		+			
3	Cytoplasm																				
3.1	General coagulation		+			+++	+++			++	+++	+			+++	+++		+++	+++		
3.2	Ribosomes														+						
3.3	Nucleic acids	+																			
3.4	Thiol groups				+		+	+	+	+		+	+	+	+		+		+		
3.5	Amino groups							+	++	+			+				+			+	
4	High reactive compounds: multitarget reactors							+		+			+				+				

Crosses, indicating activity, which appear in several rows for a given compound, demonstrate the multiple actions for the compound concerned. This activity is nearly always concentration-dependent, and the number of crosses indicates the order of concentration at which the effect is elicited, i.e. +, elicited at low concentrations; +++, elicited at high concentrations.

When a cross appears in only one target row, this is the only known site of action of the drug.

QAC, quaternary ammonium compound.

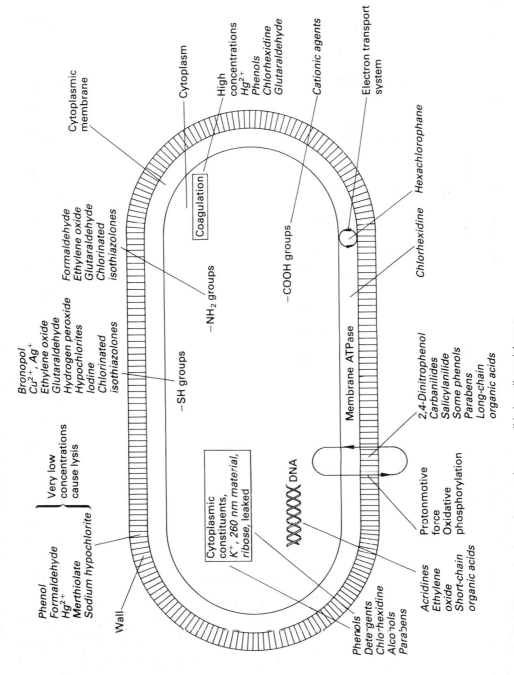

Fig. 12.1 Diagram showing main targets for non-antibiotic antibacterial agents.

Phenol
Formaldehyde
Hg²⁺
Merthiolate
Sodium hypochlorite

Very low
concentrations
cause lysis

Bronopol
Cu²⁺, Ag⁺
Ethylene oxide
Glutaraldehyde
Hydrogen peroxide
Hypochlorites
Iodine
Chlorinated
isothiazolones

Formaldehyde
Ethylene oxide
Glutaraldehyde
Chlorinated
isothiazolones

Cytoplasmic
membrane

Cytoplasm

High
concentrations
Hg²⁺
Phenols
Chlorhexidine
Glutaraldehyde

Cationic agents

Electron transport
system

Hexachlorophane

Chlorhexidine

Coagulation

−NH₂ groups

−SH groups

−COOH groups

Wall

Cytoplasmic
constituents,
K⁺, 260 nm material,
ribose, leaked

DNA

Membrane ATPase

2,4-Dinitrophenol
Carbanilides
Salicylanilide
Some phenols
Parabens
Long-chain
organic acids

Protonmotive
force
Oxidative
phosphorylation

Acridines
Ethylene
oxide
Short-chain
organic acids

Phenols
Detergents
Chlorhexidine
Alcohols
Parabens

that they have a very wide spectrum of cell interactions and it is difficult to pin-point the fatal reaction. In fact, it is safe to say that there is no single fatal reaction but that death results from the accumulated effects of many reactions; one or two specific reactions of compounds in this category have already been referred to.

β-Propiolactone is one example. It will alkylate amino, imino, hydroxyl and carboxyl groups, all of which occur in proteins, and react also with thiol and disulphide groups responsible for the secondary structure of proteins and the activity of some enzymes.

Another example is ethylene oxide, which has a very similar range of chemical activity.

Sulphur dioxide, sulphites and bisulphites, used as preservatives in fruit juices, ciders and perrys are yet other examples.

5   Conclusions

The above account, Table 12.1 and Fig. 12.1 all indicate the range and complexity of the reactions involved in the action of some non-antibiotic antibacterial agents.

The concentration-dependent dual or even multiple role of many of these substances should be noted. For a more detailed treatment the reader is directed to the references given below.

6   Further reading

Ayres H., Furr J.R. & Russell A.D. (1993) A rapid method of evaluating permeabilizing activity against *Pseudomonas aeruginosa. Lett Appl Microbiol*, **17**, 149–187.

Collier P.J., Ramsey A.J., Austin P. & Gilbert P. (1991) Uptake and distribution of some isothiazolone biocides in *Escherichia coli* and *Schizosaccharomyces pombe* NCYC 1354. *Int J Pharm*, **66**, 201–206 and preceding two papers.

Denyer S.P. & Hugo W.B. (eds) (1991) *Mechanisms of Action of Chemical Biocides: their Study and Exploitation.* Society for Applied Bacteriology Technical Series No. 27. Oxford: Blackwell Scientific Publications.

Fuller S.J., Denyer S.P., Hugo W.B., Pemberton D., Woodcock P.M., & Buckley A.J. (1985) The mode of action of 1,2-benzisothiazolin-3 one on *Staphylococcus aureus. Lett Appl Microbiol*, **1**, 13–15.

Hugo W.B. (1967) The mode of action of antiseptics. *J Appl Bacteriol*, **30**, 17–50.

Hugo W.B. (ed.) (1971) *The Inhibition and Destruction of the Microbial Cell.* London: Academic Press.

Hugo W.B. (1976a) Survival of microbes exposed to chemical stress. In: *The Survival of Vegetative Microbes* (eds T.R.G. Gray & J.R. Postgate), pp. 383–413. 26th Symposium of the Society for General Microbiology. Cambridge: Cambridge University Press.

Hugo W.B. (1976b) The inactivation of vegetative bacteria by chemicals. In: *The Inactivation of Vegetative Bacteria* (eds F.A. Skinner & W.B. Hugo), pp. 1–11. Symposium of the Society of Applied Bacteriology. London: Academic Press.

Hugo W.B. (1980) The mode of action of antiseptics. In: *Wirkungmechanisma von Antiseptica* (eds H. Wigert & W. Weufen), pp. 39–77. Berlin: VEB Verlag.

Hugo W.B. (1992) Disinfection mechanisms. In: *Principles and Practice of Disinfection, Preservation and Sterilization*, 2nd edn. (eds A.D. Russell, W.B. Hugo & G.A.J. Ayliffe), pp. 187–210. Oxford: Blackwell Scientific Publications.

Russell A.D. & Chopra I. (1996) *Understanding Antibacterial Action and Resistance* 2nd edn. Chichester: Ellis Horwood.

Russell A.D. & Hugo W.B. (1994) Antimicrobial activity and action of silver. In *Progress in Medicinal Chemistry* (eds G.P. Ellis & D.K. Luscombe), vol. 39, pp. 351–370. Amsterdam: Elsevier.

Vaara M. (1992) Agents that increase the permeability of the outer membrane. *Microbiol Rev*, **56**, 395–411.

13 Resistance to non-antibiotic antimicrobial agents

1   Introduction

2   Relative microbial responses to biocides

3   Bacterial resistance to biocides: general mechanisms

4   Intrinsic bacterial resistance
4.1 Gram-positive cocci
4.2 Gram-negative bacteria
4.2.1 Enterobacteriaceae
4.2.2 Pseudomonads
4.3 Mycobacteria
4.4 Bacterial spores
4.4.1 Spore structure
4.4.2 Spore development (sporulation) and resistance
4.4.3 Mature spores and resistance
4.4.4 Germination, outgrowth and susceptibility
4.5 Physiological (phenotypic) adaptation to intrinsic resistance

5   Acquired bacterial resistance to biocides
5.1 Resistance acquired by mutation
5.2 Plasmid-encoded resistance
5.2.1 Resistance to cations and anions
5.2.2 Resistance to other biocides

6   Sensitivity and resistance of fungi
6.1 General comments
6.2 Mechanisms of fungal resistance

7   Sensitivity and resistance of protozoa

8   Sensitivity and resistance of viruses

9   Activity of biocides against prions

10   Pharmaceutical and medical relevance

11   Further reading

1   Introduction

Biocides are widely used as antiseptics, disinfectants and preservatives in a variety of fields, e.g. industrial, medical and pharmaceutical, dental, veterinary, food microbiology.

Several factors are known to influence biocidal activity: these include the period of contact, biocide concentration, pH, temperature, the presence of organic matter and the nature and condition of the microorganisms being treated. Bacterial resistance to antibiotics is a well-established phenomenon and has been widely studied for many years. By contrast, the mechanisms of insusceptibility to non-antibiotic chemical agents are less well understood.

2   Relative microbial responses to biocides

Different types of microbes show varying responses to biocides. This is demonstrated clearly in Table 13.1. Additionally, it must be noted that Gram-positive bacteria such as staphylococci and streptococci are generally more sensitive to biocides than are Gram-negative bacteria. Enterococci are frequently antibiotic-resistant, but are not necessarily more resistant to biocides than are streptococci. Methicillin-resistant *Staphylococcus aureus* (MRSA) strains are rather more resistant to biocides, especially cationic ones, than are methicillin-sensitive *Staph. aureus* (MSSA) strains. Amongst Gram-negative

Table 13.1 Comparative responses of microorganisms to biocides

Type of microorganism	Biocide susceptibility or resistance
Bacteria	Non-sporing most susceptible, acid-fast bacteria intermediate, spores most resistant
Fungi	Fungal spores may be resistant
Viruses	Non-enveloped more resistant than enveloped
Parasites	Coccidia may be highly resistant
Prions	Usually highly resistant

bacteria, the most marked resistance is shown by *Pseudomonas aeruginosa*, *Providencia stuartii* and *Proteus* species.

Mycobacteria are more resistant than other non-sporulating bacteria to a wide range of biocides. Examples of such organisms are *Mycobacterium tuberculosis*, the *M. avium-intracellulare* (MAI) group and *M. chelonae* (*M. chelonei*). Of the bacteria, however, the most resistant of all to biocides are bacterial spores, e.g. *Bacillus subtilis*, *B. cereus*.

Moulds and yeasts show varying responses to biocides. These organisms are often important in the pharmaceutical context because they may cause spoilage of formulated products. Various types of protozoa are potentially pathogenic and inactivation by biocides may be problematic. Viral response to biocides depends upon the type and structure of the virus particle and on the nature of the biocide.

The most resistant of all infectious agents to chemical inactivation are the prions, which cause transmissible degenerative encephalopathies.

These different types of microorganisms are considered below; whenever possible, the mechanisms of resistance will be considered and the clinical or pharmaceutical relevance discussed.

3 Bacterial resistance to biocides: general mechanisms

Bacterial resistance to biocides (Table 13.2) is usually considered as being of two types: (a) intrinsic (innate, natural), a natural property of an organism, or (b) acquired, either by chromosomal mutation or by the acquisition of plasmids or transposons. Intrinsic resistance to biocides is usually demonstrated by Gram-negative bacteria, mycobacteria and bacterial spores whereas acquired resistance can result by mutation or, more frequently, by the acquisition of genetic elements, e.g. plasmid- (or transposon-) mediated resistance to mercury compounds. Intrinsic resistance may also be exemplified by physiological (phenotypic) adaptation, a classical example of which is biofilm production.

4 Intrinsic bacterial resistance

As already pointed out, staphylococci and streptococci are generally more sensitive to biocides than are Gram-negative bacteria; examples are provided in Table 13.3. On the

Table 13.2 Intrinsic and acquired bacterial resistance to biocides

Distinguishing feature	Intrinsic resistance	Acquired resistance
General property	Natural property	Achieved by mutation or by acquisition of plasmid or transposon (Tn)
Mechanisms*		
(1) Alteration of biocide (enzymatic inactivation)	Chromosomally mediated, but not usually relevant	Plasmid/Tn-mediated e.g. mercurials
(2) Impaired uptake	Applies to several biocides	Less important
(3) Efflux	Not known	Cationic biocides and antibiotic-resistant staphylococci
Biofilm production	Phenotypic adaptation	Plasmid transfer may occur within biofilms
Pharmaceutical/clinical significance	High	Could be high in certain circumstances

* See Table 13.4 for additional information.

Table 13.3 Sensitivity of microorganisms to chlorhexidine

Organism	Minimum inhibitory concentration *($\mu g\,ml^{-1}$)
Gram-negative bacteria	
Pseudomonas aeruginosa	10–500
Proteus mirabilis	25–100
Pseudomonas cepacia	5–100
Serratia marcescens	3–50
Salmonella typhimurium	14
Klebsiella aerogenes	1–12
Escherichia coli	1–5
Gram-positive bacteria	
Staphylococcus aureus	1–2
Enterococcus faecalis	1–3
Bacillus subtilis	1–3
Streptococcus mutans	0.1
Mycobacterium tuberculosis	0.7–6
Fungi	
Candida albicans	7–15
Trichophyton mentagrophytes	3
Penicillium notatum	200

* The minimum inhibitory concentration (MIC) is the lowest concentration of an antimicrobial agent that prevents growth. The lower the MIC value, the more active the agent.

other hand, mycobacteria and especially bacterial spores are much more resistant. A major reason for this variation in response is associated with the chemical composition and structure of the outer cell layers such that there is restricted uptake of a biocide. In consequence of this cellular impermeability, a reduced concentration of the antimicrobial compound is available at the target site(s) so that the cell may escape severe injury. Another, less frequently observed, mechanism is the presence of constitutive, biocide-degrading enzymes.

Intrinsic resistance may than be defined as a natural, chromosomally controlled property of a bacterial cell that enables it to circumvent the action of a biocide (see Table 13.2). A summary of intrinsic resistance mechanisms is provided in Table 13.4.

4.1 Gram-positive cocci

The cell wall of staphylococci is composed essentially of peptidoglycan and teichoic acids. Substances of high molecular weight can traverse the wall, a ready explanation for the sensitivity of these organisms to most biocides. However, the plasticity of the bacterial cell envelope is well known and the growth rate and any growth-limiting nutrient will affect the physiological state of the cells. The thickness and degree of crosslinking of peptidoglycan may be modified and hence the sensitivity of the cells to antibacterial agents. Likewise 'fattened' cells of *Staph. aureus* which have been trained in the laboratory to contain much higher levels of cell wall lipid than normal cells, are less sensitive to higher phenols. Normally, staphylococci contain little or no cell wall lipid and consequently the lipid-enriched cells represent physiologically adapted cells which present an intrinsic resistance to certain biocidal agents.

4.2 Gram-negative bacteria

4.2.1 *Enterobacteriaceae*

A great deal of our current understanding of the structure and function of the outer membrane of Gram-negative bacteria has come from studies with *Escherichia coli* and *Salmonella typhimurium*. The permeability barrier function of the outer membrane can

Table 13.4 Examples of intrinsic resistance mechanisms to biocides in bacteria

Type of resistance	Bacteria	Mechanism	Examples
Impermeability	Gram-negative	OM barrier	QACs, triclosan, diamidines
	Mycobacteria	Waxy cell wall	QACs, chlorhexidine, organomercurials
	Bacterial spores	Spore coats and cortex	QACs, chlorhexidine, organomercurials, phenols
	Other Gram-positive	Phenototypic adaptation	Chlorhexidine
Enzymatic	Gram-negative	Chemical inactivation	Chlorhexidine

OM, outer membrane; QAC, quaternary ammonium compound.

be demonstrated by treatment of *E. coli* cells with ethylenediamine tetra-acetic acid (EDTA), which greatly enhances their permeability and sensitivity towards antimicrobial agents. By binding metal ions such as magnesium, which is essential for the stability of the outer membrane, EDTA releases 30–50% of the lipopolysaccharide (LPS) from the outer membrane together with some phospholipid and protein. The permeability barrier is effectively removed and the cells, which retain their viability, then become sensitive to large hydrophobic antibiotics such as fucidin and rifampicin against which they are normally resistant. More complete removal of the outer membrane and peptidoglycan with EDTA and lysozyme (a muramidase enzyme which degrades peptidoglycan) produces spheroplasts in Gram-negative bacteria. These osmotically fragile, but viable, cells are equivalent to protoplasts of Gram-positive bacteria, which are cells where the wall has been completely removed with lysozyme. Both spheroplasts and protoplasts are equally sensitive to lysis by membrane-active agents such as quaternary ammonium compounds (QACs), phenols and chlorhexidine. This demonstrates that the difference in sensitivities of whole cells to these agents is not due to a difference in sensitivity of the target cytoplasmic membrane but in the different permeability properties of the overlying wall or envelope structures.

The outer membrane of Gram-negative bacteria plays an important role in limiting access of susceptible target sites to antibiotics and biocides. This means that, as pointed out earlier (see Table 13.3), Gram-negative bacteria are usually less sensitive to many antibacterial agents than are Gram-positive organisms. This is particularly marked with inhibitors such as hexachlorophane, diamidines, QACs, triclosan and some lipophilic acids.

The surface of deep rough (heptose-less) mutants of *E. coli* and *Sal. typhimurium* is more hydrophobic than the surface of smooth, wild-type bacteria because of the presence of phospholipid patches on the surface of the former. Deep rough mutants are hypersensitive to hydrophobic drugs and biocides. In wild-type bacteria, the porins and intact LPS molecules prevent ready access of hydrophobic molecules to the underlying phospholipid molecules. Studies with a homologous series of parabens (the methyl, ethyl, propyl and butyl esters of *p*-hydroxybenzoic acid) of increasing lipophilicity have demonstrated that activity increases from methyl to butyl against smooth strains and considerably more against rough strains of both *E. coli* and *Sal. typhimurium*. The butyl ester has the greatest, and the methyl ester the least, effect on the cytoplasmic membrane.

The hydrated nature of amino acid residues lining the porin channels presents an energetically unfavourable barrier to the passage of hydrophobic molecules. In the rough strains the reduction in the amount of polysaccharide on the cell surface allows hydrophobic molecules to approach the surface of the outer membrane and cross the outer membrane lipid bilayer by passive diffusion. This process is greatly facilitated in the deep rough and heptose-less strains which have phospholipid molecules on the outer face of their outer membranes as well as on the inner face. The exposed areas of phospholipids favour the absorption and penetration of the hydrophobic agents.

Two pathways now emerge for penetration of antibacterial agents across the outer membrane:

1 hydrophilic, which is porin-mediated;
2 hydrophobic, involving diffusion.

This picture holds for all Gram-negative bacteria. It is especially important for the Enterobacteriaceae which survive the antibacterial action of hydrophobic bile salts and fatty acids in the gut by the combined effects of the penetration barrier of their smooth LPS and the small size of their porin channels (which restricts passage of hydrophilic molecules to those of molecular weight less than 650). By contrast, an organism like *Neisseria gonorrhoeae*, which does not produce an O-antigen polysaccharide on its LPS and is naturally rough, is very sensitive to hydrophobic molecules. Natural fatty acids help to defend the body against these organisms.

Cationic biocides which have strong surface-active properties and which attack the inner (cytoplasmic) membrane, e.g. chlorhexidine and QACs, also damage the outer membrane and thus are believed to mediate their own uptake into the cells. Segments of the outer membrane are removed, thereby allowing access of these antibacterial agents to the periplasm and vulnerable cytoplasmic membrane. Their effect can be seen quite dramatically under the electron microscope. Small bulges or blebs appear on the outer face of the outer membrane. The blebs increase in size and are released from the cells as vesicles containing LPS, protein and phospholipid. The outer membrane has a limited capacity to reassemble itself; this it does with phospholipids spontaneously re-forming into a bilayer. If the amount of outer membrane material released is too great to be compensated for by phospholipid, the cells lose their protective barrier, and the agents penetrate to the cytoplasmic membrane and cause irreversible damage.

It must also be pointed out that the QACs are considerably less active against wild-type than against deep rough strains of *E. coli* and *Sal. typhimurium*. It is clear, then, that the outer membrane must act as a permeability barrier against these compounds.

Studies with porin-deficient mutants of many Gram-negative species have confirmed that detergents do not use the porin channels to gain access to the cytoplasmic membrane. Porin-deficient strains in general show no difference in sensitivity to detergents compared with their parent strains, even though the permeability of their outer membrane to small hydrophilic molecules is reduced up to 100-fold. Other mutations affecting the stability of the outer membrane, such as loss of the lipoprotein which anchors it to the peptidoglycan, are associated with extreme sensitivity to membrane-active agents. Some mutants of *E. coli* are highly permeable and sensitive to a wide range of antimicrobial agents, but have no major defect in envelope composition. The explanation presumably lies in the way the individual components are organized in the envelope. Since components are not covalently linked together, ionic interactions mediated by divalent metal ions play an important part in maintaining the integrity of the outer membrane. For this reason, EDTA is particularly effective in destabilizing the outer membrane and making it permeable to agents. EDTA potentiates the action of many antimicrobials and for this purpose is a valuable additive to preservatives, especially QACs. One disinfectant formulation that has been available commercially has EDTA and the phenolic agent chloroxylenol as its active constituents.

Hospital isolates of *Serratia marcescens* may be highly resistant to chlorhexidine, hexachlorophane liquid soaps and detergent creams. The outer membrane probably determines resistance to biocides.

Members of the genus *Proteus* are unusually resistant to high concentrations of chlorhexidine and other cationic biocides and are more resistant to EDTA than most other types of Gram-negative bacteria. A less acidic type of LPS may be responsible for reduced binding of, and hence increased resistance to, cationic biocides. Decreased susceptibility to EDTA may result from the reduced divalent cation content of the *Proteus* outer membrane.

4.2.2   *Pseudomonads*

Pseudomonas aeruginosa is notorious for its ability to survive in the environment, particularly in moist conditions. It is a dangerous contaminant of medicines, surgical equipment, clothing and dressings, with the ability to cause serious infections in immunocompromised patients. The intrinsic resistance of Gram-negative bacteria is especially apparent with *Ps. aeruginosa*; many disinfectants and preservatives possess insufficient activity against it to be of any use. Added to the problem of natural resistance to antimicrobials is the organism's extensive repertoire of phenotypic variation.

The basis of the greater resistance of *Ps. aeruginosa* compared with other Gram-negative bacteria (see Table 13.3) is not at all clear. The answer presumably lies in the properties of the envelope because when this is removed, the resulting spheroplasts are just as sensitive as those of other organisms. The outer membrane is not significantly different from that of other organisms in terms of overall composition. The same components (LPS, proteins, phospholipid, peptidoglycan) are present. One difference is the number of phosphate groups present in the lipid A region of the LPS. This is significantly higher in *Ps. aeruginosa* than in members of the Enterobacteriaceae and might account for the unusual sensitivity of the organism to EDTA. The high phosphate content means that the outer membrane is unusually dependent upon divalent metal ions for stability; their removal by EDTA therefore has a dramatic effect upon cell integrity. Magnesium-depleted cells of *Ps. aeruginosa* are extremely resistant to EDTA. Presumably the lower magnesium content of the cell envelope reflects a decreased phosphorylation of lipid A. Other effects follow from magnesium depletion, including complex changes in lipid composition and increased production of an outer membrane protein known as H1, which is believed to replace magnesium ions in binding together LPS molecules on the cell surface.

Burkholderia (formerly *Pseudomonas*) *cepacia* is intrinsically resistant to a number of biocides, notably benzalkonium chloride and chlorhexidine. Again, the outer membrane is likely to act as a permeability barrier. By contrast, *Ps. stutzeri* (an organism implicated in eye infections caused by some cosmetic products) is invariably intrinsically sensitive to a range of biocides, including QACs and chlorhexidine. This organism contains less wall muramic acid than other pseudomonads but it is unclear as to whether this could be a contributory factor in its enhanced biocide susceptibility.

4.3   Mycobacteria

Mycobacteria consist of a fairly diverse group of acid-fast bacteria. The best-known members are *M. tuberculosis* and *M. leprae*, the causative agents of tuberculosis and leprosy, respectively. Other mycobacteria can also cause serious infection, e.g. members of the MAI group, and there are many opportunistic species.

Mycobacteria show a high level of resistance to inactivation by biguanides (e.g. chlorhexidine), QACs and organomercurials. Phenols may or may not be mycobactericidal. Alkaline glutaraldehyde exerts a lethal effect but more slowly than against other non-sporulating bacteria, but MAI is more resistant than *M. tuberculosis*. Recently, glutaraldehyde-resistant *M. chelonae* strains have been isolated from endoscope washers.

The mycobacterial cell wall is highly hydrophobic, with a mycoylarabinogalactan-peptidoglycan skeleton composed of two covalently linked polymers, an arabinagalactan mycolate (mycolic acid, D-arabinose and D-galactose) and a peptidoglycan containing *N*-glycomuramic acid instead of *N*-acetylmuramic acid. The mycolic acids have an important role to play in reducing cell wall permeability to hydrophilic molecules. However, porins are present which are similar to those found in *Ps. aeruginosa* cell envelopes so that only low molecular weight hydrophilic substances can enter the cell via this route.

Overall, the mechanisms involved in the role of the mycobacterial cell wall as a permeability barrier are poorly understood and it is not known why MAI and *M. chelonae*, in particular, are more resistant than other species of mycobacteria.

4.4   Bacterial spores

Bacterial spores, of the genera *Bacillus* and *Clostridium*, are invariably the most resistant of all types of bacteria to biocides. Many biocides, e.g. biguanides and QACs, will kill (or at low concentrations be bacteriostatic to) non-sporulating bacteria but not bacterial spores. Other biocides such as alkaline glutaraldehyde are sporicidal, although higher concentrations for longer contact periods may be necessary than for a bactericidal effect.

4.4.1   Spore structure

A typical bacterial spore has several components (Chapter 1, see Fig. 1.8). The germ cell (protoplast or core) and germ cell wall are surrounded by the cortex, external to which are the inner and outer spore coats. An exosporium is present in some spores but may surround just one spore coat. The protoplast is the location of RNA, DNA, dipicolinic acid (DPA) and most of the calcium, potassium, manganese and phosphorus present in the spore. Also present are substantial amounts of low molecular weight basic proteins, the small acid-soluble spore proteins (SASPs) which are rapidly degraded during germination. The cortex consists largely of peptidoglycan, some 45–60% of the muramic acid residues not having either a peptide or an *N*-acetyl substituent but instead forming an internal amide known as muramic lactam. The cortical membrane (germ cell wall, primordial cell wall) is a dense inner layer of the cortex that develops into the cell wall of the emergent cell when the cortex is degraded during germination. Two membranes, the inner and outer forespore membranes, surround the forespore during germination. The inner forespore membrane eventually becomes the cytoplasmic membrane of the germinating spore, whereas the outer forespore membrane persists in the spore integuments.

The spore coats make up a major portion of the spore, consisting mainly of protein with smaller amounts of complex carbohydrates and lipid and possibly large amounts of phosphorus. The outer spore coat contains the alkali-resistant protein fraction and is associated with the presence of disulphide-rich bonds. The alkali-soluble fraction is found in the inner spore coats and consists predominantly of acidic polypeptides which can be dissociated to their unit components by treatment with sodium dodecyl sulphate.

4.4.2 *Spore development (sporulation) and resistance*

Response to a biocide depends upon the cellular stage of development. Sporulation, a process in which a bacterial spore develops from a vegetative cell, involves seven stages (I–VII; Chapter 1, see Fig. 1.9); of these, stages IV–VII (cortex and coat development) are the most important in relation to the development of biocide resistance. Resistance to biocidal agents develops during sporulation and may be an early, intermediate or late/very late event. For example, resistance to chlorhexidine occurs at an intermediate stage, at about the same time as heat resistance, whereas decreasing susceptibility to glutaraldehyde is a very late event.

4.4.3 *Mature spores and resistance*

Spore coatless forms, produced by treatment of spores under alkaline conditions with UDS (urea plus dithiothreitol plus sodium lauryl sulphate), have been of value in estimating the role of the coats in limiting access of biocides to their target sites. However, this treatment removes a certain amount of spore cortex also. The amount of cortex remaining can be further reduced by subsequent use of lysozyme. These findings, taken as a whole, demonstrate that the spore coats have an undoubted role to play in conferring resistance of spores to biocides and that the cortex, also, is an important barrier especially since (UDS + lysozyme)-treated spores are much more sensitive to chlorine- and iodine-releasing agents than are UDS-exposed spores.

SASPs comprise about 10–20% of the protein in the dormant spore, exist in two forms (α/β and γ) and are degraded during germination. They are essential for expression of spore resistance to ultraviolet radiation and also appear to be involved in resistance to some biocides, e.g. hydrogen peroxide. Spores ($\alpha^- \beta^-$) deficient in α/β-type SASPs are much more peroxide-sensitive than are wild-type (normal) spores. It has been proposed that in wild-type spores DNA is saturated with α/β-type SASPs and is thus protected from free radical damage.

4.4.4 *Germination, outgrowth and susceptibility*

During germination and/or outgrowth, cells regain their sensitivity to antibacterial agents. Some inhibitors act at the germination stage (e.g. phenolics, parabens), whereas others such as chlorhexidine and the QACs do not affect germination but inhibit outgrowth. Glutaraldehyde, at low concentrations, is an effective inhibitor of both stages. During germination, several degradative changes occur in the spore, e.g. loss of dry weight, decrease in optical density, loss of dipicolinic acid, increase in stainability, increase in oxygen consumption; whereas biosynthetic processes (RNA, DNA, protein, cell wall syntheses) become apparent during outgrowth. It is difficult, at present, to put forward a theory that will account for the relatively specific activity of most biocides during these two very dissimilar cellular changes.

4.5 Physiological (phenotypic) adaptation to intrinsic resistance

Bacteria grown under different conditions may show wide response to biocides. For example, fattened cells of *Staph. aureus* obtained by repeated subculturing in glycerol-containing media are more resistant to benzylpenicillin and higher phenols.

Both nutrient limitation and reduced growth rates may alter the sensitivity of bacteria to biocides. These changes in susceptibility can be considered as the expression of intrinsic resistance brought about by exposure to environmental conditions. These aspects assume greater importance when organisms existing as biofilms are considered. The association of microorganisms with solid surfaces leads to the generation of biofilms, which may be considered as consortia of bacteria organized within an extensive exopolysaccharide polymer (glycocalyx). The physiology of bacteria existing at different parts of biofilm is affected because the cells experience different nutrient conditions. Growth rates are likely to be reduced within the depths of a biofilm, one reason being the growth-limiting concentrations of essential nutrients that are available. Consequently, the sessile organisms present differ phenotypically from the planktonic-type cells found in liquid cultures. Frequently, bacteria within a biofilm are less sensitive to a biocide than planktonic cells.

Apart from nutrient limitation and diminished growth rates, another reason for this decreased susceptibility is the prevention of access of a biocide to the underlying cells. Thus, in this mechanism, the glycocalyx as well the rate of growth of the biofilm micro-colony in relation to the diffusion rate of the biocide across the biofilm, can affect susceptibility. A possible third mechanism involves the increased production of degradative enzymes by attached cells, but the importance of this has yet to be determined.

The non-random distribution of bacteria in biofilms has important applications for industry (biofouling, corrosion) and in medical practice (use of appliances within the human body).

5 Acquired bacterial resistance to biocides

Acquired resistance to biocides results from genetic changes in a cell and arises either by mutation or by the acquisition of genetic material (plasmids, transposons) from another cell (Table 13.5).

5.1 Resistance acquired by mutation

Acquired, non-plasmid-encoded resistance to biocides can result when bacteria are exposed to gradually increasing concentrations of a biocide. Examples are provided by highly QAC-resistant *Serratia marcescens*, and chlorhexidine-resistant *Ps. mirabilis*, *Ps. aeruginosa* and *Ser. marcescens*.

5.2 Plasmid-encoded resistance

5.2.1 Resistance to cations and anions

Amongst the Enterobacteriaceae, plasmids may carry genes specifying resistance to

Table 13.5 Examples of acquired resistance mechanisms to biocides in bacteria

Type of resistance	Bacteria	Mechanism	Examples
Enzymatic	Gram-positive* Gram-negative	Plasmid/Tn-encoded inactivation	Mercury compounds Mercury compounds, formaldehyde
Impaired uptake	Gram-negative	Plasmid-encoded porin modification	QACs
Efflux	Gram-positive*	Plasmid-encoded expulsion from cells	QACs Chlorhexidine?

QAC, quaternary ammonium compound.
* Non-mycobacterial, non-sporing bacteria.

antibiotics and in some instances to mercury, organomercury and other cations and some anions. Mercury resistance is inducible and is not the result of training or tolerance. Transposon (Tn) 501 conferring mercury resistance has been widely studied. Plasmids conferring resistance to mercury are of two types:

1 'narrow spectrum', conferring resistance to Hg(II) and to a few specified organomercurials;

2 'broad spectrum', encoding resistance to those in (1) plus other organomercury compounds.

There is enzymatic reduction of mercury to Hg metal and its vaporization in 1, and enzymatic hydrolysis followed by vaporization in 2. Plasmid-encoded resistance to other metallic ions has also been described but, apart from silver, is probably of little clinical relevance.

Plasmid-mediated resistance to silver salts is of particular importance in the hospital environment, because silver nitrate and silver sulphadiazine may be used topically for preventing infections in severe burns. Silver reduction is not a primary resistance mechanism since sensitive and resistant cells can equally convert Ag^+ to metallic silver. Plasmid-mediated resistance to silver salts is, in fact, difficult to demonstrate, but where it has been shown to occur, decreased accumulation rather than silver reduction is believed to be the mechanism involved.

5.2.2 Resistance to other biocides

Plasmid-mediated resistance to other biocides has not been widely studied and the results to date may be somewhat conflicting. Plasmid-encoded resistance to formaldehyde has been described in *Ser. marcescens*, presumably due to aldehyde degradation. There is evidence that some plasmids are responsible for producing surface changes in cells and that the response depends not only on the plasmid but also on the host cell. Gram-negative bacteria showing high resistance to QACs and chlorhexidine as well as to antibiotics have been isolated but it has not been possible to establish a linked association of resistance in these organisms.

MRSA strains are a frequent problem in hospital infection, such strains often showing multiple antibiotic resistance. Furthermore, increased resistance to some cationic biocides (chlorhexidine, QACs, diamidines and the now little-used crystal violet and acridines) and to another cationic agent, ethidium bromide, is found in MRSA strains carrying genes encoding gentamicin resistance. At least three determinants have been identified as being responsible for biocide resistance in clinical isolates of *Staph. aureus*: *qac*A, which encodes resistance to QACs, acridines, ethidium bromide and low-level resistance to chlorhexidine; *qac*B, which is similar but specifies resistance to the intercalating dyes and QACs; and the genetically unrelated *qac*C which specifies resistance to QACs and low-level resistance to ethidium bromide.

Evidence has been presented to show the expulsion (efflux) of acridines, ethidium bromide, crystal violet and diamidines (and possibly chlorhexidine). Recombinant *Staph. aureus* plasmids transferred into *E. coli* cells are responsible for conferring resistance in the latter organisms to these agents. Multidrug resistance to antibiotics and cationic biocides has also been described in coagulase-negative staphylococci (*Staph. epidermidis*) mediated by multidrug export genes *qac*A and *qac*C.

The clinical relevance of biocide resistance of antibiotic-resistant staphylococci is, however, unclear. It has been claimed that the resistance of these organisms to cationic-type biocides confers a selective advantage, i.e. survival, when such disinfectants are employed clinically. However, the in-use concentrations are several times higher than those to which the organisms are resistant.

6 Sensitivity and resistance of fungi

6.1 General comments

Surprisingly little is known about the resistance of yeasts, fungi and fungal spores to disinfectants and preservatives. They are a major source of potential contamination in pharmaceutical product preparation and aseptic processing since they abound in the environment. It is, however, possible to make some general observations:

1 moulds are often, but not invariably, more resistant than yeasts, e.g. to chlorhexidine and organomercurials;

2 fungicidal concentrations are often much higher than those needed to inhibit growth, and inactivation may be comparatively slow;

3 biocides are often considerably less active against yeasts and moulds than against non-sporulating bacteria.

For example, *Candida albicans* and (especially) *Aspergillus niger* are much more resistant to a variety of biocides than Gram-positive and Gram-negative bacteria.

6.2 Mechanisms of fungal resistance

By analogy with bacteria, two basic mechanisms of fungal resistance to biocides can be envisaged:

1 Intrinsic (natural, innate) resistance. In one form of intrinsic resistance, the fungal cell wall (see Chapter 2) is considered to present a barrier to exclude or, more likely, to reduce the penetration by biocide molecules. The evidence to date is sketchy but the available information tentatively links cell wall glucan, wall thickness and consequent relative porosity to the sensitivity of *Saccharomyces cerevisiae* to chlorhexidine.

Another type of intrinsic resistance is shown by organisms that are capable of producing constitutive enzymes which degrade biocide molecules. Heavy metal activity is reduced by some strains of *Sacch. cerevisiae* which produce hydrogen sulphide; this combines with heavy metals (e.g. copper, mercury) to form insoluble sulphides thereby rendering the organisms less tolerant than non-enzyme-producing counterparts. Inactivation of other fungitoxic agents has also been described, e.g. the role of formaldehyde dehydrogenase in resistance to formaldehyde and the degradation of potassium sorbate by a *Penicillium* species. Degradation by fungi of biocides such as chlorhexidine, QACs and other aldehydes does not appear to have been recorded.

2 Acquired resistance. This term is used to denote resistance arising as a consequence of mutation or via the acquisition of genetic material. There is no evidence linking the presence of plasmids in fungal cells and the ability of the organisms to acquire resistance to fungicidal or fungistatic agents. The development of resistance to antiseptic-type agents has not been widely studied, but acquired resistance to organic acids has been demonstrated, presumably by mutation.

7 Sensitivity and resistance of protozoa

Several distinct types of protozoa (e.g. *Giardia, Cryptosporidium, Naegleria, Entamoeba* and *Acanthamoeba*) are potentially pathogenic and may be acquired from water. A resistant cyst stage is included in their life cycle, the trophozoite form being sensitive to biocides. Little is known about mechanisms of inactivation by chemical agents and there appear to have been few significant studies linking excystment and encystment with the development of sensitivity and resistance, respectively.

From the evidence currently available, it is likely that the cyst cell wall acts in some way as a permeability barrier, thereby conferring intrinsic resistance to the cyst form.

8 Sensitivity and resistance of viruses

An important hypothesis was put forward in the USA by Klein and Deforest in 1963 and modified in 1983. Essentially the original concept was based on whether viruses could be classified as:

1 'lipophilic', i.e. those, such as herpes simplex virus, which possessed a lipid envelope; and

2 'hydrophilic', e.g. poliovirus, which did not contain a lipid envelope.

In the later (1983) modification, three groups were considered (Fig. 13.1):

1 lipid-enveloped viruses, which were inactivated by lipophilic biocides;

2 non-lipid picornaviruses (pico = very small, e.g. polio and Coxsackie viruses all of which are RNA viruses);

3 other, larger, non-lipid viruses, e.g. adenoviruses.

Viruses in groups 2 and 3 are much more resistant to biocides.

Although many papers have been published on the virucidal (viricidal) activity of biocides there is little information available about the uptake of biocides and their penetration into viruses of different types, or of their interaction with viral protein and nucleic acid.

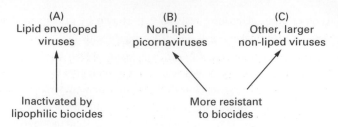

Fig. 13.1 Viral responses to biocides.

9 Activity of biocides against prions

Prions are responsible for the so-called 'slow virus diseases', a distinct group of unusual neurological disorders. They are believed to be markedly resistant to inactivation by many chemical and physical agents but because they have not been purified, it is at present difficult to state whether this is an intrinsic property of prions or whether it results from the protective effect of host tissue present. Certainly very high concentrations of a biocide acting for long periods may be necessary to produce inactivation.

10 Pharmaceutical and medical relevance

The inherent variability in biocidal sensitivity of microorganisms has several important practical implications. For example, the population of bacteria making up the normal flora of organisms contaminating the working surfaces, floor, air or water supply in an environment such as a hospital pharmacy will probably contain a very low number of naturally resistant organisms. These might be resistant to the agent used as a disinfectant because they have acquired additional genetic information or lost, by mutation, genes involved in controlling the expression of other genes. In the absence of the antimicrobial agent, the resistant strains would have no competitive advantage over the sensitive strains, and in fact they might grow more slowly and would not predominate in the population. Under the selective pressure introduced by continual use of one kind of disinfectant, resistant strains would predominate as the sensitive strains are eliminated. Eventually the entire population would be resistant to the disinfectant and a serious contamination hazard would arise. This fact is of significance in the design of suitable hospital disinfection policies.

Tuberculosis is on the increase in developed countries such as the USA and UK; furthermore, MAI may be associated with AIDS sufferers. Hospital-acquired opportunistic mycobacteria may cause disseminated infection and also lung infections, endocarditis and pericarditis. Transmission of mycobacterial infection by endoscopy is rare, despite a marked increase in the use of flexible fibreoptic endoscopes, but bronchoscopy is probably the greatest hazard for the transmission of *M. tuberculosis* and other mycobacteria. Thus, biocides used for bronchoscope disinfection must be chosen carefully to ensure that such transmission does not occur.

11   Further reading

Bloomfield S.F. & Arthur M. (1994) Mechanisms of inactivation and resistance of spores to chemical biocides. *J Appl Bact Symp Suppl*, **76**, 91S–104S.

Brown M.R.W. & Gilbert P. (1993) Sensitivity of biofilms to antimicrobial agents. *J Appl Bact Symp Suppl*, **74**, 87S–97S.

Klein M. & Deforest A. (1983) Principles of viral inactivation. In: *Disinfection, Sterilization and Preservation* (ed. S.S. Block), 3rd edn, pp. 422–434. Philadelphia: Lea & Febiger.

Nikaido H., Kim S.-H. & Rosenberg E.Y. (1993) Physical organization of lipids in the cell wall of *Mycobacterium chelonae*. *Mol Microbiol*, **8**, 1025–1030.

Nikaido H. & Vaara M. (1985) Molecular basis of bacterial outer membrane permeability. *Microbiol Rev*, **49**, 1–32.

Russell A.D. (1995) Mechanisms of bacterial resistance to biocides. *Int Biodet Biodeg*, **36**, 247–265.

Russell A.D. & Chopra I. (1996) *Understanding Antibacterial Action and Resistance*, 2nd edn. Chichester: Ellis Horwood.

Russell A.D. & Day M.J. (1996) Antibiotic and biocide resistance in bacteria. *Microbios*, **85**, 45–65.

Russell A.D. & Furr J.R. (1996) Biocides: mechanisms of antifungal action and fungal resistance. *Sci Progr*, **79**, 27–48.

Russell A.D. & Russell N.J. (1995) Biocides: activity, action and resistance. In: *Fifty Years of Antimicrobials: Past Perspectives and Future Trends* (eds P.A. Hunter, G.K. Derby & N.J. Russell) 53rd Symposium of the Society for General Microbiology, pp. 327–365. Cambridge: Cambridge University Press.

Russell A.D., Hugo W.B. & Ayliffe G.A.J. (eds) (1998) *Principles and Practice of Disinfection, Preservation and Sterilization*, 3rd edn. Oxford: Blackwell Science.

Setlow P. (1994) Mechanisms which contribute to the long-term survival of spores of *Bacillus* species. *J Appl Bact Symp Suppl*, **76**, 49S–60S.

Stickler D.J. & King J.B. (1998) Intrinsic resistance to non-antibiotic antibacterial agents. In: *Principles and Practice of Disinfection, Preservation and Sterilisation* (eds A.D. Russell, W.B. Hugo & G.A.J. Ayliffe), 3rd edn. Oxford: Blackwell Science.

Taylor D.M. (1998) Inactivation of unconventional agents of the transmissible degenerative encephalopathies. In: *Principles and Practice of Disinfection, Preservation and Sterilization* (eds A.D. Russell, W.B. Hugo & G.A.J. Ayliffe), 3rd edn. Oxford: Blackwell Science.

14 Fundamentals of immunology

1   **Introduction**
1.1   Historical aspects of immunology
1.2   Definitions

2   **Non-specific defence mechanisms (innate immune system)**
2.1   Skin and mucous membranes
2.2   Phagocytosis
2.2.1   Role of phagocytosis
2.3   The complement system and other soluble factors
2.4   Inflammation
2.5   Host damage
2.5.1   Exotoxins
2.5.2   Endotoxins

3   **Specific defence mechanisms (adaptive immune system)**
3.1   Antigenic structure of the microbial cell

4   **Cells involved in immunity**
4.1   Humoral immunity
4.2   Monoclonal antibodies
4.2.1   Uses of monoclonal antibodies
4.3   Immunoglobulin classes
4.3.1   Immunoglobulin M (IgM)
4.3.2   Immunoglobulin G (IgG)
4.3.3   Immunoglobulin A (IgA)
4.3.4   Immunoglobulin D (IgD)
4.3.5   Immunoglobulin E (IgE)
4.4   Humoral antigen–antibody reactions
4.5   Complement
4.5.1   The classical pathway

4.5.2   The alternative pathway
4.5.3   Regulation of complement activity
4.6   Cell-mediated immunity (CMI)
4.6.1   Helper T cells (TH cells)
4.6.2   Suppressor T cells (Ts cells)
4.6.3   Cytotoxic T cells (Tc cells)
4.7   Immunoregulation
4.8   Natural killer (NK) cells
4.9   Immunological tolerance
4.10   Autoimmunity

5   **Hypersensitivity**
5.1   Type I (anaphylactic) reactions
5.2   Type II (cytolytic or cytotoxic) reactions
5.3   Type III (complex-mediated) reactions
5.4   Type IV (delayed hypersensitivity) reactions
5.5   Type V (stimulatory hypersensitivity) reactions

6   **Tissue transplantation**
6.1   Immune response to tumours

7   **Immunity**
7.1   Natural immunity
7.1.1   Species immunity
7.1.2   Individual immunity
7.2   Acquired immunity
7.2.1   Active acquired immunity
7.2.2   Passive acquired immunity

8   **Further reading**

1   Introduction

The science of immunology is one of the most rapidly expanding sciences and represents a vast area of knowledge and research; thus, in a short chapter it is impossible to deal in depth with its theory and application and a list of further reading is given at the end of the chapter.

1.1   Historical aspects of immunology

From almost the first written observations by man it was recognized that persons who had contracted and recovered from certain diseases were not susceptible (i.e. were immune) to further attacks. Thucydides, over 2500 years ago, described in detail an epidemic in Athens (which could have been typhus or plague) and noted that sufferers were 'touched by the pitying care of those who had recovered because they were themselves free of apprehension, for no-one was ever attacked a second time or with a fatal result'.

Many attempts were made to induce this immune state. In ancient times the process of variolation (the inoculation of live organisms of smallpox obtained from diseased pustules from patients who were recovering from the disease) was practised extensively in India and China. The success rate was very variable and often depended on the skill of the variolator. The results were sometimes disastrous for the recipient. The father of immunology was Edward Jenner, an English country doctor who lived from 1749 to 1823. He had observed on his rounds the similarity between the pustules of smallpox and those of cowpox, a disease that affected cows' udders. He also observed that milkmaids who had contracted cowpox by handling the diseased udders were immune to smallpox. Deliberate inoculation of a young boy with cowpox and a later subsequent challenge, after the boy had recovered, with the contents of a pustule taken from a person who was suffering from smallpox failed to induce the disease and subsequent rechallenges also failed. The process of vaccination (Latin, *vacca*, cow) was adopted as a preventative measure against smallpox, even though the mechanism by which this immunity was induced was not understood.

In 1801, Jenner prophesied the eradication of smallpox by the practice of vaccination. In 1967 the disease infected 10 million people. The World Health Organization (WHO) initiated a programme of confinement and vaccination with the object of eradicating the disease. In Somalia in 1977 the last case of naturally acquired smallpox occurred, and in 1979 the WHO announced the total eradication of smallpox, thus fulfilling Jenner's prophecy.

The science of immunology not only encompasses the body's immune responses to bacteria and viruses but is extensively involved in: tumour recognition and subsequent rejection; the rejection of transplanted organs and tissues; the elimination of parasites from the body; allergies; and autoimmunity (the condition when the body mounts a reaction against its own tissues).

1.2 Definitions

Disease in humans and animals may be caused by a variety of microorganisms, the three most important groups being bacteria, rickettsia and viruses.

An organism which has the ability to cause disease is termed a *pathogen*. The term *virulence* is used to indicate the degree of pathogenicity of a given strain of microorganism. Reduction in the normal virulence of a pathogen is termed *attenuation*; this can eventually result in the organism losing its virulence completely and it is then termed *avirulent*. Conversely, any increase in virulence is termed *exaltation*.

The body possesses an efficient natural defence mechanism which restricts microorganisms to areas where they can be tolerated. A breach of this mechanism, allowing them to reach tissues which are normally inaccessible, results in an infection. Invasion and multiplication of the organism in the infected host may result in a pathological condition, the clinical entity of disease.

2   Non-specific defence mechanisms (innate immune system)

The body possesses a number of non-specific antimicrobial systems which are operative at all times against potentially pathogenic microorganisms. Prior contact with the infectious agent has no intrinsic effect on these systems.

2.1   Skin and mucous membranes

The intact skin is virtually impregnable to microorganisms and only when damage occurs can invasion take place. Furthermore, many microorganisms fail to survive on the skin surface for any length of time due to the inhibitory effects of fatty acids and lactic acid in sweat and sebaceous secretions. Mucus, secreted by the membranes lining the inner surfaces of the body, acts as a protective barrier by trapping microorganisms and other foreign particles and these are subsequently removed by ciliary action linked, in the case of the respiratory tract, with coughing and sneezing.

Many body secretions contain substances that exert a bactericidal action, for example the enzyme lysozyme which is found in tears, nasal secretions and saliva; hydrochloric acid in the stomach which results in a low pH; and basic polypeptides such as spermine which are found in semen.

The body possesses a normal bacterial flora which, by competing for essential nutrients or by the production of inhibitory substances such as monolactams or colicins, suppresses the growth of many potential pathogens.

2.2   Phagocytosis

Metchnikoff (1883) recognized the role of cell types (phagocytes) which were responsible for the engulfment and digestion of microorganisms. They are a major line of defence against microbes that breach the initial barriers described above. Two types of phagocytic cells are found in the blood, both of which are derived from the totipotent bone marrow stem cell.

1   The monocytes, which constitute about 5% of the total blood leucocytes. They migrate into the tissues and mature into macrophages (see below).

2   The neutrophils (also called polymorphonuclear leucocytes, PMNs), which are the professional phagocytes of the body. They constitute >70% of the total leucocyte population, remaining in the circulatory system for less than 48 hours before migrating into the tissues, in response to a suitable stimulus, where they phagocytose material. They possess receptors for Fc and activated C3 which enhance their phagocytic ability (see later in chapter).

Another group of phagocytic cells are the macrophages. These are large, long-lived cells found in most tissues and lining serous cavities and the lung. Other macrophages recirculate through the secondary lymphoid organs, spleen and lymph nodes where they are advantageously placed to filter out foreign material. The total body pool of macrophages constitutes the so-called reticuloendothelial system (RES). Macrophages are also involved with the presentation of antigen to the appropriate lymphocyte population (see later).

Role of phagocytosis

The microorganism initially adheres to the surface of the phagocytic cell, and this is then followed by engulfment of the particle so that it lies within a vacuole (phagosome) within the cell. Lysosomal granules within the phagocyte fuse with the vacuole to form a phagolysosome. These granules contain a variety of bactericidal components which destroy the ingested microorganism by systems that are oxygen-dependent or oxygen-independent.

When a microorganism breaches the initial barriers and enters the body tissues, the phagocytes form a formidable defence barrier. Phagocytosis is greatly enhanced by a family of proteins called *complement*.

2.3 The complement system and other soluble factors

Complement comprises a group of heat-labile serum proteins which, when activated, are associated with the destruction of bacteria in the body in a variety of ways. It is present in low concentrations in serum but, as its action is linked intimately with a second (specific) set of defence mechanisms, its composition and role will be dealt with later in the chapter.

Proteins produced by virally infected cells have been shown to interfere with viral replication. They also activate leucocytes that can recognize these infected cells and subsequently kill them. These leucocytes are known as natural killer (NK) cells and the proteins are termed *interferons* (see also Chapters 3, 5 and 24).

The serum concentration of a number of proteins increases dramatically during infection. Their levels can increase by up to 100-fold compared with normal levels. They are known collectively as acute phase proteins and certain of them have been shown to enhance phagocytosis in conjunction with complement.

2.4 Inflammation

One early symptom of injury to tissue due to a microbial infection is inflammation. This begins with the dilatation of local arterioles and capillaries which increases the blood flow to the area and causes characteristic reddening. Fluid accumulates in the area of the injury due to an increase in the permeability of the capillary walls and this leads to localized oedema, which creates a pressure on nerve endings resulting in pain. This early oedema may actually promote bacterial growth. Fibrin is deposited which tends to limit the spread of the microorganisms. Blood phagocytes adhere to the inside of the capillary walls and penetrate through into the surrounding tissue. They are attracted to the focus of the infection by chemotactic substances in the inflammatory exudate originating from complement.

Inflammation is a non-specific reaction which can be induced by a variety of agents apart from microorganisms. Lymphokines and derivatives of arachidonic acid, including prostaglandins, leukotrienes and thromboxanes are probable mediators of the inflammatory response. The release of vasoactive amines such as histamine and serotonin (5-hydroxytryptamine) from activated or damaged cells also contribute to inflammation.

Fever is the most common manifestation. The thermoregulatory centre in the hypothalamus regulates body temperature and this can be affected by endotoxins (heat-stable lipopolysaccharides) of Gram-negative bacteria and also by a monokine secreted by monocytes and macrophages called interleukin-1 (IL-1) which is also termed endogenous pyrogen. Antibody production and T-cell proliferation have been shown to be enhanced at elevated body temperatures and thus are beneficial effects of fever.

Host damage

Microorganisms that escape phagocytosis in a local lesion may now be transported to the regional lymph nodes via the lymphatic vessels. If massive invasion occurs with which the resident macrophages are unable to cope, microorganisms may be transported through the thoracic duct into the bloodstream. The appearance of viable microorganisms in the bloodstream is termed bacteraemia and is indicative of an invasive infection and failure of the primary defences.

Pathogenic organisms possess certain properties which enable them to overcome these primary defences. They produce metabolic substances, often enzymic in nature, which facilitate the invasion of the body. The following are examples of these.

1 Hyaluronidase and streptokinase are produced by the haemolytic streptococci and enable the organism to spread rapidly through the tissue. Hyaluronidase dissolves hyaluronic acid (intercellular cement), whereas streptokinase (Chapter 25) dissolves blood clots.

2 Coagulase is produced by many strains of staphylococci and causes the coagulation of plasma surrounding the organism. This can act as a barrier protecting the organism against phagocytosis. The presence of a capsule outside the cell wall serves a similar function. The production of coagulase (Chapter 1) is used as an indication of the pathogenicity of the strain.

3 Lecithinase is produced by *Clostridium perfringens*. This is a calcium-dependent lecithinase whose activity depends on the ability to split lecithin. Since lecithin is present in the membrane of many different kinds of cells, damage can occur throughout the body. Lecithinase causes the hydrolysis of erythrocytes and the necrosis of other tissue cells.

4 Collagenase is also produced by *Cl. perfringens* and this degrades collagen, which is the major protein of fibrous tissue. Its destruction promotes the spread of infection in tissues.

5 Leucocidins kill leucocytes and are produced by many strains of streptococci, most strains of *Staphylococcus aureus* and likewise most strains of pathogenic Gram-negative bacteria, isolated from sites of infection.

Damage to the host may arise in two ways. First, multiplication of the microorganisms may cause mechanical damage to the tissue cells through interference with the normal cell metabolism, as seen in viral and some bacterial infections. Second, a toxin associated with the microorganism may adversely affect the tissues or organs of the host. Two types of toxins, called exotoxins and endotoxins, are associated with bacteria.

Exotoxins

These are produced inside the cell and diffuse out into the surrounding environment. They are produced by both Gram-positive and Gram-negative bacteria. They are extremely toxic and are responsible for the serious effects of certain diseases; for example, the toxin produced by *Cl. tetani* (the causal organism of tetanus) is neurotoxic and causes severe muscular spasms due to impairment of neural control. Examples of other toxins identified are necrotoxins (causing tissue damage), enterotoxins (causing intestinal damage) and haemolysins (causing haemolysis of erythrocytes). Gram-positive bacteria producing exotoxins are certain members of the genera *Clostridium*, *Streptococcus* and *Staphylococcus* whilst an example of a Gram-negative bacterium is *Vibrio cholerae* (the causal organism of cholera). Several exotoxins consist of two moieties: one aids entrance of the exotoxin into the target cell whilst the toxic activity is associated with the other fraction.

2.5.2

Endotoxins

These are lipopolysaccharide–protein complexes associated mainly with the cell envelope of Gram-negative bacteria (see Chapter 1). They are responsible for the general non-specific toxic and pyrogenic reactions (Chapters 1 and 18) common to all organisms in this group. The specific toxic reactions for different pathogenic Gram-negative bacteria are due to the production of a toxin *in vivo*. Organisms of interest in this group are those causing cholera, plague, typhoid and paratyphoid fever, and whooping-cough.

3 Specific defence mechanisms (adaptive immune system)

Microorganisms which successfully overcome the non-specific defence mechanisms then have to contend with a second line of defence, the specific defence mechanisms. These involve the stimulation of a specific immune response by the invading microorganism and are evoked by what are termed *immunogens*. These may cause the appearance in the serum of modified serum globulins called immunoglobulins. The term *antigen* is given to a substance that stimulates immunoglobulins that have the ability to combine with the antigen that stimulated their production. These immunoglobulins are then termed *antibodies*. All antibodies are immunoglobulins but it is not certain that all immunoglobulins have antibody function. Antigens associated with microorganisms consist of proteins, polysaccharides, lipids or mixtures of the three and invariably have a high molecular weight. The antigen–antibody reaction is a highly specific one and this specificity is due to differences in the chemical composition of the outer surfaces of the organism. Bacteria, rickettsia and viruses all have the ability to induce antibody formation. The synthesis and release of free antibody into the blood and other body fluid is termed the *humoral immune response*.

Antigens, however, can induce a second type of response which is known as the *cell-mediated immune response*. The antigenic agent stimulates the appearance of 'sensitized' lymphocytes in the body which confer protection against organisms that have the ability to live and replicate inside the cells of the host. Certain of these lymphocytes are also involved in the rejection of tissue grafts.

Antigenic structure of the microbial cell

The microbial cell surface constitutes a multiplicity of different antigens. These antigens may be common to different species or types of microorganisms or may be highly specific for that one type only.

Three groups of antigens are found in the intact bacterial cell.

H-antigens. These are associated with the flagella and are therefore only found on motile bacteria (H, *Hauch*, a film, and refers to the film-like swarming seen originally in cultures of flagellated *Proteus*). The precise chemical composition of flagella can vary between bacteria, resulting in a range of different antibodies being produced and use is made of these differences in the typing of different strains of *Salmonella*.

O-antigens. These are associated with the surface of the bacterial cell wall and are often referred to as the somatic antigens (O, *ohne Hauch*, without film, and refers to non-swarming cultures, i.e. absence of flagella). The specificity of the reaction between these antigens and the corresponding antibodies in Gram-negative bacteria is due to the nature and number of the type-specific polysaccharide side-chains attached to the lipid A and core polysaccharide portion of the lipopolysaccharide (LPS) (see Chapter 1). This group of organisms is, however, very liable to mutate during cultivation in artificial media and the resultant mutant may lose the O-specific side-chain antigens, resulting in the exposure of the more deep-seated core polysaccharide, the R (rough) antigens, which may share a common structure with other unrelated Gram-negative bacteria and so are no longer type-specific. This change is known as the S → R change and is so called because of an alteration in the appearance of the colonies of the organism from the normal, smooth, glistening colony to a rough-edged, matt colony. This S → R change represents a loss of the type-specific O-antigens with a concomitant loss in the specificity of the antigen–antibody reaction.

The major type-specific antigens of Gram-positive bacteria are the teichoic acid moieties associated with the cell wall (see Chapter 1).

Surface antigens. Many bacteria possess a characteristic polysaccharide capsule external to the cell wall and this too has antigenic properties. Over 80 serological types of the Gram-positive *Pneumococcus* group have been differentiated by immunologically distinct polysaccharides in the capsule. Certain Gram-negative organisms of the enteric bacteria, e.g. salmonellae, may possess a polysaccharide microcapsule which is also antigenic and is thought to be responsible for the virulence of the bacteria. It is termed the Vi antigen and its presence is important in relation to the production of the typhoid vaccines.

4   **Cells involved in immunity**

The cells that make up the immune system are distributed throughout the body but are found mainly in the lymphoreticular organs, which may be divided into the primary lymphoid organs, i.e. the thymus and bone marrow, and the secondary or peripheral organs, e.g. lymph nodes, spleen, Peyer's patches (which are collections of lymphoid tissue in the submucosa of the small intestine) and the tonsils.

A large number of cells are involved in the immune response and all are derived from the multipotential stem cells of the bone marrow. The predominant cell is the lymphocyte but monocytes–macrophages, endothelial cells, eosinophils and mast cells are also involved with certain immune responses. The two types of immunity (humoral and cell-mediated) are dependent on two distinct populations of lymphocytes, the B cells and the T cells respectively. Both the humoral and the cell-mediated systems interact to achieve an effective immune response.

4.1   Humoral immunity

Humoral immunity, known as antibody-mediated immunity, is due directly to a reaction between circulating antibody and inducing antigen and may involve complement. The B cells originate in the bone marrow. In chickens, a lymphoid organ embryonically derived from gut epithelium and known as the bursa of Fabricius is responsible for the maturation of the B cells into immunocompetent cells, which subsequently can synthesize antibody after stimulation by antigen. The bursal equivalent in humans is the bone marrow itself. An antigen (e.g. a bacterium) may possess multiple determinants (epitopes) and each one of these epitopes will stimulate an antibody which will subsequently react with that epitope and with closely related epitopes only. Each B cell is only capable of recognizing one epitope via a specific receptor on its surface. This receptor has been shown to be antibody itself. Activation of the B cell occurs by binding of the antigen to the receptor and the resultant complex is endocytosed. For activation to proceed, additional signals are now required.

These are supplied by the secretion of peptide molecules (termed cytokines or lymphokines) from a subset of the T-cell family (the helper T cells, TH cells). These peptide molecules (interleukins (IL) 2,4,5 and 6) stimulate the B cells to proliferate, undergo clonal expansion and mature into plasma cells which secrete antibody and also into the longer-living, non-dividing memory cells.

Antigens requiring the assistance of TH cells are termed T-dependent (TD) antigens.

Subsequent antigenic stimulation results in high antibody titres (secondary or memory response) as there is now an expanded clone of cells with memory of the original antigen available to proliferate into mature plasma cells (Fig. 14.1).

Some antigens, such as type 3 pneumococcal polysaccharide, LPS and other polymeric substances such as dextrans (poly-D-glucose) and levan (poly-D-fructose) can induce antibody synthesis without the assistance of TH cells. These are known as T-independent (TI) antigens. Only one class of immunoglobulin (IgM) is synthesized and there is a weak memory response.

Immunoglobulins are associated with the γ-globulin fraction of plasma proteins but, as stated earlier, not all immunoglobulins exhibit antibody activity.

The immunoglobulin (Ig) molecules can be subdivided into different classes on the basis of their structure, and in humans five major structural types can be distinguished. Each type has been distinguished on the basis of a polypeptide chain structure consisting of one pair of heavy (large) chains and one pair of light (small) chains joined by disulphide bonds. The heavy chains are given the name of the corresponding Greek

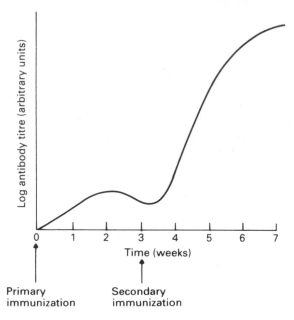

Fig. 14.1 Antibody response to primary and secondary immunization doses.

letter (γ chain in IgG, μ in IgM, α in IgA, δ in IgD and ε in IgE). All classes have similar sets of light chains consisting of one of two types, the kappa (κ) or lambda (λ) chains. A suggested ground plan for the most abundant Ig, IgG, is illustrated in Fig. 14.2.

IgG consists of four polypeptide subunits held together by disulphide bonds. Native immunoglobulins are rather resistant to proteolytic digestion but certain enzymes have been useful in elucidating their structure. Papain cleaves the molecule into three fragments of similar size:

1 two Fab fragments each carrying a single antigen-combining site and comprising the variable regions of both chains, the constant region of the light chains and the first constant domain of the heavy chain;

2 one Fc fragment composed of the terminal halves of the heavy chains which have no affinity for antigen but can be crystallized.

Cleavage with pepsin yields two fragments only, one consisting of two Fab fragments and the other an Fc fragment which is partially degraded by the enzyme. The variable regions on both the heavy and light chains contribute towards antigen recognition, whilst the constant regions of the heavy chain, particularly the Fc part of the heavy-chain backbone, direct the biological activity of the molecule, e.g. complement fixation (see later) and the interaction with a variety of tissue cells, via membrane receptors for the Fc region.

Intrastrand bonding via disulphide links cause the molecule to fold into 'globular domains' and it is these that direct the biological activity of the molecule.

4.2   **Monoclonal antibodies**

After antigenic stimulation, the normal antibody response involves the activation of a

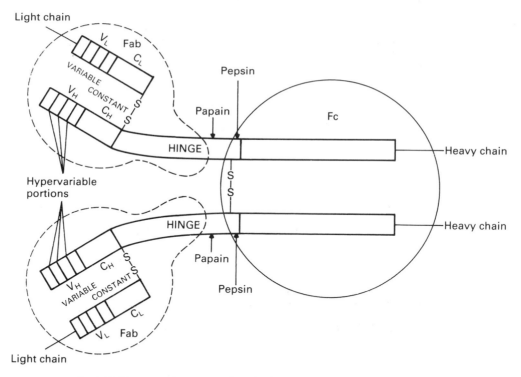

Fig. 14.2 Diagrammatic representation of IgG.

large number of clones of antibody-secreting cells (i.e. it is polyclonal). This is due to the fact that antigens possess multiple epitopes. In 1975 Kohler and Milstein successfully developed cell fusion techniques which enabled them to isolate clones of cells which synthesized identical antibody molecules (Fig. 14.3).

The principles of the technique rely on the fact that an antibody-secreting cell can become cancerous and the unchecked proliferation of such a cell is called a *myeloma*. Progeny of the original transformed cell will continue to secrete a single kind of antibody molecule only. Myeloma cells, like other malignant cells, grow indefinitely in tissue culture. However, the specificity of the antibody is unknown. Mutant myeloma cells have been isolated which have lost the ability to secrete antibody while still retaining their cancerous growth properties.

Mouse myeloma cells are fused with an antibody-secreting cell from the spleen of a mouse immunized with the required antigen. The technique is called somatic cell hybridization and the resultant cell is termed a 'hybridoma'. The rate of successful hybrid formation is low and a technique is necessary which can select these successful fusions. The standard technique is to use a myeloma cell line that has lost the capacity to synthesize hypoxanthine-guanine phosphoribosyl-transferase (HGPRT). This enzyme enables cells to synthesize nucleotides using an extracellular source of hypoxanthine as a precursor. The absence of HGPRT is normally no problem as cells can use an alternative pathway. When, however, these cells are exposed to aminopterin (a folic acid analogue; see Chapter 8) they are unable to use this other pathway and become fully dependent on HGPRT.

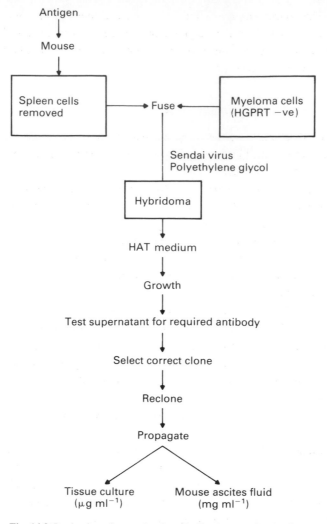

Fig. 14.3 Production of monoclonal antibodies (see text for details).

The cell fusion mixture is transferred to a culture medium containing hypoxanthine, aminopterin and thymidine (HAT medium). Unfused myeloma cells are unable to grow as they lack HGPRT. Unfused normal spleen cells can grow but their proliferation is limited and they eventually die out. The hybridoma cell can proliferate in the HAT medium as the normal spleen cell supplies the enzyme which enables the hybridoma to utilize extracellular hypoxanthine.

The hybridoma is now screened for the production of the desired antibody by testing the supernatant from each culture. A single culture, even though positive for antibody production, can contain the progeny of two or more successful fusions. Therefore, it is necessary to dilute positive cultures so that fresh cultures can be started with a single hybridoma cell. When successful, such cultures are truly monoclonal and the antibody is directed against a single epitope on a preselected antigen. Once established, these cell lines are immortal.

The concentration of antibody in tissue cultures of the hybridoma is low (10–60 μg ml^{-1}) but the use of large culture vessels can obviate this. The hybridoma can also be propagated in mice where the antibody concentration in the serum and other body fluids can reach 10 mg ml^{-1}.

4.2.1   *Uses of monoclonal antibodies*

Monoclonal antibodies are very sensitive, specific reagents and have applications in many areas of the biological sciences. They revolutionized immunology within a few years of their discovery.

The investigation and characterization of cell surfaces by probing with monoclonal antibodies is one of the most vital areas of application. In this context they have been used in the following ways:

1   To study the ABO and rare blood groups.

2   To detect HLA antigens and consequently to type tissues for transplantation.

3   To classify cell lines, e.g. the T-cell subsets, and thence to separate these cell subpopulations.

4   To study cell–cell interactions and differentiation, e.g. embryology.

5   In oncology, to study the relationship between the normal and the tumour cell, to detect tumour-associated antigens (CEA, carcino-embryonic antigen, and AFP, α-fetoprotein) and subsequently to enable cancer therapy to be monitored, to locate tumour metastases, and to deliver cytotoxic drugs, toxins, radionuclides, or liposomes to tumour cells.

6   To identify and characterize bacterial and viral antigens which can then be purified and used to prepare subunit vaccines.

Monoclonal antibodies have further been employed for studying drug and hormone receptors, enzymes and proteins. A whole range of immunoassay techniques using monoclonals have been developed to detect low levels of materials in body fluids, e.g. oxytocin can be detected in human blood using a radioimmunoassay down to 1 pmol l^{-1}. Similar assays are used to monitor antibiotic therapy using potentially toxic drugs, e.g. gentamicin. The future of monoclonal antibodies continues to be one of enormous potential and excitement.

4.3   Immunoglobulin classes

The synthesis of antibodies belonging to the various classes of immunoglobulin proceeds at different rates after the initial and subsequent antigenic stimuli.

4.3.1   *Immunoglobulin M (IgM)*

Synthesis of this class occurs after the primary antigenic stimulus. IgMs are polymers of five four-peptide subunits and have a theoretical valency of 10, although against large antigens such as bacteria their effective valency is five. They are extremely effective agglutinating agents and, as they are largely confined to the bloodstream and they appear early in the response to infection, they are of particular importance in bacteraemia.

Serum concentrations lie between 0.5 and 2.5 mg ml^{-1}. IgM can fix complement and a single molecule can initiate the complement cascade. IgM (with IgD) is the major immunoglobulin expressed on the surface of B cells where it acts as an antigen receptor.

4.3.2   *Immunoglobulin G (IgG)*

This is the major immunoglobulin synthesized during the secondary response and in normal human adults is present at serum concentrations between 10 and 15 mg ml^{-1}. Within this class there are four subclasses, designated IgG$_1$, IgG$_2$, IgG$_3$ and IgG$_4$.

It has the ability to cross the placenta and therefore provides a major line of defence against infection for the newborn. This can be reinforced by transfer of colostral IgG across the gut mucosa of the neonate. It diffuses readily into the extravascular spaces where it can act in the neutralization of bacterial toxins and can bind to microorganisms enhancing the process of phagocytosis (opsonization). This is due to the presence on the phagocytic cell surface of a receptor for Fc.

Complexes of IgG with the bacterial cell activate complement with the resultant advantages to the host.

4.3.3   *Immunoglobulin A (IgA)*

This occurs in the seromucous secretions such as saliva, tears, nasal secretions, sweat, colostrum and secretions of the lung, urinogenital and gastrointestinal tracts. Its purpose appears to be to protect the external surfaces of the body from microbial attack. It occurs as a dimer in these secretions but as a monomer in human plasma, where its function is not known. The function of IgA appears to be to prevent the adherence of microorganisms to the surface of mucosal cells thus preventing them entering the body tissues. It is protected from proteolysis by combination with another protein—the secretory component.

It is present at serum levels between 0.5 and 3 mg ml^{-1} but higher concentrations are found in secretions. There are two subclasses of this immunoglobulin.

4.3.4   *Immunoglobulin D (IgD)*

This occurs in normal serum at very low levels (30–50 μg ml^{-1}) but is the predominant surface component of B cells. Immature B cells express surface IgM without IgD but as these cells mature IgD is also expressed. After activation of the B cells, surface IgD can no longer be detected and it would appear that IgD may be involved with the differentiation of B cells.

4.3.5   *Immunoglobulin E (IgE)*

This is a very minor serum component (0.1–0.3 μg ml^{-1}) but is a major class of immunoglobulins. It binds with very high affinity to mast cells and basophils via a site in the Fc region of the molecule. Crosslinking of the cell-bound IgE antibodies by antigen triggers the degranulation of these cells with the release of histamine, leukotrienes and other vasoactive compounds. This class may play a role in immunity to helminthic parasites but in the western world it is more commonly associated with immediate hypersensitivity reactions such as hay fever and extrinsic asthma.

4.4	**Humoral antigen–antibody reactions**

Antibody molecules are bivalent whilst antigens can be multivalent. The resultant combination may result in either small, soluble complexes, or large insoluble aggregates, depending on the nature of the two molecules in the system. The following are examples of the reactions that can occur.

1 Neutralization. Small soluble complexes neutralize microbial toxins.

2 Precipitation. The formation of insoluble precipitates which enable the phagocytes to eliminate soluble antigen from the body.

3 Agglutination. The aggregation of bacterial cells into agglutinates enabling phagocytes to eliminate these cells rapidly from the body.

4 Cytotoxic reactions. The antibody and cell react, with resultant lysis of the cell. It was found that the presence of a third component, called complement, was necessary for this reaction to take place.

4.5	**Complement**

Complement activity was first recognized by Bordet, who showed that the lytic activity of rabbit anti-sheep erythrocyte serum was lost on heating to 56°C but was restored by the addition of fresh serum from an unimmunized rabbit. Thus, two factors were necessary, a heat-stable factor, antibody, plus a heat-labile factor, complement, which is present in all sera.

Complement is not a single protein but comprises a group of functionally linked proteins that interact with each other to provide many of the effector functions of humoral immunity and inflammation. Most of the components of the system are present in the serum as proenzymes, i.e. enzyme precursors. Activation of a complement molecule occurs as a result of proteolytic cleavage of the molecule, which in itself confers proteolytic activity on the molecule. Thus, many components of the system serve as the substrate of a prior component and, in turn, activate a subsequent component. This pattern of sequential activation results in the system being called the 'complement cascade'.

Complement can be activated by two pathways, the classical pathway and the alternative pathway (Fig. 14.4).

4.5.1	*The classical pathway*

The first component of complement is C1. This is a complex of three molecules designated C1q, C1r and C1s. The classical pathway is only initiated by an immune complex (antibody bound to antigen) when C1q binds to the Fc portion of the complexed antibody (IgM or IgG). The binding of C1q activates the C1r and C1s molecules associated with it to yield activated C1 which now cleaves C4 and then C2 (subunits of

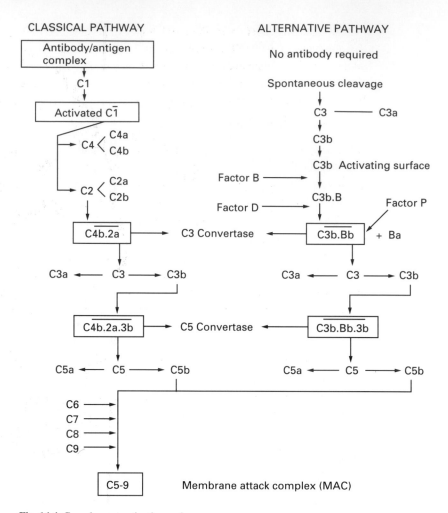

Fig. 14.4 Complement activation pathways.

complement that possess enzymatic activity have a bar over the subunits name). Cleavage of C4 yields a small fragment (C4a) and a large fragment, designated C4b, which binds to the cell surface near the C1 molecule.

Cleavage of C2 yields two fragments: a larger one, C2a, and a smaller one, C2b. C2a binds to a site on C4b to yield $\overline{\text{C4b2a}}$, which is a C3 convertase as it can now cleave C3 into C3a and C3b. C3b is bound to the $\overline{\text{C4b2a}}$ complex to yield $\overline{\text{C4b2a3b}}$. This complex is enzymatically active against C5 and for this reason is described as a C5 convertase. C5 is cleaved into C5a and C5b; it is the latter molecule that serves as a locus for the assembly of a single molecule each of C6, C7 and C8. The resulting C5b.6.7.8 complex allows the polymerization of C9 into a tubular hydrophobic structure that is inserted into the lipid bilayer of the cell membrane which forms a transmembrane channel through which ions and small molecules are able to diffuse freely. This structure is termed the membrane attack complex (MAC).

C3a and C5a are released into the fluid surroundings where they serve as potent anaphylotoxins in that they cause vasoactive substances such as histamines to be released from mast cells and basophils. C5a is also strongly chemotactic for neutrophils.

Free C3b fragments bind to the surface of the target cell. There are specific receptors for membrane-bound C3b on polymorphs and macrophages. This allows immune adherence of the complexes to these cells, thus facilitating subsequent phagocytosis. While antibodies alone bring about phagocytosis of antibody-coated particles through Fc receptors that are also found on phagocytes, the presence of C3b markedly enhances the phagocytic process.

4.5.2   *The alternative pathway*

The cleavage of C3 and the activation of the remainder of the complement cascade can be triggered, in the absence of complement-fixing antibody, by agents such as bacterial polysaccharide. C3 in the serum cleaves spontaneously and the C3b generated is rapidly inactivated (factors I and H). However, C3b bound to the surface of many microbes is able to bind to a serum protein designated factor B, which is now, in turn, cleaved by another serum protease, factor D. The resulting complex, $\overline{C3b.B}b$, is stabilized by another protein called *properdein* (P). The resultant stable complex, $\overline{C3b.Bb}$, is a C3 convertase, analogous to $\overline{C4b.2a}$. It cleaves C3 to form a multimolecular complex, $C3b.Bb.3b$, which is a C5 convertase and can generate C5b which is the focal point for the assembly of the MAC.

Proteins B, D and P also amplify the effects of the classical pathway in that some of the 3b generated by this pathway interacts with these proteins to form additional C3 convertase that supplements that provided by $\overline{C4b.2a}$. Likewise, enhanced cleavage of C5 occurs due to the dual activity of $\overline{C4.2a.3b}$ and $C3b.Bb.C3b$ complexes.

4.5.3   *Regulation of complement activity*

The spontaneous generation of C3b creates the potential for the triggering of the entire complement cascade. Two regulatory proteins prevent this. Factor I inactivates C3b unless it is bound to a surface. This action is enhanced by factor H, which also removes Bb from the $\overline{C3b.Bb}$ complex, thus inactivating the C3 convertase. The classical pathway is also under regulatory control as activated C1 could theoretically continue to cleave C4 and C2 molecules until they were entirely consumed. The presence in the serum of a C1 inhibitor (C1 INH) prevents this by binding to activated C1, allowing only a brief interval during which it can cleave C4 and C2 before it is deactivated by C1 INH.

Complement plays a significant part in the defence of the body. It can cause lysis of Gram-negative organisms by allowing lysozyme to reach the peptidoglycan layer of the organism. The generation of the C3b complex on the surface of the cell facilitates phagocytosis as the phagocytes possess a receptor for C3b, whilst C3a and C5a cause the release of histamine with the resultant increase in vascular permeability increasing the flow of serum antibody into the infected area. C3a and C5a also attract phagocytic cells to the focus of the infection.

4.6   Cell-mediated immunity (CMI)

The term cell-mediated immunity is used to describe the localized reactions that occur to those microorganisms that have the ability to live and multiply within the cells of the host, e.g. the tubercle bacillus, viruses and protozoal parasites. These reactions are mediated by lymphocytes and phagocytes and antibody plays a subordinate role.

When immunologists recognized that there were different classes of lymphocytes that were functionally and developmentally different, attempts were made to develop methods to distinguish them. This was initially done by raising antibodies to the cell surface proteins using animals of a different strain or type, i.e. 'alloantibodies'. The advent of hybridoma technology allowed the production of monoclonal antibodies that reacted specifically with defined populations of lymphocytes via cell surface molecules which acted as antigens (markers). Some of these markers are specific for cells of a particular lineage, whereas others indicate the state of activation or differentiation of the same cells. Thus, a marker that is recognized by a group ('cluster') of monoclonal antibodies is called a member of a cluster of differentiation and given a 'CD' designation.

The lymphocytes involved in CMI originate from the multipotential stem cell and are processed by the thymus gland; hence the name 'T' cells. The role of the thymus is to rearrange the genes associated within the T cell receptor (TCR) so that the mature T cells recognize foreign but not self antigens. This receptor has been isolated using monoclonal antibody probes and has been shown to consist of two disulphide-linked polypeptide chains termed the α and β chain. This receptor is associated with a characteristic cell surface marker, CD3. Antigen recognition occurs via this membrane structure CD3/TCR. Mature T cells also express other antigenic markers, notably CD4 or CD8. Thymectomized neonate mice do not exhibit the CMI response indicating the importance of the thymus gland.

Infection with a human immunodeficiency virus (HIV-1 and HIV-2; see Chapter 3) can cause the destruction of the TH cell, which is the critical cell of the immune system. This leads to the condition known as acquired immune deficiency syndrome (AIDS). At present, it is still not known why, in some cases, infection with HIV leaves the immune system intact whereas in others it is irreversibly destroyed, giving rise to AIDS.

The immune system must be able to distinguish between antigens against which an immune response would be beneficial and those where such a response would be harmful to the host, i.e. it must be able to distinguish between 'self' and 'non-self'. This is achieved via molecules of the major histocompatibility complex (MHC). The human MHC is located on chromosome 6 and is known as the HLA (human leucocyte antigen). It is divided into four main regions, designated A, B, C and D. Products of this region are expressed on the surface of cells and these enable cells of the immune system to recognize and signal to each other. Three main groups of these molecules have been identified.

1   Class 1 MHC molecules are integral membrane proteins found on the surface of all nucleated cells and platelets. They are the classical antigens involved in graft rejection.

2   Class 2 MHC molecules are expressed on the surface of B cells, macrophages, monocytes, various antigen-presenting cells (APCs) and certain cells of the T-cell family.

3   Class 3 MHC molecules consist of several complement components.

T cells only respond to protein antigens when the antigen has been processed by the APCs. The resultant small peptide molecules are then bound to the Class 2 molecules on the surface of the APCs. Monocytes, macrophages, B cells, dendritic cells and some

T cells all have the ability to internalize and degrade proteins into peptide fragments and can all therefore act as APCs.

The major T cell classes and their functions are listed below.

Helper T cells (TH cells)

These are the central cells of the immune system as they are essential for activation of the other cells associated with an effective immune response by the secretion of peptide mediators termed cytokines. Cytokines produced by macrophages and monocytes are termed monokines whilst those produced by lymphocytes are termed lymphokines. TH cells express CD4 on their surface.

CD4 is a transmembrane glycoprotein, approximately 55 kDa in size; it serves as a cell–cell adhesion molecule by virtue of its specific affinity for Class 2 MHC molecules. Likewise, it may transduce signals or facilitate TCR complex-mediated signal transduction upon binding Class 2 MHC molecules. CD4 is also the receptor for HIV (see Chapter 3).

Activation of the TH cells requires two signals. The first is the binding of CD3/TCR to the Class 2 MHC-antigen complex on the surface of the APC. This stimulates the APC to secrete a monokine (IL-1). This represents the second signal as the now activated TH cell secretes a lymphokine (IL-2) together with a series of other cytokines associated with cell growth and differentiation. IL-2 induces the growth of cells expressing IL-2 receptors which include the TH cells actually producing it, i.e. an autocatalytic effect. Cytokines secreted by activated TH cells are also associated with the proliferation and differentiation of B cells associated with the humoral response.

T cells responsible for delayed-type hypersensitivity secrete lymphokines which recruit and activate non-specific cells like macrophages into the area of the reaction. Examples of some of these lymphokines are listed below.

1 A macrophage chemotactic factor (MAC) which causes an accumulation of mononuclear phagocytes at the site of the antigen-mediated lymphokine release.

2 A macrophage migration inhibitory factor (MIF) which encourages the macrophages to remain in the area.

3 A macrophage-activating factor (MAF) which enhances the cell's ability to kill ingested intracellular organisms.

Suppressor T cells (Ts cells)

These are a class of lymphocytes thought to be distinct from helper and cytolytic T cells. Their function is to inhibit the activation phase of the immune responses. Their existence as a distinct population of cells has been doubted by many investigators, but they may be lymphocytes that can inhibit immune responses in different ways.

This may occur by the production of cytokines with inhibitory function; the ability to absorb necessary growth and differentiation factors; the possible lysis of cells bearing the stimulatory antigens in association with MHC molecules (Class I and Class II); the possible release of specific soluble factors (TsF) which may be directed at either the TH cell or the B cell.

The receptors on the Ts cell may recognize antigen which will then act as a bridge between the Ts and its target (the antigen receptor) or, alternatively, the Ts receptor may be a mirror image of the receptor on the target cell and produce direct suppression by binding to it. This recognition is termed 'idiotype recognition'. Ts cells express CD8 on their surface.

4.6.3   *Cytotoxic T cells (Tc cells)*

Virally infected host cells, and also tissue grafts from a genetically dissimilar donor, have been shown to stimulate the formation of T cells that are cytotoxic for these cells (Tc cells). Tc cells express CD8 on their cell surface.

On human Tc cells, the C8 molecules consist of two distinct glycoproteins, called CD8α and CD8β. The molecule may be a homodimer of CD8α chains or a disulphide-linked heterodimer. Like the CD4 molecule on TH cells, it is thought to serve as an adhesion molecule, but now binding to MHC Class 1 molecules which would be on the target cell. The CD8 molecule may transduce signals or facilitate TCR:CD3-mediated transduction upon binding Class 1 MHC molecules.

These T cells recognize peptide antigens bound to Class 1 MHC molecules on the surface of the target cell. During viral infections, viral peptides bind to self MHC1 molecules and are subsequently expressed on the cell surface. The MHC1 molecules of transplanted tissues are themselves recognized by the Tc cells.

Like TH cells, two signals are required to activate the Tc cell. The first is an interaction between the TCRs and the Class 1 MHC molecule/foreign epitope complex on the surface of the target cell. The second signal is that of IL-2 produced by the activated TH cell with the resultant release of cytotoxins which destroy the target cell.

4.7   **Immunoregulation**

An ongoing immune response can be regulated by three mechanisms.

Suppressor T cells. These cells can be specific for the antigen receptors on both B and T cells and thereby can suppress the activity of these two groups of cells.

Antibody feedback. Antibodies produced in response to an antigen are capable of inhibiting further immune responses to that antigen. This may occur due to diminishing antigen levels as a result of its combination with antibody or through an idiotypic network.

Idiotypic network. Idiotypic determinants (idiotypes) are unique antigenic epitopes characteristic of the antigen receptors on the surface of T and B cells. They are associated with the variable regions of these receptors. Antibodies produced by B cells as the result of antigenic stimulation can themselves stimulate the production of auto-anti-idiotypic antibodies which have the ability to combine with the B-cell receptor (Ig) and thus can dampen down the immune response. Idiotypes may likewise stimulate the production of T cells specific for idiotypic determinants. Jerne (1974) postulated his network hypothesis consisting of a series of complementary anti-idiotypic responses which modulate the immune response.

4.8 Natural killer (NK) cells

NK cells are a subset of lymphocytes found in blood and lymphoid tissues, especially the spleen. They are about 15 μm in diameter, possess a kidney-shaped nucleus and have two or three large granules in the cytoplasm. They are derived from the bone marrow. NK cells have the ability to kill certain tumour lines and normal cells infected by virus. Killing by NK cells is not specific for viral antigenic epitopes, and is not restricted by MHC molecules. They do not possess CD3 but do express CD2, CD16 and CD56, together with a low-affinity receptor for the Fc portion of IgG.

The most important role of NK cells is to provide a first line of defence against viral infections as they do not require prior exposure to antigen in order to respond. They are therefore effective against virally infected cells prior to the development of antibodies and antigen-specific Tc cells. NK cells operate independently of MHC antigens on the target cell and their activity is markedly enhanced by IL-2, α-interferon and other agents that activate macrophages, such as BCG vaccine. They may play an important part in controlling the development of neoplastic cells in the body.

NK cells possess a receptor for Fcγ and this enables them to adhere to target cells coated in antibody with the resultant destruction of that cell. This phenomenon is known as antibody-dependent cell-mediated cytotoxicity (ADCC). This was attributed to a separate cell population known as killer (K) cells but these have now been shown to be in effect NK cells.

4.9 Immunological tolerance

The administration of antigenic material does not always evoke an immunological response, a condition termed 'tolerance'. The classic example of this is the exposure of the immature lymphoid system of neonates to antigen, inducing a state of unresponsiveness to later challenge by the same antigen after the animal has reached immunological maturity. This could be the means whereby, during gestation, the body becomes unresponsive to its own constituents enabling the mature lymphoid system to distinguish in later life between 'self' and 'non-self'.

Tolerance can also be induced in adults, but higher doses of the antigen are required where it has been shown that both T and B cells are made unresponsive. As most antibody responses are T-dependent it is likely that it is these cells which are the ones affected. In order to maintain this state of tolerance it is necessary for the antigen to persist in the animal, as in its absence immunocompetent cells which are being produced throughout life are not being rendered tolerant.

Tolerance can occur in several ways.

1 Genetic unresponsiveness. If the animal lacks the necessary genetic ability to recognize antigenic material it will be 'immunologically' silent.

2 T-suppression. Ts cells may be activated more effectively than Th cells, thereby suppressing the immune response.

3 Helplessness. T cells are more readily tolerated than B cells and if they are unable to activate the B cells these cells could be described as 'helpless'.

4 Clonal deletion. Contact with antigen in the neonate results in death or permanent inactivation of the developing lymphocytes.

4.10   Autoimmunity

One fundamental property of an animal's immune system is that it does not normally react against its own body constituents, i.e. it exhibits tolerance. However, clinical and experimental evidence shows that certain diseases exist in which the patient apparently destroys his/her own cells. The reactions could involve Tc cells, B cells or NK cells, and the result of the reaction with antigen may result in a pathological condition arising (autoimmune disease). Autoimmunity is the mirror-image of tolerance and reflects the loss of tolerance to 'self'.

Autoimmunity can arise by the following.

1 Evasion of tolerance to self antigens. Hidden or sequestered antigens do exist, for instance spermatozoa and eye-lens tissue. These are confined to anatomical sites which do not have access to lymphoid tissue, and exposure of the above to lymphoid cells as a result of surgery or accident results in the production of the corresponding antibodies.

Drugs frequently bind to blood elements directly (e.g. penicillin to erythrocytes) and the antibodies to the resultant complex react with, and damage, cells coated with the drug. Viruses, especially those that bud, become associated with the host cell surface antigens with the resultant generation of Tc cells.

2 Breakdown of tolerance mechanisms. There are at least two mechanisms for maintaining unresponsiveness to self. The first is by specific deletion of self-reactive clones and the second by suppression. A failure of either of these two may result in an autoimmune disease. In normal, healthy individuals, antigen-binding, self-reactive B cells and the resultant low titres of autoantibodies are not uncommon. The origin of the self-reactive B cells is not clear, but there are four ways in which they may become activated.

    (a) Polyclonal activation. High concentrations of polyclonal activators, such as LPS and high molecular weight dextrans, activate B cells irrespective of the immunoglobulin receptor on the B cell surface. Polyclonal activation occurs in parasitic infections and in certain viral infections with the production of a wide spectrum of autoantibodies.

    (b) Non-specific helper factors. T-cell activation results in the production of a variety of lymphokines which can activate these B cells.

    (c) Cross-reactive antigens. These are shared by host and microorganism and this cross-reaction can activate autoreactive B cells.

    (d) Absence of T-cell suppression. The sudden depletion or elimination of Ts cells can lead to the spontaneous development of autoantibodies due to the maturation of the autoreactive B cells.

Types of autoimmune diseases vary widely, from 'organ-specific' diseases such as thyroiditis where there may be stimulation (thyrotoxicosis) by antibody against the receptor for pituitary thyroid-stimulating hormone (TSH) or inhibition (myxoedema) by cell destruction probably mediated by NK cells and autoantibody, through to 'nonorgan-specific' diseases such as systemic lupus erythematosus (SLE), where both lesions and autoantibodies are not confined to any one organ. In SLE, antibodies have been detected to DNA, erythrocytes and platelets, and cytotoxic antibodies to T lymphocytes have also been demonstrated. A strong case can be made for rheumatoid arthritis resulting from an autoimmune response to the Fc portion of IgG which gives rise to complexes which are ultimately responsible for the pathological changes characteristic of the rheumatoid joint.

5 Hypersensitivity

Not all antigen–antibody reactions are of benefit to the body, as sometimes the complexes (or their subsequent interaction with body tissues) may result in tissue damage. This must be regarded as a malfunction of the immune system and is known as a hypersensitive reaction. These reactions can be categorized into five main types. The first three involve the interaction between antigen and humoral antibody, and as the onset of the reaction is rapid, the condition is termed *immediate* hypersensitivity. The fourth type (*delayed* hypersensitivity) involves T cells and the symptoms of the reaction appear after 24 hours. The fifth type is where antibody stimulates cell function.

5.1 Type I (anaphylactic) reactions

In these reactions the antigen reacts with antibodies that are bound to the surface of mast cells through the Fc portion. This leads to the degranulation of the mast cells with the resultant release of vasoactive amines which give rise to the characteristic reactions of inflammation. The symptoms of the reaction that appear depend on the distribution of the cell-bound antibody, for example allergic reactions affecting the skin (urticaria), nasal mucosa (rhinitis), eyes (angioneurotic oedema), bronchioles (extrinsic asthma) and the cardiovascular system (anaphylactic shock). Antibodies involved in these reactions are mainly IgE but sometimes IgG. They are called homocytotropic or reaginic antibodies and are responsible for the common allergic reactions that affect nearly 10% of the population.

5.2 Type II (cytolytic or cytotoxic) reactions

These reactions involve damage to particular cells or tissues. The combination of circulating antibody with the antigen on the cell surface results in the destruction of the cell by phagocytosis either by opsonic adherence through Fc or by immune adherence through C3b. Activation of the full complement system results in lysis. ADCC reactions involving NK cells may also occur. Type II reactions include the destruction of erythrocytes by cytolytic antibodies induced by incompatible blood transfusion; Rhesus incompatibility; autoimmune reactions which result in autoantibodies being produced against the patient's own red cells; and cells whose surface has been altered by sensitizing drugs. Antibodies involved in these reactions are of the IgG and IgM classes.

5.3   Type III (complex-mediated) reactions

These reactions are due to the presence of immune complexes either in the circulation or extravascular space. The complexes may localize in capillary networks (lungs, kidney, joints) where, together with complement and polymorphs, they may produce extensive tissue damage. Two main types of reactions fall into this group.

1   The Arthus reaction. The phenomenon is a local one and occurs if a soluble antigen is introduced into the body when there is a great excess of antibody. The union between the two results in an acute inflammatory reaction which may involve complement, polymorphs, lymphokines or platelet aggregation, all of which enhance the inflammatory response.

2   Serum sickness. This occurs when there is an excess of antigen to antibody, resulting in the formation of soluble complexes. These may circulate and cause systemic reactions or be widely deposited in the kidneys, joints and skin. A rise in temperature, swollen lymph nodes, a generalized urticarial rash and painful swollen joints occur. The repeated administration of foreign serum (e.g. antidiphtheria serum or antitetanus serum prepared in horses) can lead to this condition due to antibodies being produced to the horse protein material.

5.4   Type IV (delayed hypersensitivity) reactions

These reactions are slow to manifest themselves (1–3 days after contact with antigen). Many allergic reactions to bacteria, viruses and fungi, sensitization to simple chemicals and the rejection of transplanted tissues result. The reactions are initiated by reaction between antigen-specific T cells and antigen, with the resultant release of lymphokines that affect a variety of accessory cells, especially macrophages. Antibody and complement are not involved. The classic example of this type of reaction may arise in persons subjected to the tuberculin test. Subjects who have previously been in contact with *Mycobacterium tuberculosis* have T cells sensitized to a protein extract of the tubercle bacillus. Intradermal injections of this protein extract induce an inflammatory response in the skin, at the site of the injection, which appears after 24 hours and may persist for several months. It is taken as an indication of immunity to the disease due to prior exposure to the organism, and a rough indication of the quality of this immunity can be interpreted according to the response to varying concentrations of the protein.

Reaction against virally infected or transplanted cells results in stimulated lymphocytes transforming into Tc cells which can eliminate target cells bearing the sensitizing antigen.

5.5   Type V (stimulatory hypersensitivity) reactions

Cells possess surface receptor sites for the chemical messengers of the body. Should an autoantibody be produced against this site, it can combine with it and cause the same effect as the chemical messenger, e.g. thyrotoxicosis caused by autoantibody to the receptor site to TSH as previously described (section 4.10).

6   Tissue transplantation

The replacement of certain diseased or damaged organs by healthy ones is now a fairly routine occurrence, but the immunological nature of graft rejection was only accepted when it was shown that second grafts from the same donor were more rapidly rejected than first grafts. Tissue transferred from one site to another within the same individual (*autografts*) or between genetically identical individuals, e.g. uniovular twins (*isografts*), are invariably successful. Grafts between genetically different individuals of the same species (*allografts*) or between different species (*xenografts*) evoke an intense immunological response and are rejected.

The specificity of transplantation antigens is under genetic control and these genes can be divided into two categories. The first are those that control the 'strong' transplantation antigens which induce intense allograft reactions where incompatibility between donor and recipient leads to rapid graft rejection. In mice this locus is termed the H-2 complex and in humans the HLA system. These constitute the MHC, which dominates all transplantation reactivity.

As previously described, four principal loci have been identified in the HLA system, namely HLA-A, B, C and D, and their products occur as transmembrane glycoprotein antigens. The second category of histocompatibility genes codes for 'minor' transplantation antigens where differences between donor and recipient lead to relatively slow graft rejection. Successful organ grafting relies on matching donor and recipient antigens as closely as possible but often the clinical urgency of the transplant does not permit this. Graft rejection is mediated by T and/or B cells with their usual associated systems such as complement, NK cells, etc., and the time taken for rejection to occur depends on whether the recipient has previously been sensitized to the antigens of the donor. The major routine measures to prevent graft rejection are the use of anti-inflammatory and immunosuppressive drugs such as steroids, azathioprine and cyclosporin A, where the rationale is to destroy cells responding to antigen. The use of antibodies to host lymphocytes (antilymphocyte serum, ALS) in conjunction with chemotherapy has proved successful in heart grafts.

Tissue-typing studies have revealed that there is a large range of diseases, mostly of presumed immunologic origin, that are associated with the presence of a specific HLA antigen. The most overwhelming relationship occurs in the disease ankylosing spondylitis, where 95% of sufferers possess the HLA-B27 antigen compared with an incidence of only 5% in the controls. The precise reason for the relationship is not known but many divergent theories have been postulated.

6.1   Immune response to tumours

It is suggested that altered cells which could be potentially malignant are recognized by the immune system and eliminated. This must mean that cancer cells possess new antigens on their cell surface. These antigens have been identified and can be categorized into three groups.

1   Virally induced antigens result from a malignant transformation occurring in the cell, due to an oncogenic virus. These evoke powerful immune responses in experimental animals.

2 Cells transformed by chemical carcinogens possess antigens that evoke a weak response.

3 Naturally occurring tumours evoke little or no immune response in experimental animals. This is disappointing but it must be remembered that these cells have already escaped the normal immune surveillance.

The possible use of immunotherapy for the prevention or treatment of malignant disease relies on the stimulation of the natural immune response and this is an area of exciting research, but has, as yet, proved to have limited success.

7   Immunity

Immunity, the state of relative resistance to an infection, can be divided into two main groups, natural and acquired immunity.

7.1   Natural immunity

This is subdivided into the following.

7.1.1   *Species immunity*

Humans are susceptible to diseases to which other animals are immune and vice versa. This is due to body temperature, biochemical differences, etc.

7.1.2   *Individual immunity*

Variation in natural immunity between individuals can depend on the state of health, age, hormonal balance, etc.

7.2   Acquired immunity

This is subdivided into actively acquired and passively acquired immunity, each of which may be induced naturally or artificially.

7.2.1   *Active acquired immunity*

This is produced as a result of an antigenic stimulus. This stimulus may occur naturally by means of a clinical or subclinical infection, or artificially by the deliberate introduction into the body of the appropriate antigen in the form of a vaccine or toxoid (Chapter 16). This type of immunity is normally long-lasting.

7.2.2   *Passive acquired immunity*

Passively acquired immunity involves no 'work' on the part of the body's defence mechanisms, and produces immediate protection of short duration.

It involves the transfer into the recipient of preformed antibody, i.e. there is no antigenic stimulus. This can occur (a) naturally, by transplacental passage of antibody from mother to child and also by antibodies being transmitted in breast milk; or (b) artificially, by means of the administration of antibodies preformed in another human (human γ-globulin) or in animals, e.g. horses, which are used for the production of antitoxic sera (antitoxins such as tetanus, diphtheria, etc.; see Chapter 15). The length of the immunity depends on the rate of degradation of the antibody and is only short-lived.

8   Further reading

Abbas A.K., Lichtman A.H. & Pober J.S. (1994) *Cellular and Molecular Immunology*, 2nd edn. London: W.B. Saunders.

Alzari P.M., Lascombe M. & Poljak R.J. (1988) Three-dimensional structure of antibodies. *Ann Rev Immunol*, **6**, 555–580.

Arai K., Lee F., Miyajima A., Miyatake S., Arai N. & Yokota T. (1990) Cytokines: coordinators of immune and inflammatory responses. *Ann Rev Biochem*, **59**, 783–836.

Baldwin R.W. (1985) Monoclonal antibody targeting of anti-cancer agents. *Eur J Cancer Clin Oncol*, **21**, 1281–1285.

Bloom B.R., Salgame P. & Diamond B. (1992) Revisiting and revising suppressor T cells. *Immunol Today*, **13**, 131–136.

Campbell R.D. & Trowsdale J. (1993) Map of the human MHC. *Immunol Today*, **14**, 349–352.

Germain R.H. & Marguiles D.M. (1993) The biochemistry and cell biology of antigen processing and presentation. *Ann Rev Immunol*, **11**, 403–450.

Ikuta K., Uchida N., Friedman J. & Weissman I.L. (1992) Lymphocyte development from stem cells. *Ann Rev Immunol*, **10**, 759–783.

Jerne N.K. (1974) Towards a network theory of the immune system. *Ann Immunol (Instit Pasteur)*, **125C**, 373–389.

Kohler G. & Milstein C. (1975) Continuous cultures of fused cells secreting antibody of predefined specificity. *Nature*, **256**, 495–497.

Leder P. (1982) The genetics of antibody diversity. *Sci Am*, **246**, 72–83.

Liddell J.E. & Cryer A. (1991) *A Practical Guide to Monoclonal Antibodies*. Chichester: John Wiley.

Micell M.C. & Parnes J.R. (1993) The role of CD4 and CD8 in T cell activation and differentiation. *Adv Immunol*, **53**, 59–122.

Morgan B.P. & Walport M.J. (1991) Complement deficiency and disease. *Immunol Today*, **12**, 301–306.

Muller G. (Ed.) (1984) Idiotype networks. *Immunol Rev*, 79.

Parker D.C. (1993) T cell-dependent B cell activation. *Ann Rev Immunol*, **11**, 331–360.

Playfair J.H.L. (1992) *Immunology at a Glance*, 5th edn. Oxford: Blackwell Scientific Publications.

Roitt I.M. (1994) *Essential Immunology*, 8th edn. Oxford: Blackwell Scientific Publications.

Schreiber S.L. & Crabtree G.R. (1992) The mechanisms of action of cyclosporin A and FK506. *Immunol Today*, **13**, 136–142.

Sprent J.E., Gao E.-K. & Webb S.R. (1990) T cell reactivity to MHC molecules: immunity versus tolerance. *Science*, **248**, 1357–1363.

Tomlinson E. & Davis S.S. (eds) (1986) *Site Specific Drug Delivery*. Chichester: John Wiley. (This deals in part with monoclonal antibodies.)

Tonegawa S. (1993) Somatic generation of antibody diversity. *Nature*, **302**, 575–581.

Trinchieri G. (1989) Biology of natural killer cells. *Adv Immunol*, **47**, 187–376.

Weiss R.A. (1993) How does HIV cause AIDS? *Science*, **260**, 1273–1279.

15 The manufacture and quality control of immunological products

1	**Introduction**		2.4	Blending
			2.5	Filling and drying
2	**Vaccines**		2.6	Quality control
2.1	The seed lot system		2.6.1	In-process control
2.2	Production of the bacteria and the		2.6.2	Final-product control
	bacterial components of bacterial			
	vaccines		**3**	**Immunosera**
2.2.1	Fermentation			
2.2.2	Processing of bacterial harvests		**4**	**Human immunoglobulins**
2.3	Production of the viruses and the viral			
	components of viral vaccines		**5**	**Tailpiece**
2.3.1	Growth of viruses			
2.3.2	Processing of viral harvests		**6**	**Further reading**

1 Introduction

Immunological products comprise a group of pharmaceutical preparations with diverse origins but with a common pharmacological purpose: the enhancement of a recipient's immune status in a manner that provides immunity to infectious disease. The immunological products that are generally available today are of three types: vaccines, immunosera and human immunoglobulins.

Vaccines are by far the most important immunological products. They induce immunity to many diseases and in so doing they have provided benefits for humankind, and for its animals, comparable with the benefits provided by anaesthetics and antibiotics. Smallpox vaccine, relentlessly deployed under the aegis of the World Health Organization, has made possible the eradication of one of the world's most terrible infections. Diphtheria, tetanus, whooping-cough, poliomyelitis, measles, and German measles vaccines have been wonderfully effective in those countries in which there have been the resources and the will to deploy them in health care programmes. Vaccines that provide protection against many other infections are available for use in appropriate circumstances.

Immunosera, which were once very widely used in the prophylaxis and treatment of many infections, are little used today, as vaccines have made some immunosera unnecessary and lack of proven therapeutic benefit has caused others to be relegated to immunological history. Tetanus antitoxin is an exception in that it is a very effective prophylactic that is still used in countries where there are inadequate supplies of tetanus immunoglobulin. Human immunoglobulins have important but limited uses.

Vaccines achieve their protective effects by stimulating a recipient's immune system to synthesize antibodies that promote the destruction of infecting microbes or neutralize bacterial toxins. This form of protection, known as active immunity, develops in the course of days and in the cases of many vaccines develops adequately only after two or three doses of vaccine have been given at intervals of days or weeks. Once established, this immunity lasts for years but it may need to be reinforced by 'booster' doses of vaccine given at relatively long intervals.

Immunosera and human immunoglobulins depend for their protective effects on their content of antibodies derived, in the case of immunosera, from immunized animals and, in the case of immunoglobulins, from humans who have been immunized or who have high antibody titres consequent upon prior infection. This form of immunity, known as passive immunity, is achieved immediately but is limited in its duration to the time that protective levels of antibodies remain in the circulation: see also Chapter 16.

A feature that is common to vaccines, immunosera and human immunoglobulins is the marked specificity of their actions. Each provides immunity to only one infection. This specificity has led to the development of vaccines and immunosera with several different components such as are present in the widely used diphtheria/tetanus/pertussis vaccines that are used to prevent the infectious diseases that commonly afflict infants and young children.

In addition to the three types of immunological product that are generally available there are two further types: synthetic peptide vaccines and monoclonal antibodies. Both have been extensively investigated but neither has, as yet, a place in conventional prophylaxis or therapeutics.

Principles of immunity were discussed in Chapter 14, whereas Chapter 16 describes a vaccination and immunization programme.

2 Vaccines

The vaccines currently used for the prevention of the infectious diseases of humans all originate, albeit in a variety of ways, from pathogenic microbes. The essence of vaccine manufacture thus consists of procedures which produce from dangerous pathogens, their components or their products, the immunogens that are devoid of pathogenic properties but which, nonetheless, retain the property of inducing a protective response in those to whom they are administered. The methods that are used by vaccine manufacturers are constrained by costs, by problems of delivery to the vaccinee and, most of all, by the biological properties of the pathogens from which vaccines are derived. Even so, the vaccines used in conventional vaccination programmes today are of only five readily recognizable types.

1 *Live vaccines.* Live vaccines are preparations of live bacteria or viruses which, when administered in an appropriate way, cause symptomless or almost symptomless infections. In the course of such an infection the constituents of the microbes in a vaccine evoke an immune response which provides protection against a serious natural disease. Live vaccines have a long history. The very first vaccine, smallpox vaccine, was a live vaccine. It was introduced in 1796 by the Gloucestershire doctor, Edward Jenner, who recognized that an attack of the mild condition known as cowpox protected milkmaids from smallpox during epidemics of this dreaded disease. He therefore took some fluid, the lymph, from a cowpox pustule on the hand of a milkmaid and used it to inoculate a small boy. A little later he courageously inoculated the boy with lymph from a case of smallpox—and nothing happened! The boy, protected as he was by the cowpox infection, remained well. Jenner's use of the causative organism of one disease

to provide protection against another is paralled by the use of the bacille Calmette–Guérin (BCG) strain of bovine tubercle bacilli to protect against infections with the human strain. However, in this case, there is the difference that the ability of the BCG strain to cause disease, its pathogenicity or virulence, has been reduced by many sequential subcultivations on laboratory media. Live vaccines such as smallpox and BCG vaccines that rely on the phenomenon of 'cross-protection' are exceptions to the generality that most vaccines are derived from the causative organisms of the diseases against which each is intended to provide protection. Thus, a virulent typhoid bacillus that was enzymically crippled by the action of nitrosoguanosine on its DNA gave rise to the live typhoid vaccine Ty21a. Likewise polioviruses from human infections were grown in the laboratory in such a way that it was possible to select infectious but innocuous progeny viruses suitable for use in live (oral) poliovaccines. Comparable procedures have been used to obtain the viruses that are currently used in live measles, mumps, rubella and yellow fever vaccines. The microbes with the reduced ability to cause disease that are used in live vaccines are said to have attenuated virulence and are often referred to as attenuated or vaccine strains.

2   *Killed vaccines.* Killed vaccines are suspensions of bacteria or of viruses that have been killed by heat or by disinfectants such as phenol or formaldehyde. Killed microbes do not replicate and cause an infection and so it is necessary that, in each dose of a killed vaccine, there are sufficient microbes to stimulate a vaccinee's immune system. Killed vaccines have therefore to be relatively concentrated suspensions. Even so, such preparations are rather poor antigens and, at the same time, tend to be somewhat toxic. It is thus necessary to divide the total amount of vaccine that is needed to induce protection into two or three doses that are given at intervals of a few days or weeks. Such a course of vaccination takes advantage of the enhanced 'secondary' response that occurs when a vaccine is administered to a person whose immune system has been sensitized by a previous dose of the same vaccine. The best known killed vaccines are whooping-cough (pertussis), typhoid, cholera, Salk type poliovaccine and rabies vaccine.

3   *Toxoid vaccines.* Toxoid vaccines are preparations derived from the toxins that are secreted by certain species of bacteria. In the manufacture of such vaccines, the toxin is separated from the bacteria and treated in a way that eliminates toxicity without eliminating immunogenicity. Formalin (*ca*. 38% of formaldehyde gas in water) is used for this purpose and consequently the treated toxins are often referred to as formol toxoids. Toxoid vaccines are very effective in the prevention of those diseases such as diphtheria and tetanus in which the harmful effects of the infecting bacteria are due to the deleterious action of bacterial toxins on physiology and biochemistry.

4   *Bacterial cell component vaccines.* Several bacterial vaccines that consist, not of whole bacterial cells as in conventional whooping-cough vaccine, but of components of the bacterial cells, are now available. The potential advantage of such vaccines is that they evoke an immune response only to the component, or components, in the vaccine and thus induce a response that is more specific and effective. At the same time, the amount of adventitous material in the vaccine is reduced and with it the likelihood of adverse reactions. Among the vaccines prepared from cell components are various acellular whooping-cough (pertussis) vaccines which have either a single component or several bacterial components. Other vaccines based on bacterial components, in each case on one or more capsular polysaccharides, are the *Haemophilus influenzae*

Type B vaccine, the *Neisseria meningitidis* Type A and C vaccine, the 23-valent pneumococcal polysaccharide vaccine and an acellular typhoid vaccine.

5 *Viral subunit vaccines*. Three viral subunit vaccines are widely available, two influenza vaccines and a hepatitis B vaccine. The influenza vaccines are prepared by treating intact influenza virus particles from embryonated hens' eggs infected with influenza virus with a surface acting agent. The virus particles are disrupted and release the two virus subunits, haemagglutinin and neuraminidase, that are required in the vaccine. The hepatitis B vaccine was, at one time, prepared from hepatitis B surface antigen (HBsAg) obtained from the blood of the victims of hepatitis B. This very constrained source of antigen has been replaced by yeast cells that have been genetically engineered to express HBsAg during fermentation.

2.1 The seed lot system

The starting point for the production of all microbial vaccines is the isolation of the appropriate microbe. Such isolates have been mostly derived from human infections and in some cases have yielded strains suitable for vaccine production very readily; in other cases a great deal of manipulation and selection in the laboratory have been needed before a suitable strain has been obtained.

Once a suitable strain is available, the practice is to grow, often from a single organism, a sizeable culture which is distributed in small amounts in a large number of ampoules and then stored at −70°C or freeze-dried. This is the seed lot. From this seed lot, one or more ampoules are taken and used as the seed to originate a limited number of batches of vaccine which are first examined exhaustively in the laboratory and then, if found to be satisfactory, tested for safety and efficacy in clinical trials. Satisfactory results in the clinical trials validate the seed lot as the seed from which batches of vaccine for routine use can subsequently be produced.

2.2 Production of the bacteria and the bacterial components of bacterial vaccines

The bacteria and bacterial components needed for the manufacture of bacterial vaccines are readily prepared in laboratory media by well-recognized fermentation methods. The end-product of the fermentation, the harvest, is processed to provide a concentrated and purified vaccine component that may be conveniently stored for long periods or even traded as an article of commerce.

2.2.1 Fermentation

The production of a bacterial vaccine batch begins with the resuscitation of the bacterial seed contained in an ampoule of the seed lot stored at −70°C or freeze dried. The resuscitated bacteria are first cultivated through one or more passages in preproduction media. Then, when the bacteria have multiplied sufficiently, they are used to inoculate a batch of production medium. This is usually contained in a large fermenter, the contents of which are continuously stirred. Usually the pH and the oxidation–reduction potential of the medium are monitored and adjusted throughout the growth period in a manner intended to obtain the greatest bacterial yield. In the case of rapidly growing bacteria the maximum yield is obtained after about a day but in the case of bacteria that grow slowly the maximum yield may not be reached before 2 weeks. At the end of the growth period the contents of the fermenter, which are known as the harvest, are ready for the next stage in the production of the vaccine.

2.2.2   *Processing of bacterial harvests*

The harvest is a very complex mixture of bacterial cells, metabolic products and exhausted medium. In the case of a live attenuated vaccine it is innocuous and all that is necessary is for the bacteria to be separated and resuspended in an appropriate menstruum, possibly for freeze-drying. In a vaccine made from a pathogen the harvest may be intensely dangerous and great care is necessary in the following procedures.

1   *Killing*. The process by which the live bacteria in the culture are killed and thus rendered harmless. Heat and disinfectants are employed. Heat and/or formalin are required to kill the cells of *Bordetella pertussis* used to make whooping-cough vaccines, and phenol is used to kill the *Vibrio cholerae* in cholera vaccine and the *Salmonella typhi* in typhoid vaccine.

2   *Separation*. The process by which the bacterial cells are separated from the culture fluid. Centrifugation using either a batch or continuous flow process is commonly used, but precipitation of the cells by reducing the pH is an alternative. In the case of vaccines prepared from cells, the fluid is discarded and the cells are resuspended in a saline mixture; where vaccines are made from a constituent of the fluid, the cells are discarded.

3   *Fractionation*. The process by which components are extracted from bacterial cells or from the medium in which the bacteria are grown and obtained in a purified form. The polysaccharide antigens of *Neisseria meningitidis* are separated from the bacterial cells by treatment with hexadecyltrimethylammonium bromide and those of *Streptococcus pneumoniae* with ethanol. The purity of an extracted material may be improved by resolubilization in a suitable solvent and precipitation. After purification, a component may be dried to a powder, stored indefinitely and, as required, incorporated into a vaccine in precisely weighed amounts at the blending stage.

4   *Detoxification*. The process by which bacterial toxins are converted to harmless toxoids. Formalin is used to detoxify the toxins of both *Corynebacterium diphtheriae* and *Clostridium tetani*. The detoxification may be performed either on the whole culture in the fermenter or on the purified toxin after fractionation.

5   *Adsorption*. The adsorption of the components of a vaccine on to a mineral adjuvant. The mineral adjuvants, or carriers, most often used are aluminium hydroxide, aluminium phosphate and calcium phosphate and their effect is to increase the immunogenicity and decrease the toxicity, local and systemic, of a vaccine. Diphtheria vaccine, tetanus vaccine, diphtheria/tetanus vaccine and diphtheria/tetanus/pertussis vaccine are generally prepared as adsorbed vaccines.

6   *Conjugation*. The linking of a vaccine component that induces only a poor immune response, with a vaccine component that induces a good immune response. The immunogenicity for infants of the capsular polysaccharide of *H. influenzae* Type b is greatly enhanced by the conjugation of the polysaccharide with diphtheria and tetanus toxoids, and with the outer membrane protein of *Neisseria meningitidis*.

2.3 Production of the viruses and the viral components of viral vaccines

Viruses replicate only in living cells so the first viral vaccines were necessarily made in animals: smallpox vaccine in the dermis of calves and sheep; and rabies vaccines in the spinal cords of rabbits and the brains of mice. Such methods are no longer used in advanced vaccine production and the only intact animal hosts that are used are embryonated hens' eggs. Almost all of the virus that is needed for viral vaccine production is obtained from cell cultures infected with virus of the appropriate strain.

2.3.1 *Growth of viruses*

Embryonated hens' eggs are still the most convenient hosts for the growth of the viruses that are needed for influenza and yellow fever vaccines. Influenza viruses accumulate in high titre in the allantoic fluid of the eggs and yellow fever virus accumulates in the nervous systems of the embryos.

2.3.2 *Processing of viral harvests*

The processing of the virus-containing material from infected embryonated eggs may take one or other of several forms. In the case of influenza vaccines the allantoic fluid is centrifuged to provide a concentrated and partially purified suspension of virus. This concentrate is treated with ether or other disruptive agents to split the virus into its components when split virion or surface antigen vaccines are prepared. The chick embryos used in the production of yellow fever vaccine are homogenized in water to provide a virus-containing purée. Centrifugation then precipitates most of the embryonic debris and leaves much of the yellow fever virus in an aqueous suspension.

Cell cultures provide infected fluids that contain little debris and can generally be satisfactorily clarified by filtration. Because most viral vaccines made from cell cultures consist of live attenuated virus, there is no inactivation stage in their manufacture. There are, however, two important exceptions: inactivated poliomyelitis virus vaccine is inactivated with dilute formalin or β-propiolactone and rabies vaccine is inactivated with β-propiolactone. The preparation of these inactivated vaccines also involves a concentration stage, by adsorption and elution of the virus in the case of poliomyelitis vaccine and by ultrafiltration in the case of rabies vaccine. When processing is complete the bulk materials may be stored until needed for blending into final vaccine. Because of the lability of many viruses, however, it is necessary to store most purified materials at temperatures of $-70°C$.

2.4 Blending

Blending is the process in which the various components of a vaccine are mixed to form a final bulk. It is undertaken in a large, closed vessel fitted with a stirrer and ports for the addition of constituents and withdrawal of the final blend. When bacterial vaccines are blended, the active constituents usually need to be greatly diluted and the vessel is first charged with the diluent, usually containing a preservative such as thiomersal. A single-component final bulk is then made by adding bacterial suspension, bacterial component or concentrated toxoid in such quantity that it is at the desired concentration in the final product. A multiple-component final bulk of a combined vaccine is made by adding each required component in sequence. When viral vaccines are blended, the need to maintain adequate antigenicity or infectivity may preclude dilution and tissue culture fluids or concentrates made from them are often used undiluted or, in the case of multicomponent vaccines, merely diluted one with another. After thorough mixing a final bulk may be broken down into a number of moderate sized volumes to facilitate handling.

2.5 Filling and drying

As vaccine is required to meet orders, bulk vaccine is distributed into single dose ampoules or into multidose vials as necessary. Vaccines that are filled as liquids are sealed and capped in their containers, whereas vaccines that are provided as dried preparations are freeze-dried before sealing.

The single-component bacterial vaccines are listed in Table 15.1. For each vaccine, notes are provided of the basic material from which the vaccine is made, the salient production processes and tests for potency and for safety. The multicomponent vaccines that are made by blending together two or more of the single component vaccines are required to meet the potency and safety requirements for each of the single components that they contain. The best known of the combined bacterial vaccines is the adsorbed diphtheria, tetanus and pertussis vaccine (DTPer/Vac/Ads) that is used to immunize infants, and the adsorbed diphtheria and tetanus vaccine (DT/Vac/Ads) that is used to reinforce the immunity of school entrants.

The single-component viral vaccines are listed in Table 15.2 with notes similar to those provided with the bacterial vaccines. The only combined viral vaccine that is widely used is the measles, mumps and rubella vaccine (MMR Vac). In a sense, however, both the inactivated (Salk) poliovaccine (Pol/Vac (inactivated)) and the live (Sabin) poliovaccine (Pol/Vac (oral)) are combined vaccines in that they are both mixtures of virus of each of the three serotypes of poliovirus. Influenza vaccines, too, are combined vaccines in that many contain components from as many as three virus strains, usually from two strains of influenza A and one strain of influenza B.

2.6 Quality control

The quality control of vaccines is intended to provide assurances of both the efficacy and the safety of every batch of every product. It is executed in three ways:
1 in-process control;
2 final-product control; and
3 a requirement that for each product the starting materials, intermediates, final product and processing methods are consistent.

The results of all quality control tests are always recorded in detail as, in those countries in which the manufacture of vaccines is regulated by law, they are part of the evidence on which control authorities judge the suitability or otherwise of each batch of each preparation.

Table 15.1 Bacterial vaccines used for the prevention of infectious disease in humans. Vaccines marked * are those used in conventional immunization schedules; those marked † are used to provide additional protection when circumstances indicate a need

Vaccine	Source material	Processing	Potency assay	Safety tests
Anthrax*	Medium from cultures of *B. anthracis*	**1** Separation of protective antigen from medium **2** Adsorption	3 + 3 quantal assay in guinea-pigs using challenge with *B. anthracis*	Exclusion of live *B. anthracis* and of anthrax toxin
BCG*	Cultures of live BCG cells in liquid or on solid media	**1** Bacteria centrifuged from medium **2** Resuspension in stabilizer **3** Freeze-drying	Viable count; induction of sensitivity to tuberculin in guinea-pigs	Exclusion of virulent mycobacteria; absence of excessive dermal reactivity
Diphtheria (adsorbed)*	Cultures of *C. diphtheriae* in liquid medium	**1** Separation and concentration of toxin **2** Conversion of toxin to toxoid **3** Adsorption of toxoid to adjuvant	3 + 3 quantal assay in guinea-pigs using intra-dermal challenge	Inoculation of guinea-pigs to exclude residual toxin
Haemophilus influenzae type b*	Cultures of *H. influenzae* type b	**1** Separation of capsular polysaccharide **2** Conjugation with a protein	Estimation of capsular poly-saccharide content	
Neisseria meningitidis Types A and C†,	Cultures of *N. meningitidis* of serotypes A and C	**1** Precipitation with hexadecyl-trimethyammonium bromide **2** Solubilization and purification **3** Blending **4** Freeze-drying	Estimation of capsular poly-saccharide content	
Pneumococcal polysaccharide†	Cultures of 23 serotypes of *Strep. pneumoniae*	**1** Precipitation of polysaccharides with ethanol **2** Blending into polyvalent vaccine	Physico-chemical estimation of polysaccharides	
Tetanus (adsorbed)*	Cultures of *Cl. tetani* in liquid medium	**1** Conversion of toxin to toxoid **2** Separation and purification of toxoid **3** Adsorption to adjuvant	3 + 3 quantal assay in mice using subcutaneous challenge with tetanus toxin	Inoculation of guinea-pigs to exclude presence of untoxoided toxin

continued on p. 312

Table 15.1 *Continued*

Vaccine	Source material	Processing	Potency assay	Safety tests
Typhoid† whole cell	Cultures of *Sal. typhi* grown in liquid media	**1** Killing with heat or phenol **2** Separation and resuspension of bacteria in saline	Induction of antibodies in rabbits	Exclusion of live *Sal. typhi*
Typhoid Vi capsular polysaccharide antigen†	Cultures of *Sal. typhi* grown in liquid medium	Extraction of capsular antigen	Estimation of capsular antigen	
Typhoid live vaccine†	Cultures of *Sal. typhi* strain Ty21A	Encapsulation	Estimation of content of live bacteria	
Whooping-cough (Pertussis) whole cell*	Cultures of *B. pertussis* grown in liquid or on solid media	**1** Harvest **2** Killing with formalin **3** Resuspension	3 + 3 quantal assay in mice using intra-cerebral challenge with live *Bord. pertussis*	Estimation of bacteria to limit content to 20×10^9 per human dose; weight gain test in mice to exclude excess toxicity
Whooping-cough (Pertussis) (acellular)†	Cultures of *Bord. pertussis*	**1** Harvest **2** Extraction and blending of cell components	As for whole-cell whooping-cough vaccine	Weight gain test in mice to exclude excess toxicity

Notes: Diphtheria and whooping cough vaccines are seldom used as single-component preparations but as components of diphtheria/tetanus vaccines and diphtheria/tetanus/pertussis vaccines. A combined diphtheria/tetanus/pertussis/Hib vaccine is available.

Bacterial vaccines less generally available than those listed in the table include botulism vaccine, necrotizing enteritis (pigbel) vaccine, *Pseudomonas aeruginosa* vaccine and tularaemia vaccine.

2.6.1 In-process control

In-process quality control is the control exercised over starting materials and intermediates. Its importance stems from the opportunities that it provides for the examination of a product at the stages in its manufacture at which testing is most likely to provide the most meaningful information. The WHO Requirements and national authorities stipulate many in-process controls but manufacturers often perform tests in excess of those stipulated, especially sterility tests (Chapter 23) as, by so doing, they obtain assurance that production is proceeding normally and that the final product is likely to be satisfactory. Examples of in-process control abound but three of different types should suffice.

1 The quality control of both diphtheria and tetanus vaccines requires that the products are tested for the presence of free toxin, that is for specific toxicity due to inadequate detoxification with formalin, at the final-product stage. By this stage, however, the toxoid concentrates used in the preparation of the vaccines have been much diluted and, as the volume of vaccine that can be inoculated into the test animals (guinea-pigs)

Table 15.2 Viral vaccines used for the prevention of infectious disease in humans. The vaccines marked * are those used in conventional immunization programmes, those marked † are used to provide additional protection when circumstances indicate a need

Vaccine	Source material	Processing	Potency assay	Safety tests
Hepatitis A†	Human diploid cells infected with hepatitis A virus	**1** Separation of virus from cells **2** Inactivation with HCHO **3** Adsorption to Al(OH)$_3$ gel	Assay of antigen content by ELISA	Inoculation of cell cultures to exclude presence of live virus
Hepatitis B†	Yeast cells genetically modified to express surface antigen	**1** Separation of HBsAg from yeast cells **2** Adsorption to Al(OH)$_3$ gel	Immunogenicity assay or HBsAg assay by ELISA	Test for presence of yeast DNA
Influenza (split virion)†	Allantoic fluid from embryonated hens' eggs infected with influenza viruses A and B	**1** Harvest of viruses **2** Disruption with surface active agent **3** Blending of components of different serotypes	Assay of haemagglutinin content by immunodiffusion	Inoculation of embryonated hens' eggs to exclude live virus
Influenza (surface antigen)†	Allantoic fluid from embryonated hens' eggs infected with influenza viruses A and B	**1** Inactivation and disruption **2** Separation of haemagglutinin and neuraminidase **3** Blending of haemagglutinins and neuraminidase of different serotypes	Assay of haemagglutinin content by immunodiffusion	Inoculation of embryonated hens' eggs to exclude live virus
Measles*	Chick embryo cell cultures infected with attenuated measles virus	**1** Clarification **2** Freeze-drying	Infectivity titration in cell cultures	Tests to exclude presence of extraneous viruses
Mumps*	Chick embryo cell cultures infected with attenuated mumps virus	**1** Clarification **2** Freeze-drying	Infectivity titration in cell cultures	Tests to exclude presence of extraneous viruses
Poliomyelitis (inactivated)† (Salk type)	Human diploid cell cultures infected with each of the three serotypes of poliovirus	**1** Clarification **2** Inactivation with formalin **3** Concentration **4** Blending of virus of each serotype	Induction of antibodies to polioviruses in chicks or guinea-pigs	Inoculation of cell cultures and monkey spinal cords to exclude live virus

continued on p. 314

Table 15.2 *Continued*

Vaccine	Source material	Processing	Potency assay	Safety tests
Poliomyelitis (live or oral)* (Sabin type)	Cell cultures infected with attenuated poliovirus of each of the three serotypes	1 Clarification 2 Blending of virus of three serotypes in stabilizing medium	Infectivity titration of each of three virus serotypes	Test for attenuation by inoculation of spinal cords of monkeys and comparison of lesions with those produced by a reference vaccine
Rabies†	Human diploid cell cultures infected with rabies virus	1 Clarification 2 Inactivation with beta-propiolactone	3 + 3 quantal assay in mice	Inoculation of cell cultures to exclude live virus
Rubella* (German measles)	Human diploid cell cultures infected with attenuated rubella virus	1 Clarification 2 Blending with stabilizer 3 Freeze-drying	Infectivity titration in cell cultures	Tests to exclude presence of extraneous viruses
Varicella†	Human diploid cell cultures infected with attenuated varicella virus	1 Clarification 2 Freeze-drying	Infectivity titration in cell cultures	Tests to exclude presence of extraneous viruses
Yellow fever†	Aqueous homogenate of chick embryos infected with attenuated yellow fever virus 170	1 Centrifugation to remove cell debris 2 Freeze drying	Infectivity-titration in cell cultures by plaque assay	Tests to exclude extraneous viruses

Notes: Measles, mumps and rubella vaccines are generally administered in the form of a combined measles/mumps/rubella vaccine (MMR vaccine).

Viral vaccines less generally available than those listed in the table include Congo Crimean haemorrhagic fever vaccine, dengue fever vaccine, Japanese encephalitis B vaccine, smallpox vaccine, tick borne encephalitis vaccine, and Venezuelan encephalitis vaccine.

ELISA, enzyme-linked immunosorbent assay.

is limited, the tests are relatively insensitive. In-process control, however, provides for tests on the undiluted concentrates and thus increases the sensitivity of the method at least 100-fold.

2   An example from virus vaccine manufacture is the titration, prior to inactivation, of the infectivity of the pools of live poliovirus used to make inactivated poliomyelitis vaccine. Adequate infectivity of the virus from the tissue cultures is an indicator of the adequate virus content of the starting material and, since infectivity is destroyed in the inactivation process, there is no possibility of performing such an estimation after formolization.

3   A more general example from virus vaccine production is the rigorous examination of tissue cultures to exclude contamination with infectious agents from the source animal or, in the cases of human diploid cells or cells from continuous cell lines, to detect

cells with abnormal characteristics. Monkey kidney cell cultures are tested for simian herpes B virus, simian virus 40, mycoplasma and tubercle bacilli. Cultures of human diploid cells and continuous line cells are subjected to detailed karyological examination (examination of chromosomes by microscopy) to ensure that the cells have not undergone any changes likely to impair the quality of a vaccine or lead to undesirable side-effects.

2.6.2 *Final-product control*

Vaccines containing killed microbes or their products are generally tested for potency in assays in which the amount of the vaccine that is required to protect animals from a defined challenge dose of the appropriate pathogen, or its product, is compared with the amount of a standard vaccine that is required to provide the same protection. The usual format of the test is the 3 + 3 dose quantal assay that is used to estimate the potency of whooping-cough vaccine (*British Pharmacopoeia* 1993). Three logarithmic serial doses of the test vaccine and three logarithmic serial doses of the standard vaccine are made and each is used to inoculate a group of 16 mice. In the case of both the vaccine and the standard the middle dose is chosen, on the basis of experience, so that it is sufficient to induce a protective response in about 50% of the animals to which it is given. Each lower dose may then be expected to protect fewer than 50% of the mice to which it is given and each higher dose to protect more than 50% of the animals to which it is given. Fourteen days later all of the mice are infected ('challenged') with *Bordetella pertussis* and, after a further 14 days, the number of mice surviving in each of the six groups is counted. The number of survivors in each group is then used to calculate the potency of the test vaccine relative to the potency of the standard vaccine by the statistical method of probit analysis (Finney 1971). The potency of the test vaccine may be expressed either as a percentage of the potency of the standard vaccine but, as the standard vaccine will have an assigned potency in International Units (IU), the potency of the test vaccine may be expressed in similar units. Tests similar to that used to estimate the potency of whooping-cough vaccine are prescribed for the estimation of the potencies of diphtheria vaccine and of tetanus vaccine. In the cases of these two vaccines the bacterial toxins are used as the challenge material (*British Pharmacopoeia* 1993).

Vaccines containing live microorganisms are generally tested for potency by counts of their viable particles. In the case of the only live bacterial vaccine in common use, BCG vaccine, dilutions of vaccine are made and dropped in fixed volumes on to solid media capable of supporting the microorganisms' growth. After a fortnight the colonies generated by the drops are counted and the live count of the undiluted vaccine is calculated. The potency of live viral vaccines is estimated in much the same way except that a substrate of living cells is used. Dilutions of vaccine are inoculated on to tissue culture monolayers in Petri dishes or in plastic trays, and the live count of the vaccine is calculated from the infectivity of the dilutions and dilution factor involved.

Safety tests. Because many vaccines are derived from basic materials of intense pathogenicity—the lethal dose of a tetanus toxin for a mouse is estimated to be $3 \times 10^{-5} \mu g$—safety testing is of paramount importance. Effective testing provides a guarantee of the safety of each batch of every product and most vaccines in the final container must pass one or more safety tests as prescribed in a pharmacopoeial monograph. This generality does not absolve a manufacturer from the need to perform 'in-process' tests as required, but it is relaxed for those preparations which have a final formulation that makes safety tests on the final product either impractical or meaningless.

Bacterial vaccines are regulated by relatively simple safety tests. Those vaccines composed of killed bacteria or bacterial products must be shown to be completely free from the living microbes used in the production process and inoculation of appropriate bacteriological media with the final product provides an assurance that all organisms have been killed. Those containing diphtheria and tetanus toxoids require in addition, a test system capable of revealing inadequately detoxified toxins; inoculation of guinea-pigs, which are exquisitely sensitive to both diphtheria and tetanus toxins, is always used for this purpose. Inoculation of guinea-pigs is also used to exclude the presence of abnormally virulent organisms in BCG vaccine.

Viral vaccines present problems of safety testing far more complex than those experienced with bacterial vaccines. With killed viral vaccines the potential hazards are those due to incomplete virus inactivation and the consequent presence of residual live virus in the preparation. The tests used to detect such live virus consist of the inoculation of susceptible tissue cultures and of susceptible animals. The cultures are examined for cytopathic effects and the animals for symptoms of disease and histological evidence of infection at autopsy. This test is of particular importance in inactivated poliomyelitis vaccine, the vaccine being injected intraspinally into monkeys. At autopsy, sections of brain and spinal cord are examined microscopically for the histological lesions indicative of proliferating poliovirus.

With attenuated viral vaccines the potential hazards are those associated with reversion of the virus during production to a degree of virulence capable of causing disease in vaccinees. To a large extent this possibility is controlled by very careful selection of a stable seed but, especially with live attenuated poliomyelitis vaccine, it is usual to compare the neurovirulence of the vaccine with that of a vaccine known to be safe in field use. The technique involves the intraspinal inoculation of monkeys with a reference vaccine and with the test vaccine and a comparison of the neurological lesions and symptoms, if any, that are caused. If the vaccine causes abnormalities in excess of those caused by the reference it fails the test.

Tests of general application. In addition to the tests designed to estimate the potency and to exclude the hazards peculiar to each vaccine there are a number of tests of more general application. These relatively simple tests are as follows.

1 *Sterility.* In general, vaccines are required to be sterile. The exceptions to this requirement are smallpox vaccine made from the dermis of animals and bacterial vaccines such as BCG, Ty21A and tularaemia vaccine which consist of living but attenuated microbes. WHO requirements and pharmacopoeial standards stipulate, for vaccine batches of different size, the numbers of containers that must be tested and found to be sterile. The preferred method of sterility testing is membrane filtration as this technique permits the testing of large volumes without dilution of the test media. The test system must be capable of detecting aerobic and anaerobic organisms and fungi (see Chapter 23).

2 *Freedom from abnormal toxicity.* The purpose of this simple test is to exclude the presence in a final container of a highly toxic contaminant. Five mice of 17–22 g and two guinea-pigs of 250–350 g are inoculated with one human dose or 1.0 ml, whichever is less, of the test preparation. All must survive for 7 days without signs of illness.

3 *Presence of aluminium and calcium.* The quantity of aluminium in vaccines containing aluminium hydroxide or aluminium phosphate as an adjuvant is limited to 1.25 mg per dose and it is usually estimated compleximetrically. The quantity of calcium is limited to 1.3 mg per dose and is usually estimated by flame photometry.

4 *Free formalin.* Inactivation of bacterial toxins with formalin may lead to the presence of small amounts of free formalin in the final product. The concentration, as estimated by colour development with acetylacetone, must not exceed 0.02%.

5 *Phenol concentration.* When phenol is used to preserve a vaccine its concentration must not exceed 0.25% w/v or, in the case of some vaccines, 0.5% w/v. Phenol is estimated by the colour reaction with amino-phenazone and hexacyanoferrate.

3   **Immunosera**

Immunosera are preparations derived from the blood of animals, usually from the blood of horses. To prepare an immunoserum a horse is injected with a sequence of spaced doses of an antigen until a trial blood sample shows that the injections have induced a high titre of antibody to the injected antigen. A large volume of blood is then removed by venepuncture and collected into a vessel containing sufficient citrate solution to prevent clotting. The blood cells are allowed to settle and the supernatant plasma is drawn off. The plasma is then fractionated by the addition of ammonium sulphate and the globulin fraction is recovered and treated with pepsin to yield a refined immunoserum, Harms (1948). This refined immunoserum contains no more than a trace of the albumin that was present in the plasma. The refined immunoserum is titrated for the potency of its antibody content, diluted to the required concentration and transferred into ampoules. Two or more monovalent immunosera may be blended together to provide a multivalent immunoserum.

The quality of immunosera is controlled by potency tests and by conventional tests for safety and sterility. The potency tests have a common design in that, in the case of all immunosera, the potency is estimated by comparing the amount of an immunoserum that is required to neutralize an effect of an homologous antigen with the amount of a standard preparation that is required to achieve the same effect. Serial dilutions of the immunoserum and of a standard preparation are made and to each is added a constant amount of the homologous antigen. Each mixture is then inoculated into a group of animals, usually guinea-pigs or mice, and the dilutions of the immunoserum and of the standard which neutralize the effects of the antigen are noted. As the potencies of the standard preparations are expressed in IU the potencies of the immunosera are determined in corresponding units per millilitre (*British Pharmacopoeia* 1993).

Table 15.3 lists the immunosera for which there is a need, or a potential need, today and indicates the required potencies of these immunosera and the salient features of the potency assay methods.

Table 15.3 Immunosera used in the prevention of infections in humans

Immunoserum	Potency assay method	Potency requirement
Botulinum antitoxin	Neutralization of the lethal effects of botulinum toxins A, B and E in mice	500 IU ml^{-1} of type A 500 IU ml^{-1} of Type B 50 IU ml^{-1} of Type E
Diphtheria antitoxin	Neutralization of the erythrogenic effect of diphtheria toxin in the skin of guinea-pigs	1000 IU ml^{-1} if prepared in horses 500 IU ml^{-1} if prepared in other species
Tetanus antitoxin	Neutralization of the paralytic effect of tetanus toxin in mice	1000 IU ml^{-1} for prophylaxis 3000 IU ml^{-1} for treatment

In each of the assays of potency the amount of the immunoserum and the amount of a corresponding standard antitoxin that are required to neutralize the effects of a defined dose of the corresponding toxin are determined. The two determined amounts and the assigned unitage of the standard antitoxin are then used to calculate the potency of the immunoserum in International Units (IU).

4 Human immunoglobulins

Human immunoglobulins are preparations of the immunoglobulins, principally immunoglobulin G (IgG), that are present in human blood. They are derived from the plasma of donated blood and from plasma obtained by plasmapheresis. Normal immunoglobulin, that is immunoglobulin that has relatively low titres of antibodies, is prepared from pools of plasma obtained from not fewer than a thousand individuals; specific immunoglobulins, that is immunoglobulins with a high titre of a particular antibody, are usually prepared from smaller pools of plasma obtained from individuals who have suffered recent infections or who have undergone recent immunization and who thus have a high titre of a particular antibody. Each contribution of plasma to a pool is tested for the presence of hepatitis B surface antigen (HBsAg), for antibodies to human immunodeficiency viruses I and II (HIV I and II) and for antibodies to hepatitis C virus in order to identify, and to exclude from a pool, any plasmas capable of transmitting infection from donor to recipient.

The immunoglobulins are obtained from the plasma pools by fractionation methods that are based on ethanol precipitation in the cold with rigorous control of protein concentration, pH and ionic strength (Cohn *et al.* 1946; Kistler & Nitschmann 1962). Some of the fractionation steps may contribute to the safety of immunoglobulins by inactivating or removing contaminating viruses that have not been recognized by testing of the blood donations. The immunoglobulin may be presented either as a freeze-dried or a liquid preparation at a concentration that is 10 to 20 times that in plasma. Glycine may be added as a stabilizer and thiomersal as a preservative.

The quality control of immunoglobulins includes potency tests and conventional tests of safety and sterility. The potency tests consist of neutralization tests that parallel those used for the potency assay of immunosera, except that in the cases of some immunoglobulins the assays are made *in vitro*. In addition to the safety and sterility tests, total protein is determined by nitrogen estimations, the protein composition by

Table 15.4 Immunoglobulins used in the prevention and treatment of infections in humans

Immunoglobulin	Potency assay method	Potency requirement
Hepatitis B	Radioimmunoassay or enzymoimmunoassay	Not less than 100 IU ml^{-1}
Measles	Neutralization of the infectivity of measles virus for cell cultures	Not less than 50 IU ml^{-1}
Normal	Neutralization tests in cell cultures or in animals	Measurable amounts of one bacterial antibody and of one viral antibody for which there are international standards
Rabies	Neutralization of the infectivity of rabies virus for mice	Not less than 150 IU ml^{-1}
Tetanus	Neutralization of the paralytic effect of tetanus toxin in mice	Not less than 50 IU ml^{-1}
Varicella/zoster	ELISA in paralled with a standard varicella-zoster immunoglobulin	Not less than 100 IU ml^{-1}

In each of the assays of potency the amount of the immunoglobulin and the amount of a corresponding standard preparation that are required to neutralize the infectivity or other biological activity of a defined amount of virus or to neutralize a defined amount of a bacterial toxin are determined. The two determined amounts and the assigned unitage of the standard preparation are then used to calculate the potency of the immunoglobulin in International Units (IU). ELISA, enzyme-linked immunosorbent assay.

cellulose acetate electrophoresis and molecular size by liquid chromatography. The presence of immunoglobulins derived from species other than humans is excluded by precipitin tests. Table 15.4 lists six human immunoglobulins and their requisite potencies and indicates the methods in which the potencies are determined.

5   Tailpiece

Immunological products, notably vaccines, provide very secure protection from diseases caused by small pathogenic entities such as bacterial toxins and many viruses. They provide somewhat less secure protection from larger pathogens such as bacteria and little protection, if any, from much larger pathogens such as malaria parasites. There thus appears to be a rough inverse correlation between the efficacies of vaccines and the sizes of the pathogens from which each vaccine is intended to provide protection. This relationship may reflect the way in which vaccine-induced antibodies react with a toxin or pathogen. Small homogeneous tetanus toxin molecules may be completely invested by tetanus antitoxin molecules and thus wholly neutralized. In contradistinction malarial parasites may be unaffected by antibodies that attach only to a cell component that is not essential for the parasite's survival. It has recently been suggested (Beverly 1996) that in order to make effective vaccines against larger pathogens it may first be necessary to identify those molecules in the pathogens that are essential for each pathogen's survival. A vaccine containing such molecules might induce antibodies to a pathogen's essential molecules and thus provide immunity against larger pathogens comparable with that provided by the vaccines against toxins and small pathogens.

The cost of the vaccines used in the routine immunization of infants, children and adolescents is roughly equivalent to the cost of 100 loaves of bread. In the industrialized countries that is a small price to pay for what is virtually life-long protection from diphtheria, tetanus, whooping-cough, *H. Influenzae* type B infection, poliomyelitis, measles, mumps and rubella. In many developing countries it is a price far beyond the reach of either individuals or health authorities but a price that is in large part borne by the World Health Organization's Expanded Programme of Immunization.

6   Further reading

Beverley P.C.L. (1996) A job in time. *MRC News Winter*, 1996.

British Medical Association and Pharmaceutical Press (1997) *The British National Formulary*. London: BMA. (This publication contains a useful section on immunological products. New editions appear at intervals.)

British Pharmacopoeia (1993) London: Her Majesty's Stationery Office. (The *British Pharmacopoeia* contains edited versions of the monographs for immunological products that appear in the *European Pharmacopoeia*.)

Cohn E.J., Strong L.E., Hughes W.L., Hulford D.J., Ashworth J.N., Melin M. & Taylor H.I. (1946) Preparation and properties of serum proteins IV. *J Am Chem Soc*, **68**, 459–475.

Datapharm Publications Ltd (1996) *The Data Sheet Compendium*. London. (This publication contains reproductions of the Data Sheets of immunological products that are licensed by the Medicines Control Authority.)

Finney D.J. (1971) *Probit Analysis*. London: Cambridge University Press.

Harms A.J. (1948) The purification of antitoxic plasmas by enzyme treatment and heat denaturation. *Biochem J*, **42**, 340–347.

Kistler P. & Nitschmann HS. (1962) Large scale production of human plasma fractions. *Vox Sang*, **7**, 414–424.

Sheffield F. (1990) The measurement of immunity. In: *Topley and Wilson's Principles of Bacteriology, Virology and Immunity* (eds M.T. Parker & L.H. Collier), 8th edn. pp. 437–448. London: Edward Arnold.

16 Vaccination and immunization

1   **Introduction**

2   **Spread of infection**
2.1   Common source infections
2.2   Propagated source infections

3   **Objectives of a vaccine/immunization programme**
3.1   Severity of the disease
3.2   Effectiveness of the vaccine/immunogen
3.3   Safety
3.4   Cost
3.5   Longevity of the immunity

4   **Classes of immunity**
4.1   Passive acquired immunity
4.2   Active acquired immunity

5   **Classes of vaccine**
5.1   Live vaccines
5.2   Killed and component vaccines

6   **Routine immunization against infectious disease**

6.1   Poliomyelitis vaccination
6.2   Measles, mumps and rubella vaccination (MMR)
6.2.1   Measles
6.2.2   Mumps
6.2.3   Rubella
6.2.4   MMR vaccine
6.3   Tuberculosis
6.4   Diphtheria, tetanus and pertussis (DTP) immunization
6.4.1   Diphtheria
6.4.2   Tetanus
6.4.3   Pertussis (whooping-cough)
6.4.4   DTP vaccine combinations and administration
6.5   *Haemophilus influenza* Type B (HiB) immunization

7   **Juvenile immunization schedule**

8   **Immunization of special risk groups**

9   **Further reading**

1   Introduction

People rarely suffer from the same infectious disease twice. When such re-infection does occur it is usually either with an antigenically modified strain (common cold, influenza), the patient is immunocompromised (immunosuppressive drugs, immunological disorders) or a long time has elapsed since the first infection. Alternatively the patient may have failed to eliminate the primary infection which has then remained latent and emerges in a modified or similar form (herpes simplex, cold sores; herpes zoster, chickenpox). Immunity towards re-infection was recognized long before the discovery of the causal agents of infectious disease. Efforts were therefore made towards developing treatment strategies that might generate immunity to infection. An early development was the attempted control of smallpox (*Variola major*) through the deliberate introduction, into the skin of healthy individuals, of material taken from active smallpox lesions. Such treatments produced single localized lesions and commonly, but not always, protected the recipient from contracting full-blown smallpox. The process became known as variolation, and, unknown to its practitioners, attenuated the disease through changing the route of infection of the causal organism. Unfortunately, occasional cases of smallpox resulted from such treatment. Further developments recognized that immunity developed towards one disease often brings with it cross-immunity towards another related condition. Cowpox is a disease of cattle that can be transmitted to man. Symptoms are similar but less severe than those of smallpox. Material taken from active cowpox (*Vaccinia*) lesions was therefore substituted into the variolation procedures. This conferred much of the protection against smallpox that had become associated with variolation but without the associated risk. Edward Jenner's discovery, made over two centuries ago, became known as vaccination and heralded a new era in disease control. The term vaccination is now widely used to describe prophylactic measures that use live microorganisms or their products to induce immunity. The more general term immunization describes procedures that induce immunity in the recipient but which do not necessarily involve the use of microorganisms. Nowadays vaccination and immunization procedures are used not only to protect the individual against infection but also to protect communities against epidemic disease. Such public health measures have met with spectacular success as illustrated in Fig. 16.1 for the incidence of paralytic poliomyelitis. In instances, where there is no reservoir of the pathogen other than in infected individuals, and survival outside the host is limited (i.e. smallpox, poliomyelitis and measles) then such programmes, worldwide, have the potential to eradicate the disease permanently.

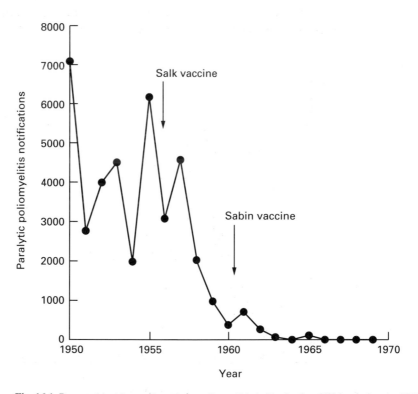

Fig. 16.1 Reported incidence of paralytic poliomyelitis in England and Wales during the 1950s and 1960s. After introduction of vaccination programmes the incidence of disease dropped from an endemic incidence of *ca*. 5000 cases per year to fewer than 10.

2   Spread of infection

Infectious diseases may either be spread from a common reservoir of the infectious agent that is distinct from diseased individuals (common source) or they might transfer directly from a diseased individual to a healthy one (propagated source).

2.1   Common source infections

In common source infections, the reservoir of infection might be animate (i.e. insect vectors of malaria and yellow fever) or they might be inanimate (infected drinking water, cooling towers, contaminated food supply). In the simplest of cases the source of infection is transient (i.e. food sourced to a single retail outlet or to an isolated event such as a wedding reception). In such instances the onset of new cases is rapid, phased over 1–1.5 incubation periods, and the decline in new cases closely follows the elimination of the source (Fig. 16.2). This leads to an acute outbreak of infection limited socially and geographically to those linked with the source. Such an incident was epitomized by the outbreak of *Escherichia coli* O157 infections, in Lanarkshire, in the winter of 1996.

If the source of the infection persists, after onset, then the incidence of new cases is maintained at a level which is commensurate with the infectivity of the pathogen and the frequency of exposure of individuals. In this manner, if cases of the variant Creutzfeldt–Jacob disease (vCJD), first recognized in the mid-1990s, relates to human exposure to bovine spongiform encephalopathy-infected beef in the early 1980s, then

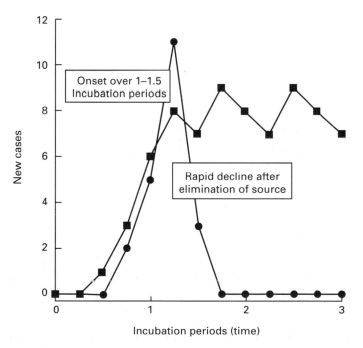

Fig. 16.2 Incidence pattern for common-source outbreaks of infection where the source persists (■) and where it is short-lived (●).

the incidence of vCJD will increase over 1–1.5 incubation periods (i.e. 10–15 years) and be sustained for many years before a decline. In such a scenario vCJD, related to a single common-source outbreak, would persist well into the next millenium.

For those infectious diseases that are transmitted to humans via insect vectors the onset and decline phases of epidemics are rarely observed other than as a reflections of the seasonal variation in the prevalence of the insect. Rather, the disease is endemic within the population group and has a steady incidence of new cases. Diseases such as these are generally controlled by public health measures and environmental control of the vector with vaccination and immunization being deployed to protect individuals (e.g. yellow fever vaccination).

2.2 Propagated source infections

Propagated outbreaks of infection relate to the direct transmission of an infective agent from a diseased individual to a healthy, susceptible one. Mechanisms of such transmission were described in Chapter 4 and include inhalation of infective aerosols (measles, mumps, diphtheria), direct physical contact (syphilis, herpes virus) and, where sanitation standards are poor, through the introduction of infected faecal material into drinking water (cholera, typhoid). The ease of transmission, and hence the rate of onset of an epidemic (Fig. 16.3) relates not only to the susceptibility status, and general state of health of the individuals but also to the virulence properties of the organism, the route of transmission, the duration of the infective period associated with the disease,

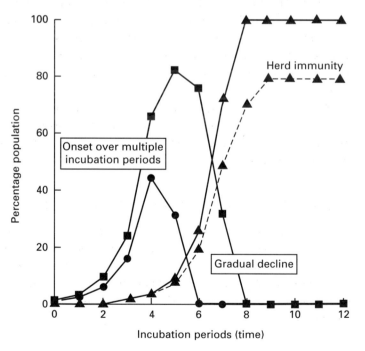

Fig. 16.3 Propagated outbreaks of infection showing the incidence of new cases (●), diseased individuals (■), and recovered immune (▲). The dotted line indicates the incidence pattern for an incompletely mixed population group.

behavioural patterns, age of the population group and population density (i.e. urban versus rural). Each infective individual will be capable of transmitting the disease to those susceptible individuals that they encounter during their infective period. The number of persons to which a single infective individual might transmit the disease, and hence the rate of occurence of the infection within the population, will depend upon the population density with respect to susceptible and infective individuals, the degree and nature of their social interaction, and the duration and timing of the infective period. Clearly if infectivity precedes the manifestation of disease then spread of the infection will be greater than if these were concurrent. Since each infected individual will, in turn, become a source of infection then this leads to a near exponential increase in the incidence of disease. Fig. 16.3 shows the incidence of disease within a theoretical population group. This hypothetical group is perfectly mixed, and all individuals are susceptible to the infection. The model infection has an incubation period of 1 day and an infective period of 2 days commencing at the onset of symptoms and recovery 1 day later. For the sake of this illustration it has been assumed that each infective individual will infect two others per day until all of the population group have contracted the disease. In practice, however, the rate of transmission will decrease as the epidemic progresses since the recovered individuals will become immune to further infection and reduce the population density with respect to susceptible individuals. Epidemics therefore often cease before all members of the community have been infected (Fig. 16.3, dotted line). If the proportion of immune individuals within a population group can be maintained above this threshold level then the likelihood of an epidemic arising from a single isolated infection incident is small (herd immunity). The threshold level itself is a function of the infectivity of the agent and the population density. Outbreaks of measles and chickenpox therefore tend to occur annually in the late summer amongst children attending school for the first time. This has the effect of concentrating all susceptible individuals in one, often confined, space and thereby reducing the proportion of immune subjects to below the threshold for propagated transmission.

An effective vaccination programme is therefore one that can maintain the proportion of individuals who are immune to a given infectious disease above the critical level. Such a programme will not prevent isolated cases of infection but will prevent these from becoming epidemic.

3   Objectives of a vaccine/immunization programme

There is the potential to develop a protective vaccine/immunization programme for each and every infectious disease. Whether or not such vaccines are developed and deployed is related to the severity and economic impact of the disease upon the community as well as the effects upon the individual. Principles of immunity and of the production and quality control of immunological products are discussed in Chapters 14 and 15, respectively.

3.1   Severity of the disease

The severity of the disease, not only in terms of its morbidity and mortality and the probability of permanent injury to its survivors, but also in the likelihood of infection, must be sufficient to warrant the development and routine deployment of a vaccine and its subsequent use. Thus, whilst influenza vaccines are constantly reviewed and stocks maintained, the control of influenza epidemics through vaccination is not recommended. Rather, those groups of individuals, such as the elderly, who are at special risk from the infection are protected.

Vaccines to be included within a national immunization and vaccination programme are chosen to reflect the infection risks within that country. Additional immunization, appropriate for persons travelling abroad, is intended not only to protect the at-risk individual, but also to prevent importing the disease into an unprotected home community.

| 3.2 | **Effectiveness of the vaccine/immunogen** |

Vaccination and immunization programmes seldom confer 100% protection against the target disease. More commonly the degree of protection is *ca*. 60–95%. In such instances whilst individuals receiving treatment will have a high probability of becoming immune, virtually all members of a community must be treated in order to reduce the proportion of susceptibles to below the threshold for epidemic spread of the disease. Antidiphtheria and antitetanus prophylaxis, which utilize toxoids, are amongst the most efficient immunization programmes whereas the performance of BCG is highly variable, and cholera vaccine (killed) gives little personal protection and is virtually useless in combating epidemics.

| 3.3 | **Safety** |

No medical or therapeutic procedure comes without some risk to the patient. All possible steps are taken to ensure safety, quality and efficacy of vaccines and immunological products (Chapter 15). The risks associated with immunization procedures must be constantly reviewed and balanced against the risks of, and associated with, contracting the disease. In this respect, smallpox vaccination in the UK was abandoned in the mid 1970s as the risks associated with vaccination then exceeded the predicted number of deaths that would follow importation of the disease. Shortly after this, in May 1980, The World Health Assembly pronounced the world to be free of smallpox. Similarly, the incidence of paralytic poliomyelitis in the USA and UK in 1996 was low but the majority of cases related to vaccine use. As the worldwide elimination of poliomyelitis approaches, there is much debate as to the value of the vaccine outside of an endemic area.

Public confidence in the safety of vaccines and immunization procedures is essential if compliance is to match the needs the community. In this respect public concern and anxiety, in the mid 1970s, over the perceived safety of pertussis vaccine led to a reduction in coverage of the target group from *ca*. 80% to *ca*. 30%. Major epidemics of whooping-cough, with over 100 000 notified cases, followed in 1977/1979 and 1981/83. By 1992, public confidence had returned, coverage had increased to 92% and there were only 4091 reported cases.

3.4 Cost

Cheap effective vaccines are an essential component of the global battle against infectious disease. It was estimated that the 1996 costs of the USA childhood vaccination programme, directed against polio, diphtheria, pertussis, tetanus, measles and tuberculosis, was $1 for the vaccines and $14 for the programme costs. The newer vaccines, particularly those that have been genetically engineered, are considerably more expensive, putting the costs beyond many budgets of developing countries.

3.5 Longevity of the immunity

The ideal of any vaccine is to provide life-long protection to the individual against disease. Immunological memory (Chapter 14) depends upon the survival of cloned populations of small B and T lymphocytes (memory cells). These small lymphocytes have a lifespan in the body of *ca*. 15–20 years. Thus, if the immune system is not boosted, either by natural exposure to the organism or by re-immunization, then immunity gained in childhood will be attenuated or lost completely by the age of 30. Those vaccines which provide only poor protection against disease have proportionately reduced time-spans of effectiveness. Yellow fever vaccination, which is highly effective, must therefore be repeated at 10-year intervals, whilst typhoid vaccines are only effective for 1–3 years. Whether or not immunization in childhood is boosted at adolescence or in adult life depends on the relative risks associated with the infection as a function of age.

4 Classes of immunity

The theoretical background which underlies immunity to infection has been discussed in detail in Chapter 14. Immunity to infection may be passively acquired through the receipt of preformed, protective antibodies or it may be actively acquired through an immune response following deliberate or accidental exposure to microorganisms or their component parts. Active acquired immunity might involve either or both humoral and cell-mediated responses.

4.1 Passive acquired immunity

Humoral antibodies of the IgG class are able to cross the placenta from mother to fetus. These antibodies will provide passive protection of the new-born against those diseases which involve humoral immunity and to which the mother is immune. In this fashion, new-born infants in the UK have passive protection against tetanus but not against tuberculosis which requires cell-mediated immunity. Secretory antibodies are also passed to the new born together with the first deliveries of breast milk (colostrum). Such antibodies provide some passive protection against infections of the gastrointestinal tract.

Maternally acquired antibodies will react not only with antigen associated with a threatening infection but also with antigens introduced to the body as part of an immunization programme. Premature immunization, i.e. before degradation and elimination of the maternal antibodies, will therefore reduce the potency of an administered vaccine. This aspect of the timing of a course of vaccinations is discussed later.

Administration of preformed antibodies, taken from animals, from pooled human serum, or from human cell-lines is often used to treat an existing infection (e.g. tetanus, diphtheria) or condition (venomous snake-bite). Pooled human serum may also be administered prophylactically, within a slow-release vehicle, for those persons entering parts of the world where diseases such as hepatitis A are endemic. Such administrations confer no long-term immunity and will interfere with concurrent vaccination procedures.

4.2   Active acquired immunity

Active acquired immunity (Chapter 14) relates to exposure of the immune system to antigenic materials. Such exposure might be related to a naturally occurring, or vaccine-associated infection, or it might be associated with direct introduction of non-viable antigenic material to the body. The latter might occur through insect or animal bites and stings, inhalation, ingestion or deliberate injection. The route of exposure to antigen will influence the nature of the subsequent immune response. Thus, injection of antigen will lead primarily to humoral (IgG, IgM) production, whilst exposure of epithelial tissues (gut, respiratory tract) will lead not only to the production of secretory antibodies (IgA, IgE) but also, through the common immune response, to a stimulation of humoral antibody.

The magnitude and specificity of an immune response depends not only upon the duration of the exposure to antigen but also upon its time–concentration profile. During a naturally occurring infection the levels of antigen are very small at onset and localized to the portal of entry to the host. Since the amounts of antigen are small they will react only with a small, highly defined group of small lymphocytes. These will undergo transformation to produce various antibody classes specific to the antigen together with cloned B and T cells. The immune responses and the infection will progress simultaneously. The microorganisms will release greater amounts of antigenic materials as the infection progresses. These will, in turn, react with an increasing number of cloned lymphocytes, to produce yet more antibody. Eventually the antibody levels will be sufficient to bring about the elimination, from the host, of the infecting organism. The net result of this encounter is that the host has developed a highly specific immunological memory of the encounter.

This situation should be contrasted with the injection of a non-replicating immunogen. Often the amount of antigen introduced is large when compared with the levels present during the initial stages of an infection. In a non-immune animal these antigens will react not only with those lymphocytes that are capable of producing antibody of high specificity but also with those of a lower specificity. Antibody (high and low specificity) produced will react with and remove the residual antigen. The immune response will cease after this initial (primary) challenge. On a subsequent (secondary) challenge the antigen will react with residual preformed antibody relating to the first challenge together with a more specific subgroup of the original cloned lymphocytes. As the number of challenges is increased the proportion of lymphocytes specific to the antigen is also increased. After a sufficient number of consecutive challenges the magnitude and specificity of the immune response matches that which would occur during a natural infection with an organism bearing the antigen. This pattern of exposure brings with it certain problems. Firstly, since introduced immunogen will react preferentially with preformed antibody rather than lymphocytes then sufficient time must elapse between exposures so as to allow the natural loss of antibody to occur. Secondly, immunity to infection will only be complete after the final challenge with immunogen. Thirdly, low specificity antibody produced during the early exposures to antigen might cross-react with host tissues to produce adverse reactions to the vaccine.

5   Classes of vaccine

Vaccines may be considered as representing live microorganisms, killed microorganisms or purified bacterial and viral components (component vaccines). These vaccine classes have been described in detail in Chapter 15. Some additional points about their use are discussed below.

5.1   Live vaccines

Vaccines may be live, infective microorganisms, attenuated with respect to their pathogenicity but retaining their ability to infect or they might be genetically engineered such that one mildly infective organism carries with it antigens from an unrelated pathogen.

Two major advantages stem from the use of live vaccines. Firstly, the immunization mimics a natural infection such that only a single exposure is required to render an individual immune. Secondly, the exposure may be mediated through the natural route of infection (e.g. oral) thereby stimulating an immune response that is appropriate to a particular disease (e.g. secretory antibody as primary defence against poliomyelitis virus in the gut).

Disadvantages associated with the use of live vaccines are also apparent. Live attenuated vaccines, administered through the natural route of infection, will be replicated in the patient and could be transmitted to others. If attenuation is lost during this replicative process then infections might result (see poliomyelitis, below). A second, major disadvantage of live vaccines is that the course of their action might be affected by the infection and immunological status of the patient.

5.2   Killed and component vaccines

Since these vaccines are unable to evoke a natural infection profile with respect to the release of antigen they must be administered on a number of occasions. Immunity is not complete until the course of immunization is complete and, with the exception of toxin-dominated diseases (diphtheria, tetanus) where the immunogen is a toxoid, will never match the performance of live vaccine delivery. Specificity of the immune response generated in the patient is initially low. This is particularly the case when the vaccine is composed of a relatively crude cocktail of killed cells where the immune response is directed only partly towards antigenic components of the cells that are associated with the infection process. This increases the possibility of adverse reactions in the patient.

Release profiles of these immunogens can be improved through their formulation with adjuvants (Chapters 14, 15), and the immunogenicity of certain purified bacterial components such as polysaccharides can be improved by their conjugation to a carrier.

6 Routine immunization against infectious disease

6.1 Poliomyelitis vaccination

Poliovirus, a picornavirus, has three immunologically distinct types (I, II & III). The first phase of poliomyelitis infection is an acute infection of the gastrointestinal tract, during which time the virus is found in the throat and in faeces. The second phase is characterized by an invasion of the bloodstream, and in the third phase the virus migrates from the bloodstream into the meninges. Infections range in severity from clinically inapparent (>90%) to paralytic. Paralytic poliomyelitis is a major illness, but only occurs in 0.1–2% of infected individuals. It is characterized by the destruction of large nerve cells in the anterior horn of the brain resulting in varying degrees of paralysis. The infection is transmitted by the faecal–oral route and unvaccinated adults are at greatest risk from paralytic infection than children.

Polio is the only disease, at present, for which both live and killed vaccines compete. Since the introduction of the killed virus (Salk) in 1956 and the live attenuated virus (Sabin) in 1962 there has been a remarkable decline in the incidence of poliomyelitis (Fig. 16.1). The inactivated polio vaccine (IPV) contains formalin-killed poliovirus of all three serotypes. On injection, the vaccine stimulates the production of antibodies of the IgM and IgG class which neutralize the virus in the second stage of infection. A course of three injections at monthly intervals produces long-lasting immunity to all three poliovirus types.

A live, oral polio vaccine (OPV) is widely used in many countries, including the UK and USA. Its main advantages over the IPV vaccine are its lower cost and easier administration. OPV contains attenuated poliovirus of each of the three types and is administered, as a liquid, onto the tongue. The vaccine strains infect the gastrointestinal mucosa and oropharynx, promoting the common immune response, and involving both humoral and secretory antibodies. IgA, secreted within the gut epithelium, provides local resistance to the first stages of poliomyelitis infection. Infection of epithelial cells with one strain of enterovirus often, however, inhibits simultaneous infection by related strains. At least three administrations of OPV are therefore required with each dosing conferring immunity to one of the vaccine serotypes. These doses must be separated by a period of at least 1 month in order to allow the previous infection to elapse. Booster vaccinations are also provided to cover the eventuality that some other enterovirus infection, present at the time of vaccination, had reduced the response to the vaccine strains.

Faecal excretion of vaccine virus will occur and may last for up to 6 weeks. Such released virus will spread to close contacts and infect/(re)immunize them. Since the introduction of OPV, notifications of paralytic poliomyelitis in the UK have dropped spectacularly. From 1985–95, 19 of the 28 notified cases of paralytic poliomyelitis were associated with vaccine strains (14 recipients, 5 contacts). Vaccine-associated poliomyelitis may occur through reversion of the attenuated strains to the virulent wild-type, particularly with types II and III and is estimated to occur once per 4 million doses. Since the wild-type virus can be isolated in faeces, infection may occur in unimmunized contacts as well as vaccine recipients. Since the risks of natural infections with poliomyelitis within developed countries has now diminished markedly, the greater risk resides with the live vaccine strains. Proposals are therefore now being considered in the USA that OPV should be replaced with IPV.

6.2 Measles, mumps and rubella vaccination (MMR)

Measles, mumps and rubella (German measles) are infectious diseases, with respiratory routes of transmission and infection, caused by members of the paramyxovirus group. Each virus is immunologically distinct and has only one serotype. Whilst the primary multiplication sites of these viruses is within the respiratory tract, the diseases are associated with viral multiplication elsewhere in the host.

6.2.1 *Measles*

Measles is a severe, highly contagious, acute infection that frequently occurs in epidemic form. After multiplication within the respiratory tract the virus is transported throughout the body, particularly to the skin where a characteristic maculopapular rash develops. Complications of the disease can occur, particularly in malnourished children, the most serious being measles encephalitis which can cause permanent neurological injury and death.

A live vaccine strain of measles (Chapter 15) was introduced in the USA in 1962 and to the UK in 1968. A single injection produces high-level immunity in over 95% of recipients. Moreover, since the vaccine induces immunity more rapidly than the natural infection, it may be used to control the impact of measles outbreaks. The measles virus cannot survive outside of an infected host. Widespread use of the vaccine therefore has the potential, as with smallpox, of eliminating the disease worldwide. Mass immunization has reduced the incidence of measles to almost nil, although a 15-fold increase in the incidence was noted in the USA between 1989 and 1991 because of poor compliance.

6.2.2 *Mumps*

Mump virus infects the parotid glands to cause swelling and a general viraemia. Complications include pancreatitis, meningitis and orchitis, the latter occasionally leading to male sterility. Infections can also cause permanent unilateral deafness at any age. In the absence of vaccination, infection occurs in >90% of individuals by age 15 years. A live attenuated mumps vaccine has been available since 1967 and has been part of the juvenile vaccination programme in the UK since 1988 when it was included as part of the MMR triple vaccine (see below).

6.2.3 *Rubella*

Rubella is a mild, often subclinical infection that is common amongst children aged between 4 and 9 years. Infection during the first trimester of pregnancy brings with it a major risk of abortion or congenital deformity in the fetus (congenital rubella syndrome (CRS)).

Rubella immunization was introduced to the UK in 1970 for pre-pubertal girls and non-immune women. The vaccine utilizes a live cold-adapted Wistar RA27/3 vaccine strain of the virus. The major disadvantage of the vaccine is that, as with the wild type, the fetus is infected. Whilst there have been no reports of CRS associated with use of the vaccine, the possible risk makes it imperative that women do not become pregnant within 1 month of vaccination. Until 1988 boys were not routinely protected against rubella. Their susceptibility to the virus was thought to maintain the natural prevalence of the disease in the community and thereby reinforce the vaccine-induced immunity in vaccinated, adult females. This proved not to be the case, rather cases of CRS could be related to incidence of the disease in children. Rubella vaccine is now given to both sexes at the age of 15 months.

6.2.4 MMR vaccine

MMR vaccine was introduced to the UK in 1988 for young children of both sexes, replacing single-antigen measles vaccine. It consists of a single dose of a lyophilized preparation of live attenuated strains of the measles, mumps and rubella viruses. Immunization results in sero-conversion to all three viruses in over 95% of recipients. For maximum effect MMR vaccine is recommended for children of both sexes aged 12–15 months but can also be given to non-immune adults. From October 1996 a second dose of MMR was recommended for children aged 4 years in order to prevent the re-accumulation of sufficient susceptible children to sustain future epidemics. Single-antigen rubella vaccine will continue to be given to girls aged 10–14 years if they have not previously received MMR vaccine.

6.3 Tuberculosis

Tuberculosis (TB) is a major cause of death and morbidity worldwide, particularly where poverty, malnutrition and poor housing prevail. Human infection is acquired by inhalation of *Mycobacterium tuberculosis* and *M. bovis*. Tuberculosis is primarily a disease of the lungs, causing chronic infection of the lower respiratory tract, but may spread to other sites or proceed to a generalized infection (miliary tuberculosis). Active disease can result either from a primary infection or from a subsequent reactivation of a quiescent infection. Following inhalation, the mycobacteria are taken up by alveolar macrophages where they survive and multiply. Circulating macrophages and lymphocytes, attracted to the site, carry the organism to local lymph nodes where a cell-mediated immune response is triggered. The host, unable to eliminate the pathogen, contains them within small granulomas or tubercles. If high numbers of mycobacteria are present then the cellular responses can result in tissue necrosis. The tubercles contain viable pathogens which may persist for the remaining life of the host. Reactivation of the healed primary lesion is thought to account for over two-thirds of all newly reported cases of the disease.

The incidence of TB in the UK declined 10-fold between 1948 and 1987, since when just over 5000 new cases have been notified each year. Those most at risk include pubescent children, health service staff and individuals intending to stay for more than 1 month in countries where TB is endemic.

A live vaccine is required to elicit protection against TB since both antibody and cell-mediated immunity are required for protective immunity. Vaccination with BCG (bacille Calmette–Guérin) derived from an attenuated *M. bovis* strain is commonly used in countries where TB is endemic. The vaccine was introduced in the UK in 1953 and was administered intradermally to children aged 13–14 years and unprotected adults. Efficacy in the UK has been shown to be greater than 70% with protection lasting at least 15 years. In other countries, where the general state of health and well-being of the population is less than in the developed world, the efficacy of the vaccine has been shown to be significantly less than this.

Because of the risks of adverse reaction to the vaccine by persons who had already been exposed to the disease a sensitivity test must be carried out prior to immunization with BCG. A Mantoux skin test assesses an individual's sensitivity to a purified protein derivative (PPD) prepared from heat-treated antigens (tuberculin) extracted from *M. tuberculosis*. A positive test implies past infection or past, successful immunization. Those with strongly positive tests may have active disease and should be referred to a chest clinic. Many people with active TB, especially disseminated TB, however, sero-convert from skin test positive to skin test negative. Results of the skin test must therefore be interpreted with care.

Much debate surrounds the use of BCG vaccine, a matter of some importance, considering that TB kills *ca.* 3 million people annually and that drug-resistant strains have emerged. Whilst the vaccine has demonstrated some efficacy in preventing juvenile TB, it has little prophylactic effect against post-primary TB in those already infected. One solution is to bring forward the BCG immunization to include neonates. Immunization at 2–4 weeks of age will ensure that immunization precedes infection, and will also negate the requirement for a skin test. Passive-acquired maternal antibody to TB is unlikely to interfere with the effectiveness of the immunization since immunity relates to a cell-mediated response. Alternative strategies involve improvement of the vaccine possibly through the introduction, into the BCG strain, of genes that encode protective antigens of *M. tuberculosis*.

6.4 Diphtheria, tetanus and pertussis (DTP) immunization

Immunization against these three, unrelated diseases, is considered together since the vaccines are all non-living and are often co-administered as a triple vaccine as part of the juvenile vaccination programme.

6.4.1 *Diphtheria*

This is an acute, non-invasive infectious disease associated with the upper respiratory tract (Chapter 4). The incubation period is from 2 to 5 days although the disease remains communicable for up to 4 weeks. A low molecular weight toxin is produced which affects myocardium, nervous and adrenal tissues. Death results in 3–5% of infected children. Diphtheria immunization protects by stimulating the production of an antitoxin. This antitoxin will protect against the disease but not against infection of the respiratory tract. The immunogen is a toxoid, prepared by formaldehyde treatment of the purified toxin (Chapter 15) and administered whilst adsorbed to an adjuvant, usually aluminium phosphate or aluminium hydroxide. The primary course of diphtheria prophylaxis consists of three doses starting at 2 months of age and separated by an interval of at least 1 month. The immune status of adults may be determined by administration of Schick test toxin, which is essentially a diluted form of the vaccine.

6.4.2   *Tetanus*

Tetanus is not an infectious disease but relates to the production of a toxin by germinating spores and vegetative cells of *Clostridium tetani* that might infect a deep puncture wound. The organism, which may be introduced into the wound from the soil, grows anaerobically at such sites. The toxin is adsorbed into nerve cells and acts like strychnine on nerve synapses (Chapter 4). Tetanus immunization employs a toxoid and protects by stimulating the production of antitoxin. This antitoxin will neutralize toxin as it is released by the organisms and before it can be adsorbed into nerves. Since the toxin is produced only slowly following infection then the vaccine, which acts rapidly, may be used prophylactically in those unimmunized persons who have recently suffered a candidate injury. The toxoid, as with diphtheria toxoid, is formed by reaction with formaldehyde and adsorbed onto an adjuvant. The primary course of tetanus prophylaxis consists of three doses starting at 2 months of age and separated by an interval of at least 1 month.

6.4.3   *Pertussis (whooping-cough)*

Caused by the non-invasive respiratory pathogen *Bordetella pertussis*, whooping-cough (Chapter 4) may be complicated by bronchopneumonia, repeated post-tussis vomiting leading to weight loss and to cerebral hypoxia associated with a risk of brain damage. Until the mid 1970s the mortality from whooping-cough was about one per 1000 notified cases with a higher rate for infants under 1 year of age. A full course of vaccine, which consists of a suspension of killed *Bord. pertussis* organisms (Chapter 15), gives complete protection in over 80% of recipients. The primary course of pertussis prophylaxis consists of three doses starting at 2 months of age and separated by an interval of at least 1 month.

6.4.4   *DTP vaccine combinations and administration*

The primary course of DTP protection consists of three doses of a combined vaccine, each dose separated by at least 1 month and commencing not earlier than 2 months of age. In such combinations the pertussis component of the vaccine acts as an additional adjuvant for the toxoid components. Monovalent pertussis and tetanus vaccines, and combined vaccines lacking the pertussis component (DT) are available. If pertussis vaccination is contraindicated or refused then DT vaccine alone should be offered. The primary course of pertussis vaccination is considered sufficient to confer life-long protection, especially since the mortality associated with disease declines markedly after infancy. The risks associated with tetanus and diphtheria infection persist throughout life. DT vaccination is therefore repeated before school entry, at 4–5 years of age, and once again at puberty.

Haemophilus influenzae Type B (HiB) immunization

Seven different capsular serotypes of *Haemophilus influenza* Type B are associated with respiratory infection in young children. The most common presentation of these infections is as meningitis, frequently associated with bacteraemia. The sequelae following HiB infection include deafness, convulsions and intellectual impairment. The fatality rate is *ca.* 4–5% with 8–11% of survivors having permanent neurological disorders. The disease, which is rare in children under 3 months, peaks both in its incidence and severity at 12 months of age. Infection is uncommon after 4 years of age. Before the introduction of HiB vaccination the incidence of the disease in the UK was estimated at 34 per 100 000. The vaccine utilizes purified preparations of the polysaccharide capsule of the major serotypes. Polysaccharides are poorly immunogenic and must be conjugated onto a protein carrier in order to enhance their efficacy. HiB vaccines are variously conjugated onto diphtheria and tetanus toxoids (above), group B meningococcal outer membrane protein and a non-toxic derivative of diphtheria toxin (CRM197) and can now be mixed and co-administered with the DTP vaccine. Three doses of the vaccine are recommended separated by 1 month. No reinforcement is recommended at 4 years of age since the risks from infection are negligible at this time.

7 Juvenile immunization schedule

The timing of the various components of the juvenile vaccination programme is subject to continual review. In the 1960s, the primary course of DTP vaccination consisted of three doses given at 3, 6 and 12 months of age, together with OPV. This separation gave adequate time for the levels of induced antibody to decline between successive doses of the vaccines. Current recommendations (Table 16.1) accelerate the vaccination programme with no reductions in its efficacy. Thus, MMR vaccination has replaced separate measles and rubella prophylaxis and BCG vaccination may now be given at

Table 16.1 Children's immunization schedule for UK (1996)

Vaccine	Age	Notes
BCG	Neonatal (1st month)	If not at 13–14 years
DTP and HiB Poliomyelitis	1st dose 2 months 2nd dose 3 months 3rd dose 4 months	Primary course
MMR	12–15 months	Any time over 12 months
Booster DT Poliomyelitis MMR booster	3–5 years	3 years after primary course
BCG	10–14 years	If not in infancy
Booster DT	13–18 years	

birth. DTP vaccination occurs at 2, 3 and 4 months to coincide with administration of HiB. It is imperative that as many individuals as possible benefit from the vaccination programme. Fewer visits to the doctor's surgery translate into improved patient compliance and less likelihood of epidemic spread of the diseases in question. The current recommendations minimize the number of separate visits to the clinic whilst maximizing the protection generated.

8 Immunization of special risk groups

Whilst not recommended for routine administration, vaccines additional to those represented in the juvenile programme are available for individuals in special risk categories. These categories relate to occupational risks or risks associated with travel abroad. Such immunization protocols include those directed against cholera, typhoid, meningitis (types A, C), anthrax, hepatitis A and B, influenza, Japanese encephalitis, rabies, tick-borne encephalitis, and yellow fever.

9 Further reading

Salisbury D.M. & Begg N.T. (eds) (1996) *Immunisation Against Infectious Disease*. HMSO: London. (Updated every 2–3 years).

Mims C.A. (1987) *The Pathogenesis of Infectious Disease*, 3rd edn. London: Academic Press.

Salyers A.A. & Whitt D.D. (1994) *Bacterial Pathogenesis: A Molecular Approach*. Washington: American Society for Microbiology Press.

Part 3
Microbiological Aspects of
Pharmaceutical Processing

Many failures in pharmaceutical processing have arisen because of the inability of those responsible for its design to be aware of the distribution and survival potential of microorganisms in the environment and in the raw materials and equipment used in a pharmaceutical factory.

The first chapter in this section provides a unique account of the ecology, i.e. distribution, survival and life-style, of microorganisms in the factory environment, and should enable process designers, controllers and quality control personnel to comprehend, trace and eradicate the sources of failure due to extraneous microbial contaminants in the finished product. Much of the information given here is applicable to hospital manufacture also, and this is extended in a contribution (Chapter 19) dealing with contamination in hospital pharmaceutical products and in the home.

The dire consequences of failure to heed the precepts enunciated in Chapter 17 are considered in Chapters 18 and 19 which review the spoilage wreaked upon pharmaceutical products as a consequence of microbial infestation. The wide, and at first sight bizarre, range of substrates used by contaminating microorganisms and the range of biochemical reactions that follow and which, in turn, give rise to the overall picture of spoilage are well documented; it would be no exaggeration to state that microbial spoilage and its prevention, through both good working conditions and the use of preservatives, represent the major problem of pharmaceutical microbiology.

An important group of pharmaceutical products, including those intended for parenteral administration for instillation into the eye, are required to be free from living microorganisms, and with parenteral products, from those residues of the bacterial cell which may give rise to fever. The principles of their preparation and sterilization are considered in Chapter 21, while the theory of sterilization processes is dealt with in the preceding chapter. These two chapters *in toto* cover the most exacting operation in medicine preparation, and one in which failure has given rise to several disasters ranging from patient death, for instance as a result of sterilization failure in intravenous drips, to blindness in the case of contaminated eyedrops.

Chapter 22 deals with general factory and hospital hygiene and the principles of good manufacturing practice (GMP) which if adhered to go a long way towards compounding the success of the processes described in Chapters 17 and 20.

The subject of quality control and surveillance is discussed in a chapter on sterilization control and sterility testing, which deals with aspects of in-process and post-process control.

Finally, lest it be thought that microorganisms are always harmful, two chapters (24 and 25) describe ways in which they can be harnessed for the benefit of mankind.

17 Ecology of microorganisms as it affects the pharmaceutical industry

1   Introduction

2   Atmosphere
2.1 Microbial content
2.2 Reduction of microbial count
2.3 Compressed air

3   Water
3.1 Raw or mains water
3.2 Softened water
3.3 Deionized or demineralized water
3.4 Distilled water
3.5 Water produced by reverse osmosis
3.6 Distribution system
3.7 Disinfection of water

4   Skin and respiratory-tract flora
4.1 Microbial transfer from operators
4.2 Hygiene and protective clothing

5   Raw materials

6   Packaging

7   Buildings
7.1 Walls and ceilings
7.2 Floors and drains
7.3 Doors, windows and fittings

8   Equipment
8.1 Pipelines
8.2 Cleansing
8.3 Disinfection and sterilization
8.4 Microbial checks

9   Cleaning equipment and utensils

10 Further reading

1 Introduction

The microbiological quality of pharmaceutical products is influenced by the environment in which they are manufactured and by the materials used in their formulation. With the exception of preparations which are terminally sterilized in their final container, the microflora of the final product may represent the contaminants from the raw materials, from the equipment with which it was made, from the atmosphere, from the person operating the process or from the final container into which it was packed. Some of the contaminants may be pathogenic whilst others may grow even in the presence of preservatives and spoil the product. Any microorganisms which are destroyed by in-process heat treatment may still leave cell residues which may be toxic or pyrogenic (Chapter 1), since the pyrogenic fraction, lipid A, which is present in the cell wall is not destroyed under the same conditions as the organisms.

In parallel to improvements in manufacturing technology there have been developments in Good Manufacturing Practices to minimize contamination by a study of the ecology of microorganisms, the hazards posed by them and any points in the process which are critical to their control. This approach has been distilled into the concept of Hazard Analysis of Critical Control Points (HACCP), with the objective of improving the microbiological safety of the product in a cost-effective manner, which has been assisted by the development of rapid methods for the detection of microorganisms.

2 Atmosphere

2.1 Microbial content

Air is not a natural environment for the growth and reproduction of microorganisms since it does not contain the necessary amount of moisture and nutrients in a form which can be utilized. However, almost any sample of untreated air contains suspended bacteria, moulds and yeasts, but to survive they must be able to tolerate desiccation and the continuing dry state. Microorganisms commonly isolated from air are the spore-forming bacteria *Bacillus* spp. and *Clostridium* spp., the non-sporing bacteria *Staphylococcus* spp., *Streptococcus* spp. and *Corynebacterium* spp., the moulds *Penicillium* spp., *Cladosporium* spp., *Aspergillus* spp. and *Mucor* spp., as well as the yeast *Rhodotorula* spp.

The number of organisms in the atmosphere depends on the activity in the environment and the amount of dust which is disturbed. An area containing working machinery and an active personnel will have a higher microbial count than one with a still atmosphere, and the air count of a dirty, untidy room will be greater than that of a clean room. The microbial air count is also influenced by humidity. A damp atmosphere usually contains fewer organisms than a dry one as the contaminants are carried down by the droplets of moisture. Thus, the air in a cold-store is usually free from microorganisms and air is less contaminated during the wet winter months than in the drier summer months.

Microorganisms are carried into the atmosphere suspended on particles of dust, skin or clothing, or in droplets of moisture or sputum following talking, coughing or sneezing. The size of the particles to which the organisms are attached, together with the humidity of the air, determines the rate at which they will settle out. Bacteria and moulds not attached to suspended matter will settle out slowly in a quiet atmosphere. The rate of settling out will depend upon air currents caused by ventilation, air extraction systems, convection currents above heat sources and the activity in the room.

The microbial content of the air may be increased during the handling of contaminated materials during dispensing, blending and their addition to formulations. In particular, the use of starches and some sugars in the dry state may increase the mould count. Some packaging components, for example card and paperboard, have a microflora of both moulds and bacteria, and this is often reflected in high counts around packaging machines.

Common methods for checking the microbiological quality of air include the following (see also p. 250).

1   The exposure of Petri dishes containing a nutrient agar to the atmosphere for a given length of time. This relies upon microorganisms or dust particles bearing them to settle on the surface.

2   The use of an air-sampling machine which draws a measured volume of air from the environment and impinges it on a nutrient agar surface on either a Petri dish, a plastic strip or a membrane filter which may then be incubated with a nutrient medium. This method provides valuable information in areas of low microbial contamination, particularly if the sample is taken close to the working area.

The type of formulation being prepared determines the microbiological standard of the air supply required and the hazard it poses. In areas where products for injection and ophthalmic use which cannot be terminally sterilized by moist heat are being manufactured, the air count should be very low and regarded as a critical control point in the process since although these products are required to pass a test for sterility (Chapter 23), the test itself is destructive, and therefore only relatively few samples are tested. An unsatisfactory air count may lead to the casual contamination of a few containers and be undetected by the test for sterility. In addition if the microbiological air quality is identified as a critical point, it may also give an early warning of potential contamination and permit timely correction. The manufacture of liquid or semi-solid preparations for either oral or topical use requires a clean environment for both the production and filling stages. Whilst many formulations are adequately protected by chemical preservatives or a pH unfavourable to airborne bacteria that may settle in them, preservation against mould spores is more difficult to achieve.

2.2 Reduction of microbial count

The microbial count of air may be reduced by filtration, chemical disinfection and to a limited extent by ultraviolet (UV) light. Filtration is the most commonly used method and filters may be made of a variety of materials such as cellulose, glass wool, fibreglass mixtures or polytetrafluorethylene (PTFE) with resin or acrylic binders. For the most critical aseptic work, it may be necessary to remove all particles in excess of $0.1\,\mu m$ in size, but for many operations a standard of less than 100 particles per 3.5 litres ($1.0\,ft^3$) of $0.5\,\mu m$ or larger (class 100) is adequate. Such fine filtration is usually preceded by a coarse filter stage, or any suspended matter is removed by passing the air through an electrostatic field. To maintain efficiency, all air filters must be kept dry, since microorganisms may be capable of movement along continuous wet films and may be carried through a damp filter.

Filtered air may be used to purge a complete room, or it may be confined to a specific area and incorporate the principle of laminar flow, which permits operations to be carried out in a gentle current of sterile air. The direction of the airflow may be horizontal or vertical, depending upon the type of equipment being used, the type of operation and the material being handled. It is important that there is no obstruction between the air supply and the exposed product, since this may result in the deflection of microorganisms or particulate matter from a non-sterile surface and cause contamination. Airflow gauges are essential to monitor that the correct flow rate is obtained in laminar flow units and in complete suites to ensure that a positive pressure from clean to less clean areas is always maintained.

The integrity of the air-filtration system must be checked regularly, and the most common method is by counting the particulate matter both in the working area and across the surface of the filter. For systems which have complex ducting or where the surfaces of the terminal filters are recessed, smoke tests using a chemical of known particle size may be introduced just after the main fan and monitored at each outlet. The test has a twofold application as both the terminal filter and any leaks in the ducting can be checked. These methods are useful in conjunction with those for determining the microbial air count as given earlier.

Chemical disinfectants are limited in their use as air sterilants because of their irritant properties when sprayed. However, some success has been achieved with atomized propylene glycol at a concentration of 0.05–0.5 mg l^{-1} and quaternary ammonium compounds (QACs) at 0.075% may be used. For areas which can be effectively sealed off for fumigation purposes, formaldehyde gas at a concentration of 1–2 mg l^{-1} of air at a relative humidity of 80–90% is effective.

Ultraviolet (UV) irradiation at wavelengths between 280 and 240 nm (2800 and 2400 Å) is used to reduce bacterial contamination of air, but is only active at a relatively short distance from source. Bacteria and mould spores, in particular those with heavily pigmented spore coats, are often resistant to such treatment.

2.3 Compressed air

Compressed air has many applications in the manufacture of pharmaceutical products. A few examples of its uses are the conveyance of powders and suspension, providing aeration for some fermentations and as a power supply for the reduction of particle size by impaction. Unless it is sterilized by filtration or a combination of heat and filtration, microorganisms present will be introduced into the product. The microbial content of compressed air may be assessed by bubbling a known volume through a nutrient liquid and either filtering through a membrane, which is then incubated with a nutrient agar and a total viable count made, or the microbial content may be estimated more rapidly using techniques developed to detect changes in physical or chemical characteristics in the nutrient liquid.

3 Water

The microbial ecology of water is of great importance in the pharmaceutical industry due to its multiple uses as a constituent of many products as well as for various washing and cooling processes. Two main aspects are involved: the quality of the raw water and any processing it receives and the distribution system. Both should be taken into consideration when reviewing the hazards to the finished product and any critical control points.

Microorganisms indigenous to fresh water include *Pseudomonas* spp., *Alcaligenes* spp., *Flavobacterium* spp., *Chromobacter* spp. and *Serratia* spp. Such bacteria are nutritionally undemanding and often have a relatively low optimum growth temperature. Bacteria which are introduced as a result of soil erosion, heavy rainfall and decaying plant matter include *Bacillus subtilis*, *B. megaterium*, *Klebsiella aerogenes* and *Enterobacter cloacae*. Contamination by sewage results in the presence of *Proteus* spp., *Escherichia coli* and other enterobacteria, *Streptococcus faecalis* and *Clostridium* spp. Bacteria which are introduced as a result of animal or plant debris usually die as a result of the unfavourable conditions.

An examination of stored industrial water supplies showed that 98% of the contaminants were Gram-negative bacteria; other organisms isolated were *Micrococcus* spp., *Cytophaga* spp., yeast, yeast-like fungi and actinomycetes.

3.1　Raw or mains water

The quality of the water from the mains supply varies with both the source and the local authority, and whilst it is free from known pathogens and from faecal contaminants such as *E. coli*, it may contain other microorganisms. When the supply is derived from surface water the flora is usually more abundant and faster-growing than that of supplies from a deep water source such as a well or spring. This is due to surface waters receiving both microorganisms and nutrients from soil and sewage whilst water from deep sources has its microflora filtered out. On prolonged storage in a reservoir, water-borne organisms tend to settle out, but in industrial storage tanks the intermittent through-put ensures that, unless treated, the contents of the tank serve as a source of infection. The bacterial count may rise rapidly in such tanks during summer months and reach $10^5–10^6$ ml^{-1}.

One of the uses of mains water is for washing chemicals used in pharmaceutical preparations to remove impurities or unwanted by-products of a reaction, and although the bacterial count of the water may be low, the volume used is large and the material being washed may be exposed to a considerable number of bacteria.

The microbial count of the mains water will be reflected in both softened and deionized water which may be prepared from it.

3.2　Softened water

This is usually prepared by either a base-exchange method using sodium zeolite, by a lime-soda ash process, or by the addition of sodium hexametaphosphate. In addition to the bacteria derived from the mains water, additional flora of *Bacillus* spp. and *Staphylococcus aureus* may be introduced into systems which use brine for regeneration and from the chemical filter beds which, unless treated, can act as a reservoir for bacteria.

Softened water is often used for washing containers before filling with liquid or semi-solid preparations and for cooling systems. Unless precautions are taken, the microbial count in a cooling system or jacketed vessel will rise rapidly and if faults develop in the cooling plates or vessel wall, contamination of the product may occur.

3.3　Deionized or demineralized water

Deionized water is prepared by passing mains water through anion and cation exchange resin beds to remove the ions. Thus, any bacteria present in the mains water will also be present in the deionized water, and beds which are not regenerated frequently with strong acid or alkali are often heavily contaminated and add to the bacterial content of the water. This problem has prompted the development of resins able to resist microbiological contamination. One such resin, a large-pore, strong-base, macroreticular, quaternary ammonium anion exchange resin which permits microorganisms to enter the pore cavity and then electrostatically binds them to the cavity surface, is currently being marketed. The main function is as a final cleaning bed downstream of conventional demineralizing columns.

Deionized water is used in pharmaceutical formulations, for washing containers and plant, and for the preparation of disinfectant solutions.

3.4   Distilled water

As it leaves the still, distilled water is free from microorganisms, and contamination occurs as a result of a fault in the cooling system, the storage vessel or the distribution system. The flora of contaminated distilled water is usually Gram-negative bacteria and since it is introduced after a sterilization process, it is often a pure culture. A level of organism up to $10^6 ml^{-1}$ has been recorded.

Distilled water is often used in the formulation of oral and topical pharmaceutical preparations and a low bacterial count is desirable. It is also used after distillation with a specially designed still, often made of glass, for the manufacture of parenteral preparations and a post-distillation heat sterilization stage is commonly included in the process. Water for such preparations is often stored at 80°C in order to prevent bacterial growth and the production of pyrogenic substances which accompany such growth.

3.5   Water produced by reverse osmosis

Water produced by reverse osmosis (RO) is forced by an osmotic pressure through a semi-permeable membrane which acts as a molecular filter. The diffusion of solubles dissolved in the water is impeded, and those with a molecular weight in excess of 250 do not diffuse at all. The process, which is the reverse of the natural process of osmosis, thus removes microorganisms and their pyrogens. Post-RO contamination may occur if the plant after the membrane, the storage vessel or the distribution system is not kept free from microorganisms.

3.6   Distribution system

If microorganisms colonize a storage vessel, it then acts as a microbial reservoir and contaminates all water passing through it. It is therefore important that the contents of all storage vessels are tested regularly. Reservoirs of microorganisms may also build up in booster pumps, water meters and unused sections of pipeline. Where a high positive pressure is absent or cannot be continuously maintained, outlets such as cocks and taps may permit bacteria to enter the system.

An optimum system for reducing the growth of microbial flora is one that ensures a constant recirculation of water at a positive pressure through a ring-main without 'dead-legs' (areas which due to their location are not regularly used) and only very short branches to the take-off points. In addition there should be a system to re-sterilize the water, usually by membrane filtration or UV light treatment, just prior to return to the main storage tank.

Some plumbing materials used for storage vessels, pipework and jointing may support microbial growth. Some plastics, in particular plasticized polyvinylchlorides and resins used in the manufacture of glass-reinforced plastics, have caused serious microbiological problems when used for water storage and distribution systems. Both natural and synthetic rubbers used for washers, O-rings and diaphragms are susceptible to contamination if not sanitized regularly. For jointing, packing and lubricating materials, PTFE and silicone-based compounds are superior to those based on natural products such as vegetable oils or fibres and animal fats, and petroleum-based compounds.

3.7	**Disinfection of water**

Three methods are used for treating water, namely chemicals, filtration or UV light.

1   Chemical treatment is applicable usually to raw, mains and softened water, but is also used to treat the storage and distribution systems of distilled and deionized water and of water produced by reverse osmosis (section 3.5).

Sodium hypochlorite and chlorine gas are the most common agents for treating the water supply itself, and the concentration employed depends both upon the dwell time and the chlorine demand of the water. For most purposes a free residual chlorine level of 0.5–5 p.p.m. is adequate. For storage vessels, pipelines, pumps and outlets a higher level of 50–100 p.p.m. may be necessary, but it is usually necessary to use a descaling agent before disinfection in areas where the water is hard. Distilled, deionized and RO systems and pipelines may be treated with sodium hypochlorite or 1% formaldehyde solution. With deionized systems it is usual to exhaust the resin beds with brine before sterilization with formaldehyde to prevent its inactivation to paraformaldehyde. If only local contamination occurs, live steam is often effective in eradicating it. During chemical sterilization it is important that no 'dead-legs' remain untreated and that all instruments such as water meters are treated.

2   Membrane filtration is useful where the usage is moderate and a continuous circulation of water can be maintained. Thus, with the exception of that drawn off for use, the water is continually being returned to the storage tank and refiltered. As many water-borne bacteria are small, it is usual to install a 0.22-μm pore-size membrane as the terminal filter and to use coarser prefilters to prolong its life. Membrane filters require regular sterilization to prevent microbial colonization and 'grow through'. They may be treated chemically with the remainder of the storage/distribution system or removed and treated by moist heat. The latter method is usually the most successful for heavily contaminated filters.

3   UV light at a wavelength of 254 nm is useful for the disinfection of water of good optical clarity. Such treatment has an advantage over chemical disinfection as there is no odour or flavour problem and, unlike membrane filters, is not subject to microbial colonization. The siting in the distribution system is important since any insanitary fittings downstream of the unit will recontaminate the water. Industrial in-line units with sanitary type fittings which replace part of the water pipeline are manufactured.

One of the most useful techniques for checking the microbial quality of water is by membrane filtration, since this permits the concentration of a small number of organisms from a large volume of water. When chlorinated water supplies are tested it is necessary to add an inactivating agent such as sodium thiosulphate. Although an incubation temperature of 37°C may be necessary to recover some pathogens or faecal contaminants from water, many indigenous species fail to grow at this temperature, and it is usual to incubate at 20–26°C for their detection.

4 Skin and respiratory-tract flora

4.1 Microbial transfer from operators

Microorganisms may be transferred to pharmaceutical preparations from the process operator. This is undesirable in the case of tablets and powders, and may result in spoilage of solutions or suspensions, but in the case of parenterals it may have serious consequences for the patient. Of the natural skin flora organisms, *Staph. aureus* is perhaps the most undesirable. It is common on the hands and face and, since it resides in the deep layers of the skin, is not eliminated by washing. Other bacteria present are *Sarcina* spp. and diphtheroids, but occasionally Gram-negative rods such as *Mima* spp. (*Acinetobacter*) and *Alcaligenes* spp. achieve resident status in moist regions. In the fatty and waxy sections of the skin, lipophilic yeast are often present, *Pityrosporum ovale* on the scalp and *P. orbiculare* on glabrous skin. Various dermatophytic fungi such as *Epidermophyton* spp., *Microsporon* spp. and *Trichophyton* spp. may be present. Ear secretions may also contain saprophytic bacteria.

Bacteria other than the natural skin flora may be transferred from the operator as a result of poor personal hygiene, such as faecal organisms from the anal region or bacteria from a wound. Open wounds without clinical manifestation of bacterial growth often support pathogenic bacteria and *Staph. aureus* has been found in 20%; other contaminants include micrococci, enterococci, *a*-haemolytic and non-haemolytic streptococci, *Clostridium* spp., *Bacillus* spp. and Gram-negative intestinal bacteria. *Clostridium perfringens* in such circumstances is usually present as a saprophyte and dies fairly rapidly. Wounds showing signs of infection may support *Staph. aureus*, *Strep. pyogenes*, enterococci, coliforms, *Proteus* spp. and *Pseudomonas aeruginosa*.

The nasal passages may contain large numbers of *Staph. aureus* and a limited number of *Staph. albus*, whilst the nasopharynx is often colonized by streptococci of the viridans group, *Strep. salivarius* or *Neisseria pharyngis*. Occasionally, pathogens such as *Haemophilus influenzae* and *K. pneumoniae* may be present. The most common organisms secreted during normal respiratory function and speech are saprophytic streptococci of the viridans group.

The hazard of the transfer of microorganisms from humans to pharmaceutical preparations may be reduced by comprehensive training in personal hygiene coupled with regular medical checks to prevent carriers of pathogenic organisms from coming in contact with any product.

4.2 Hygiene and protective clothing

Areas designed for the manufacture of products intended for injection and eye or ear preparations usually have washing facilities with foot-operated taps, antiseptic soap and hot-air hand driers at the entrance to the suite, which must be used by all process operators. For the manufacture of such products it is also necessary for the operators to wear sterilized clothing including gowns, trousers, boots, hoods, face masks and gloves. For the production of products for oral and topical use, staff should be made to wash their hands before entering the production area. The requirements for protective clothing are usually less stringent but include clean overalls, hair covering and gloves, and where possible, face masks are an advantage.

5   Raw materials

Raw materials account for a high proportion of the microorganisms introduced during the manufacture of pharmaceuticals, and the selection of materials of a good microbiological quality aids in the control of contamination levels in both products and the environment. It is, however, common to have to accept raw materials which have some non-pathogenic microorganisms present and an assessment must be made as to the risk of their survival to spoil the finished product by growing in the presence of a preservative system, or the efficacy of an in-process treatment stage to destroy or remove them. Whatever the means of prevention of growth or survival by chemical or in-process treatment, it should be regarded as critical and controlled accordingly.

Untreated raw materials which are derived from a natural source usually support an extensive and varied microflora. Products from animal sources such as gelatine, desiccated thyroid, pancreas and cochineal may be contaminated with animal-borne pathogens. For this reason some statutory bodies such as the *British Pharmacopoeia* (1993) require freedom of such materials from *Escherichia coli* and *Salmonella* spp. at a stated level before they can be used in the preparation of pharmaceutical products. The microflora of materials of plant origin such as gum acacia and tragacanth, agar, powdered rhubarb and starches may arise from that indigenous to plants and may include bacteria such as *Erwinia* spp., *Pseudomonas* spp., *Lactobacillus* spp., *Bacillus* spp. and streptococci, moulds such as *Cladosporium* spp., *Alternaria* spp. and *Fusarium* spp., and non-mycelated yeasts, or those introduced during cultivation. For example, the use of untreated sewage as a fertilizer may result in animal-borne pathogens such as *Salmonella* spp. being present. Some refining processes modify the microflora of raw materials, for example drying may concentrate the level of spore-forming bacteria and some solubilizing processes may introduce water-borne bacteria such as *E. coli*.

Synthetic raw materials are usually free from all but incidental microbial contamination.

The storage condition of raw materials, particularly hygroscopic substances, is important, and since a minimum water activity (A_w) of 0.70 is required for osmophilic yeasts, 0.80 for most spoilage moulds and 0.91 for most spoilage bacteria, precautions should be taken to ensure that dry materials are held below these levels. Some packaging used for raw materials, such as unlined paper sacks, may absorb moisture and may itself be subject to microbial deterioration and so contaminate the contents. For this reason polythene-lined sacks are preferable. Some liquid or semi-solid raw materials contain preservatives, but others such as syrups depend upon osmotic pressure to prevent the growth of osmophiles which are often present. With this type of material it is important that they are held at a constant temperature since any variation may result in evaporation of some of the water content followed by condensation and dilution of the surface layers to give an A_w value which may permit the growth of osmophiles and spoil the syrup.

The use of natural products with a high non-pathogenic microbial count is possible if a sterilization stage is included either before or during the manufacturing process.

Such sterilization procedures (see also Chapter 20) may include heat treatment, filtration, irradiation, recrystallization from a bactericidal solvent such as an alcohol, or for dry products where compatible, ethylene oxide gas. If the raw material is only a minor constituent and the final product is adequately preserved either by lack of A_w chemically or by virtue of its pH, sugar or alcohol content, an in-process sterilization stage may not be necessary. If, however, the product is intended for parenteral or ophthalmic use a sterilization stage is essential.

The handling of contaminated raw materials as described previously may increase the airborne contamination level, and if there is a central dispensing area precautions may be necessary to prevent airborne cross-contamination, as well as that from infected measuring and weighing equipment. This presents a risk for all materials but in particular those stored in the liquid state where contamination may result in the bulk being spoiled.

6   Packaging

Packaging material has a dual role and acts both to contain the product and to prevent the entry of microorganisms or moisture which may result in spoilage, and it is therefore important that the source of contamination is not the packaging itself. The microflora of packaging materials is dependent upon both its composition and storage conditions. This, and a consideration of the type of pharmaceutical product to be packed, determine whether a sterilization treatment is required.

Glass containers are sterile on leaving the furnace, but are often stored in dusty conditions and packed for transport in cardboard boxes. As a result they may contain mould spores of *Penicillium* spp., *Aspergillus* spp. and bacteria such as *Bacillus* spp. It is commonplace to either airblow or wash glass containers to remove any glass spicules or dust which may be present, and it is often advantageous to include a disinfection stage if the product being filled is a liquid or semi-solid preparation. Plastic bottles which are either blow- or injection-moulded have a very low microbial count and may not require disinfection. They may, however, become contaminated with mould spores if they are transported in a non-sanitary packaging material such as unlined cardboard.

Packaging materials which have a smooth, impervious surface, free from crevices or interstices, such as cellulose acetate, polyethylene, polypropylene, polyvinylchloride, and metal foils and laminates, all have a low surface microbial count. Cardboard and paperboard, unless treated, carry mould spores of *Cladosporium* spp., *Aspergillus* spp. and *Penicillium* spp. and bacteria such as *Bacillus* spp. and *Micrococcus* spp.

Closure liners of pulpboard or cork, unless specially treated with a preservative, foil or wax coating, are often a source of mould contamination for liquid or semi-solid products. A closure with a plastic flowed-in linear is less prone to introduce or support microbial growth than one stuck in with an adhesive, particularly if the latter is based on a natural product such as casein. If required, closures can be sterilized by either formaldehyde or ethylene oxide gas.

In the case of injectables and ophthalmic preparations which are manufactured aseptically but do not receive a sterilization treatment in their final container the packaging has to be sterilized. Dry heat at 170°C is often used for vials and ampoules. Containers and closures may also be sterilized by moist heat, chemicals and irradiation, but consideration for the destruction or removal of bacterial pyrogens may be necessary.

Regardless of the type of sterilization, the process must be validated and critical control points established.

7 Buildings

7.1 Walls and ceilings

Moulds are the most common flora of walls and ceilings and the species usually found are *Cladosporium* spp., *Aspergillus* spp., in particular *A. niger* and *A. flavus*, *Penicillium* spp. and *Aurebasidium* (*Pullularia*) spp. They are particularly common in poorly ventilated buildings with painted walls. The organisms derive most of their nutrients from the plaster on to which the paint has been applied and a hard gloss finish is more resistant than a softer, matt one. The addition of up to 1% of a fungistat such as pentachlorophenol, 8-hydroxyquinoline or salicylanilide is an advantage. To reduce microbial growth, all walls and ceilings should be smooth, impervious and washable and this requirement may be met by cladding with a laminated plastic. In areas where humidity is high, glazed bricks or tiles are the optimal finish, and where a considerable volume of steam is used, ventilation at ceiling level is essential.

To aid cleaning, all electrical cables and ducting for other services should be installed deep in cavity walls where they are accessible for maintenance but do not collect dust. All pipes which pass through walls should be sealed flush to the surface.

7.2 Floors and drains

To minimize microbial contamination, all floors should be easy to clean, impervious to water and laid on a flat surface. In some areas it may be necessary for the floor to slope towards a drain, in which case the gradient should be such that no pools of water form. Any joints in the floor, necessary for expansion, should be adequately sealed. The floor-to-wall junction should be coved.

The finish of the floor usually relates to the process being carried out and in an area where little moisture or product is liable to be split, polyvinylchloride welded sheeting may be satisfactory, but in wet areas or where frequent washing is necessary, brick tiles, sealed concrete or a hard ground and polished surface like terazzo is superior. In areas where acid or alkaline chemicals or cleaning fluids are applied, a resistant sealing and jointing material must be used. If this is neglected the surface becomes pitted and porous and readily harbours microorganisms.

Where floor drainage channels are necessary they should be open if possible, shallow and easy to clean. Connections to drains should be outside areas where sensitive products are being manufactured and, where possible, drains should be avoided in areas where aseptic operations are being carried out. If this cannot be avoided, they must be fitted with effective traps, preferably with electrically operated heat-sterilizing devices.

7.3 Doors, windows and fittings

To prevent dust from collecting, all ledges, doors and windows should fit flush with walls. Doors should be well fitting to reduce the entry of microorganisms, except where a positive air pressure is maintained. Ideally, all windows in manufacturing areas should serve only to permit light entry and not be used for ventilation. In areas where aseptic operations are carried out, an adequate air-control system, other than windows, is essential.

Overhead pipes in all manufacturing areas should be sited away from equipment to prevent condensation and possible contaminants from falling into the product. Unless neglected, stainless steel pipes support little microbial growth, but lagged pipes present a problem and unless they are regularly treated with a disinfectant they will support mould growth.

8 Equipment

Each piece of equipment used to manufacture or pack pharmaceuticals has its own peculiar area where microbial growth may be supported, and knowledge of its weak points may be built up by regular tests for contamination. The type and extent of growth will depend on the source of the contamination, the nutrients available and the environmental conditions, in particular the temperature and pH.

The following points are common to many pieces of plant and serve as a general guide to reduce the risk of microbial colonization.

1   All equipment should be easy to dismantle and clean.

2   All surfaces which are in contact with the product should be smooth, continuous and free from pits, with all sharp corners eliminated and junctions rounded or coved. All internal welding should be polished out and there should be no dead ends. All contact surfaces require routine inspection for damage, particularly those of lagged equipment, and double-walled and lined vessels, since any crack or pinholes in the surface may allow the product to seep into an area where it is protected from cleaning and sterilizing agents, and where microorganisms may grow and contaminate subsequent batches of product.

3   There should be no inside screw threads and all outside threads should be readily accessible for cleaning.

4   Coupling nuts on all pipework and valves should be capable of being taken apart and cleaned.

5   Agitator blades and the shaft should preferably be of one piece and be accessible for cleaning. If the blades are bolted onto the shaft, the product may become entrained between the shaft and blades and support microorganisms. If the shaft is packed into a housing and this fitting is within a manufacturing vessel it also may act as a reservoir of microorganisms.

6   Mechanical seals are preferable to packing boxes since packing material is usually difficult to sterilize and often requires a lubricant which may gain access to the product. The product must also be protected from lubricant used on other moving parts.

7   Valves should be of a sanitary design, and all contact parts must be treated during cleaning and sanitation, and a wide variety of plug type valves are available for general purpose use. For aseptically manufactured and filled products valves fitted with steam barriers are available. If diaphragm valves are used, it is essential to inspect the diaphragm routinely. Worn diaphragms can permit seepage of the product into the seat

of the valve, where it is protected from cleaning and sterilizing agents and may act as a growth medium for microorganisms, in addition if diaphragm valves are used in very wet area, a purpose-made cover may be useful to prevent access of water and potential microbial growth occurring under the diaphragm.

8　All pipelines should slope away from the product source and all process and storage vessels should be self-draining. Run-off valves should be as near to the tank as possible and sampling through them should be avoided, since any nutrient left in the valve may encourage microbial growth which could contaminate the complete batch. A separate sampling cock or hatch is preferable.

9　If a vacuum exhaust system is used to remove the air or steam from a vessel, it is necessary to clean and disinfect all fittings regularly. This prevents residues which may be drawn into them from supporting microbial growth, which may later be returned to the vessel in the form of condensate and contaminate subsequent batches of product. If air is bled back into the vessel it should be passed through a sterilizing filter.

10　If any filters or straining bags made from natural materials such as canvas, muslin or paper are used, care must be taken to ensure that they are cleaned and sterilized regularly to prevent the growth of moulds such as *Cladosporium* spp., *Stachybotrys* spp., and *Aureobasidium (Pullularia) pullulans*, which utilize cellulose and would impair them.

8.1　　　Pipelines

The most common materials used for pipelines are stainless steel, glass and plastic, and the latter may be rigid or flexible. Continuous sections of pipework are often designed to be cleaned and sterilized in place by the flow of cleansing and sterilizing agents at a velocity of not less than $1.5\,\mathrm{m\,s^{-1}}$ through the pipe of the largest diameter in the system. The speed of flow coupled with a suitable detergent removes microorganisms by a scouring action. To be successful, stainless steel pipes must be welded to form a continuous length and must be polished internally to eliminate any pits or crevices which would provide a harbour for microorganisms. However, as soon as joints and cross-connections are introduced they provide a harbour for microorganisms, particularly behind rubber or teflon O-rings. In the case of plastic pipes, bonded joints can form an area where microorganisms are protected from cleaning and sterilizing agents.

The 'in-place' cleaning system described for pipelines may also be used for both plate and tubular types of heat exchange units, pumps and some homogenizers. However, valves and all T-piece fittings for valves and temperature and pressure gauges may need to be cleaned manually. Tanks and reaction vessels may be cleaned and sterilized automatically by rotary pressure sprays which are sited at a point in the vessel where the maximum area of wall may be treated. If spray balls are incorporated into a system which re-uses the cleansing in-place (CIP) fluids, then it may be necessary to incorporate a filter to remove particles which may block the pores of the spray ball. Fixtures such as agitators, pipe inlets, outlets and vents may have to be cleaned manually. The nature of many products or the plant design often renders cleaning in place impracticable and the plant has to be dismantled for cleaning and sterilizing.

8.2   Cleansing

There are several cleansing agents available to suit the product to be removed, and the agents include acids, alkalis and anionic, cationic and non-ionic detergents. The agent selected must fulfil the following criteria.

1   It must suit the surface to be cleaned and not cause corrosion.
2   It must remove the product without leaving a residue.
3   It must be compatible with the water supply.

Sometimes a combined cleansing and sterilizing solution is desirable, in which case the two agents must be compatible.

8.3   Disinfection and sterilization

Equipment may be sterilized or disinfected by heat, chemical disinfection or a combination of both. Many tanks and reaction vessels are sterilized by steam under pressure, and small pieces of equipment and fittings may be autoclaved, but it is important that the steam has access to all surfaces. Equipment used to manufacture and pack dry powder is often sterilized by dry heat. Chemical disinfectants commonly include sodium hypochlorite and organochlorines at 50–100 p.p.m. free residual chlorine, QACs (0.1–0.2%), 70% (v/v) ethanol in water and 1% (v/v) formaldehyde solution. The method of disinfection may be by total immersion for small objects or by spraying the internal surfaces of larger equipment. When plant is dismantled for cleaning and sterilizing, all fittings such as couplings, valves, gaskets and O-rings also require treatment. The removal of chemical disinfectants is very important in fermentation processes where residues may affect sensitive cultures.

All disinfection and sterilization processes for equipment should be validated, for preference using a microbiological challenge with an organism of appropriate resistance to the disinfectant, sterilant or sterilizing conditions. Once the required log reduction of the challenge organism has been achieved, physical and/or chemical parameters can be set which form the critical control points for the process.

8.4   Microbial checks

Either as part of an initial validation or as an ongoing exercise, the efficacy of CIP systems can be checked by plating out a sample of the final rinse water with a nutrient agar, or by swab tests. Swabs may be made of either sterile cotton wool or calcium alginate. The latter is used in conjunction with a diluent containing 1% sodium hexametaphosphate which dissolves the swab and releases the organisms removed from the equipment; these organisms may then be plated out with a nutrient agar or alternative methods of evaluation used. Swabs are useful for checking the cleanliness of curved pieces of equipment, pipes, orifices, valves and connections, but unless a measuring guide is used the results cannot be expressed quantitatively. Such measurement can be made by pressing a nutrient agar against a flat surface. The agar is usually poured into specially designed Petri dishes or contact plates, or is in the form of a disc sliced from a cylinder of a solid nutrient medium. The nutrient agar or plate or section, when incubated, replicates the contamination on the surface tested. Since this technique leaves a nutrient residue on the surface tested, the equipment must be washed and resterilized before use. The development of methods for the rapid detection of microorganisms has advantages over more traditional methods if quantitative results are used as part of a critical control programme, but not all methods lend themselves to identifying the contaminant, and it may be necessary to use a combination of methods if qualitative determinations are required.

9 Cleaning equipment and utensils

The misuse of brooms and mops can substantially increase the microbial count of the atmosphere by raising dust or by splashing with water-borne contaminants. To prevent this, either a correctly designed vacuum cleaner or a broom made of synthetic material, which is washed regularly, may be used. Hospital trials have shown that, when used, a neglected dry mop redistributes microorganisms which it has picked up, but a neglected wet mop redistributes many times the number of organisms it picked up originally, because it provides a suitable environment for their growth. In order to maintain mops and similar non-disposable cleaning equipment in a good hygienic state, it was found to be necessary first to wash and then to boil or autoclave the items, and finally to store them in a dry state. Disinfectant solutions were found to be inadequate.

Many chemical disinfectants (see also Chapter 10), in particular the halogens, some phenolics and QACs, are inactivated in the presence of organic matter and it is essential that all cleaning materials such as buckets and fogging sprays are kept clean. Halogens rapidly deteriorate at their use-dilution levels and QACs are liable to become contaminated with *Ps. aeruginosa* if stored diluted. For such reasons it is preferable to store the bulk of the disinfectant in a concentrated form and to dilute it to the use concentration only as required.

10 Further reading

Anderson J.D. & Cox C.S. (1967) Microbial survival. In: *Airborne Microbes* (eds P.H. Gregory & J.L. Monteith), pp. 203–226. Seventeenth Symposium of the Society for General Microbiology, Cambridge: Cambridge University Pres.

Burman N.P. & Colbourne J.S. (1977) Techniques for the assessment of growth of microorganisms on plumbing materials used in contact with potable water supplies. *J Appl Bacteriol*, **43**, 137–144.

Chambers C.W. & Clarke N.A. (1968) Control of bacteria in non-domestic water. *Adv Appl Microbiol*, **8**, 105–143.

Collings V.G. (1964) The freshwater environment and its significance in industry. *J Appl Bacteriol*, **27**, 143–150.

Denyer S.P. & Baird R.M. (Eds) (1990) *Guide to Microbiological Control in Pharmaceuticals*. Chichester: Ellis Horwood.

Favero M.S., McDade J.J., Robertson J.A., Hoffman R.V. & Edward R.W. (1968) Microbiological sampling of surfaces. *J Appl Bacteriol*, **31**, 336–343.

Gregory P.H. (1973) *Microbiology of the Atmosphere*, 2nd edn. London: Leonard Hill.

Maurer I.M. (1985) *Hospital Hygiene*, 3rd edn. London: Edward Arnold.

Nishannon A. & Pokja M.S. (1977) Comparative studies of microbial contamination of surfaces by the contact plate and swab methods. *J Appl Bacteriol*, **42**, 53–63.

Packer M.E. & Litchfield J.H. (1972) *Food Plant Sanitation*. London: Chapman & Hall.

Russell A.D., Hugo W.B. & Ayliffe G.A.J. (eds) (1998) *Principles and Practice of Disinfection. Preservation and Sterilization*, 3rd edn. Oxford: Blackwell Scientific Publications.

Skinner F.A. & Carr F.G. (eds) (1974) *The Normal Microbial Flora of Man*. Society for Applied Bacteriology Symposium No. 5. London: Academic Press.

Underwood E. (1998) Good manufacturing practice. In: *Principles and Practice of Disinfection, Preservation and Sterilization* (eds A.D. Russell, W.B. Hugo & G.A.J. Ayliffe), 3rd edn. Oxford: Blackwell Scientific Publications.

18 Microbial spoilage and preservation of pharmaceutical products

1 **Microbial spoilage**
1.1 Introduction
1.2 Types of spoilage
1.2.1 Infection induced by contaminated medicines
1.2.2 Chemical and physico-chemical deterioration of pharmaceutical products
1.2.3 Pharmaceutical ingredients susceptible to microbial attack
1.2.4 Observable effects of microbial attack on pharmaceutical products
1.3 Factors affecting microbial spoilage of pharmaceutical products
1.3.1 Types, and size, of contaminant inoculum
1.3.2 Nutritional factors
1.3.3 Moisture content: water activity (A_w)
1.3.4 Redox potential
1.3.5 Storage temperature
1.3.6 pH
1.3.7 Packaging design
1.3.8 Protection of microorganisms within pharmaceutical products

2 **Preservation of medicines using antimicrobial agents: basic principles**
2.1 Introduction
2.2 Effect of preservative concentration, temperature and size of inoculum
2.3 Factors affecting the 'availability' of preservatives
2.3.1 Effect of product pH
2.3.2 Efficiency in multiphase systems
2.3.3 Effect of container or packaging

3 **Quality assurance and the control of microbial risk in medicines**
3.1 Introduction
3.2 Quality assurance in formulation design and development
3.3 Good pharmaceutical manufacturing practice
3.4 Quality control procedures
3.5 Post-market surveillance

4 **Further reading**

1 Microbial spoilage

1.1 Introduction

Many medicines contain a wide variety of ingredients, often in quite complex physico-chemical states, included to create formulations which are efficacious, stable and sufficiently elegant to be acceptable to patients. Should microbial contaminants survive manufacture, or enter during storage or use they are likely to meet conditions which are often conducive to survival and even replication of an appreciable assortment of non-fastidious bacteria, fungi and yeasts, and microbial spoilage may ensue unless steps are taken to control it. Microbial spoilage may include:

1 survival of low levels of acutely pathogenic microorganisms, or higher levels of opportunist pathogens;

2 the presence of toxic microbial metabolites; or

3 microbial growth and initiation of chemical and physico-chemical deterioration of the formulation.

Such spoilage usually results in major financial problems for the manufacturer, either through direct loss of the faulty product or, possibly, expensive litigation with aggrieved users of the medicine.

1.2 Types of spoilage

1.2.1 Infection induced by contaminated medicines

Although infrequently reported as pharmaceutical contaminants, acute human pathogens attract considerable attention when they are present. For example, *Salmonella* spp. infections have arisen from contaminated tablets and capsules of yeast, carmine, pancreatin, thyroid extract and powdered vegetable drugs, where low levels of pathogens encountered in the finished medicines were traced to the raw ingredients used. A cholera outbreak in a West African country was traced to an oral liquid medicine which had been prepared with contaminated water. Of commoner practical concern are a wide variety of common saprophytic and non-fastidious opportunist contaminants which, although of limited pathogenicity to healthy individuals, may replicate readily in some medicines and present a significant infective hazard to certain groups of compromised patients. For example, whilst the intact cornea is quite resistant to infection, it offers little resistance to pseudomonads and related bacteria when scratched, or damaged by irritant chemicals, and numerous eyes have been lost following the use of inadequately designed ophthalmic solutions which had become contaminated by *Pseudomonas aeruginosa* and even supported its active growth. Pseudomonads contaminating 'antiseptic' solutions have infected the skin of badly burnt patients, resulting in the failure of skin grafts and even death from Gram-negative septicaemia. Infections of eczematous skin and respiratory infections in neonates have been traced to ointments and creams contaminated with Gram-negative bacteria. Oral mixtures and antacid suspensions can support the growth of Gram-negative bacteria and there are reports of serious consequences when administered to patients who were immuno-compromised as a result of antineoplastic chemotherapy. *Candida* spp. in intravenous medicines have also been reported to have caused fatal septicaemia in transplant patients receiving supportive immunosuppressant therapy. Growth of Gram-negative bacteria in bladder washout solutions have been responsible for very painful infections. Recently, several children died in the UK from *Pseudomonas* septicaemia caused by contamination of parenteral nutritional fluids during their aseptic compounding.

Fatal viral infections are well recorded resulting from the use of contaminated human tissue or fluids as components of medicines. Examples of this include human immunodeficiency virus (HIV) infection of haemophiliacs by contaminated and inadequately treated Factor VIII products made from pooled human blood, and Creutzfeld–Sakob disease (CJD) from injections of human growth hormone made with human pituitary glands, some of which were infected.

Gram-negative bacteria contain lipopolysaccharides (endotoxins) in their outer membranes that can remain in an active condition in products even after cell death and some can survive moist heat sterilization. Although inactive by the oral route, endotoxins can induce acute and often fatal febrile shock if they enter the bloodstream via contaminated infusion fluids, even in nanogram quantities, or via diffusion across membranes from contaminated haemodialysis solutions.

The acute bacterial toxins associated with food poisoning episodes are not commonly reported in pharmaceutical products, although aflatoxin-producing aspergilli have been detected in some vegetable ingredients. However, many of the metabolites of microbial deterioration have quite unpleasant tastes and smell even at low levels, and would deter most from using such a medicine.

Chemical and physico-chemical deterioration of pharmaceutical products

Microorganisms form a major part of the natural recycling processes for biological matter in the environment. As such, they possess a wide variety of degradative capabilities, which they are able to exert under relatively mild physico-chemical conditions. Mixed natural communities are often far more effective co-operative biodeteriogens than the individual species alone, and sequences of attack of complex substrates occur where initial attack by one group of microorganisms renders them susceptible to further deterioration by secondary, and subsequent, microorganisms. Under suitable environmental selection pressures even novel degradative pathways emerge, able to attack newly introduced synthetic chemicals (xenobiotics). However, the rates of degradation of materials released into the environment can vary greatly, from half lives of hours (phenol) to months ('hard' detergents) to years (halogenated pesticides). The overall rate of deterioration of a chemical will depend upon:

1 its chemical structure;

2 the physico-chemical properties of a particular environment;

3 the type and quantity of microbes present;

4 whether the metabolites produced can serve as sources of usable energy and precursors for biosynthesis of cellular components, and hence the creation of more microorganisms.

Pharmaceutical formulations may be considered as specialized micro-environments and their susceptibility to microbial attack assessed using conventional ecological criteria. Some naturally-occurring ingredients are particularly sensitive to attack, and quite a few synthetic components, such as modern surfactants, have been deliberately constructed to be readily degraded after disposal into the environment. Crude vegetable and animal drug extracts often contain wide assortments of microbial nutrients besides the therapeutic agents. This, combined with frequently conducive and unstable physico-chemical characteristics, leaves many formulations with a high potential for microbial attack, unless steps are taken to minimize it.

Pharmaceutical ingredients susceptible to microbial attack

Surface-active agents. Anionic surfactants such as the alkali metal and amine soaps of fatty acids are generally stable due to the slightly alkaline pH of the formulations, although readily degraded once diluted out into sewage. Alkyl and alkylbenzene sulphonates and sulphate esters are metabolized by ω-oxidation of their terminal methyl groups followed by sequential β-oxidation of the alkyl chains and fission of the aromatic rings. The presence of chain branching involves additional α-oxidative processes. Generally, ease of degradation decreases with increasing chain length and complexity of branching of the alkyl chain. Sulphonate and sulphate ester residues are converted to sulphate, although sulphonate residues are significantly more recalcitrant than the esters.

Non-ionic surfactants such as alkylpolyoxyethylene alcohol emulsifiers are readily metabolized by a wide variety of microorganisms. Increasing chain lengths and branching again decreases ease of attack. Alkylphenol polyoxyethylene alcohols are similarly attacked, but are significantly more resistant. Lipolytic cleavage of the fatty acids from sorbitan esters, polysorbates and sucrose esters is often followed by degradation of the cyclic nuclei, producing numerous small molecules readily utilizable for microbial growth.

Ampholytic surfactants based on phosphatides, betaines and alkylamino-substituted amino acids are an increasingly important group of surfactants and are generally reported to be reasonably biodegradable.

The cationic surfactants used as antiseptics and preservatives in pharmacy are usually only slowly degraded, at high dilution, in sewage. Pseudomonads have been found growing readily in quaternary ammonium antiseptic solutions, largely at the expense of other ingredients such as buffering materials, although some metabolism of the surfactant has also been observed.

Organic polymers. Many of the thickening and suspending agents used in pharmacy are subject to microbial depolymerization by specific classes of extracellular enzymes, yielding nutritive fragments and monomers. Examples of such enzymes, with their substrates in parentheses are: amylases (starches), pectinases (pectins), cellulases (carboxymethylcelluloses, but not alkylcelluloses), uronidases (polyuronides such as in tragacanth and acacia), dextranases (dextrans) and proteases (proteins). Agar (complex polysaccharides) is an example of a relatively inert polymer and, as such, is used as a support for solidifying microbiological culture media. The lower molecular weight polyethylene glycols are readily degraded by sequential oxidation of the hydrocarbon chain, but the larger congeners are rather more recalcitrant. Synthetic packaging polymers such as nylon, polystyrene and polyester are extremely resistant to attack, although cellophane (modified cellulose) is susceptible under some humid conditions.

Humectants. Low molecular weight materials such as glycerol and sorbitol are included in some products to reduce water loss and are usually readily metabolized unless present in high concentrations (see section 1.3.3).

Fats and oils. These hydrophobic materials are usually attacked extensively when dispersed in aqueous formulations such as oil-in-water emulsions, although fungal attack is reported in condensed moisture films on the surface of oils in bulk, or where water droplets have contaminated the bulk oil phase. Oil-in-water emulsion-based medicines are less commonly encountered than in food formulations where their microbial attack can also occur, aided by the high solubility of oxygen in many oils. Lipolytic rupture of triglycerides liberates glycerol and fatty acids, the latter often then undergoing β-oxidation of the alkyl chains and the production of odiferous ketones. While the microbial metabolism of pharmaceutical hydrocarbon oils is rarely reported, this is a problem in engineering and fuel technology when water droplets have accumulated in oil storage tanks and subsequent fungal colonization has catalysed serious corrosion.

Sweetening, flavouring and colouring agents. Many of the sugars and other sweetening agents used in pharmacy are ready substrates for microbial growth. However, some are used in very high concentrations to reduce water activity in some aqueous products and inhibit microbial attack (see section 1.3.3). At one time, a variety of colouring agents (such as tartrazine and amaranth) and flavouring agents (such as peppermint water) were kept as stock solutions for extemporaneous dispensing purposes but they frequently supported the growth of *Pseudomonas* spp. including *Ps. aeruginosa*. It is now recommended that such stock solutions contain preservatives or are made freshly as required by dilution of alcoholic solutions which are much less susceptible to microbial attack.

Therapeutic agents. It is possible to demonstrate that a variety of microorganisms under laboratory conditions can metabolize a wide assortment of drugs, resulting in loss of activity. Materials as diverse as alkaloids (morphine, strychnine, atropine), analgesics (aspirin, paracetamol), thalidomide, barbiturates, steroid esters and mandelic acid can be metabolized and serve as substrates for growth. Indeed the use of microorganisms to carry out subtle transformations on steroid molecules forms the basis of the commercial production of potent therapeutic steroidal agents (see Chapter 25). Reports of drug destruction in actual medicines are less frequent. However, examples include the metabolism of atropine in eye drops by contaminating fungi, inactivation of penicillin injections by β-lactamase-producing bacteria (see Chapter 5), steroid metabolism in damp tablets and creams by fungi, the microbial hydrolysis of aspirin in suspension by esterase-producing bacteria, and chloramphenicol deactivation in an oral medicine by a chloramphenicol acetylase-producing contaminant.

Preservatives and disinfectants. Many preservatives and disinfectants can be metabolized by a wide variety of Gram-negative bacteria, although more commonly at concentrations below their effective 'use' levels. However, quaternary ammonium antimicrobial agents are only slowly attacked. Organomercurial preservatives discharged into rivers from paper mills have been extensively converted to insidiously toxic alkylmercury compounds which could reach humans via an ascending food chain. Degradation of agents at 'use' concentrations in pharmacy and medicine is less commonly reported, but there are incidents of the growth of pseudomonads in stock solutions of quaternary ammonium antiseptics and chlorhexidine with resultant infection of patients. *Pseudomonas* spp. have metabolized 4-hydroxybenzoate ester preservatives contained in eye-drops and caused serious eye infections, and metabolized them in oral suspensions and solutions. It is important to remember this possibility when selecting preservatives for formulations.

1.2.4   *Observable effects of microbial attack on pharmaceutical products*

Microbial contaminants will usually need to be able to attack ingredients of a medicine and create substrates necessary for biosynthesis and energy production before they can replicate to levels where obvious spoilage becomes apparent since, for example, 10^6 microbes will have an overall degradative effect around 10^6 time faster than one cell. However, growth and attack may well be localized in surface moisture films or very unevenly distributed within the bulk of viscous formulations such as creams. Early

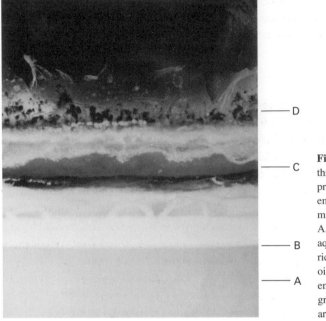

Fig. 18.1 Section (×1.5) through an inadequately preserved olive oil, oil-in-water, emulsion in an advanced state of microbial spoilage showing: A, discoloured, oil-depleted, aqueous phase; B, oil globule-rich creamed layer; C, coalesced oil layer from 'cracked' emulsion; D, fungal mycelial growth on surface. Also present are a foul taste and evil smell!

indications of spoilage are often organoleptic, with the release of very unpleasant smelling and tasting metabolites such as 'sour' fatty acids, 'fishy' amines, 'bad eggs', bitter, 'earthy' or sickly tastes and smells. Products frequently become unappealingly discoloured by microbial pigments of various shades. Thickening and suspending agents such as tragacanth, acacia or carboxymethylcellulose can be depolymerized, resulting in loss of viscosity, and sedimentation of suspended ingredients. Alternatively, microbial polymerization of sugars and surfactant molecules can produce slimy, viscous, masses in syrups, shampoos and creams, and fungal growth in creams has produced 'gritty' textures. Changes in product pH can occur depending on whether acidic or basic metabolites are released, and become so modified as to permit secondary attack by microbes previously inhibited by the initial product pH. Gaseous metabolites may be seen as trapped bubbles within viscous formulations.

When a complex formulation such as an oil-in-water emulsion is attacked, a gross and progressive spoilage sequence may be observed. Metabolism of surfactants will reduce stability and accelerate 'creaming' of the oil globules. Lipolytic release of fatty acids from oils will lower pH and encourage coalescence of oil globules and 'cracking' of the emulsion. Fatty acids and their ketonic oxidation products will provide a sour taste and unpleasant smell, whilst bubbles of gaseous metabolites may be visible, trapped in the product, and pigments may discolour the product (see Fig. 18.1).

1.3   Factors affecting microbial spoilage of pharmaceutical products

An understanding of the influence of the chemical and physico-chemical parameters of an environment on microorganisms might allow for subtle manipulation of a formulation to create conditions which are as unfavourable as possible for growth and spoilage, within the limitations of patient acceptability and therapeutic efficacy. Additionally, the overall characteristics of a particular formulation will indicate its susceptibility to attack by various classes of microorganisms.

<table>
<tr><td>1.3.1</td><td>*Types, and size, of contaminant inoculum*</td></tr>
</table>

Whilst there will be some chance that a particularly aggressive microbe may enter and contaminate a medicine, some element of prediction is possible if one considers the environment and usage to which the product is likely to be subjected during its life and the history of similar medicines (see Chapters 17 and 19). A formulator can then build in as much protection as possible against non-standard encounters, such as additional preservation for a syrup if osmotolerant yeast contamination is particularly likely.

Should failure subsequently occur, a knowledge of microbial ecology and careful identification of the contaminant(s) can be most useful in tracking down the defective steps in the design or production process. Very low levels of contaminants which are unable to replicate in a product might not cause appreciable spoilage but, should an unexpected surge in the contaminant bioburden occur, the built-in protection could become swamped and spoilage ensue. This might arise if:

1 raw materials were unusually contaminated;
2 a lapse of the plant-cleaning protocol occurred;
3 large microbial growths detached themselves from within supplying pipework;
4 a change in production procedures allowed unexpected growth of contaminants during the modified operation;
5 there was demolition work in the vicinity of the manufacturing site or;
6 there had been gross misuse of the product during administration.

However, inoculum size alone is not always a reliable indicator of likely spoilage potential. A very low level of, say, aggressive pseudomonads in a weakly preserved solution may suggest a greater risk than tablets containing fairly high numbers of fungal and bacterial spores.

When an aggressive contaminant enters a medicine, there may be an appreciable lag period before significant spoilage begins, the duration of which decreases disproportionately with increasing contaminant loading. It is possible to provide some control over extemporaneously dispensed formulations by specifying short shelf-lives of, say, 2 weeks. However, since there is usually a long delay between manufacture and administration of factory-made medicines, growth and attack could ensue during this period unless additional steps are taken to prevent it.

The isolation of a particular microorganism from a markedly spoiled product does not necessarily mean that it was the initiator of the attack. It could be a secondary opportunist contaminant which has overgrown the primary spoilage organism once the physico-chemical properties had been favourably modified by the primary spoiler

<table>
<tr><td>1.3.2</td><td>*Nutritional factors*</td></tr>
</table>

The simple nutritional requirements and metabolic adaptability of many common saprophytic spoilage microorganisms enable them to utilize many of the components of medicines as substrates for biosynthesis and growth, including not only the intended ingredients but also the wide array of trace materials contained in them. The use of crude vegetable or animal products in a formulation provides an additionally nutritious environment. Even demineralized water prepared by good ion-exchange methods will normally contain sufficient nutrients to allow significant growth of many water-borne Gram-negative bacteria such as *Pseudomonas* spp. When such contaminants fail to grow in a medicine it is unlikely to be as a result of nutrient limitation but due to other, non-supportive, physico-chemical or toxic properties.

Most acute pathogens require specific growth factors normally associated with the tissues they infect but which are often normally absent in pharmaceutical formulations. They are thus unlikely to multiply in them, although they may remain viable and infective for an appreciable time in some dry products where the conditions are suitably protective.

1.3.3   *Moisture content: water activity (A_w)*

Microorganisms require ready access to water in appreciable quantities for growth. Although some solute-rich medicines such as syrups may appear to be 'wet', microbial growth in them may be difficult since the microbes have to compete for water molecules with the vast numbers of sugar and other molecules of the formulation which also readily interact with water via hydrogen bonding. An estimate of the proportion of the uncomplexed water in a formulation available to equilibrate with any microbial contaminants and facilitate growth can be obtained by measuring its water activity (A_w). (This can be calculated from: A_w = vapour pressure of formulation ÷ vapour pressure of water under similar conditions). The greater the solute concentration, the lower is the water activity. With the exception of halophilic bacteria, most microorganisms grow best in dilute solutions (high A_w) and, as solute concentration rises (lowering A_w), growth rates decline until a minimal, growth-inhibitory A_w is reached. Limiting A_w values are of the order of: Gram-negative rods, 0.95; staphylococci, micrococci and lactobacilli, 0.9; and most yeasts, 0.88. Syrup-fermenting osmotolerant yeasts have been found spoiling products with A_w levels as low as 0.73, whilst some filamentous fungi can grow at even lower values, with *Aspergillus glaucus* as low as 0.61.

The A_w of aqueous formulations can be lowered to increase resistance to microbial attack by the addition of high concentrations of sugars or polyethylene glycols. However, even Syrup BP (66% sucrose; A_w = 0.86) has been reported to fail occasionally to inhibit osmotolerant yeasts and additional preservation may be necessary. With a trend towards the elimination of sucrose from medicines continuing, alternative solutes are being investigated, such as sorbitol and fructose, which are not thought to encourage dental caries. The use of brine to preserve some meats would be organoleptically unacceptable for medicines. A_w can also be reduced by drying, although the dry, often hygroscopic medicines (tablets, capsules, powders, vitreous 'glasses') will require suitable packaging to prevent resorption of water and consequent microbial growth (Fig. 18.2). Tablet film coatings are now available which greatly reduce water vapour uptake during storage whilst allowing ready dissolution in bulk water. These might contribute to increased microbial stability during storage in particularly humid climates, although suitable foil strip packing may be more effective, if also more expensive.

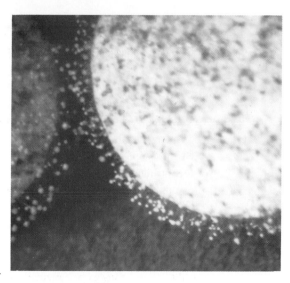

Fig. 18.2 Fungal growth on a tablet which has become damp (raised A_w) during storage under humid conditions. Note the sparseness of mycelium, and conidiophores. The contaminant is thought to be a *Penicillium* sp.

Condensed water films can accumulate on the surface of otherwise 'dry' products such as tablets or bulk oils following storage in damp atmospheres with fluctuating temperatures, resulting in sufficiently high localized A_w to initiate fungal growth. More water, produced from respiration, may then raise A_w even further, encouraging growth. Dilute aqueous films similarly formed on the surface of viscous products such as syrups and creams, or exuded by syneresis from hydrogels, can and do reach sufficiently high A_w to permit surface yeast and fungal spoilage.

Inhibition of microbial growth by reduction of A_w is more complex than by a simple binding of water molecules alone as some solutes are more effective than others at inhibiting microbial attack by particular types of microorganisms even when used to generate similar A_w levels. Mechanisms are thought to involve interference with cellular osmoregulation and energy production.

1.3.4   Redox potential

The ability of microbes to grow in an environment is influenced by its oxidation–reduction balance (redox potential) since they will require compatible terminal electron acceptors to permit function of their respiratory pathways. Vacuum packing of foodstuffs, or the inclusion of oxygen absorbers in the package to minimize oxygen levels, reduces attack by some of the obligate aerobic spoilage bacteria, but does not eliminate all spoilage. Oxygen removal to control spoilage in medicines is not a practical proposition although it is used to control non-biological oxidation. The use of pressurized carbon dioxide for soft drinks preservation relies more on the specific antimicrobial action of carbonic acid than to removal of oxygen. Some viscous foodstuffs, particularly those containing meat, have sufficiently low redox potentials to permit growth of dangerous anaerobic clostridia, but this is unlikely in most pharmaceuticals. The redox potential even in fairly viscous emulsions may be quite high due the appreciable solubility of oxygen in most fats and oils.

Storage temperature

Spoilage of pharmaceuticals could occur over the range of about –20° to 60°C, although much less likely at the extremes. The actual storage temperature may selectively determine spoilage by particular types of microorganisms. Storage in a deep freeze at –20°C or lower is used for long-term storage of foodstuffs and some pharmaceutical raw materials, and dispensed total parenteral nutrition (TPN) feeds have been stored in hospitals for short periods at –20°C to even further minimize the risk of growth of any contaminants which might have been introduced during their aseptic compounding. Reconstituted syrups and multi-dose eyedrop packs are sometimes dispensed with the instruction to 'store in a cool place' such as a domestic fridge (8°–12°C), partly to reduce the risk of in-use contamination growing before the expiry date. Conversely, pharmacopoeial Water for Injections is recommended to be held at 80°C or above after distillation and prior to packing and sterilization to prevent possible regrowth of Gram-negative bacteria, and the release of endotoxins.

1.3.6 *pH*

Extremes of pH prevent microbial attack, although feeble mould growth even in dilute hydrochloric acid necessitates the preservation of analytical acid standards. Around neutrality bacterial spoilage is more likely, with reports of pseudomonads and related Gram-negative bacteria growing in antacid mixtures, flavoured mouth washes and in distilled or demineralized water. Above pH 8, for instance with soap-based emulsions, spoilage is rare. For products with low pH levels such as the fruit juice-flavoured syrups (*ca.* pH 3–4) mould or yeast attack is more likely. Yeasts can metabolize organic acids and raise the pH to levels where secondary bacterial growth can occur. Although the use of low pH adjustment to preserve foodstuffs is well established (pickling, coleslaw, yoghurt etc.) it is not practicable to make deliberate use of this for medicines.

1.3.7 *Packaging design*

Packaging can have a major influence on microbial stability of some formulations, to control the entry of contaminants during both storage and use. Enormous efforts have gone into the design of containers to prevent the ingress of contaminants into medicines for parenteral administration because of the high risks of infection by this route. Self-sealing rubber wads must be used to prevent microbial entry into multi-dose injection containers (Chapter 21) following withdrawals with a hypodermic needle. Wide-mouthed cream jars will allow the entry of fingers with their concomitant high bioburden of contamination, and this can be reduced by replacement with narrow nozzle and flexible screw capped tubes. Where medicines rely on their low A_w to prevent spoilage, packaging such as strip foils must be of water vapour-proof materials with fully efficient seals. Cardboard outer packaging and labels themselves can become substrates for microbial attack under humid conditions, and preservatives are often included to reduce their risk of damage.

The survival of microorganisms in particular environments is influenced by the presence of various relatively inert materials. Thus, microbes can be more resistant to heat or desiccation in the presence of some polymers such as starch, acacia or gelatin. Adsorption onto naturally occurring particulate material may aid establishment and survival in some environments. There is a belief, but limited hard evidence, that the presence of suspended particles such as kaolin, magnesium trisilicate or aluminium hydroxide gel may influence contaminant longevity in medicines containing them, and that the presence of some surfactants, suspending agents and proteins can increase the resistance of microorganisms to preservatives, over and above their direct inactivating effect on the agents.

2   Preservation of medicines using antimicrobial agents: basic principles

2.1   Introduction

An antimicrobial 'preservative' may be included in a formulation to further reduce the risk of spoilage and, preferably, kill any anticipated low levels of contaminants remaining in a non-sterile medicine after manufacture or which might enter while stored, or during the repeated withdrawal of doses from a multi-dose container. If a medicine is unlikely to encourage growth or survival of contaminants and the infective risk is low, such as with tablets, capsules and dry powders, then a preservative might be pointless. Preservatives should not be added to deal with erratic failures in poorly controlled manufacturing processes, due to the uncertainty of success, and their possible depletion before fulfilling their intended role (see section 2.2). The bad practice of including preservatives in medicines sterilized by filtration to guard against undetected failure of the filter did not tackle the real problem of the need for properly validated filtration systems.

Ideally, such preservatives should:

1   be able to kill rapidly all microbial contaminants as they enter the medicine;
2   not be irritant or toxic to the patient;
3   be stable and effective throughout the life of the medicine; and,
4   be selective in reacting with the contaminants and not the ingredients of the medicine.

Unfortunately, the most active antimicrobial agents are often generally non-selective in action, inter-reacting significantly with formulation ingredients and patients as well as microorganisms. Once the more toxic, irritant and reactive agents are excluded, those remaining generally have only modest antimicrobial efficacy, and there are now no preservatives considered sufficiently non-toxic for use in highly sensitive areas, e.g. for injection into central nervous system tissues or for use within the eye. A number of microbiologically effective preservatives used in cosmetics are reported to cause significant incidences of contact dermatitis, and are thus precluded from use in pharmaceutical creams. Although it may be preferable to rapidly kill all contaminants as they enter a medicine, this may only be possible for relatively simple aqueous solutions such as eye-drops or injections. For physico-chemically complex systems such as emulsions and creams, only inhibition of growth and rather slow, or no, rates of killing may be realistically achieved.

In order to maximize what preservative efficiency is possible, an appreciation of those parameters which influence antimicrobial activity within medicines is essential.

2.2   Effect of preservative concentration, temperature and size of inoculum

Changes in the efficacy of preservatives vary exponentially with changes in concentration (see concentration exponent, η, Chapter 11), the extent of variation depending upon the type of agent. For example, halving the concentration of phenol ($\eta = 6$) gives a 64-fold (2^6) reduction in activity, whilst a similar dilution for chlorhexidine ($\eta = 2$) reduces killing power by only fourfold (2^2). Changes in product temperature will alter efficacy in proportions, related to different types of preservative and certain groups of microorganisms (see temperature coefficient, Q_{10}, Chapter 11). Thus, a drop in temperature from 30 to 20°C could result in fivefold and 45-fold losses of killing power towards *Escherichia coli* by phenol ($Q_{10} = 5$) or ethanol ($Q_{10} = 45$), respectively. If both temperature and concentration vary concurrently, the situation is more complex, but it has been suggested, for example, that if a 0.1% chlorocresol ($\eta = 6$, $Q_{10} = 5$) solution completely killed a suspension of *E. coli* at 30°C in 10 minutes, it would require around 90 minutes to achieve a similar effect if the temperature was lowered to 20°C and slight overheating during production had resulted in a 10% loss by vaporization in the chlorocresol concentration (other factors remaining constant).

Preservative molecules are used up as they inactivate microorganisms and as they interact non-specifically with the significant quantities of contaminant 'dirt' also introduced during use. This will result in a progressive and exponential decline in the efficiency of the remaining preservative. Preservative 'capacity' is a term used to describe the cumulative level of contamination that a preserved formulation is likely to cope with before becoming so depleted as to become ineffective. This will vary with preservative type and complexity of the formulation.

2.3   Factors affecting the 'availability' of preservatives

Most preservatives interact in solution with many of the commonly used ingredients of pharmaceutical formulations to varying extents via a number of weak bonding attractions as well as with any microorganisms present. This can result in unstable equilibria in which only a small proportion of the total preservative present is 'available' to inactivate the relatively small microbial mass, and the resultant rate of killing may be far lower than might be anticipated from the performance of simple aqueous solutions. The 'unavailable' preservative may still, however, contribute to the general irritancy of the product. It is commonly believed that where the solute concentrations are very high, and A_w is appreciably reduced, the efficiency of preservatives is often appreciably reduced and may be virtually inactive at very low A_w. A practice of including preservatives in very low A_w products such as tablets and capsules misses the point. This would only offer minimal protection for the dry tablets, and if they should become damp they will be spoiled for other, non-microbial, reasons.

Effect of product pH

In the weakly acidic preservatives, activity resides primarily in the unionized molecules and they only have significant efficacy at pHs where ionization is low. Thus, benzoic and sorbic acids (pK_a = 4.2 and 4.75, respectively) have limited preservative usefulness above pH 5, while the 4(p)-hydroxybenzoate esters with their non-ionizable ester group and poorly ionizable hydroxyl substituent (pK_a *ca.* 8.5) have moderate protective effect even at neutral pH levels. The activity of quaternary ammonium preservatives and chlorhexidine probably resides with their cations and are effective in products of neutral pH. Formulation pH can also directly influence the sensitivity of microorganisms to preservatives (see Chapter 11).

2.3.2   *Efficiency in multiphase systems*

In a multiphase formulation, such as an oil-in-water emulsion, preservative molecules will distribute themselves in an unstable equilibrium between the bulk aqueous phase and (i) the oil phase by partition, (ii) the surfactant micelles by solubilization, (iii) polymeric suspending agents and other solutes by competitive displacement of water of solvation, (iv) particulate and container surfaces by adsorption and, (v) any microorganisms present. Generally, the overall preservative efficiency can be related to the small proportion of preservative molecules remaining unbound in the bulk aqueous phase, although as this becomes depleted some slow re-equilibration between the components can be anticipated. The loss of neutral molecules into oil and micellar phases may be favoured over ionized species, although considerable variation in distribution is found between different systems.

In view of these potentials for major reductions in preservative efficacy, considerable effort has gone into attempts to devise equations in which one might substitute variously derived system parameters such as partition coefficients, surfactant and polymer binding constants and oil:water ratios in order to obtain estimates of residual preservative levels in aqueous phases. Although some modestly successful predictions have been obtained for very simple laboratory systems, they have proved of limited practical value as data for many of the required parameters are unavailable for technical grade ingredients or for the more complex commercial systems.

2.3.3   *Effect of container or packaging*

Preservative availability may be appreciably reduced by interaction with packaging materials. Examples include the permeation of phenolic preservatives into the rubber wads and teats of multi-dose injection or eye-drop containers and by their interaction with flexible nylon tubes for creams. Quaternary ammonium preservative levels in formulations have been significantly reduced by adsorption onto the surfaces of plastic and glass containers. Volatile preservatives such as chloroform are so readily lost by the routine opening and closing of containers that their usefulness is somewhat restricted to preservation of medicines in sealed, impervious containers during storage, with quite short use lives once opened.

3 Quality assurance and the control of microbial risk in medicines

3.1 Introduction

Quality assurance (QA) relates to a scheme of management which embraces *all* the procedures necessary to provide a high probability that a medicine will conform consistently to a specified description of quality (a formalized measure of its fitness for the purpose intended) on every occasion. It includes formulation design and development (R & D), good pharmaceutical manufacturing practice (GPMP), which includes quality control (QC), and post-marketing surveillance. Since many microorganisms may be hazardous to patients and/or spoil formulations if they enter and remain active in medicines it is necessary to perform a contamination risk assessment for each product by examining every stage of its anticipated life from raw materials to administration, and develop strategies calculated to reduce the overall risk(s) to acceptably low levels. Risk assessments concerning microorganisms are complicated by uncertainties about the exact infective and spoilage hazards and risks likely for many contaminants, and by difficulties in measuring their precise performance in complex systems. As the consequences of product failure and patient damage will be severe for a manufacturing company, it is usual to make worst-case presumptions and design strategies to cover them fully; lesser problems are also then encompassed. Since, for example, it is impossible to guarantee that any particular microorganism will not be infective, the presumption is made that all microbes are potentially infective for routes of administration where the likelihood of infection from contaminants is high; such medicines are then supplied in a sterile form. One must also presume that those administering medicines may not be highly skilled or motivated in contamination control techniques, and incorporate additional safeguards to control risks more appropriate to these situations. This may include detailed information on administration and even training, in addition to providing a high quality formulation.

3.2 Quality assurance in formulation design and development

Possibly, the majority of risks of microbial infection and spoilage arising from microbial contamination during manufacture, storage and use could be eliminated by presenting all medicines in sterile, impervious, single dosage units. However, the high cost of this strategy restricts its use to situations where there is a high risk of consequent infection from any contaminant microbes. Where the infective risk is assessed as much lower, less efficient, but less expensive, strategies are adopted. The high risk of infection by contaminants in parenteral medicines, combined with concerns about the systemic toxicity of preservatives almost always demands sterile single dosage units. With eyedrops for domestic use the risks are perceived to be lower, and sterile multi-dose products containing a preservative to combat the anticipated in-use contamination are accepted, although for the higher risk environment of hospitals sterile single dose units are more common. Oral and topical routes of administration are generally perceived to present relatively low risks of infection and the emphasis is more on the control of microbial content during manufacture and protection of the formulation from chemical and physico-chemical spoilage.

As part of the design process, it is necessary to include features in the formulation and delivery system to provide as much protection as possible against microbial contamination and spoilage. Because of potential toxicity and irritancy problems, antimicrobial preservatives should only be considered where there is clear evidence of positive benefit. Manipulation of physico-chemical parameters, such as A_w, the elimination of particularly susceptible ingredients, the selection of a preservative or the choice of container may contribute significantly to overall medicine stability. For 'dry' dosage forms, since it is their very low A_w which is their protection against microbial attack, the moisture vapour properties of packaging materials requires careful examination.

Preservatives are intended to offer further protection against environmental microbial contaminants. However, since they are relatively non-specific in their reactivity (see section 2), it is difficult to calculate with any certainty what proportion of preservative added to all but the simplest medicine will be available for inactivating such contamination. The only realistic solution to deciding whether a formulation is likely to be adequately preserved, without exposing it to the rigours of the real world over a fair period of time, is to devise a laboratory test where it is challenged with viable microorganisms, and see whether they are inactivated. Such tests should form part of formulation development and stability trials to ensure that suitable activity is likely to remain throughout the life of the medicine. They would not normally be used for routine manufacturing quality control.

Some 'preservative challenge tests' add relatively large inocula of various laboratory cultures to aliquots of the medicine and determine their rate of inactivation by viable counting methods (single challenge tests), whilst others re-inoculate repeatedly at set intervals, monitoring the efficiency of inactivation until the system fails (multiple challenge test). This latter technique may give a better estimate of the preservative capacity of the system than the single challenge approach, but is very time consuming and expensive. The problems arise when deciding whether performance in such tests gives reliable predictions of real in-use efficacy. Although the test organisms should bear some similarity in type and spoilage potential to those to be met in use, it is known that repeated cultivation on conventional microbiological media (nutrient agar etc.) frequently results in marked reductions in aggressiveness. Attempts to maintain spoilage activity by inclusion of formulation ingredients in the culture media gives varied results. Some manufacturers have been able to maintain active spoilage strains by cultivation in unpreserved, or diluted aliquots, of formulations.

The *British Pharmacopoeia* and the *European Pharmacopoeia* contain a preservative single challenge test which uses four stock cultures of bacteria, a yeast and a mould, none of which has any significant history of spoilage potential and which are to be cultivated on conventional media. However, extension of the basic test is recommended in some situations, such as the inclusion of an osmotolerant yeast if it is thought such in-use spoilage might be a problem. Despite its limitations and the cautious indications given as to what the tests might suggest about the formulation, several manufacturers have indicated that the test does provide some basic, but useful, indicators of likely in-use stability. UK Product Licence applications for preserved medicines must demonstrate that the formulation at least meets the preservative efficacy criteria of the *British Pharmacopoeia*, or similar, test.

Orth has applied the concepts of the D-value as used in sterilization technology (Chapter 20) to the interpretation of challenge testing. Expressing of the rate of microbial inactivation in a preserved system in terms of a D-value enables estimation of the nominal time to achieve a prescribed proportionate level of kill. Problems arise when trying to predict the behaviour of very low levels of survivors, and the method has its detractors as well as its advocates.

3.3   **Good pharmaceutical manufacturing practice**

GPMP is concerned with the manufacture of medicines, and includes control of ingredients, plant construction, process validation, production, and cleaning (see also Chapter 22). QC is that part of GPMP dealing with specification, documentation and assessing conformance to specification.

With traditional QC, a high reliance was placed on testing samples of finished products to determine the overall quality of a batch. This practice can, however, result in considerable financial loss if non-compliance is detected only at this late stage, leaving the expensive options of discarding, or reworking (often not possible), the batch. Additionally, a few microbiological test methods have poor precision and/or accuracy. Validation can be complex or impossible, and interpretation of results can prove difficult. For example, although a sterility assurance level of less than one failure in 10^6 items submitted to a terminal sterilization process is considered appropriate, conventional 'tests for sterility' for finished products (such as in the *British Pharmacopoeia*) could not possibly be relied upon to find one damaged, but not dead, microbe somewhere in 10^6 items let alone allow for its cultivation with any precision (Chapter 23). End-product testing may also not prevent or even detect the isolated rogue processing failure.

It is now generally accepted that a high assurance of overall product quality can only come from a detailed specification, control and monitoring of *all* the stages which contribute to the manufacturing process. More realistic decisions about conformance to specification can then be made using information for *all* relevant parameters (parametric release method), not just results from the selective testing of finished products. Thus, a more realistic estimate of the microbial quality of a batch of tablets would be achieved from a knowledge of such parameters as the microbial bioburden of the starting materials, temperature records from granule drying ovens, the moisture level of the dried granules, compaction data, validation records for the foil strip sealing machine and microbial levels in the finished tablets than from the contaminant content of the finished tablets alone.

It may be necessary to exclude certain undesirable contaminants from starting materials, such as pseudomonads from bulk aluminium hydroxide gel, or to include pre-treatment to reduce overall bioburdens by irradiation, such as for ispaghula husk and spices. For biotechnology-derived drugs produced in human or animal tissue culture, considerable investigation is made to exclude cell lines contaminated with latent host viruses. Official guidelines to limit the risk of prion contamination in medicines require bovine-derived ingredients to be obtained from sources where bovine spongiform encephalopathy (BSE) is not endemic.

If one considers manufacturing plant and its environs from the ecological and physiological viewpoint of microorganisms it should be possible to identify areas where contaminants might accumulate and even thrive to create hazards for subsequent batches of medicine, and then manipulate design and operating conditions to discourage such colonization. The ability to clean and dry equipment thoroughly is a very useful deterrent to growth. Design considerations must include the reductions of obscure nooks and crannies and the ability to be able to clean thoroughly into all areas. Some larger equipment now has cleansing-in-place (CIP) and sterilization-in-place (SIP) systems installed in place to improve decontamination capabilities.

It may be necessary to include intermediate steps within processing to reduce the bioburden and improve the efficiency of lethal sterilization cycles, or to prevent swamping of the preservative in a non-sterile medicine after manufacture. With some of the newer and fragile biotechnology-derived products processing may include chromatographic and/or ultrafiltration stages to ensure adequate reductions of viral contamination levels rather than conventional sterilization cycles.

In a validation exercise, it must be demonstrated that each stage of the system is capable of providing the degree of intended efficiency within the limits of variation for which it was designed. Microbial spoilage aspects of process validation might include examination of the cleaning system for its ability to remove deliberately introduced contamination. Chromatographic removal of viral contaminants would be validated by determining the log reduction achievable against a known titre of added viral particles.

3.4   Quality control procedures

Whilst there is general agreement on the need to control total microbial levels in non-sterile medicines and to exclude certain species which have proved troublesome previously, the precision and accuracy of current methods for counting (or even detecting) some microbes in complex products is poor. Acute pathogens, present in low numbers, and often damaged by processing, can be very difficult to isolate. Products showing active spoilage can yield surprisingly low viable counts on testing; although present in high numbers, a particular organism may be neither pathogenic nor the primary spoilage agent, but may be relatively inert, e.g. ungerminated spores or a secondary contaminant which has outgrown the initiating spoiler. Very unevenly distributed growth in viscous formulations will present serious sampling problems. The type of culture media (even different batches of the same media) and conditions of incubation may greatly influence any viable counts obtained from products.

A major problem is that of when to sample. If an antacid suspension contains, say, two pseudomonad cells per $100\,cm^3$ shortly after manufacture does this represent a spoilage hazard? If they die out slowly as a consequence of the preservative present then it might not, but if on the other hand they grow slowly during storage over a year levels might be attained when spoilage will be significant.

Recognizing these problems, UK food regulatory authorities have generally abandoned the use of quantitative microbial counts as enforceable standards of food quality. Despite this, the *European Pharmacopoeia* has introduced both quantitative and qualitative microbial standards for non-sterile medicines, which might become enforceable in some member states. It prescribes varying maximum total microbial levels and exclusions of particular species according the routes of administration. The *British Pharmacopoeia* has now included these tests, but suggest they should be used to assist in validating GPMP processing procedures and not as conformance standards for routine end-product testing. Thus, for a medicine to be administered orally, there should not be more than 10^3 aerobic bacteria or more than 10^2 fungi per gram or cm^3 of product, and there should be an absence of *Escherichia coli*. Higher levels may be permissible if the product contains raw materials of natural origin.

Most manufacturers perform periodic tests on their products for total microbial bioburden and for the presence of known problem microorganisms, to be used for in-house confirmation of the continuing efficiency of their GPMP systems, rather than as conventional end-product conformance tests. Fluctuation in values, or the appearance of specific and unusual species, can warn of defects in procedure and impending problems.

In order to reduce the costs of testing and shorten quarantine periods, there is considerable interest in alternatives to conventional test methods for the detection and determination of microorganisms, preferably which could be automated. Although none would appear to be in widespread use at present, some of promise include electrical impedance, microcalorimetry, use of fluorescent dyes and epi-fluorescence, and the use of 'vital' stains. Considerable advances in the sensitivity of methods for estimating microbial adenosine triphosphate (ATP) using luciferase now allows the estimation of extremely low bioburdens. The recent development of highly sensitive laser scanning devices for detecting bacteria variously labelled with selective fluorescent probes enable the apparent detection even of single cells.

Endotoxin (pyrogen) levels in parenteral and similar products must be phenomenally low in order to prevent serious endotoxic shock on administration. Formerly, this was checked by injecting rabbits and noting any febrile response. Most determinations are now performed using the *Limulus* test in which an amoebocyte lysate from the horse-shoe crab (*Limulus polyphemus*) reacts extremely specifically with microbial lipopolysaccharides to give a gel and opacification even at very high dilutions. A variant of the test using a chromogenic substrate gives a coloured end-point which can be detected spectroscopically. Tissue culture tests are under development where the ability of endotoxins to directly induce cytokine release is measured.

Sophisticated and very sensitive methods have been developed in the food industry for detecting many other microbial toxins. For example, aflatoxin detection in seedstuffs and their oils is performed by solvent extraction, adsorption onto columns containing selective antibodies for them, and detected by exposure to ultraviolet light.

Although it would be unusual to test for signs of active physico-chemical or chemical spoilage of products as part of routine quality control procedures for medicines, this may be necessary in order to examine an incident of anticipated product failure, or during formulation development. Many volatile and unpleasant-tasting metabolites are generated during active spoilage which are readily apparent. Their characterization by HPLC or GC can be used to distinguish microbial spoilage from other, non-biological deterioration. Spoilage often results in physico-chemical changes which can be monitored by conventional methods. Thus, emulsion spoilage may be followed by monitoring changes in creaming rates, pH changes, particle sedimentation and viscosity.

3.5 Post-market surveillance

Despite extensive development and a rigorous adherence to procedures, one cannot guarantee absolutely that a medicine will never fail under the harsh abuses of real-life usage. A proper quality assurance system must include procedures for monitoring in-use performance and for responding to customer complaints. These must be followed up in great detail in order to decide whether one's carefully constructed schemes for product safety require modification, to prevent the incident recurring.

4 Further reading

The chapter sections to which each reference is particularly relevant are indicated in parentheses at the end of the reference, although this section is also intended as a general suggestion of routes to material for those who wish to develop the topic in more detail.

Anon. (1997) *Rules and Guidance for Pharmaceutical Manufacturers*. London: The Stationery Office and Distributors. (3)

Attwood D. & Florence A.T. (1983) *Surfactant Systems, Their Chemistry, Pharmacy and Biology*. London: Chapman & Hall. (2.3.2)

Bloomfield S.F. & Baird R. (eds) (1996) *Microbial Quality Assurance in Pharmaceuticals, Cosmetics and Toiletries*, 2nd edn. Chichester: Ellis Horwood. (3)

Brannan D.K. (1995) Cosmetic preservation. *J Soc Cosmet Chem*, **46**, 199–220. (2)

British Pharmacopoeia (1993) Appendix XVI C: *Efficacy of Antimicrobial Preservation*, A191–A192, (and BP 1993, 1995 Addendum; Appendix XVII F, A407). London: HMSO. (3.2)

British Pharmacopoeia (1993) Appendix XVI B: *Tests for Microbial Contamination*, A184–A190 (and BP 1993, 1995 Addendum, Appendix XIV B, A405–A406). London: HMSO. (3.4)

British Pharmacopoeia (1993) (1996 Addendum) *Introduction: Microbial Contamination*, ixxxiii, and Appendix XVI D: *Microbial Quality of Pharmaceutical Preparations*, A519. London: HMSO. (3.4)

British Pharmacopoeia (1993) Appendix XVI A: *Test for Sterility*, A180–A184. London: HMSO. (3.4)

Denyer S. & Baird R. (eds) (1990) *Guide to Microbiological Control in Pharmaceuticals*. Chichester: Ellis Horwood. (3)

Gould G.W. (ed.) (1989) *Mechanisms of Action of Food Preservation Procedures*. Barking: Elsevier Science Publishers. (2)

Hugo W.B. (1995) A brief history of heat, chemical and radiation preservation and disinfectants. *Intl Biodet Biodeg*, **36**, 197–217. (2)

Martidale The Extra Pharmacopoeia, 31st edn. (1996) Disinfectants and Preservatives pp. 1111–1149. London: The Royal Pharmaceutical Society. (2)

Russell A.D., Hugo W.B. & Ayliffe G.A.J. (eds) (1998) *Principles and Practice of Disinfection, Preservation and Sterilization*, 2nd edn. Oxford: Blackwell Scientific Publications. (2)

Stebbing L. (1993) *Quality Assurance: The Route to Efficiency and Competitiveness*, 2nd edn. Chichester: Ellis Horwood. (3)

19 Contamination of non-sterile pharmaceuticals in hospital and community environments

1   Introduction

2   The significance of microbial
    contamination
2.1   Spoilage
2.2   Hazard to health

3   Sources of contamination
3.1   In manufacture
3.1.1   Water
3.1.2   Environment
3.1.3   Packaging
3.2   In use
3.2.1   Human sources
3.2.2   Environmental sources
3.2.3   Equipment sources

4   The extent of microbial contamination
4.1   Contamination in manufacture
4.2   Contamination in use

5   Factors determining the outcome of a
    medicament-borne infection
5.1   Type and degree of microbial
    contamination
5.2   The route of administration
5.3   Resistance of the patient

6   Prevention and control of
    contamination

7   Further reading

1   Introduction

Pharmaceutical products are used in a variety of ways in the prevention, treatment and diagnosis of disease. In recent years, manufacturers of pharmaceuticals have improved the quality of non-sterile products such that today the majority contain only a minimal microbial population. Nevertheless, a few rogue products with an unacceptable level and type of contamination will occasionally escape the quality control net and when used may, ironically, contribute to the spread of disease in patients.

Although the occurrence of product contamination has been well documented in medical literature, the significance for the patient has not always been clear. Evidence accumulated in the past 30 years or so has, however, enabled a better understanding of why and how contamination occurs, its extent and frequency, the factors determining the outcome for the patient and finally what preventive steps may be taken to control the problems.

2   The significance of microbial contamination

2.1   Spoilage

It has been known for many years that microbial contaminants may effect the spoilage of pharmaceutical products through chemical, physical or aesthetic changes in the nature of the product, thereby rendering it unfit for use (see Chapter 18). Active drug constituents may be metabolized to less potent or chemically inactive forms. Physical changes commonly seen are the breakdown of emulsions, visible surface growth on solids and the formation of slimes, pellicles or sediments in liquids, sometimes accompanied by the production of gas, odours or unwanted flavours, thereby rendering the product unacceptable and possibly even dangerous to the patient. It may, indeed, affect patient compliance with the prescribed course of therapy. Finally, spoilage and subsequent wastage of a product have serious economic implications for the manufacturer.

2.2   **Hazard to health**

Nowadays, it is well recognized that a contaminated pharmaceutical product may also present a potential health hazard to the patient. Although isolated outbreaks of medicament-related infections have been reported since the early part of this century, it is only in the past three decades or so that the significance of this contamination to the patient has been more fully understood. Recognition of these infections presents its own problems. It is a fortunate hospital physician who can, at an early stage, recognize contamination manifest as a cluster of infections of rapid onset, such as that following the use of a contaminated intravenous fluid in a hospital ward. The chances of a general practitioner recognizing a medicament-related infection of insidious onset, perhaps spread over several months, in a diverse group of patients in the community, are much more remote. Once recognized, there is of course a moral obligation to withdraw the offending product, and subsequent investigations of the incidence therefore become retrospective.

Pharmaceutical products of widely differing forms are susceptible to contamination by a variety of microorganisms, as shown by a few examples given in Table 19.1. Disinfectants, antiseptics, powders, tablets and other products providing an inhospitable

Table 19.1 Contaminants found in pharmaceutical products

Year	Product	Contaminant
1907	Plague vaccine	*Clostridium tetani*
1943	Fluorescein eye-drops	*Pseudomonas aeruginosa*
1946	Talcum powder	*Clostridium tetani*
1948	Serum vaccine	*Staphylococcus aureus*
1955	Chloroxylenol disinfectant	*Pseudomonas aeruginosa*
1966	Thyroid tablets	*Salmonella muenchen*
1966	Antibiotic eye ointment	*Pseudomonas aeruginosa*
1966	Saline solution	*Serratia marcescens*
1967	Carmine powder	*Salmonella cubana*
1967	Hand cream	*Klebsiella pneumoniae*
1969	Peppermint water	*Pseudomonas aeruginosa*
1970	Chlorhexidine–cetrimide antiseptic solution	*Pseudomonas cepacia*
1972	Intravenous fluids	*Pseudomonas, Erwinia* and *Enterobacter* spp.
1972	Pancreatin powder	*Salmonella agona*
1977	Contact-lens solution	*Serratia* and *Enterobacter* spp.
1981	Surgical dressings	*Clostridium* spp.
1982	Iodophor solution	*Pseudomonas aeruginosa*
1983	Aqueous soap	*Pseudomona stutzeri*
1984	Thymol mouthwash	*Pseudomonas aeruginosa*
1986	Antiseptic mouthwash	Coliforms

environment to invading contaminants are known to be at risk, as well as products with more nutritious components, such as creams and lotions with carbohydrates, amino acids, vitamins and often appreciable quantities of water. Contaminants isolated from products have ranged from true pathogens, such as *Cl. tetani*, to opportunist pathogens, such as *Ps. aeruginosa* and other free-living Gram-negative organisms, which are capable of causing disease under special circumstances. The outcome of using a contaminated product may vary from patient to patient, depending on the type and degree of contamination and how the product is to be used. Undoubtedly the most serious effects have been seen with contaminated injected products where generalized bacteraemic shock and in some cases death of patients have been reported. More likely, a wound or sore in broken skin may become locally infected or colonized by the contaminant; this may in turn result in extended hospital bed occupancy, with ensuing economic consequences. It must be stressed, however, that the majority of cases of medicament-related infections are probably not recognized or reported as such.

3   Sources of contamination

3.1   In manufacture

The same principles of contamination control apply whether manufacture takes place in industry (Chapter 17) or on a smaller scale in the hospital pharmacy. As discussed in Chapter 22, quality must be built into the product at all stages of the process and not simply assessed at the end of manufacture; (i) raw materials, particularly water and those of animal origin, must be of a high microbiological standard; (ii) all processing equipment should be subject to planned preventive maintenance and should be properly cleaned after use to prevent cross-contamination between batches; (iii) manufacture should take place in suitable premises in a clean, tidy work area supplied with filtered air; (iv) staff involved in manufacture should not only have good health but also a sound knowledge of the importance of personal and production hygiene; and (v) the end-product requires suitable packaging which will protect it from contamination during its shelf-life and is itself free from contamination.

Manufacture in hospital premises raises certain additional problems with regard to contamination control.

3.1.1   *Water*

Mains water in hospitals is frequently stored in large roof tanks, some of which may be relatively inaccessible and poorly maintained. Water for pharmaceutical manufacture requires some further treatment, usually by distillation, reverse osmosis (Chapter 17, section 3.5) or deionization or a combination of these, depending on the intended use of water. Such processes need careful monitoring, as does the microbiological quality of the water after treatment. Storage of water requires particular care, since some Gram-negative opportunist pathogens can survive on traces of organic matter present in treated water and will readily multiply at room temperature; water should therefore be stored at a temperature in excess of 80°C and circulated in the distribution system at a flow rate of 1–2 m/sec to prevent the build-up of bacterial biofilms in the piping.

Environment

The microbial flora of the pharmacy environment is a reflection of the general hospital environment and the activities undertaken there. Free-living opportunist pathogens, such as *Ps. aeruginosa* can normally be found in all wet sites, such as drains, sinks and taps. Cleaning equipment, such as mops, buckets, cloths and scrubbing machines, may be responsible for distributing these organisms around the pharmacy; if stored wet they provide a convenient niche for microbial growth, resulting in heavy contamination of equipment. Contamination levels in the production environment may, however, be minimized by observing good manufacturing practices, by installing heating traps in sink U-bends, thus destroying one of the main reservoirs of contaminants, and by proper maintenance and storage of equipment, including cleaning equipment. Additionally, cleaning of production units by contractors should be carried out to a pharmaceutical specification.

3.1.3

Packaging

Sacking, cardboard, card liners, corks and paper are unsuitable for packaging pharmaceuticals, as they are heavily contaminated, for example with bacterial or fungal spores. These have now been replaced by non-biodegradable plastic materials. Packaging in hospitals is frequently re-used for economic reasons. Large numbers of containers may be returned to the pharmacy, bringing with them microbial contaminants introduced during use in the wards. Particular problems have been encountered in the past with disinfectant solutions where residues of old stock have been 'topped up' with fresh supplies, resulting in the issue of contaminated solutions to wards. Re-usable containers must, therefore, be thoroughly washed and dried, and never refilled directly.

Another common practice in hospitals is the repackaging of products purchased in bulk into smaller containers. Increased handling of the product inevitably increases the risk of contamination, as shown by one survey when hospital-repacked items were found to be contaminated twice as often as those in the original pack (Public Health Laboratory Service Report 1971).

3.2

In use

Pharmaceutical manufacturers may justly argue that their responsibility ends with the supply of a well-preserved product of high microbiological standard in a suitable pack and that the subsequent use, or indeed abuse, of the product is of little concern to them. Although much less is known about how products become contaminated during use, there is reasonable evidence that continued use of such products is undesirable, particularly in hospitals where it may result in the spread of cross-infection.

All multidose products are subject to contamination from a number of sources during use. The sources of contamination are the same whether products are used in hospital or in the community environment, but opportunities for observing it are, of course, greater in the former.

During normal usage, the patient may contaminate his/her medicine with his/her own microbial flora; subsequent use of the product may or may not result in self-infection (Fig. 19.1). Topical products are considered to be most at risk, since the product will probably be applied by hand thus introducing contaminants from the resident skin flora of staphylococci, *Micrococcus* spp. and diphtheroids but also perhaps transient contaminants, such as *Pseudomonas*, which would normally be removed during effective handwashing. Opportunities for contamination may be reduced by using disposable applicators for topical products or by taking oral products by disposable spoon.

In hospitals, multidose products, once contaminated, may serve as a vehicle of cross-contamination or cross-infection between patients. Zinc-based products packed in large stock-pots and used in the treatment and prevention of bed-sores in long-stay and geriatric patients may become contaminated during use with organisms such as *Ps. aeruginosa* and *Staphylococcus aureus*. These unpreserved products will allow multiplication of contaminants, especially if water is present either as part of the formulation, for example in oil/water (o/w) emulsions, as a film in w/o emulsions which have undergone local cracking, or as a condensed film from atmospheric water, and appreciable numbers may then be transferred to other patients when re-used. Clearly the economics and convenience of using stock-pots need to be balanced against the risk of spreading cross-infection between patients and the inevitable increase in length of the patients' stay in hospital. The use of stock-pots in hospitals has noticeably declined over the past decade or so.

A further potential source of contamination in hospitals is the nursing staff responsible for medicament administration. During the course of their work, nurses' hands become contaminated with opportunist pathogens which are not part of the normal skin flora but are easily removed by thorough handwashing and drying. In busy wards, handwashing between attending to patients may be omitted and any contaminants may subsequently be transferred to medicaments during administration. Hand lotions and creams used to prevent chapping of nurses' hands may similarly become contaminated, especially when packaged in multidose containers and left at the side of the handbasin, frequently without a lid. The importance of thorough handwashing cannot be over-emphasized in the control of hospital cross-infection. Hand lotions and creams should be well preserved and, ideally, packaged in disposable dispensers. Other effective control methods include the supply of products in individual patient's packs and the use of a non-touch technique for medicament administration.

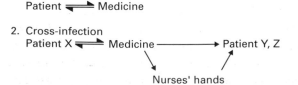

Fig. 19.1 Mechanisms of contamination during use of medicinal products.

Environmental sources

Small numbers of airborne contaminants may settle out in products left open to the atmosphere. Some of these will die during storage, with the rest probably remaining at a static level of about 10^2–10^3 colony forming units (cfu) g^{-1} or ml^{-1}. Larger numbers of water-borne contaminants may be accidentally introduced into topical products by wet hands or by a 'splash-back mechanism', if left at the side of a basin. Such contaminants generally have simple nutritional requirements and, following multiplication, levels of contamination may often exceed 10^6 cfu g^{-1} or ml^{-1}. This problem is encountered particularly when the product is stored in warm hospital wards or in hot steamy bathroom cupboards at home. Products used in hospitals as soap substitutes for bathing patients are particularly at risk, and soon not only become contaminated with opportunist pathogens such as *Pseudomonas* spp., but also provide conditions conducive for their multiplication. The problem is compounded by using stocks in multidose pots for use by several patients in the same ward over an extended period of time.

The indigenous microbial population is quite different in the home and in hospitals. Pathogenic organisms are found much more frequently in the latter and consequently are isolated more often from medicines used in hospital. Usually, there are fewer opportunities for contamination in the home, as patients are generally issued with individual supplies in small quantities.

Equipment sources

Patients and nursing staff may use a range of applicators (pads, sponges, brushes, spatulas) during medicament administration, particularly for topical products. If re-used, these easily become contaminated and may be responsible for perpetuating contamination between fresh stocks of product, as has indeed been shown in studies of cosmetic products. Disposable applicators or swabs should therefore always be used.

In hospitals today a wide variety of complex equipment is used in the course of patient treatment. Humidifiers, incubators, ventilators, resuscitators and other apparatus require proper maintenance and decontamination after use. Chemical disinfectants used for this purpose have in the past through misuse become contaminated with opportunist pathogens, such as *Ps. aeruginosa*, and ironically have contributed to, rather than reduced, the spread of cross-infection in hospital patients. Disinfectants should only be used for their intended purpose and directions for use must be followed at all times.

4   The extent of microbial contamination

Detailed examination of reports in the literature of medicament-borne contamination reveals that the majority of these are anecdotal in nature, referring to a specific product and isolated incident. Little information is available, however, as to the overall risk of products becoming contaminated and causing patient infections when subsequently used. As with risk analysis in food microbiology (assessment of the hazards of consumption of a contaminated preparation) this information is considered invaluable not only because it indicates the effectiveness of existing practices and standards, but also because the value of potential improvements in quality from a patient's point of view can be balanced against the inevitable cost of such processes. Thus, the old argument that all pharmaceutical products, regardless of their use, should be produced as sterile products, although sound in principle, is kept in perspective by the fact that it cannot be justified on economic grounds alone.

4.1 Contamination in manufacture

Investigations carried out by the Swedish National Board of Health in 1965 revealed some startling findings on the overall microbiological quality immediately after manufacture of non-sterile products made in Sweden. A wide range of products was routinely found to be contaminated with *Bacillus subtilis, Staph. albus*, yeasts and moulds, and in addition large numbers of coliforms were found in a variety of tablets. Furthermore, two nationwide outbreaks of infection were subsequently traced to the inadvertent use of contaminated products. Two hundred patients were involved in an outbreak of salmonellosis, caused by thyroid tablets contaminated with *Salmonella bareilly* and *Sal. muenchen*; and eight patients had severe eye infections following the use of hydrocortisone eye ointment contaminated with *Ps. aeruginosa*. The results of this investigation have not only been used as a yardstick for comparing the microbiological quality of non-sterile products made in other countries, but also as a baseline upon which international standards could be founded.

In the UK, the microbiological and chemical quality of pharmaceutical products made by industry has since been governed by the Medicines Act 1968. The majority of products have been found to be made to a high standard, although spot checks have occasionally revealed medicines of unacceptable quality and so necessitated product recall. By contrast, the manufacture of pharmaceutical products in hospitals has in the past been much less rigorously controlled, as shown by the results of surveys in the 1970s in which significant numbers of preparations were found to be contaminated with *Ps. aeruginosa*. In 1974, hospital manufacture also came under the terms of the Medicines Act and, as a consequence, considerable improvements have been seen in recent years not only in the conditions and standard of manufacture, but also in the chemical and microbiological quality of finished products.

Furthermore, in the past decade hospital manufacturing operations have been rationalized. Economic restraints have resulted in a critical evaluation of the true cost of these activities; competitive purchasing from industry has in many cases produced cheaper alternatives and small-scale manufacturing has been largely discouraged. Where licensed products are available, NHS policy now dictates that these are purchased from a commercial source and not made locally. Hospital manufacturing is at present concentrated on the supply of bespoke products from a regional centre or small-scale specialist manufacture of those items currently unobtainable from industry. Repacking of commercial products into more convenient pack sizes is still, however, common practice.

Removal of Crown immunity from the NHS in 1991 meant that manufacturing operations in hospitals were then subject to the full licensing provisions of the Medicines

Act 1968, i.e. hospital pharmacies intending to manufacture were required to obtain a manufacturing licence and to comply fully with the EC Guide to Good Pharmaceutical Manufacturing Practice (1989, revised in 1992); amongst other requirements, this included the use of appropriate environmental manufacturing conditions and associated environmental monitoring. Subsequently, the Medicines Control Agency (MCA) issued guidance in 1992 on certain manufacturing exemptions, by virtue of the product batch size or frequency of manufacture. At the same time the need for extemporaneous dispensing of 'one-off' special formulae continues in hospital pharmacies today, although this work has largely been transferred from the dispensing bench to dedicated preparative facilities with appropriate environmental control.

4.2 Contamination in use

Higher rates of contamination are invariably seen in products after opening and use, and, amongst these, medicines used in hospitals are more likely to be contaminated than those used in the general community. The Public Health Laboratory Service Report of 1971 expressed concern at the overall incidence of contamination in non-sterile products used on hospital wards (327 of 1220 samples) and the proportion of samples found to be heavily contaminated (18% in excess of 10^4 cfu g^{-1} or ml^{-1}). The presence of *Ps. aeruginosa* in 2.7% of samples (mainly oral alkaline mixtures) was considered to be highly undesirable.

By contrast, medicines used in the home are not only less often contaminated but also contain lower levels of contaminants and fewer pathogenic organisms. Generally, there are fewer opportunities for contamination here since smaller quantities are used by individual patients. Medicines in the home may, however, be hoarded and used for extended periods of time. Additionally, storage conditions may be unsuitable and expiry dates ignored and thus problems other than those of microbial contamination may be seen in the home.

5 Factors determining the outcome of a medicament-borne infection

A patient's response to the microbial challenge of a contaminated medicine may be diverse and unpredictable, perhaps with serious consequences. In one patient, no clinical reactions may be evident, yet in another these may be indisputable, illustrating one problem in the recognition of medicament-borne infections. Clinical reactions may range from inconvenient local infections of wounds or broken skin, caused possibly from contact with a contaminated cream, to gastrointestinal infections from the ingestion of contaminated oral products, to serious widespread infections, such as a bacteraemia or septicaemia, leading perhaps to death, as have resulted from infusion of contaminated fluids. Undoubtedly, the most serious outbreaks of infection have been seen in the past where contaminated products have been injected directly into the bloodstream of patients whose immunity is already compromised by their underlying disease or therapy. The outcome of any episode is determined by a combination of several factors, amongst which the type and degree of microbial contamination, the route of administration and the patient's resistance are of particular importance.

5.1 Type and degree of microbial contamination

Microorganisms that contaminate medicines and cause disease in patients may be classified as true pathogens or opportunist pathogens. Pathogenic organisms like *Clostridium tetani* and *Salmonella* spp. rarely occur in products, but when present cause serious problems. Wound infections from using contaminated dusting powders have been reported, including several cases of neonatal death from talcum powder containing *Cl. tetani*. Outbreaks of salmonellosis have followed the inadvertent ingestion of contaminated thyroid and pancreatic powders. On the other hand, opportunist pathogens like *Ps. aeruginosa*, *Klebsiella*, *Serratia* and other free-living organisms are more frequently isolated from medicinal products and, as their name suggests, may be pathogenic if given the opportunity. The main concern with these organisms is that their simple nutritional requirements enable them to survive in a wide range of pharmaceuticals, and thus they tend to be present in high numbers, perhaps in excess of 10^6–10^7 cfu g^{-1} or ml^{-1}; nevertheless, the product itself may show no visible sign of contamination. Opportunist pathogens can survive in disinfectants and antiseptic solutions which are normally used in the control of hospital cross-infection but which when contaminated may even perpetuate the spread of infection. Compromised hospital patients, i.e. the elderly, burned, traumatized or immunosuppressed, are considered to be particularly at risk from infection with these organisms, whereas healthy patients in the general community have given little cause for concern.

The critical dose of microorganisms which will initiate an infection is largely unknown and varies not only between species but also within a species. Animal and human volunteer studies have indicated that the infecting dose may be reduced significantly in the presence of trauma or foreign bodies or if accompanied by a drug having a local vasoconstrictive action.

5.2 The route of administration

As stated previously, contaminated products injected directly into the bloodstream or instilled into the eye cause the most serious problems. Intrathecal and epidural injections are potentially hazardous procedures. In practice, epidural injections are frequently given through a bacterial filter. Injectable and ophthalmic solutions are often simple solutions and provide Gram-negative opportunist pathogens with sufficient nutrients to multiply during storage; if contaminated, numbers in excess of 10^6 cfu and endotoxins should be expected. Total parenteral nutrition fluids, formulated for individual patients' nutritional requirements, can also provide more than adequate nutritional support for invading contaminants. *Pseudomonas aeruginosa*, the notorious contaminant of eye-drops, has caused serious ophthalmic infections, including the loss of sight in some cases. The problem is compounded when the eye is damaged through the improper use of contact lenses or scratched by fingernails or cosmetic applicators.

The fate of contaminants ingested orally in medicines may be determined by several factors, as is seen with contaminated food. The acidity of the stomach may provide a successful barrier, depending on whether the medicine is taken on an empty or full stomach and also on the gastric emptying time. Contaminants in topical products may cause little harm when deposited on intact skin. Not only does the skin itself provide an excellent mechanical barrier but, furthermore, few contaminants normally survive in competition with its resident microbial flora. Skin damaged during surgery or trauma or in patients with burns or pressure sores may, however, be rapidly colonized and subsequently infected by opportunist pathogens. Patients treated with topical steroids are also prone to local infections, particularly if contaminated steroid drugs are inadvertently used.

5.3 Resistance of the patient

A patient's resistance is crucial in determining the outcome of a medicament-borne infection. Hospital patients are more exposed and susceptible to infection than those treated in the general community. Neonates, the elderly, diabetics and patients traumatized by surgery or accident may have impaired defence mechanisms. People suffering from leukaemia and those treated with immunosuppressants are most vulnerable to infection; there is a strong case for providing all medicines in a sterile form for these patients.

6 Prevention and control of contamination

Prevention is undoubtedly better than cure in minimizing the risk of medicament-borne infections. In manufacture the principles of good manufacturing practice must be observed, and control measures must be built in at all stages. Initial stability tests should show that the proposed formulation can withstand an appropriate microbial challenge; raw materials from an authorized supplier should comply with in-house microbial specifications; environmental conditions, appropriate to the production process, require regular microbiological monitoring; finally, end-product analysis should indicate that the product is microbiologically suitable for its intended use and conforms to accepted in-house and international standards.

Based on present knowledge, contaminants, by virtue of their type or number, should not present a potential health hazard to patients when used.

Contamination during use is less easily controlled. Successful measures in the hospital pharmacy have included the packaging of products as individual units, thereby discouraging the use of multidose containers. Unit packaging (one dose per patient) has clear advantages, but economic constraints prevent this desirable procedure from being realized. Ultimately, the most fruitful approach is through the training and education of patients and hospital staff, so that medicines are used only for their intended purpose. The task of implementing this approach inevitably rests with the clinical and community pharmacists of the future.

7 Further reading

Baird R.M. (1981) Drugs and cosmetics. In: *Microbial Biodeterioration* (ed. A.H. Rose), pp. 387–426. London: Academic Press.

Baird R.M. (1985) Microbial contamination of pharmaceutical products made in a hospital pharmacy. *Pharm J*, **234**, 54–55.

Baird R.M. (1985) Microbial contamination of non-sterile pharmaceutical products made in hospitals in the North East Regional Health Authority. *J Clin Hosp Pharm*, **10**, 95–100.

Baird R.M. & Shooter R.A. (1976) *Pseudomonas aeruginosa* infections associated with the use of contaminated medicaments. *Br Med J*, **2**, 349–350.

Baird R.M., Brown W.R.L. & Shooter R.A. (1976) *Pseudomonas aeruginosa* in hospital pharmacies. *Br Med J*, **1**, 511–512.

Baird R.M., Elhag K.M. & Shaw E.J. (1976) *Pseudomonas thomasii* in a hospital distilled water supply. *J Med Microbiol*, **9**, 493–495.

Baird R.M., Parks A. & Awad Z.A. (1977) Control of *Pseudomonas aeruginosa* in pharmacy environments and medicaments. *Pharm J*, **119**, 164–165.

Baird R.M., Crowden C.A., O'Farrell S.M. & Shooter R.A. (1979) Microbial contamination of pharmaceutical products in the home. *J Hyg*, **83**, 277–283.

Baird R.M. & Bloomfield S.F.L. (eds) (1996) *Microbial Quality Assurance of Cosmetics, Toiletries and Non-sterile Pharmaceuticals*. London: Taylor and Francis.

Bassett D.C.J. (1971) Causes and prevention of sepsis due to Gram-negative bacteria: common sources of outbreaks. *Proc R Soc Med*, **64**, 980–986.

Crompton D.O. (1962) Ophthalmic prescribing. *Australas J Pharm*, **43**, 1020–1028.

Denyer S.P. & Baird R.M. (eds) (1990) *Guide to Microbiological Control in Pharmaceuticals*. Chichester: Ellis Horwood.

EC Guide to Good Manufacturing Practice (1992).

Hills S. (1946) The isolation of *Cl. tetani* from infected talc. *N Z Med J*, **45**, 419–423.

Kallings L.O., Ringertz O., Silverstolpe L. & Ernerfeldt F. (1966) Microbiological contamination of medicinal preparations. 1965 Report to the Swedish National Board of Health. *Acta Pharm Suecica*, **3**, 219–228.

Maurer I.M. (1985) *Hospital Hygiene*, 3rd edn. London: Edward Arnold.

Meers P.D., Calder M.W., Mazhar M.M. & Lawrie G.M. (1973) Intravenous infusion of contaminated dextrose solution: the Devonport incident. *Lancet*, **ii**, 1189–1192.

Morse L.J., Williams H.I., Grenn F.P., Eldridge E.F. & Rotta J.R. (1967) Septicaemia due to *Klebsiella pneumoniae* originating from a handcream dispenser. *N Engl J Med*, **277**, 472–473.

Myers G.E. & Pasutto F.M. (1973) Microbial contamination of cosmetics and toiletries. *Can J Pharm Sci*, **8**, 19–23.

Noble W.C. & Savin J.A. (1966) Steroid cream contaminated with *Pseudomonas aeruginosa*. *Lancet*, **i**, 347–349.

Parker M.T. (1972) The clinical significance of the presence of microorganisms in pharmaceutical and cosmetic preparations. *J Soc Cosm Chem*, **23**, 415–426.

Report of the Public Health Laboratory Service Working Party (1971) Microbial contamination of medicines administered to hospital patients. *Pharm J*, **207**, 96–99.

Russell A.D., Hugo W.G. & Ayliffe G.A.J. (eds) (1998) *Principles and Practice of Disinfection, Preservation and Sterilization*, 3rd edn. Oxford: Blackwell Science.

Smart R. & Spooner D.F. (1972) Microbiological spoilage in pharmaceuticals and cosmetics. *J Soc Cosm Chem*, **23**, 721–737.

20 Principles and practice of sterilization

1   **Introduction**

2   **Sensitivity of microorganisms**
2.1   Survivor curves
2.2   Expressions of resistance
2.2.1   *D*-value
2.2.2   *z*-value
2.3   Sterility assurance

3   **Sterilization methods**

4   **Heat sterilization**
4.1   Sterilization process
4.2   Moist heat sterilization
4.2.1   Steam as a sterilizing agent
4.2.2   Sterilizer design and operation
4.3   Dry heat sterilization
4.3.1   Sterilizer design
4.3.2   Sterilizer operation

5   **Gaseous sterilization**
5.1   Ethylene oxide

5.1.1   Sterilizer design and operation
5.2   Formaldehyde
5.2.1   Sterilizer design and operation

6   **Radiation sterilization**
6.1   Sterilizer design and operation
6.1.1   Gamma-ray sterilizers
6.1.2   Electron accelerators
6.1.3   Ultraviolet irradiation

7   **Filtration sterilization**
7.1   Filtration sterilization of liquids
7.2   Filtration sterilization of gases

8   **Conclusions**

9   **Acknowledgements**

10   **Appendix**

11   **Further reading**

1   Introduction

Sterilization is an essential stage in the processing of any product destined for parenteral administration, or for contact with broken skin, mucosal surfaces or internal organs, where the threat of infection exists. In addition, the sterilization of microbiological materials, soiled dressings and other contaminated items is necessary to minimize the health hazard associated with these articles.

Sterilization processes involve the application of a biocidal agent or physical microbial removal process to a product or preparation with the object of killing or removing all microorganisms. These processes may involve elevated temperature, reactive gas, irradiation or filtration through a microorganism-proof filter. The success of the process depends upon a suitable choice of treatment conditions, e.g. temperature and duration of exposure. It must be remembered, however, that with all articles to be sterilized there is a potential risk of product damage, which for a pharmaceutical preparation may result in reduced therapeutic efficacy or patient acceptability. Thus, there is a need to achieve a balance between the maximum acceptable risk of failing to achieve sterility and the maximum level of product damage which is acceptable. This is best determined from a knowledge of the properties of the sterilizing agent, the properties of the product to be sterilized and the nature of the likely contaminants. A suitable sterilization process may then be selected to ensure maximum microbial kill/removal with minimum product deterioration.

1   Sensitivity of microorganisms

The general pattern of resistance of microorganisms to biocidal sterilization processes is independent of the type of agent employed (heat, radiation or gas), with vegetative forms of bacteria and fungi, along with the larger viruses, showing a greater sensitivity to sterilization processes than small viruses and bacterial or fungal spores. The choice of suitable reference organisms for testing the efficiency of sterilization processes (see Chapter 23) is therefore made from the most durable bacterial spores, usually represented by *Bacillus stearothermophilus* for moist heat, certain strains of *B. subtilis* for dry heat and gaseous sterilization, and *B. pumilus* for ionizing radiation.

Ideally, when considering the level of treatment necessary to achieve sterility a knowledge of the type and total number of microorganisms present in a product, together with their likely response to the proposed treatment, is necessary. Without this information, however, it is usually assumed that organisms within the load are no more resistant than the reference spores or than specific resistant product isolates. In the latter case, it must be remembered that resistance may be altered or lost entirely by laboratory subculture and the resistance characteristics of the maintained strain must be regularly checked.

A sterilization process may thus be developed without a full microbiological background to the product, instead being based on the ability to deal with a 'worst case' condition. This is indeed the situation for official sterilization methods which must be capable of general application, and modern pharmacopoeial recommendations are derived from a careful analysis of experimental data on bacterial spore survival following treatments with heat, ionizing radiation or gas.

However, the infectious agents responsible for spongiform encephalopathies such as bovine spongiform encehalopathy (BSE) and Creutzfeldt–Jacob disease (CJD) exhibit exceptional degrees of resistance to all known lethal agents. Recent work has even cast doubts on the adequacy of the process of 18 min exposure to steam at 134–138°C which has been officially recommended for the destruction of these agents (and which far exceeds the lethal treatment required to achieve adequate destruction of bacterial spores).

2.1   Survivor curves

When exposed to a killing process, populations of microorganisms generally lose their viability in an exponential fashion, independent of the initial number of organisms. This can be represented graphically with a 'survivor curve' drawn from a plot of the logarithm of the fraction of survivors against the exposure time or dose (Fig. 20.1). Of the typical curves obtained, all have a linear portion which may be continuous (plot A), or may be modified by an initial shoulder (B) or by a reduced rate of kill at low survivor levels (C). Furthermore, a short activation phase, representing an initial increase in viable count, may be seen during the heat treatment of certain bacterial spores. Survivor curves have been employed principally in the examination of heat sterilization methods, but can equally well be applied to any biocidal process.

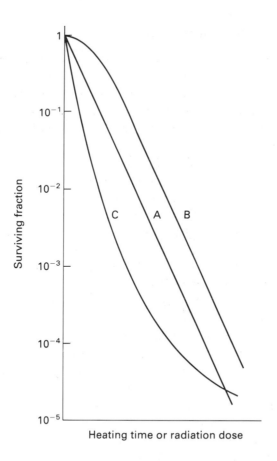

Fig. 20.1 Typical survivor curves for bacterial spores exposed to moist heat or gamma-radiation.

2.2 Expressions of resistance

2.2.1 *D-value*

The resistance of an organism to a sterilizing agent can be described by means of the *D*-value. For heat and radiation treatments, respectively, this is defined as the time taken at a fixed temperature or the radiation dose required to achieve a 90% reduction in viable cells (i.e. a 1 log cycle reduction in survivors; Fig. 20.2A). The calculation of the *D*-value assumes a linear type A survivor curve (Fig. 20.1), and must be corrected to allow for any deviation from linearity with type B or C curves. Some typical *D*-values for resistant bacterial spores are given in Table 23.2 (Chapter 23).

2.2.2 *z-value*

For heat treatment, a *D*-value only refers to the resistance of a microorganism at a particular temperature. In order to assess the influence of temperature changes on thermal resistance a relationship between temperature and log *D*-value can be developed leading to the expression of a *z*-value, which represents the increase in temperature needed to reduce the *D*-value of an organism by 90% (i.e. 1 log cycle reduction; Fig. 20.2B). For bacterial spores used as biological indicators for moist heat (*B. stearothermophilus*)

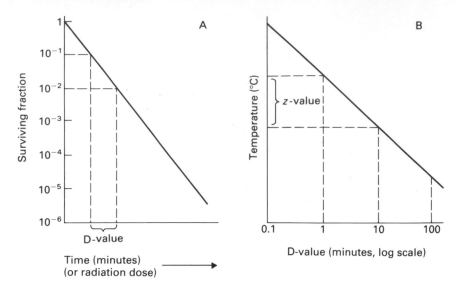

Fig.20.2 Calculation of: (A) D-value; (B) z-value.

and dry heat (*B. subtilis*) sterilization processes, mean z-values are given as 10°C and 22°C, respectively. The z-value is not truly independent of temperature but may be considered essentially constant over the temperature ranges used in heat sterilization processes.

2.3 Sterility assurance

The term 'sterile', in a microbiological context, means no surviving organisms whatsoever. Thus, there are no degrees of sterility; an item is either sterile or it is not, and so there are no levels of contamination which may be considered negligible or insignificant and therefore acceptable.

From the survivor curves presented, it can be seen that the elimination of viable microorganisms from a product is a time-dependent process, and will be influenced by the rate and duration of biocidal action and the initial microbial contamination level. It is also evident from Fig. 20.2A that true sterility, represented by zero survivors, can only be achieved after an infinite exposure period or radiation dose. Clearly, then, it is illogical to claim, or expect, that a sterilization procedure will *guarantee* sterility. Thus, the likelihood of a product being produced free of microorganisms is best expressed in terms of the probability of an organism surviving the treatment process, a possibility not entertained in the absolute term 'sterile'. From this approach has arisen the concept of sterility assurance or a microbial safety index which gives a numerical value to the probability of a single surviving organism remaining to contaminate a processed product. For pharmaceutical products, the most frequently applied standard is that the probability, post-sterilization, of a non-sterile unit is ≤ 1 in 1 million units processed (i.e. $\leq 10^{-6}$). The sterilization protocol necessary to achieve this with any given organism of known D-value can be established from the inactivation factor (IF) which may be defined as:

$$IF = 10^{t/D}$$

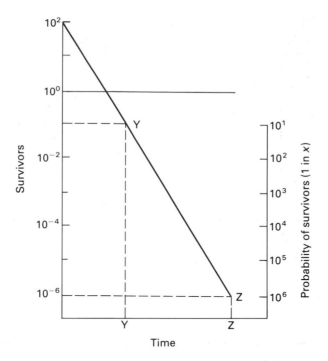

Fig. 20.3 Sterility assurance. At Y, there is (literally) 10^{-1} bacterium in one bottle, i.e. in 10 loads of single containers, there would be one chance in 10 that one load would be positive. Likewise, at Z, there is (literally) 10^{-6} bacterium in one bottle, i.e. in 1 million (10^6) loads of single containers, there is one chance in 1 million that one load would be positive.

where t is the contact time (for a heat or gaseous sterilization process) or dose (for ionizing radiation) and D is the D-value appropriate to the process employed.

Thus, for an initial burden of 10^2 spores an inactivation factor of 10^8 will be needed to give the required sterility assurance of 10^{-6} (Fig. 20.3). The sterilization process will therefore need to produce sufficient lethality to achieve an 8 log cycle reduction in viable organisms; this will require exposure of the product to eight times the D-value of the reference organism ($8D$). In practice, it is generally assumed that the contaminant will have the same resistance as the test spores unless full microbiological data are available to indicate otherwise. The inactivation factors associated with certain sterilization protocols and their biological indicator organisms (Chapter 23) are given in Table 20.1.

3 Sterilization methods

The *British Pharmacopoeia* (1993) recognizes five methods for the sterilization of pharmaceutical products. These are: (i) dry heat; (ii) heating in an autoclave (steam sterilization); (iii) filtration; (iv) ethylene oxide gas; and (v) gamma or electron radiation. In addition, other approaches involving steam and formaldehyde and ultraviolet (UV) light have evolved for use in certain situations. For each method, the possible permutations of exposure conditions are numerous, but experience and product stability

Table 20.1 Inactivation factors (IF) for selected sterilization protocols and their corresponding biological indicator (BI) organisms

Sterilization protocol	BI organism	D-value	IF
Moist heat (121°C for 15 minutes)	B. stearothermophilus	1.5 min	10
Dry heat (160°C for 2 hours)	B. subtilis var. niger	Max. 10 min	Min. 12
Irradiation (25 kGy; 2.5 Mrad)	B. pumilus	3 kGy (0.3 Mrad)	8.3

requirements have generally served to limit this choice. Nevertheless, it should be remembered that even the recommended methods and regimens do not necessarily demonstrate equivalent biocidal potential, but simply offer alternative strategies for application to a wide variety of product types. Thus, each should be validated in their application to demonstrate that the minimum required level of sterility assurance can be achieved (section 2.3 and Chapter 23).

In the following sections, factors governing the successful use of these sterilizing methods will be covered and their application to pharmaceutical and medical products considered. Methods for monitoring the efficacy of these processes are discussed in Chapter 23.

4 Heat sterilization

Heat is the most reliable and widely used means of sterilization, affording its antimicrobial activity through destruction of enzymes and other essential cell constituents. These lethal events proceed at their most rapid in a fully hydrated state, thus requiring a lower heat input (temperature and time) under conditions of high humidity where denaturation and hydrolysis reactions predominate, rather than in the dry state where oxidative changes take place. This method of sterilization is limited to thermostable products, but can be applied to both moisture-sensitive and moisture-resistant products for which the *British Pharmacopoeia* (1993) recommends dry (160–180°C) and moist (121–134°C) heat sterilization, respectively. Where thermal degradation of a product might possibly occur, it can usually be minimized by selecting the higher temperature range since the shorter exposure times employed generally result in a lower fractional degradation.

4.1 Sterilization process

In any heat sterilization process, the articles to be treated must first be raised to sterilization temperature and this involves a heating-up stage. In the traditional approach, timing for the process (the holding time) then begins. It has been recognized, however, that during both the heating-up and cooling-down stages of a sterilization cycle (Fig. 20.4), the product is held at an elevated temperature and these stages may thus contribute to the overall biocidal potential of the process.

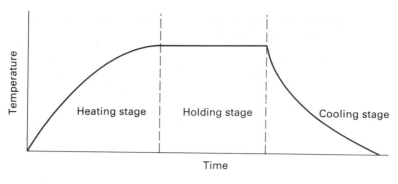

Fig. 20.4 Typical temperature profile of a heat sterilization process.

A method has been devised to convert all the temperature–time combinations occurring during the heating, sterilizing and cooling stages of a moist heat (steam) sterilization cycle to the equivalent time at 121°C. This involves following the temperature profile of a load, integrating the heat input (as a measure of lethality), and converting it to the equivalent time at the standard temperature of 121°C. Using this approach the overall lethality of any process can be deduced and is defined as the *F*-value, which expresses heat treatment at any temperature as equal to that of a certain number of minutes at 121°C. In other words, if a moist heat sterilization process has an *F*-value of *x*, then it has the same lethal effect on a given organism as heating at 121°C for *x* minutes, irrespective of the actual temperature employed or of any fluctuations in the heating process due to heating and cooling stages. The *F*-value of a process will vary according to the moist heat resistance of the reference organism; when the reference spore is that of *B. stearothermophilus* with a *z*-value of 10°C, then the *F*-value is known as the F_0-value.

A relationship between *F*- and *D*-values, leading to an assessment of the probable number of survivors in a load following heat treatment, can be established from the following equation:

$$F = D (\log N_0 - \log N)$$

in which *D* is the *D*-value at 121°C, and N_0 and *N* represent, respectively, the initial and final number of viable cells per unit volume.

The *F*-concept has evolved from the food industry and principally relates to the sterilization of articles by moist heat. Because it permits calculation of the extent to which the heating and cooling phases contribute to the overall killing effect of the autoclaving cycle, the *F*-concept enables a sterilization process to be individually developed for a particular product. This means that adequate sterility assurance can be achieved in autoclaving cycles in which the traditional pharmacopoeial recommendation of 15 min at 121°C is not achieved. The holding time may be reduced below 15 min if there is a substantial killing effect during the heating and cooling phases, and an adequate cycle can be achieved even if the 'target' temperature of 121°C is not reached. Thus, *F*-values offer both a means by which alternative sterilizing cycles can be compared in terms of their microbial killing efficiency, and a mechanism by which over-processing of marginally thermolabile products can be reduced without compromising sterility assurance. They have found application in the sterilization of medical and pharmaceutical products by moist heat where, for aqueous preparations, the *British Pharmacopoeia* (1993) generally requires a minimum F_0-value of 8 from a steam sterilization process.

There is an apparent anomaly in that it also states that the 'preferred' combination of temperature and time is a minimum of 121°C maintained for 15 minutes, which, by definition, equates to an F_0 value of 15. The latter, however, is applicable where the material to be sterilized may contain relatively large numbers of thermophilic bacterial spores, and an F_0 of 8 is appropriate for a 'microbiologically validated' process where the bioburden is low and the spores likely to be present are those of (the generally more heat sensitive) mesophilic species.

F_0 values may be calculated either from the 'area under the curve' of a plot of autoclave temperature against time constructed using special chart paper on which the temperature scale is modified to take into account the progressively greater lethality of higher temperatures, or by use of the equation below:

$$F_0 = \Delta t \, \Sigma 10^{(T-121)/z}$$

where Δt = time interval between temperature measurements; T = product temperature at time t; z is (assumed to be) 10°C.

Thus, if temperatures were being recorded from a thermocouple at 1.00 minute intervals then $\Delta t = 1.00$, and a temperature of, for example, 115°C maintained for 1 minute would give an F_0 value of 1 minute $\times 10^{(115-121)/10}$ which is equal to 0.251 minutes. In practice, such calculations could easily be performed on the data from several thermocouples within an autoclave using PC-driven software, and, in a manufacturing situation, these would be part of the batch records. Such a calculation facility is offered as an optional extra by most autoclave manufacturers.

Application of the F-value concept has been largely restricted to steam sterilization processes although there is a less frequently employed, but direct parallel in dry heat sterilization (see section 4.3).

4.2   Moist heat sterilization

Moist heat has been recognized as an efficient biocidal agent from the early days of bacteriology, when it was principally developed for the sterilization of culture media. It now finds widespread application in the processing of many thermostable products and devices. In the pharmaceutical and medical sphere it is used in the sterilization of dressings, sheets, surgical and diagnostic equipment, containers and closures, and aqueous injections, ophthalmic preparations and irrigation fluids, in addition to the processing of soiled and contaminated items (Chapter 21).

Sterilization by moist heat usually involves the use of steam at temperatures in the range 121–134°C, and while alternative strategies are available for the processing of products unstable at these high temperatures, they rarely offer the same degree of sterility assurance and should be avoided if at all possible. The elevated temperatures generally associated with moist heat sterilization methods can only be achieved by the generation of steam under pressure.

By far the most commonly employed standard temperature/time cycles for bottled fluids and porous loads (e.g. surgical dressings) are 121°C for 15 minutes and 134°C

Table 20.2 Pressure–temperature relationships and antimicrobial efficacies of alternative steam sterilization cycles

Temperature (°C)	Holding time (minutes)	Steam pressure		Inactivation factor* (decimal reductions)
		(kPa)	(psi)	
115	30	69	10	5.2
121	15	103	15	10
126	10	138	20	21
134	3	207	30	40

* Calculated for a spore suspension having a D_{121} of 1.5 minutes and a Z value of 10°C.

for 3 minutes, respectively. Not only do high temperature–short time cycles often result in lower fractional degradation (see section 4), they also afford the advantage of achieving higher levels of sterility assurance due to greater inactivation factors (Table 20.2). The 115°C for 30 minute cycle was considered an acceptable alternative to 121°C for 15 minutes prior to the publication of the 1988 *British Pharmacopoeia*, but it is no longer considered sufficient to give the desired sterility assurance levels for products which may contain significant concentrations of thermophilic spores.

4.2.1 Steam as a sterilizing agent

To act as an efficient sterilizing agent, steam should be able to provide moisture and heat efficiently to the article to be sterilized. This is most effectively done using saturated steam, which is steam in thermal equilibrium with the water from which it is derived, i.e. steam on the phase boundary (Fig. 20.5). Under these circumstances, contact with a cooler surface causes condensation and contraction drawing in fresh steam and leading to the immediate release of the latent heat, which represents approximately 80% of the heat energy. In this way heat and moisture are imparted rapidly to articles being sterilized and dry porous loads are quickly penetrated by the steam.

Steam for sterilization can either be generated within the sterilizer, as with portable bench or 'instrument and utensil' sterilizers, in which case it is constantly in contact with water and is known as 'wet' steam, or can be supplied under pressure (350–400 kPa) from a separate boiler as 'dry' saturated steam with no entrained water droplets. The killing potential of 'wet' steam is the same as that of 'dry' saturated steam at the same temperature, but it is more likely to soak a porous load creating physical difficulties for further steam penetration. Thus, major industrial and hospital sterilizers are usually supplied with 'dry' saturated steam and attention is paid to the removal of entrained water droplets within the supply line to prevent introduction of a water 'fog' into the sterilizer.

If the temperature of 'dry' saturated steam is increased, then, in the absence of entrained moisture, the relative humidity or degree of saturation is reduced and the steam becomes superheated (Fig. 20.5). During sterilization this can arise in a number of ways, for example by overheating the steam jacket (see section 4.2.2), by using too dry a steam supply, by excessive pressure reduction during passage of steam from the boiler to the sterilizer chamber, and by evolution of heat of hydration when steaming

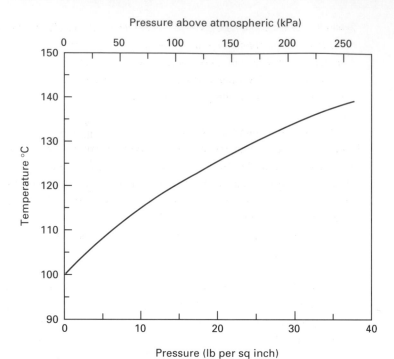

Fig. 20.5 Pressure-temperature diagram for water vapour.

over-dried cotton fabrics. Superheated steam behaves in the same manner as hot air since condensation and release of latent heat will not occur unless the steam is cooled to the phase boundary temperature. Thus, it proves to be an inefficient sterilizing agent, and although a small degree of transient superheating can be tolerated, a maximum acceptable level of 5°C superheat is set, i.e. the temperature of the steam is never greater than 5°C above the phase boundary temperature at that pressure.

The relationship between temperature and pressure holds true only in the presence of pure steam; adulteration with air contributes to a partial pressure but not to the temperature of the steam. Thus, in the presence of air the temperature achieved will reflect the contribution made by the steam and will be lower than that normally attributed to the total pressure recorded. Addition of further steam will raise the temperature but residual air surrounding articles may delay heat penetration or, if a large amount of air is present, it may collect at the bottom of the sterilizer, completely altering the temperature profile of the sterilizer chamber. It is for these reasons that efficient air removal is a major aim in the design and operation of a boiler-fed steam sterilizer.

4.2.2   *Sterilizer design and operation*

Steam sterilizers, or autoclaves as they are sometimes known, are stainless steel vessels designed to withstand the steam pressures employed in sterilization. They can be: (i) 'portable' sterilizers, where they generally have internal electric heaters to produce steam and are used for small pilot or laboratory-scale sterilization and for the treatment of instruments and utensils; or (ii) large-scale sterilizers for routine hospital or industrial use, operating on 'dry' saturated steam from a separate boiler (Fig. 20.6). Because of their widespread use within pharmacy this latter type will be considered in greatest detail.

There are two main types of large sterilizers, those designed for use with porous loads (i.e. dressings) and generally operated at a minimum temperature of 134°C, and those designed as bottled-fluid sterilizers employing a minimum temperature of 121°C. The stages of operation are common to both and can be summarized as air removal and steam admission, heating-up and exposure, and drying or cooling. Many modifications of design exist and in this section only general features will be considered. Fuller treatments of sterilizer design and operation can be found in Health Technical Memorandum 2010 (1994).

General design features. Steam sterilizers are constructed with either cylindrical or oblong chambers, with preferred capacities ranging from 400 to 800 litres. They can be sealed by either a single door or by doors at both ends (to allow through-passage of processed materials; see Chapter 22, section 3.2.3). During sterilization the doors are held closed by a locking mechanism which prevents opening when the chamber is under pressure and until the chamber has cooled to a pre-set temperature, typically 80°C.

In the larger sterilizers the chamber may be surrounded by a steam-jacket which can be used to heat the autoclave chamber and promote a more uniform temperature throughout the load. The same jacket can also be filled with water at the end of the cycle to facilitate cooling and thus reduce the overall cycle time. The chamber floor slopes towards a discharge channel through which air and condensate can be removed. Temperature is monitored within the opening of the discharge channel and by thermocouples in dummy packages; jacket and chamber pressures are followed using pressure gauges. In hospitals and industry, it is common practice to operate sterilizers on an automatic cycle, each stage of operation being controlled by a timer responding to temperature- or pressure-sensing devices.

Operation

1 *Air removal and steam admission.* Air can be removed from steam sterilizers either by downward displacement with steam, evacuation or a combination of the two. In the downward displacement sterilizer, the heavier cool air is forced out of the discharge channel by incoming hot steam. This has the benefit of warming the load during air removal which aids the heating-up process. It finds widest application in the sterilization of bottled fluids where bottle breakage may occur under the combined stresses of evacuation and high temperature. For more air-retentive loads (i.e. dressings), however, this technique of air removal is unsatisfactory and mechanical evacuation of the air is essential before admission of the steam. This can either be to an extremely high level (e.g. 2.5 kPa) or can involve a period of pulsed evacuation and steam admission, the latter approach improving air extraction from dressings packs. After evacuation, steam penetration into the load is very rapid and heating-up is almost instantaneous. It is

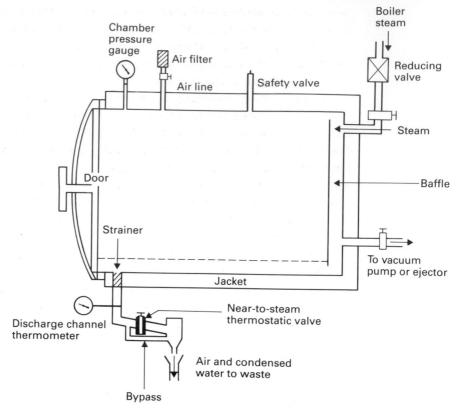

Fig. 20.6 Main constructional features of a large-scale steam sterilizer (autoclave).

axiomatic that packaging and loading of articles within a sterilizer be so organized as to facilitate air removal.

During the sterilization process, small pockets of entrained air may still be released, especially from packages, and this air must be removed. This is achieved with a near-to-steam thermostatic valve incorporated in the discharge channel. The value operates on the principle of an expandable bellows containing a volatile liquid which vaporizes at the temperature of saturated steam thereby closing the valve, and condenses on the passage of a cooler air–steam mixture, thus reopening the valve and discharging the air. Condensate generated during the sterilization process can also be removed by this device. Small quantities of air will not, however, lower the temperature sufficiently to operate the valve and so a continual slight flow of steam is maintained through a bypass around the device in order to flush away residual air.

It is common practice to package sterile fluids, especially intravenous fluids, in flexible plastic containers. During sterilization these can develop a considerable internal pressure in the airspace above the fluid and it is therefore necessary to maintain a proportion of air within the sterilizing chamber to produce sufficient overpressure to prevent these containers from bursting (air ballasting). In sterilizers modified or designed to process this type of product, air removal is therefore unnecessary but special attention must be paid to the prevention of air 'layering' within the chamber. This is overcome by the inclusion of a fan or through a continuous spray of hot water within the chamber to mix the air and steam. Air ballasting can also be employed to prevent bottle breakage.

2 *Heating-up and exposure.* When the sterilizer reaches its operating temperature and pressure the sterilization stage begins. The duration of exposure may include a heating-up time in addition to the holding time and this will normally be established using thermocouples in dummy articles.

3 *Drying or cooling.* Dressings packs and other porous loads may become dampened during the sterilization process and must be dried before removal from the chamber. This is achieved by steam exhaust and application of a vacuum, often assisted by heat from the steam-filled jacket if fitted. After drying, atmospheric pressure within the chamber is restored by admission of sterile filtered air.

For bottled fluids the final stage of the sterilization process is cooling, and this needs to be achieved as rapidly as possible to minimize thermal degradation of the product and to reduce processing time. In modern sterilizers, this is achieved by circulating water in the jacket which surrounds the chamber or by spray-cooling with retained condensate delivered to the surface of the load by nozzles fitted into the roof of the sterilizer chamber. This is often accompanied by the introduction of filtered, compressed air to minimize container breakage due to high internal pressures (air ballasting). Containers must not be removed from the sterilizer until the internal pressure has dropped to a safe level, usually indicated by a temperature of less than 80°C. Occasionally, spray-cooling water may be a source of bacterial contamination and its microbiological quality must be carefully monitored.

4.3 Dry heat sterilization

The lethal effects of dry heat on microorganisms are due largely to oxidative processes which are less effective than the hydrolytic damage which results from exposure to steam. Thus, dry heat sterilization usually employs higher temperatures in the range 160–180°C and requires exposure times of up to 2 hours depending upon the temperature employed (section 10).

Again, bacterial spores are much more resistant than vegetative cells, and their recorded resistance varies markedly depending upon their degree of dryness. In many early studies on dry heat resistance of spores their water content was not adequately controlled, so conflicting data arose regarding the exposure conditions necessary to achieve effective sterilization. This was partly responsible for variations in recommended exposure temperatures and times in different pharmacopoeias.

Its application is generally restricted to glassware and metal surgical instruments (where its good penetrability and non-corrosive nature are of benefit), non-aqueous thermostable liquids and thermostable powders (see Chapter 21). In practice, the range of materials which are actually subjected to dry heat sterilization is quite limited, and consists largely of items used in hospitals. The major industrial application is in the sterilization of glass bottles which are to be filled aseptically, and here the attraction of the process is that it not only achieves an adequate sterility assurance level, but that it also destroys bacterial endotoxins (products of Gram-negative bacteria, also known as pyrogens, that cause fever when injected into the body). These are difficult to eliminate by other means. For the purposes of depyrogenation of glass, temperatures of approximately 250°C are used.

The F-value concept which was developed for steam sterilization processes has an equivalent in dry heat sterilization although its application has been limited. The F_H designation describes the lethality of a dry heat process in terms of the equivalent number of minutes exposure at 170°C, and in this case a z value of 20°C has been found empirically to be appropriate for calculation purposes; this contrast with the value of 10°C which is typically employed to describe moist heat resistance.

4.3.1   *Sterilizer design*

Dry heat sterilization is usually carried out in a hot air oven which comprises an insulated polished stainless steel chamber, with a usual capacity of up to 250 litres, surrounded by an outer case containing electric heaters located in positions to prevent cool spots developing inside the chamber. A fan is fitted to the rear of the oven to provide circulating air, thus ensuring more rapid equilibration of temperature. Shelves within the chamber are perforated to allow good air flow. Thermocouples can be used to monitor the temperature of both the oven air and articles contained within. A fixed temperature sensor connected to a chart recorder provides a permanent record of the sterilization cycle. Appropriate door-locking controls should be incorporated to prevent interruption of a sterilization cycle once begun.

Recent sterilizer developments have led to the use of dry-heat sterilizing tunnels where heat transfer is achieved by infra-red irradiation or by forced convection in filtered laminar airflow tunnels. Items to be sterilized are placed on a conveyer belt and pass through a high-temperature zone (250 – 300 + °C) over a period of several minutes.

4.3.2   *Sterilizer operation*

Articles to be sterilized must be wrapped or enclosed in containers of sufficient strength and integrity to provide good post-sterilization protection against contamination. Suitable materials are paper, cardboard tubes or aluminium containers. Container shape and design must be such that heat penetration is encouraged in order to shorten the heating-up stage; this can be achieved by using narrow containers with dull non-reflecting surfaces. In a hot-air oven, heat is delivered to articles principally by radiation and convection; thus, they must be carefully arranged within the chamber to avoid obscuring centrally placed articles from wall radiation or impending air flow. The temperature variation within the chamber should not exceed ±5°C of the recorded temperature. Heating-up times, which may be as long as 4 hours for articles with poor heat-conducting properties, can be reduced by preheating the oven before loading. Following sterilization, the chamber temperature is usually allowed to fall to around 40°C before removal of sterilized articles; this can be accelerated by the use of forced cooling with filtered air.

5   Gaseous sterilization

The chemically reactive gases ethylene oxide ($(CH_2)_2O$), and formaldehyde (methanal, H.CHO) possess broad-spectrum biocidal activity, and have found application in the sterilization of re-usable surgical instruments, certain medical, diagnostic and electrical equipment, and the surface sterilization of powders. Sterilization processes using ethylene oxide sterilization are far more commonly used on an international basis than those employing formaldehyde.

Ethylene oxide treatment can also be considered as an alternative to radiation sterilization in the commercial production of disposable medical devices (Chapter 21). These techniques do not, however, offer the same degree of sterility assurance as heat methods and are generally reserved for temperature-sensitive items.

The mechanism of antimicrobial action of the two gases is assumed to be through alkylation of sulphydryl, amino, hydroxyl and carboxyl groups on proteins and imino groups of nucleic acids. At the concentrations employed in sterilization protocols, type A survivor curves (section 2.1, Fig. 20.1) are produced, the lethality of these gases increasing in a non-uniform manner with increasing concentration, exposure temperature and humidity. For this reason, sterilization protocols have generally been established by an empirical approach using a standard product load containing suitable biological indicator test strips (Chapter 23). Concentration ranges (given as weight of gas per unit chamber volume) are usually in the order of $800-1200\,mg\,l^{-1}$ for ethylene oxide and $15-100\,mg\,l^{-1}$ for formaldehyde, with operating temperatures in the region of $45-63°C$ and $70-75°C$, respectively. Even at the higher concentrations and temperatures, the sterilization processes are lengthy and therefore unsuitable for the resterilization of high-turnover articles. Further delays occur because of the need to remove toxic residues of the gases before release of the items for use. In addition, because recovery of survivors in sterility tests is more protracted with gaseous sterilization methods than with other processes, an extended quarantine period may also be required.

As alkylating agents, both gases are potentially mutagenic and carcinogenic (as is the ethylene chlorohydrin which results from ethylene oxide reaction with chlorine), they also produce symptoms of acute toxicity including irritation of the skin, conjunctiva and nasal mucosa; consequently, strict control of their atmospheric concentrations is necessary and safe working protocols are required to protect personnel. Formaldehyde can normally be detected by smell at concentrations lower than those permitted in the atmosphere, whereas this is not true for ethylene oxide. Table 20.3 summarizes the comparative advantages afforded by ethylene oxide and low-temperature steam formaldehyde (LTSF) processes.

5.1   Ethylene oxide

Ethylene oxide gas is highly explosive in mixtures of >3.6% v/v in air; in order to reduce this explosion hazard it is usually supplied for sterilization purposes as a 10% mix with carbon dioxide, or as an 8.6% mixture with HFC 124 (2 chloro-1,1,1,2 tetrafluoroethane) which has replaced fluorinated hydrocarbons (freons). Alternatively, pure ethylene oxide gas can be used at below atmospheric pressure in sterilizer chambers from which all air has been removed.

The efficacy of ethylene oxide treatment depends upon achieving a suitable concentration in each article and this is assisted greatly by the good penetrating powers of the gas, which diffuses readily into many packaging materials including rubber, plastics, fabric and paper. This is not without its drawbacks, however, since the level of

Table 20.3 Relative merits of ethylene oxide and low-temperature steam formaldehyde (LTSF) processes

Advantages of ethylene oxide over LTSF	Advantage of LTSF over ethylene oxide
Wider international regulatory acceptance	Less hazardous because formaldehyde is not flammable and is more readily detected by smell
Better gas penetration into plastics and rubber	Cycle times may be shorter
Relatively slow to form solid polymers (with the potential to block pipes etc.)	The gas is obtained readily from aqueous solution (formalin) which is a more convenient source than gas in cylinders
With long exposure times it is possible to sterilize at ambient temperatures	
Very low incidence of product deterioration	

ethylene oxide in a sterilizer will decrease due to absorption during the process and the treated articles must undergo a desorption stage to remove toxic residues. Desorption can be allowed to occur naturally on open shelves, in which case complete desorption may take many days, e.g. for materials like PVC, or it may be encouraged by special forced aeration cabinets where flowing, heated air assists gas removal, reducing desorption times to between 2 and 24 hours.

Organisms are more resistant to ethylene oxide treatment in a dried state, as are those protected from the gas by inclusion in crystalline or dried organic deposits. Thus, a further condition to be satisfied in ethylene oxide sterilization is attainment of a minimum level of moisture in the immediate product environment. This requires a sterilizer humidity of 30–70% and frequently a preconditioning of the load at relative humidities of greater than 50%.

5.1.1 Sterilizer design and operation

An ethylene oxide sterilizer consists of a leak-proof and explosion-proof steel chamber, normally of 100–300 litre capacity, which can be surrounded by a hot-water jacket to provide a uniform chamber temperature. Successful operation of the sterilizer requires removal of air from the chamber by evacuation, humidification and conditioning of the load by passage of subatmospheric pressure steam followed by a further evacuation period and the admission of preheated vaporized ethylene oxide from external pressurized canisters or single-charge cartridges. Forced gas circulation is often employed to minimize variations in conditions throughout the sterilizer chamber. Packaging materials must be air-, steam- and gas-permeable to permit suitable conditions for sterilization to be achieved within individual articles in the load. Absorption of ethylene oxide by the load is compensated for by the introduction of excess gas at the beginning or by the addition of more gas as the pressure drops during the sterilization process. The same may also be true for moisture absorption, which is compensated for by supplementary addition of water to maintain appropriate relative humidity.

After treatment, the gases are evacuated either directly to the outside atmosphere or through a special exhaust system. Filtered, sterile air is then admitted either for a repeat of the vacuum/air cycle or for air purging until the chamber is opened. In this way, safe removal of the ethylene oxide is achieved reducing the toxic hazard to the operator. Sterilized articles are removed directly from the chamber and arranged for desorption.

The operation of an ethylene oxide sterilizer should be monitored and controlled automatically. A typical operating cycle for pure ethylene oxide gas is given in Fig. 20.7, and general conditions are summarized in section 10.

| 5.2 | **Formaldehyde** |

Formaldehyde gas for use in sterilization is produced by heating formalin (37% w/v aqueous solution of formaldehyde) to a temperature of 70–75°C with steam, leading to the process known as LTSF. Formaldehyde has a similar toxicity to ethylene oxide and although absorption to materials appears to be lower similar desorption routines are recommended. A major disadvantage of formaldehyde is low penetrating power and this limits the packaging materials that can be employed to principally paper and cotton fabric.

| 5.2.1 | *Sterilizer design and operation* |

An LTSF sterilizer is designed to operate with subatmospheric pressure steam. Air is removed by evacuation and steam admitted to the chamber to allow heating of the load and to assist in air removal. The sterilization period starts with the release of formaldehyde by vaporization from formalin (in a vaporizer with a steam jacket) and continues through either a simple holding stage or through a series of pulsed evacuations and steam and formaldehyde admission cycles. The chamber temperature is maintained by a thermostatically controlled water jacket, and steam and condensate are removed via a drain channel and an evacuated condenser. At the end of the treatment period formaldehyde vapour is expelled by steam flushing and the load dried by alternating stages of evacuation and admission of sterile, filtered air. A typical pulsed cycle of operation is shown in Fig. 20.8 and general conditions are summarized in section 10.

| 6 | **Radiation sterilization** |

Several types of radiation find a sterilizing application in the manufacture of pharmaceutical and medical products, principal among which are accelerated electrons (particulate radiation), gamma-rays and ultraviolet (UV) light (both electromagnetic radiations). The major target for these radiations is believed to be microbial DNA, with damage occurring as a consequence of ionization and free radical production (gamma-rays and electrons) or excitation (UV light). This latter process is less damaging and less lethal than ionization, and so UV irradiation is not as efficient a sterilization method as electron or gamma-irradiation. As mentioned earlier (section 2), vegetative bacteria

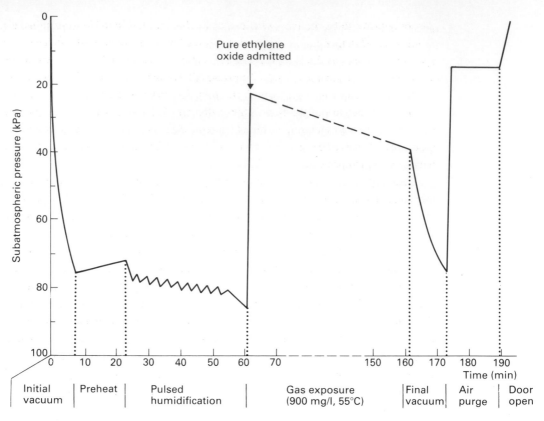

Fig. 20.7 Typical operating cycle for pure ethylene oxide gas.

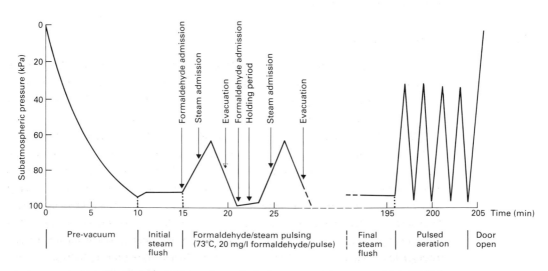

Fig. 20.8 Typical operating cycle for low-temperature steam and formaldehyde treatment.

generally prove to be the most sensitive to irradiation (with notable exceptions, e.g. *Deinococcus* (*Micrococcus*) *radiodurans*), followed by moulds and yeasts, with bacterial spores and viruses as the most resistant (except in the case of UV light where mould spores prove to be most resistant). The extent of DNA damage required to produce cell death can vary and this, together with the ability to carry out effective repair, probably decides the resistance of the organism to radiation. With ionizing radiations (gamma-ray and accelerated electrons), microbial resistance decreases with the presence of moisture or dissolved oxygen (as a result of increased free radical production) and also with elevated temperatures.

Radiation sterilization with high-energy gamma-rays or accelerated electrons has proved to be a useful method for the industrial sterilization of heat-sensitive products. However, undesirable changes can occur in irradiated preparations, especially those in aqueous solution where radiolysis of water contributes to the damaging processes. In addition, certain glass or plastic (e.g. polypropylene, PTFE) materials used for packaging or for medical devices can also suffer damage. Thus, radiation sterilization is generally applied to articles in the dried state; these include surgical instruments, sutures, prostheses, unit-dose ointments, plastic syringes and dry pharmaceutical products (Chapter 21). With these radiations, destruction of a microbial population follows the classic survivor curves (see Fig. 20.1) and a *D*-value, given as a radiation dose, can be established for standard bacterial spores (e.g. *Bacillus pumilus*) permitting a suitable sterilizing dose to be calculated. In the UK it is usual to apply a dose of 25 kGy (2.5 Mrad) for pharmaceutical and medical products, although lower doses are employed in the USA and Canada.

UV light, with its much lower energy, causes less damage to microbial DNA. This, coupled with its poor penetrability of normal packaging materials, renders UV light unsuitable for sterilization of pharmaceutical dosage forms. It does find applications, however, in the sterilization of air, for the surface sterilization of aseptic work areas, and for the treatment of manufacturing-grade water.

6.1   Sterilizer design and operation

6.1.1   *Gamma-ray sterilizers*

Gamma-rays for sterilization are usually derived from a cobalt-60 (^{60}Co) source (caesium-137 may also be used), with a half-life of 5.25 years, which on disintegration emits radiation at two energy levels of 1.33 and 1.17 MeV. The isotope is held as pellets packed in metal rods, each rod carefully arranged within the source and containing up to 20 kCi (740×10^{12} Bq) of activity; these rods are replaced or rearranged as the activity of the source either drops or becomes unevenly distributed. A typical ^{60}Co installation may contain up to 1 MCi (3.7×10^{16} Bq) of activity. For safety reasons, this source is housed within a reinforced concrete building with walls some 2 m thick, and it is only raised from a sunken water-filled tank when required for use. Control devices operate to ensure that the source is raised only when the chamber is locked and that it is immediately lowered if a malfunction occurs. Articles being sterilized are passed through the irradiation chamber on a conveyor belt or monorail system and move around the raised source, the rate of passage regulating the dose absorbed (Fig. 20.9).

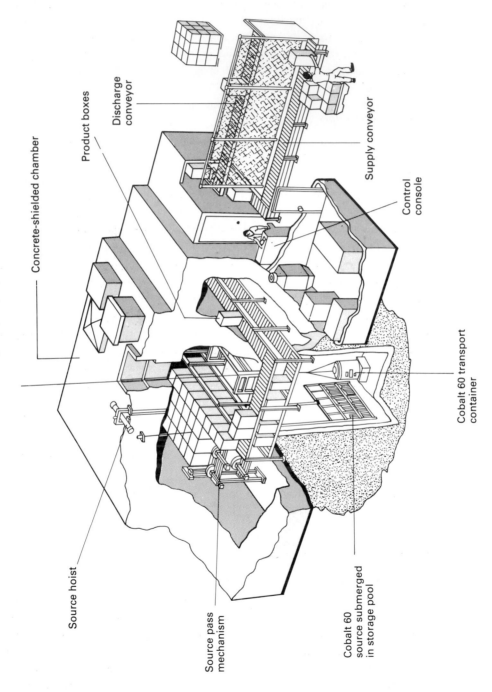

Concrete-shielded chamber

Product boxes

Discharge conveyor

Supply conveyor

Control console

Source hoist

Source pass mechanism

Cobalt 60 source submerged in storage pool

Cobalt 60 transport container

Fig. 20.9 Diagram of a typical cobalt-60 irradiation plant.

Radiation monitors are continually employed to detect any radiation leakage during operation or source storage, and to confirm a return to satisfactory background levels within the sterilization chamber following operation. The dose delivered is dependent upon source strength and exposure period, with dwell times typically up to 20 hours duration.

The difference in radiation susceptibilities of microbial cells and humans may be gauged from the fact that a lethal human dose would be delivered by an exposure of seconds or minutes.

6.1.2 Electron accelerators

Two types of electron accelerator machine exist, the electrostatic accelerator and the microwave linear accelerator, producing electrons with maximum energies of 5 MeV and 10 MeV, respectively. Although higher energies would achieve better penetration into the product, there is a risk of induced radiation, and so they are not used. In the first, a high-energy electron beam is generated by accelerating electrons from a hot filament down an evacuated tube under high potential difference, while in the second, additional energy is imparted to this beam in a pulsed manner by a synchronized travelling microwave. Articles for treatment are generally limited to small packs and are arranged on a horizontal conveyor belt, usually for irradiation from one side but sometimes from both. The sterilizing dose is delivered more rapidly in an electron accelerator than in a ^{60}Co plant, with exposure times for sterilization usually amounting to only a few seconds or minutes. Varying extents of shielding, depending upon the size of the accelerator, are necessary to protect operators from X-rays generated by the bremsstrahlung effect.

6.1.3 Ultraviolet irradiation

The optimum wavelength for UV sterilization is around 260 nm. A suitable source for UV light in this region is a mercury lamp giving peak emission levels at 254 nm. These sources are generally wall- or ceiling-mounted for air disinfection, or fixed to vessels for water treatment. Operators present in an irradiated room should wear appropriate protective clothing and eye shields.

7 Filtration sterilization

The process of filtration is unique amongst sterilization techniques in that it removes, rather than destroys, microorganisms. Further, it is capable of preventing the passage of both viable and non-viable particles and can thus be used for both the clarification and sterilization of liquids and gases. The principal applications of sterilizing-grade filters are the treatment of heat-sensitive injections and ophthalmic solutions, biological products and air and other gases for supply to aseptic areas (see Chapters 21 and 22).

They may also be required in industrial applications where they become part of venting systems on fermenters, centrifuges, autoclaves and freeze-dryers. Certain types of filter (membrane filters) also have an important role in sterility testing, where they can be employed to trap and concentrate contaminating organisms from solutions under

Table 20.4 Some characteristics of membrane and depth filters

Characteristic	Membrane	Depth
Absolute retention of microorganisms greater than rated pore size	+	−
Rapid rate of filtration	+	−
High dirt-handling capacity	−	+
Grow-through of microorganisms	Unlikely	+
Shedding of filter components	−	+
Fluid retention	−	+
Solute adsorption	−	+
Good chemical stability	Variable (depends on membrane)	+
Good sterilization characteristics	+	+

+, applicable; −, not applicable.

test. These filters are then placed on the surface of a solid nutrient medium and incubated to encourage colony development (Chapter 23).

The major mechanisms of filtration are sieving, adsorption and trapping within the matrix of the filter material. Of these, only sieving can be regarded as absolute since it ensures the exclusion of all particles above a defined size. It is generally accepted that synthetic membrane filters, derived from cellulose esters or other polymeric materials, approximate most closely to sieve filters, while fibrous pads, sintered glass and sintered ceramic products can be regarded as depth filters relying principally on mechanisms of adsorption and entrapment. Some of the characteristics of filter media are summarized in Table 20.4. The potential hazard of microbial multiplication within a depth filter and subsequent contamination of the filtrate (microbial grow-through) should be recognized.

7.1 Filtration sterilization of liquids

In order to compare favourably with other methods of sterilization, the microorganism removal efficiency of filters employed in the processing of liquids must be high. For this reason, membrane filters of 0.2–0.22 μm nominal pore diameter are chiefly used, while sintered filters are used only in restricted circumstances, i.e. for the processing of corrosive liquids, viscous fluids or organic solvents. It may be tempting to assume that the pore size is the major determinant of filtration efficiency and two filters of 0.2 μm pore diameter from different manufacturers will behave similarly. This is not so because, in addition to the sieving effect, trapping within the filter matrix, adsorption and charge effects all contribute significantly towards the removal of particles. Consequently, the depth of the membrane, its charge and the tortuosity of the channels are all factors which can make the performance of one filter far superior to that of another. The major criterion by which filters should be compared, therefore, is their titre reduction values, i.e. the ratio of the number of organisms challenging a filter under defined conditions to the number penetrating it. In all cases, the filter medium employed must be sterilizable, ideally by steam treatment; in the case of membrane filters this may be for once-only use, or, in the case of larger industrial filters, a small

Table 20.5 Effect of membrane
disc filter diameter on filtration
volumes

Filter diameter (mm)	Effective filtration area (cm²)	Typical batch volume (litres)
13	0.8	<0.01
25	3.9	0.05–0.1
47	11.3	0.1–0.3
90	45	0.3–5
142	97	5–20
293	530	>20

fixed number of resterilizations; sintered filters may be resterilized many times. Filtration sterilization is an aseptic process and careful monitoring of filter integrity is necessary as well as final product sterility testing (Chapter 23).

Membrane filters, in the form of discs, can be assembled into pressure-operated filter holders for syringe mounting and in-line use or vacuum filtration tower devices. Filtration under pressure is generally considered most suitable since filling at high flow rates directly into the final containers is possible without problems of foaming, solvent evaporation or air leaks. The filtration capacity of a range of membrane filter discs is given in Table 20.5. To increase the filtration area, and hence process volumes, several discs can be used in parallel in multiple-plate filtration systems or, alternatively, membrane filters can be fabricated into plain or pleated cylinders and installed in cartridges. Membrane filters are often used in combination with a coarse-grade fibreglass depth prefilter to improve their dirt-handling capacity.

7.2 Filtration sterilization of gases

The principal application for filtration sterilization of gases is in the provision of sterile air to aseptic manufacturing suites, hospital isolation units and some operating theatres. Filters employed generally consist of pleated sheets of glass microfibres separated and supported by corrugated sheets of Kraft paper or aluminium; these are employed in ducts, wall or ceiling panels, overhead canopies, or laminar airflow cabinets (Chapter 22). These high-efficiency particulate air (HEPA) filters can remove up to 99.997% of particles greater than 0.3 µm in diameter and thus are acting as depth filters. In practice their microorganism removal efficiency is rather better since the majority of bacteria are found associated with dust particles and only the larger fungal spores are found in the free state. Air is forced through HEPA filters by blower fans, and prefilters are used to remove larger particles to extend the lifetime of the HEPA filter. The operational efficiency and integrity of a HEPA filter can be monitored by pressure differential and airflow rate measurements, and dioctylphthalate smoke particle penetration tests.

Other applications of filters include sterilization of venting or displacement air in tissue and microbiological culture (carbon filters and hydrophobic membrane filters); decontamination of air in mechanical ventilators (glass fibre filters); treatment of exhausted air from microbiological safety cabinets (HEPA filters); and the clarification and sterilization of medical gases (glass wool depth filters and hydrophobic membrane filters).

8   Conclusions

A sterilization process should always be considered a compromise between achieving good antimicrobial activity and maintaining product stability. It must, therefore, be validated against a suitable test organism and its efficacy continually monitored during use. Even so, a limit will exist as to the type and size of microbial challenge which can be handled by the process without significant loss of sterility assurance. Thus, sterilization must not be seen as a 'catch-all' or as an alternative to good manufacturing practices but must be considered as only the final stage in a programme of microbiological control.

9   Acknowledgements

The assistance of the following is gratefully acknowledged: F.J. Ley, Isotron plc, Swindon (for discussions and permission to reproduce Fig. 20.9); M.S. Copson, Albert Browne Ltd, Leicester (for discussions and permission to reproduce Fig. 20.6).

10   Appendix

Examples of typical conditions employed in the sterilization of pharmaceutical and medical products

Sterilization method	Conditions
Moist heat (autoclaving)	121°C for 15 min 134°C for 3 min
Dry heat	160°C for 120 min 170°C for 60 min 180°C for 30 min
Ethylene oxide	Gas concentration: 800–1200 mg l^{-1} 45–63°C 30–70% relative humidity 1–4 hours sterilizing time
Low-temperature steam and formaldehyde	Gas concentration: 15–100 mg l^{-1} Steam admission to 73°C 40–180 min sterilizing time depending on type of process

Irradiation
  Gamma-rays or accelerated
  electrons
	25 kGy (2.5 Mrad) dose

Filtration	≤0.22 μm pore size, sterile membrane filter

Further reading

Baird R.M. & Bloomfield S.F. (eds) (1996) *Microbial Quality Assurance in Cosmetics, Toiletries and Non-sterile Pharmaceuticals*. London: Taylor & Francis.

British Pharmacopoeia (1993) London: HMSO.

British Standards Institution (1991) *Specification for Steam Sterilizers for Aqueous Fluids in Rigid Sealed Containers*: BS 3970. London: BSI.

British Standards Institution (1990) *Sterilizing and Disinfecting Equipment for Medical Products*. BS 3970, Parts, 1, 3, 4, 5. London: BSI.

Denyer S.P. & Baird R.M. (eds) (1990) *Guide to Microbiological Control in Pharmaceuticals*. Chichester: Ellis Horwood. (Chapters 7, 8 and 9 provide additional information.)

European Pharmacopoeia, 3rd edn. (1997) Maisonneure: SA.

Gardner J.F. & Peel M.M. (1991) *Introduction to Sterilisation, Disinfection and Infection Control*. Melbourne: Churchill Livingstone.

Gilbert P. & Allison D. (1996) Redefining the 'sterility' of sterile products. *Eur J Parenteral Sci*, **1**, 19–23.

Health Technical Memorandum (1994) *Sterilisers*. HTM 2010. London: Department of Health.

Russell A.D. (1982) *The Destruction of Bacterial Spores*. London: Academic Press.

Russell A.D., Hugo W.B. & Ayliffe G.A.J. (eds) (1998) *Principles and Practice of Disinfection, Preservation and Sterilization*, 3rd edn. Oxford: Blackwell Scientific Publications.

Stumbo C.R. (1973) *Thermobacteriology in Food Processing*, 2nd edn. London: Academic Press.

United States Pharmacopeia (1995) 23rd revision. Rockville MD: US Pharmacopeial Convention.

21 Sterile pharmaceutical products

1	**Introduction**	4.5	Contact-lens solutions
		4.5.1	Wetting solutions
2	**Injections**	4.5.2	Cleaning solutions
2.1	Design philosophy	4.5.3	Soaking solutions
2.2	Intravenous infusions		
2.2.1	Intravenous additives	**5**	**Dressings**
2.2.2	Total parenteral nutrition (TPN)		
2.3	Small-volume aqueous injections	**6**	**Implants**
2.3.1	Problems of drug stability		
2.4	Small-volume oily injections	**7**	**Absorbable haemostats**
		7.1	Oxidized cellulose
3	**Non-injectable sterile fluids**	7.2	Absorbable gelatin foam
3.1	Non-injectable water	7.3	Human fibrin foam
3.2	Urological (bladder) irrigation solutions	7.4	Calcium alginate
3.3	Peritoneal dialysis and haemodialysis		
	solutions	**8**	**Surgical ligatures and sutures**
3.4	Inhaler solutions	8.1	Sterilized surgical catgut
		8.2	Non-absorbable types
4	**Ophthalmic preparations**		
4.1	Design philosophy	**9**	**Instruments and equipment**
4.2	Eye-drops		
4.3	Eye lotions	**10**	**Further reading**
4.4	Eye ointments		

1   Introduction

Certain forms of drug administration and other pharmaceutical products, such as dressings and sutures, must be sterile in order to avoid the possibility of nosocomial (hospital-induced) infection arising from their usage. This applies particularly to medicines which are administered parenterally but also to any material or instrument likely to contact broken skin or internal organs. While inoculation of human pathogenic bacteria, fungi or viruses poses the most obvious danger to the patient, it should also be realized that microorganisms usually regarded as non-pathogenic which inadvertently gain access to body cavities in sufficiently large numbers can also result in a severe, often fatal, infection. Consequently, injections, ophthalmic preparations, irrigation fluids, dialysis solutions, sutures and ligatures, implants, certain surgical dressings, as well as instruments necessary for their use or administration, must be presented for use in a sterile condition and in such a way that they remain sterile throughout the period of use.

Principles of the methods employed to sterilize pharmaceutical products are described in Chapter 20. The *British Pharmacopoeia* (1993) recommends autoclaving and filtration as suitable methods applicable to aqueous liquids, and dry heat for non-aqueous and dry solid preparations. The choice is determined largely by the ability of the formulation and container to withstand the physical stresses applied by moist heat treatment. The use of ionizing radiation or ethylene oxide is also appropriate in specific instances. The primary considerations relate to the ability of active ingredients to withstand the applied stress and of the container to maintain the product in a sterile condition until use. It should be realized that all products intended to be sterilized must be rendered and kept thoroughly clean and therefore of low microbial content prior to sterilization. Thus, the process itself is not overtaxed and is generally well within safety limits to guarantee sterility with minimal stress applied to the product. Because of the clinical consequences (such as granuloma in the lung) of injecting solid particles into the bloodstream, the numbers of particles present in injections and in other solutions used in body cavities must be restricted. *The British Pharmacopoeia* (1993) set limits for injections based on operation of a particle-detecting apparatus. *The European Pharmacopoeia* (1997) describes a microscope method for particulate contamination of injections and intravenous infusions, i.e. extraneous, mobile, undissolved particles, other than bubbles, unintentionally present in the solutions. The test method provides a qualitative method for identifying and detecting the characteristics of such particles together with an indication of their possible origin. It might then be possible to develop means of avoiding such contamination. Limits are given in the *United States Pharmacopoeia* (1995) for large-volume injections, using this method.

2 Injections

2.1 Design philosophy

Any injectable product must be designed and produced to the highest possible pharmaceutical standards. Not only must the product have the minimum possible levels of particles and pyrogenic substances, but also the formulation and packaging must maintain product integrity throughout the production processes, the shelf-life and during administration. The formulation must be such as to ensure that the product remains physically and chemically stable over the designated shelf-life. To achieve this, excipients such as buffers and antioxidants may be required to ensure chemical stability, and solubilizers, such as propylene glycol or polysorbates, may be necessary for drugs with poor aqueous solubility to maintain the drug in solution. The packaging must prevent water, excipient or drug loss during sterilization and storage and, in addition, retain microbiological integrity. Axiomatically, ingress of microorganisms must be prevented. The packaging must not contribute any significant amounts of extractable chemicals to the contents, for example vulcanizing agents from rubber or plasticizers from polyvinyl chloride (PVC) infusion containers.

Most injections are formulated as aqueous solutions, with Water for Injections BP as the vehicle. The formulation of injections depends upon several factors, namely the aqueous solubility of the active ingredient, the dose to be employed, thermal stability of the solution, the route of injection and whether the product is to be prepared as a multidose one (i.e. with a dose or doses removed on different occasions) or in a single-dose form (as the term suggests, only one dose is contained in the injection). Nowadays, most injections are prepared as single-dose forms and this is mandatory for certain routes, e.g. spinal injections such as the intrathecal route and large-volume intravenous infusions (section 2.2). Multidose injections may require the inclusion of a suitable preservative to prevent contamination following the removal of a dose on different occasions. Single-dose injections are usually packed in glass ampoules containing 1, 2 or 5 ml of product; to ensure removal of the correct volume by syringe, it is necessary to add an appropriate overage to an ampoule. Thus, a 1-ml ampoule will actually contain 1.1 ml of product, with 2.15 ml in a 2-ml ampoule. Full details are to be found in the *British Pharmacopoeia* (1993).

Some types of injections must be made iso-osmotic with blood serum. This applies particularly to large-volume intravenous infusions if at all possible; hypotonic solutions cause lysis of red blood corpuscles and thus must not be used for this purpose. Conversely, hypertonic solutions can be employed: these induce shrinkage, but not lysis, of red cells which recover their shape later. Intraspinal injections must also be isotonic, and to reduce pain at the site of injection so should intramuscular and subcutaneous injections. Adjustment to isotonicity can be determined by the following methods.

1 Depression of freezing-point, which depends on the number of dissolved particles present in solution. A useful equation is given by:

$$W = \frac{0.52 - a}{b}$$

in which W is the percentage (w/v) of adjusting substance, a the freezing-point of unadjusted solution and b the depression of the freezing-point of water by 1% w/v of adjusting substance.

2 Sodium chloride equivalent, which is produced by dividing the value for the depression of freezing-point produced by a solution of the substance by the corresponding value of a solution of sodium chloride of the same strength.

For details of these and other methods, the *Pharmaceutical Codex* (1993) should be consulted.

2.2 **Intravenous infusions**

These consist of large-volume injections or drips (500 ml or more) that are infused at various rates (e.g. 50–500 ml h^{-1}) into the venous system; they are sterilized in an autoclave (see Chapter 20). The most commonly used infusions are isotonic sodium chloride and glucose. These are used to maintain fluid and electrolyte balance, for replacement of extracellular body fluids (e.g. after surgery or during prolonged periods of fluid loss), as a supplementary energy source (1 litre of 5% w/v glucose = 714 kJ) and as a vehicle for drugs. Such solutions are prepared using freshly distilled water as a vehicle under rigidly controlled conditions to minimize pyrogen (see Chapters 1 and 18) and particle content, and filtered to remove remaining particles immediately before distribution to the final clean container.

Other important examples are blood and blood products, which are collected and processed in sterile containers, and plasma substitutes, for example dextrans and degraded gelatin. Dextrans, glucose polymers consisting essentially of $(1 \rightarrow 6)$ α-links, are produced as a result of the biochemical activities of certain bacteria of the genus *Leuconostoc*, e.g. *L. mesenteroides* (see Chapter 25).

A small range of intravenous infusions, e.g. those containing amino acids or chlormethiazole, are prepared in glass containers. These are sealed with a rubber closure held on by an aluminium screw cap or crimp-on ring. The rubber should be non-fragmenting, not release soluble extractives, and be sufficiently soft and pliable to seal around the giving set needle inserted immediately prior to use. Although bottles are sterilized by autoclaving, it is still possible for the infusion in glass bottles to become contaminated with microorganisms before use. For instance, during the final part of the autoclave process, bottles may be spray-cooled with water to hasten the cooling process and therefore reduce the total autoclaving time. However, due to the poor fit between bottle lip and rubber plug (a skirted insert type is used) it is possible for the spray-cooling water to spread by capillary movement between bottle thread and screw cap and even enter the bottle contents. This process is encouraged if the bottle contains a vacuum as a consequence of rubber seal failure during heating-up. It should also be remembered that autoclaving leads to considerable heat and pressure stresses on the container. Failure may result from any imperfection in the bottle or plug. Microbes may also gain access to the contents of bottles during storage if hair-line cracks (a result of bad handling and rough treatment) are present, through which fluid may seep outwards and microorganisms inwards to contaminate the fluid. Finally, contamination may occur during use due to poor aseptic techniques when setting up the infusion, via an ineffective air inlet (allowing replacement of infused fluid with air) or when changing the giving set or bottle.

Most infusions are now packed in plastic containers. The plastic material should be pliable, thermoresistant, transparent and non-toxic. Plasticized PVC and polyethylene are commonly used. The former is transparent and very pliable, allowing the pack to collapse as the contents are withdrawn (consequently no air inlet is required). These packs are also amenable to the inclusion of ports into the bag, allowing greater safety during use. Such ports can be protected by sterile overseals. Two problems arise: (i) the possibility of toxic extractives, e.g. diethyl phthalate, from the plastic entering the fluid if poor quality PVC is used; and (ii) moisture permeability leading to loss of water if the packs are not protected by a water-impermeable outer wrap. Bags of high-quality polyethylene are readily moulded (although separate ports cannot be included), translucent and free from potential toxic extractives. As stated, these packs normally collapse readily during infusion. An important advantage of all plastic packs is that the containers are hermetically sealed prior to autoclaving and, therefore, spray-cooling water cannot enter the pack unless there is seal failure, an easily detected occurrence. However, the autoclaving of plastic bags is more complex than that of bottled fluids because a steam–air mixture is necessary to prevent bursting of the bags when heated (air-ballasting); adequate mixing of the steam and air is therefore required to prevent layering of gases inside the chamber.

2.2.1 Intravenous additives

A common practice in hospitals is to add drugs to infusions immediately prior to, or during, administration. The most common additives are potassium chloride, lignocaine, heparin, certain vitamins and antibiotics.

Potentially, this can be a hazardous practice. For instance, the drug may precipitate in the infusion fluid because of the pH (e.g. amphotericin) or the presence of calcium salts (e.g. thiopentone). The drug may degrade rapidly (e.g. ampicillin in 5% w/v glucose). Multiple additions may lead to precipitation of one or both of the drugs or to accelerated degradation. Finally, drug loss may occur because of absorption by the container. For instance, insulin is absorbed by glass or PVC, glyceryl trinitrate and diazepam are absorbed by PVC. Apart from these problems, if the addition is not carried out under strict aseptic conditions the fluid can become contaminated with microorganisms during the procedure. Thus, any addition should be made in a laminar-flow work station or isolator, preferably in the pharmacy, and the fluid administered within 24 hours, unless prepared under strict aseptic conditions.

Another approach to the problem of providing an intravenous drug additive service is to add the drug to a small-volume (50–100 ml) infusion in a collapsible plastic container and store the preparation at –20°C in a freezer. The infusion can be removed when required and thawed rapidly by microwave. Many antibiotics are stable for several months when stored in minibags at –20°C and are unaffected by the thawing process in a suitable microwave oven. Other antibiotics, e.g. ampicillin, are degraded when frozen.

2.2.2   *Total parenteral nutrition (TPN)*

Total parenteral nutrition is the use of concentrated mixtures of amino acids, vitamins, inorganic salts and an energy source (carbohydrate or fat emulsion, e.g. soyabean oil with lecithin as emulsifying agent) for the long-term feeding of patients who are unconscious or unable to take food. Many hospital pharmacies operate a TPN service. All or most of the ingredients to feed a patient for 1 day are combined in one large (3-litre capacity) collapsible plastic bag. The contents are infused over a 12–24 hour period. Transfer of amino acid, glucose and electrolyte infusions, and the addition of vitamins and trace elements, must be carried out with great care under aseptic conditions to avoid microbial contamination. These solutions often provide good growth conditions for bacteria and moulds. Fats are administered as oil-in-water emulsions, comprising small droplets of a suitable vegetable oil (e.g. soyabean) emulsified with egg lecithin and sterilized by autoclaving. In many cases, the fat emulsion may be added to the 3-litre bag.

2.3   **Small-volume aqueous injections**

This category comprises single-dose injections, usually of 1–2 ml but as high as 50 ml, dispensed in borosilicate glass ampoules, plastic (polyethylene or polypropylene) ampoules or, rarely, multidose glass vials of 5–15 ml capacity stoppered with a rubber closure through which a hypodermic needle can be inserted, e.g. insulins, vaccines. The closure is designed to reseal after withdrawal of the needle. It is unwise to include too many doses in a multidose container because of the risk of microbial contamination during repeated use. Bactericides must be added to injections in multidose containers to prevent contamination during withdrawal of successive doses, except as detailed below. Bactericides may not be used in injections in which the total volume to be injected at one time exceeds 15 ml. This may occur if the solubility of a drug is such that a therapeutic dose is only soluble in this order of volume (e.g. Bemegride Injection). There is also an absolute prohibition on the inclusion of bactericides in injections of the following categories: intra-arterial, intracardiac, intrathecal or subarachnoid, intracisternal and peridural.

Small-volume injections may be sterilized by the following methods.

1 Heating in an autoclave for injections packed in glass ampoules.

2 Filtration followed by aseptic sealing (plastic containers). Since the product is not sterilized in its final container, a bactericide may be included to reduce the risks of contamination.

<table>
<tr><td>2.3.1</td><td>*Problems of drug stability*</td></tr>
</table>

1 Thermostability. The choice of sterilization method depends on the thermostability of the active ingredient, autoclaving being applied only to drugs that are heat stable in aqueous solution.

2 Chemical stability. Some medicaments undergo chemical change in aqueous solutions. If the change is due to oxidation, a reducing agent such as sodium metabisulphite is included (e.g. Adrenaline Injection BP).

Aqueous solutions of some drugs are so unstable that chemical stabilization is impossible. In this case the drug itself, not its aqueous solution, is sterilized by dry heat (160°C for 2 hours or its equivalent at higher temperatures) in its final container and dissolved immediately before use by the addition of sterile water (Water for Injections BP). For drugs which are both thermolabile and unstable in aqueous solution, a sterile solution of the drug is freeze-dried in the final container and is reconstituted as above just before use (e.g. many antibiotics, Hyaluronidase BP).

Details of time–temperature regimens as dictated by injection volume and heat transfer to the whole of the product (section 2.2) and of possible interactions between active ingredients and containers must be considered (see also Chapter 20).

2.4 Small-volume oily injections

Certain small-volume injections are available where the drug is dissolved in a viscous oil because it is insoluble in water; non-aqueous solvent must be used. In addition, drugs in non-aqueous solvents provide a depot effect, for example for hormonal compounds. The intramuscular route of injection must be used. The vehicle may be a metabolizable fixed oil such as arachis or sesame oil (but not a mineral oil) or an ester such as ethyl oleate which is also metabolizable. The latter is less viscous and therefore easier to administer but the depot effect is of shorter duration. The drug is normally dissolved in the oil, filtered under pressure and distributed into ampoules. After sealing, the ampoules are sterilized by dry heat, for example, at 160°C for 2 hours. A bactericide is probably ineffective in such a medium and therefore offers very little protection against contamination in a multidose oily injection.

3 Non-injectable sterile fluids

There are many other types of solution required in a sterile form for use particularly in hospitals.

3.1 Non-injectable water

This is sterile water, not necessarily of injectable water standards, which is used widely during surgical procedures for wound irrigation, moistening of tissues, washing of surgeons' gloves and instruments during use and, when warmed, as a haemostat. Isotonic saline may also be used. Topical water (as it is often called) is prepared in 500-ml and 1-litre polyethylene or polypropylene containers with a wide neck, to allow for ease for pouring, and tear-off cap. Hospitals in the UK probably use larger quantities of topical fluids than of intravenous infusions.

3.2 Urological (bladder) irrigation solutions

These are used for the rinsing of the urinary tract to aid tissue integrity and cleanliness during or after surgery. Either water or glycine solution is used, the latter eliminating the risk of intravascular haemolysis when electrosurgical instruments are used. These are sterile solutions produced in collapsible or semi-rigid plastic containers of up to 3-litre capacity.

3.3 Peritoneal dialysis and haemodialysis solutions

Peritoneal dialysis solutions are admitted into the peritoneal cavity as a means of removing accumulated waste or toxic products following renal failure or poisoning. They contain electrolytes and glucose (1.4–7% w/v) to provide a solution equivalent to potassium-free extracellular fluid. Lactate or acetate is added as a source of bicarbonate ions. Slightly hypertonic solutions are usually employed to avoid increasing the water content of the intravascular compartment. A more hypertonic solution, containing a higher glucose concentration, is used to achieve a more rapid removal of water. In fact, the peritoneal cavity behaves as if it were separated from the body organs by a semi-permeable membrane. Warm peritoneal solution (up to 5 litres) is perfused into the cavity for 30–90 minutes and then drained out completely. This procedure can then be repeated as often as required. Since the procedure requires large volumes, these fluids are commonly packed in 2.5-litre containers. It is not uncommon to add drugs (for instance potassium chloride or heparin) to the fluid prior to use.

Haemodialysis is the process of circulating the patient's blood through a machine via tubing composed of a semi-permeable material such that waste products permeate into the dialysing fluid and the blood then returns to the patient. Haemodialysis solutions need not be sterile but must be free from heavy bacterial contamination.

3.4 Inhaler solutions

In cases of severe acute asthmatic attacks, bronchodilators and steroids for direct delivery to the lungs may be needed in large doses. This is achieved by direct inhalation via a nebulizer device; this converts a liquid into a mist or fine spray. The drug is diluted in small volumes of Water for Injections BP before loading into the reservoir of the machine. This vehicle must be sterile and preservative-free and is therefore prepared as a terminally sterilized unit dose in polyethylene nebules.

4 Ophthalmic preparations

4.1 Design philosophy

Medication intended for instillation on to the surface of the eye is formulated in aqueous solution as eye-drops or lotion or in an oily base as an ointment. Because of the possibility of eye infection occurring, particularly after abrasion or damage to the corneal surface, all ophthalmic preparations must be sterile. Since there is a very poor blood supply to the anterior chamber, defence against microbial invasion is minimal; furthermore, it appears to provide a particularly good environment for growth of bacteria. As well as being sterile, eye products should also be relatively free from particles which might cause damage to the cornea. However, unlike aqueous injections, the recommended vehicle is purified water since the presence of pyrogens (Chapter 1) is not clinically significant.

Another type of sterile ophthalmic product is the contact lens solution (section 4.5); however, unlike the other types, this is not used for medication purposes but merely as wetting, cleaning and soaking solutions for contact lenses.

4.2 Eye-drops

Eye-drops are presented for use in: (i) sterile single-dose plastic sachets containing 0.3–0.5 ml of liquid; (ii) multidose amber fluted eye-dropper bottles including the rubber teat as part of the closed container or supplied separately (*British Pharmacopoeia* 1993); or (iii) plastic bottles with integral dropper. It should be covered with a breakable seal to indicate that the dropper or cap has not been removed prior to initial use. Although a standard design of bottle is used in hospitals, many proprietory products are manufactured in plastic bottles designed to improve safety and care of use. The maximum volume in each container is limited to 10 ml. Because of the likelihood of microbial contamination of eye-dropper bottles during use (arising from repeated opening or contact of the dropper with infected eye tissue or the hands of the patient), it is essential to protect the product against inopportune contamination. Eye-drops for surgical theatre use should be supplied in single-dose containers (*British Pharmacopoeia* 1993).

Examples of preservatives are: phenylmercuric nitrate or acetate (0.002% w/v), chlorhexidine acetate (0.01% w/v), thiomersal (0.01% w/v) and benzalkonium chloride (0.01% w/v). Chlorocresol is too toxic to the corneal epithelium, but 8-hydroxyquinoline and thiomersal may be used in specific instances. The principal consideration in relation to antimicrobial properties is the activity of the bactericide against *Pseudomonas aeruginosa*, a major source of serious nosocomial eye infections. Although benzalkonium chloride is probably the most active of the recommended preservatives, it cannot always be used because of its incompatibility with many compounds commonly used to treat eye diseases, nor should it be used to preserve eye-drops containing anaesthetics. Since benzalkonium chloride reacts with natural rubber, silicone or butyl rubber teats should be substituted. Since silicone rubber is permeable to water vapour, products should not be stored for more than 3 months after manufacture. As with all rubber components, the rubber teat should be pre-equilibrated with the preservative prior to use. Thermostable eye-drops and lotions are sterilized at 121°C for 15 minutes. For thermolabile drugs, filtration sterilization followed by aseptic filling into sterile containers is necessary. Eye-drops in plastic bottles are prepared aseptically.

In order to lessen the risk of eye-drops becoming heavily contaminated either by repeated inoculation or growth of resistant organisms in the solution, use is restricted, after the container is first opened, to 1 month. This is usually reduced to 7 days for hospital ward use on one eye of a single patient. The period is shorter in the hospital environment because of the greater danger of contamination by potential pathogens, particularly pseudomonads.

Finally, eye-drops for use during open-eye surgery must *not* contain a preservative because of their cytotoxicity. Single-dose preparations are, therefore, ideally suited for this purpose.

4.3   Eye lotions

Eye lotions are isotonic solutions used for washing or bathing the eyes. They are sterilized in relatively large-volume containers (100 ml or greater). Eye lotions are sterilized by autoclaving in coloured fluted glass bottles with a rubber closure and screw cap, or plastic container with screw cap or tear-off seal. They may contain a bactericide if intended for intermittent domiciliary use for up to 7 days. If intended for first aid or similar purposes, however, no bactericide is included and any remaining solution discarded after 24 hours.

4.4   Eye ointments

Eye ointments are prepared in a semi-solid base (e.g. Simple Eye Ointment BP, which consists of yellow soft paraffin, eight parts; liquid paraffin, one part; wool fat, one part). The base is filtered when molten to remove particles and sterilized at 160°C for 2 hours. The drug is incorporated prior to sterilization if heat stable, or added aseptically to the sterile base. Finally, the product is aseptically packed in clear sterile aluminium or plastic tubes. Since the product contains virtually no water, the danger of bacteria proliferating in the ointment is negligible. Therefore, there is no recommended maximum period during which they can be used.

4.5   Contact-lens solutions

Most contact lenses are worn for optical reasons as an alternative to spectacles. Contact lenses are of two types, namely hard lenses, which are hydrophobic, and soft lenses, which may be either hydrophilic or hydrophobic. The surfaces of lenses must be wetted before use, and wetting solutions (section 4.5.1) are used for this purpose. Hard and, more especially, soft lenses become heavily contaminated with protein material during use and must therefore be cleaned (section 4.5.2) before disinfection (section 4.5.3). Contact lenses are potential sources of eye infection and consequently microorganisms should be removed before the lens is again inserted into the eye. Lenses must also be clean and easily wettable by the lacrimal secretions. Contact-lens solutions are thus sterile solutions of the various types described below. Apart from achieving their stated functions, either singly or in combination, all solutions must be non-irritating and must protect against microbial contamination during use and storage.

4.5.1 Wetting solutions

These are used to hydrate the surfaces of hard lenses after disinfection. Since they must also cope with chance contamination, they must contain a preservative as well as a wetting agent. They may be isotonic with lacrimal secretions and be formulated to a pH of about 7.2 for compatibility with normal tears.

4.5.2 Cleaning solutions

These are responsible for the removal of ocular debris and protein deposits, and contain a cleaning agent that consists of a surfactant and/or an enzyme product. Since they must also cope with chance contamination, they contain a preservative, are isotonic, and have a pH of about 7.2.

4.5.3 Soaking solutions

These are responsible for disinfection of lenses but also maintain the lenses in a hydrated state. The antimicrobial agents used for disinfecting hard lenses are those used in eye-drops (benzalkonium, chlorhexidine, phenylmercuric acetate or nitrate, thiomersal and chlorbutol). Ethylene diamine tetra-acetic acid (EDTA) is usually present as a synergist (see Chapter 12). Benzalkonium chloride and chlorbutol are strongly bound to hydrophilic soft contact lenses and therefore cannot be used in storage solutions for these. Chlorhexidine and thiomersal are usually employed. It must be added that the concentrations of all preservatives used in contact-lens solutions are lower than those employed in eye-drops, in order to minimize irritancy. Hydrogen peroxide is now becoming commonly used, but must be inactivated prior to lens insertion on to the eye.

Finally, heat may be utilized as an alternative method to disinfect soft contact lenses, especially the hydrophilic type. Lenses are boiled in isotonic saline.

5 Dressings

Dressings and surgical materials are used widely in medicine, both as a means of protecting and providing comfort for wounds and for many associated activities such as cleaning, swabbing, etc. They may or may not be used on areas of broken skin. If there is a potential danger of infection arising from the use of a dressing then it must be sterile. For instance, sterile dressings must be used on all open wounds, both surgical and traumatic, on burns and during and after catheterization at a site of injection. It is also important to appreciate that sterile dressings must be packaged in such a way that they can be applied to the wound aseptically.

Dressings are described in the *British Pharmacopoeia* (1993). Methods for their sterilization include autoclaving, dry heat, ethylene oxide and ionizing radiation. Any

Table 21.1 Uses of surgical dressings and methods of sterilization

Dressing	Uses	Method of sterilization
Required to be sterile		
Chlorhexidine gauze dressing	Medicated open-wound dressing, burns, grafts	
Framycetin gauze dressing	Medicated open wound dressing, burns, grafts	
Knitted viscose primary dressing	Ulcerative and granulating wounds	
Paraffin gauze dressing	Burns, scalds, grafts	Any combination of dry heat, gamma-radiation and ethylene oxide
Perforated film absorbent dressing	Postoperative wounds	
Polyurethane foam dressing	Burns, ulcers, grafts, granulating wounds	
Semi-permeable adhesive film	Adhesive dressing for open wounds, i.v. sites, stoma care, etc.	
Sodium fusidate gauze dressing	Medicated open wound dressing, burns, grafts	
May be sterile for use in certain circumstances		
Absorbent cotton wool	Swabbing, cleaning, medication application	Any method
Elastic adhesive dressing	Protective wound dressing	Ethylene oxide or gamma-radiation
Plastic wound dressings	Protective dressing (permeable or occlusive)	Ethylene oxide or gamma-radiation
Absorbent cotton gauze	Absorbent wound dressing	Any method
Gauze pads	Swabbing, dressing, wound packing	Any method
Absorbent viscose wadding	Wound cleaning, swabbing, skin antiseptic application	Any method

other effective method may be used. The choice is governed principally by the stability of the dressing constituents to the stress applied and the nature of their components. Most cellulosic and synthetic fibres withstand autoclaving but there are exceptions. For instance, boric acid tenderizes cellulose fibres during autoclaving, and dressings containing waxes cannot be sterilized by moist heat. Certain constituents are also adversely affected on exposure to large doses of gamma-radiation. Those dressings that are required to be sterile are listed in Table 21.1, together with other dressings and materials that may be sterilized when required.

A very important aspect of dressings production is packaging. The packaging material must allow correct sterilization conditions (for example permeation of moisture or ethylene oxide), retain the dressing in a sterile condition and allow for its removal without contamination prior to use. All dressings intended for aseptic handling and application must be double-wrapped. For steam sterilization they may be individually wrapped in fabric, paper or nylon and sterilized in metal drums, cardboard boxes or bleached Kraft paper. The choice of method also determines the design of the autoclave cycle. Dressings may be sterilized in downward displacement autoclaves, which rely on displacement of air by steam, or in the more modern high prevacuum autoclaves in which virtually all the air is removed before the admission of steam. This method ensures rapid heating-up of the dressings, reduces the time needed to achieve sterilization (e.g. 134°C for 3 minutes) and shortens the overall sterilization cycle.

A recent development is the use of spray-on dressings. A convenient type is an acrylic polymer dissolved in ethyl acetate and packed as an aerosol. This should be self-sterilizing. The film after application is able to maintain the sterility of a clean wound for up to 2 weeks. However, they can only be used on clean, relatively dry wounds.

6   Implants

Implants are small, sterile cylinders of drug, inserted beneath the skin or into muscle tissue to provide slow absorption and prolonged action therapy. This is principally based on the fact that such drugs, invariably hormones, are almost insoluble in water and yet the implant provides a rate of dissolution sufficient for a therapeutic effect. The *British Pharmacopoeia* (1993) describes one implant, testosterone. The *United States National Formulary* (1990) also includes oestradiol. Implants are made from the pure drug into tablet form by compression or fusion. No other ingredient can be included since this may be insoluble or toxic or, most importantly, may influence the rate of drug release.

Compression of sterile drugs must be conducted under aseptic conditions using sterile machine parts and materials. After manufacture, the outer surface of the implant is sterilized by immersion in 0.002% w/v phenylmercuric nitrate at 75°C for 12 hours. After the surface has been dried, each implant is placed aseptically into a sterile glass phial with a cotton-wool plug at both ends. This prevents damage and reduces the risk of glass spicules, formed when the phial is opened, adhering to the implant. This compression process is not ideal. The absence of a lubricant increases the difficulties of making tablets; the hardness of the implant is difficult to regulate, which consequently leads to variations in the rate of drug release. The alternative method, fusion, can be used provided the drug is heat-stable. The pure drug is melted at 5–10°C above its melting temperature and poured into moulds. Note that if the melting temperature is high enough the interior of the implant will automatically be sterilized by this process. It is also possible to sterilize the implant after packaging, by dry heat, provided the melting temperature is above 160°C. Clearly, it is easier to manufacture sterile implants by fusion since the process does not require presterilized ingredients or aseptic processing. The implant hardness is also very consistent.

7   Absorbable haemostats

The reduction of blood loss during or after surgical procedures where suturing or ligature is either impractical or impossible can often be accomplished by the use of sterile, absorbable haemostats. These consist of a soft pad of solid material packed around and over the wound which can be left *in situ*, being absorbed by body tissues over a period of time, usually up to 6 weeks. The principal mechanism of action of these is the ability to encourage platelet fracture because of their fibrous or rough surfaces, and to act as a matrix for complete blood clotting. Four products commonly used are: oxidized cellulose, absorbable gelatin sponge, human fibrin foam and calcium alginate.

7.1 Oxidized cellulose

This consists of cellulosic material which has been partially oxidized. White gauze is the most common form, although lint is also used. It can be absorbed by the body in 2–7 weeks, depending on the size. Its action is based principally on a mechanical effect and it is used in the dry state. Since it inactivates thrombin, its activity cannot be enhanced by thrombin incorporation.

7.2 Absorbable gelatin foam

This is an insoluble gelatin foam produced by whisking warm gelatin solution to a uniform foam, which is then dried. It can be cut into suitable shapes, packed in metal or paper containers and sterilized by dry heat (150°C for 1 hour). Moist heat destroys the physical properties of the material. Immediately before use, it can be moistened with normal saline containing thrombin. It behaves as a mechanical haemostat providing the framework on which blood clotting can occur.

7.3 Human fibrin foam

This is a dry sponge of human fibrin prepared by clotting a foam of human fibrinogen solution with human thrombin. It is then freeze-dried, cut into shapes and sterilized by dry heat at 130°C for 3 hours. Before use, it is saturated with thrombin solution. Blood coagulation occurs in contact with the thrombin in the interstices of the foam.

7.4 Calcium alginate

This is composed of the sodium and calcium salts of alginic acid formed into a powder or fibrous material and sterilized by autoclaving. It aids clotting by forming a sodium–calcium alginate complex in contact with tissue fluids, acting principally as a mechanical haemostat. It is relatively slowly absorbed and some residues may occasionally remain in the tissues.

8 Surgical ligatures and sutures

The use of strands of material to tie off blood or other vessels (ligature) and to stitch wounds (suture) is an essential part of surgery. Both absorbable and non-absorbable materials are available for this purpose.

8.1 Sterilized surgical catgut

This consists of absorbable strands of collagen derived from mammalian tissue, particularly the intestine of sheep. Because of its source, it is particularly prone to bacterial contamination, and even anaerobic spores may be found in such material.

Therefore, sterilization is a particularly difficult process. Since collagen is converted to gelatin when exposed to moist heat, autoclaving cannot be used. The official method is to pack the 'plain' catgut strands (up to 350 cm) on a metal spindle in a glass or other suitable container with a tubing fluid, the purpose of which is to maintain both flexibility and tensile strength after sterilization. Probably the most suitable method is to expose the material to gamma-radiation. There is minimal loss of tensile strength and the container can be overwrapped prior to sterilization to provide a sterile container surface for opening aseptically. The alternative method involves placing the coiled suture immersed in a tubing fluid (commonly 96% ethyl alcohol with or without 0.002% w/v phenylmercuric nitrate) and stored for sufficient time to ensure sterilization. The outer surface of the phial must be sterilized before opening to avoid contamination of the suture when removed. Therefore, the phial is immersed in 1% w/v formaldehyde in ethanol for 24 hours prior to use. It cannot be heated. A non-official method of sterilization is to immerse the catgut in a non-aqueous solvent (naphthalene or toluene) and heat at 160°C for 2 hours. The catgut becomes hard and brittle during this process, and is aseptically transferred to an aqueous tubing fluid to restore its flexibility and tensile strength.

Catgut is packed in single threads, up to 350 cm in length, of various thicknesses related to tensile strength, in single-use glass or plastic containers which cannot be resealed after use. Any remaining material should be discarded. Hardened catgut is prepared by treating strands with certain agents to prolong resistance to digestion. If hardened with chromium compounds, the material is known as 'chromicized' catgut.

8.2 Non-absorbable types

Sutures and ligatures are also made from many materials not absorbed by the body tissues. These consist of uniform strands of metal or organic material which will not cause any tissue reactions and are capable of sterilization. Depending on the physical stability of each material, they are preferably sterilized by autoclaving or gamma-radiation. They are packed in single-use glass or plastic containers which may contain a tubing fluid with or without a bactericide. The different materials are described in the *British Pharmacopoeia* (1993). These include linen (adversely affected by gamma-rays), nylon (either monofilament or plaited), silk and stainless steel (monofilament or twisted).

9 Instruments and equipment

The method chosen for sterilization of instruments (see also Table 21.2) depends on the nature of the components and the design of the item. The wide range of instruments that may be required in a sterile condition includes syringes (glass and plastic disposable), needles, giving sets, metal surgical instruments (scalpels, scissors, forceps, etc.), rubber gloves, catheters, etc. Relatively complicated equipment, such as pressure transducers, pacemakers, kidney dialysis equipment, incubators and aerosol machine parts may also be sterilized. Artificial joints could also be included in the vast range of items required in modern medical practice in a sterile condition. The choice of method depends largely on the physical stability of the items and the appropriate technique in particular

Table 21.2 Methods* commonly used to sterilize or disinfect equipment

Equipment	Method of treatment	Disinfection or sterilization	Preferred method	Comments
Syringes (glass)	Dry heat	Sterilization	Dry heat using assembled syringes	Autoclave not recommended: difficulty with steam penetration unless plungers and barrels sterilized separately
Syringes (glass), dismantled	Moist heat	Sterilization		
Syringes (disposable)	Gamma-radiation Ethylene oxide	Sterilization	Gamma-radiation	Possibility of 'crazing' of syringes after ethylene oxide
Needles (all metal)	Dry heat	Sterilization	Dry heat	
Needles (disposable)	Gamma-radiation Ethylene oxide	Sterilization	Gamma-radiation	
Metal instruments (including scalpels)	Autoclave Dry heat	Sterilization	Dry heat	Cutting edges should be protected from mechanical damage during the process
Disposable instruments	Gamma-radiation Ethylene oxide	Sterilization	Gamma-radiation	
Rubber gloves	Autoclave Gamma-radiation Ethylene oxide	Sterilization	Gamma-radiation	If autoclave used, care with drying at end of process. Little oxidative degradation when high-vacuum autoclave used
Administration (giving) sets	Gamma-radiation Ethylene oxide	Sterilization	Gamma-radiation	
Respirator parts	Moist heat (autoclave)	Sterilization	Sterilization by steam where possible	Chemicals not recommended: may be microbiologically ineffective, may present hazard to patient safety by compromising the safety devices on the machine
	Moist heat (low-temperature steam, or hot water at 80°C)	Disinfection		
Dialysis machines	Chemical	Disinfection	Formalin	Ethylene oxide not recommended in NHS for practical reasons
Fragile, heat-sensitive equipment	Ethylene oxide Chemical	Sterilization Disinfection	Ethylene oxide under expert supervision	

*1 Disposable equipment should not be resterilized or re-used.
 2 Ethylene oxide is a difficult process to control, and the Department of Health discourages its use in hospitals.
 3 Low-temperature steam with formaldehyde is of value in the disinfection/sterilization of some heat-sensitive materials (see also Chapter 20).
 4 Chemical agents, e.g. glutaraldehyde, hypochlorite.

situations. For instance, incubators necessitate a chemical method of sterilization. On the other hand, even delicate instruments like pressure transducers are now available that can withstand autoclaving. This is a new and developing field of medical technology in which many factors may have to be considered before the choice is made as to the most appropriate method of sterilization in any particular situation.

10 Further reading

Allwood M.C. (1990) Package design and product integrity. In: *Guide to Microbiological Control in Pharmaceuticals* (eds S. Denyer & R. Baird), pp. 341–355. Chichester: Ellis Horwood.

Allwood M.C. (1990) Adverse reactions to parenterals. In: *Topics in Pharmacy: Formulation Factors in Adverse Reactions* (eds A.T. Florence & A.G. Salole). London: Wright.

British Pharmacopoeia (1993) *and Addenda*. London: HMSO.

Denyer S. & Baird R. (eds) (1990) *Guide to Microbiological Control in Pharmaceuticals*. London: Ellis Horwood.

Pharmaceutical Codex (1993) London: Pharmaceutical Press.

European Pharmacopoeia (1997) 3rd edn. Strasbourg: Council of Europe.

Phillips I., Meers P.D. & D'Arcy P.F. (1976) *Microbiological Hazards of Infusion Therapy*. Lancaster: MTP Press.

Russell A.D., Hugo W.B. & Ayliffe G.A.J. (1998) *Principles and Practice of Disinfection, Preservation and Sterilization*, 3rd edn. Oxford: Blackwell Science.

Turco S. & Young R.E. (1987) *Sterile Dosage Forms*, 3rd edn. Easton, Philadelphia: Lea and Febiger.

United States Pharmacopoeia (1995) 23rd revision. Rockville, MD: US Pharmacopoeia Convention.

22 Factory and hospital hygiene and good manufacturing practice

1   Introduction
1.1   Definitions
1.1.1   Manufacture
1.1.2   Quality assurance
1.1.3   Good manufacturing practice (GMP)
1.1.4   Quality control
1.1.5   In-process control

2   Control of microbial contamination during manufacture: general aspects
2.1   Environmental cleanliness and hygiene
2.2   Quality of starting materials
2.3   Process design
2.4   Quality control and documentation
2.5   Packaging, storage and transport

3   Manufacture of sterile products
3.1   Clean and aseptic areas: general requirements
3.1.1   Design of premises

3.1.2   Internal surfaces, fittings and equipment
3.1.3   Services
3.1.4   Air supply
3.1.5   Clothing
3.1.6   Changing facilities
3.1.7   Cleaning and disinfection
3.1.8   Operation
3.2   Aseptic areas: additional requirements
3.2.1   Clothing
3.2.2   Entry to aseptic areas
3.2.3   Equipment and operation
3.2.4   Isolator and blow/fill/seal technology

4   Guide to Good Pharmaceutical Manufacturing Practice

5   Conclusions

6   Further reading

1   Introduction

The quality of a pharmaceutical product, whether manufactured in industry or in a hospital, cannot be ensured solely by examining in detail a small number of units taken from a completed batch. For instance, a low level or uneven distribution of microbial contamination may not be detected by conventional methods of sampling and sterility testing (Chapter 23). Instead, a product must be manufactured in a suitable environment by a procedure which minimizes the possibility of contamination occurring, at the end of which tests can be performed as an additional safeguard. This chapter describes measures essential for the control, during manufacture, of one important feature of product quality, the level of microbial contamination. It is designed to be read in conjunction with Chapters 17, 18, 20, 21 and 23.

1.1   Definitions

Several terms used in industrial and hospital production must be defined for an understanding of this chapter. These definitions are given in sections 1.1.1–1.1.5.

1.1.1   *Manufacture*

Manufacture is the complete cycle of production of a medical product. This cycle includes the acquisition of all raw materials, their processing into a final product and its subsequent packaging and distribution.

<table>
<tr><td>1.1.2</td><td>Quality assurance</td></tr>
</table>

| 1.1.2 | *Quality assurance* |

This term refers to the sum total of the arrangements made to ensure that the final product is of the quality required for its intended purpose. It consists of good manufacturing practice plus factors such as original product design and development.

| 1.1.3 | *Good manufacturing practice (GMP)* |

Good manufacturing practice (GMP) comprises that part of quality assurance which is aimed at ensuring that a product is consistently manufactured to a quality appropriate to its intended use. GMP requires that: (i) the manufacturing process is fully defined before it is commenced; and (ii) the necessary facilities are provided. In practice, this means that personnel must be adequately trained, suitable premises and equipment employed, correct materials used, approved procedures adopted, suitable storage and transport facilities available and appropriate records made.

| 1.1.4 | *Quality control* |

Quality control refers to that part of GMP which ensures that: (i) at each stage of manufacture the necessary tests are made; and (ii) the product is not released until it has passed these tests.

| 1.1.5 | *In-process control* |

This comprises any test on a product, the environment or the equipment that is made during the manufacturing process.

2 Control of microbial contamination during manufacture: general aspects

A pharmaceutical product may become contaminated by various means and at different points during the course of manufacture. There are several important ways in which this risk can be minimized in both industrial and hospital production, and these are considered below.

2.1 Environmental cleanliness and hygiene

Microorganisms may be transferred to a product from working surfaces, fixtures and equipment. In this context, pooled stagnant water is a frequent source of contamination. Thus, all premises, including processing areas, stores and laboratories, should be maintained in a clean, dry and tidy condition. For easy cleaning, walls and ceilings should have an impervious and washable surface, and floors should be made of impervious materials free from cracks and open joints where microorganisms could be harboured. For the same reasons, coving should be used at the junction between walls and floors or ceilings. All services, including pipelines, light fittings and ventilation points, should be sited so that inaccessible recesses are avoided. Procedures for cleaning and disinfection of premises are required and must be enforced. All equipment involved in the manufacturing process should be easy to dismantle and clean. It should be inspected for cleanliness before use.

Fall-out of dust- and droplet-borne microorganisms from the atmosphere is an obvious avenue whereby contamination of products may occur; therefore, 'clean' air is a prerequisite during manufacturing processes. In this context, the spread of dust during manufacturing or packaging must be avoided. Microorganisms may thrive in certain liquid preparations and in creams and ointments (Chapter 18). The manufacture of such products should thus, as far as possible, be in a closed system; this serves a dual purpose in that it protects the product not only against airborne microbial contamination but also against evaporative loss.

Potentially harmful organisms could be transferred to a product by its direct contact with personnel. High standards of personal hygiene are therefore very important, especially where sterile products (section 3) are being manufactured. Consequently, operatives should be free from communicable diseases and should have no open lesions on the exposed body surfaces. To ensure high standards of personal cleanliness, adequate handwashing facilities and protective garments, including headgear, must be provided. Direct contact between the materials and the operative's hands must be avoided; where necessary gloves should be worn.

Staff should be trained in the principles of GMP and in the practice (and theory) of the tasks assigned to them. Personnel employed in the manufacture of sterile products (section 3) should also receive basic training in microbiology.

2.2   Quality of starting materials

Raw materials, including water supplies, are an important source of microorganisms in the manufacturing area (Chapter 17) and can lead to the contamination of both the environment and the final product. Materials of natural origin are usually associated with an extensive microbial flora and require careful storage to prevent growth of the organisms and spoilage of the material. If stable, natural products with a high microbial count may undergo sterilization before use. Staff handling raw materials must receive adequate training to prevent the transfer of contaminants from one raw material to another or to the final product (cross-contamination).

Water for manufacturing may be potable mains water, water purified by ion-exchange or reverse osmosis or distillation, or water suitable for injection purposes. When required for parenteral products it must be pyrogen-free (apyrogenic) and is usually prepared in a specially designed still. Although pyrogens are not volatile, they are not removed by ordinary distillation since some will be carried over mechanically into the distillate with the entrainment (spray). Thus, a spray trap, consisting of a series of baffles, is fitted to the distilling flask to prevent spray and pyrogens from entering the condenser tubes. Water prepared in this manner can be used immediately for the preparation of injections, provided that these are sterilized within 4 hours of water collection. Alternatively, the water can be kept for longer periods at a temperature above 65°C (usually 80°C) to prevent bacterial growth with consequent pyrogen production. Ultraviolet irradiation (Chapter 20) may be useful in reducing the bacterial content but it is not to be regarded as a sterilizing agent.

2.3 Process design

The manufacturing process must be fully defined and capable of yielding, with the facilities available, a product that is microbiologically acceptable and conforms to its specifications. This demands that a process be sufficiently evaluated before commencement to ensure that it is suitable for routine production operations. Processes and procedures should be subject to frequent reappraisal and should be re-evaluated when any significant changes are made in the equipment or materials used.

2.4 Quality control and documentation

Selection of starting materials with a low microbial content aids in the control of contamination levels in the environment and the final product. One aspect of quality control is to set acceptable microbiological standards for all raw materials, together with microbial limits for in-process samples and the final product. Further microbiological quality control covers the validation of cleaning and disinfecting procedures and the monitoring of the production environment by microbial counts. Such monitoring should be carried out whilst normal production operations are in progress. In addition, sterile product manufacture will require extra safeguards in the form of tests on the operator's aseptic technique and the monitoring of both air filter and sterilizer efficiency (Chapter 23). Sterility testing (Chapter 23) on the finished product constitutes the final check on the sterilization process. Injectable products may also be tested for pyrogens.

A system of documentation should exist such that the history of each batch of the product, including details of starting materials, packaging materials, and intermediate, bulk and finished products, may be determined. Distribution records must be kept. This information is of paramount importance should a defective batch need to be recalled.

2.5 Packaging, storage and transport

Even when a product has been prepared under stringent conditions such as those outlined above, contamination could still arise during storage and transport. For this reason, the packaging used and the conditions employed during storage and transportation should be such as to minimize or, preferably, prevent deterioration or contamination.

3 Manufacture of sterile products

Sterilization methods have been discussed in Chapter 20 and the various types of sterile products have been described in Chapter 21. For manufacturing purposes an important distinction exists between a sterile product which is terminally sterilized and one which is not. Terminally sterilized means that, after preparation, the product is transferred to containers which are sealed and then immediately sterilized by heat (or radiation or ethylene oxide, as appropriate). In general, such a product must be prepared in a clean area (sections 3.1.1–3.1.8). A product which is not to be terminally sterilized is prepared under aseptic conditions either from previously sterilized materials or by filtration sterilization. In either case, filling into sterilized final containers is a post-sterilization manipulation. Strict aseptic conditions are needed throughout (sections 3.2.1–3.2.4).

Vaccines consisting of dead microorganisms, microbial extracts or inactivated viruses (see Chapter 16) may be filled in the same premises as other sterile medicinal products. The completeness of inactivation (or killing or removal of live organisms) must be proven before processing. Separate premises are needed for the filling of live or attenuated vaccines and for the preparation of biological medicinal products derived from live organisms (Chapter 16). Non-sterile products should not be processed in the same areas as sterile products.

3.1   Clean and aseptic areas: general requirements

3.1.1   *Design of premises*

Sterile production should be carried out in a purpose-built unit separated from other manufacturing areas and thoroughfares. The unit should be designed to encourage the segregation of each stage of production but should ensure a safe and organized workflow (Fig. 22.1). Sterilized products held in quarantine pending sterility test results (Chapter 23) must be kept separate from those awaiting sterilization.

3.1.2   *Internal surfaces, fittings and equipment*

Particulate, as well as microbial, contamination must be guarded against when sterile products are being manufactured. Thus, walls, ceilings and floors should possess smooth, impervious surfaces which will: (i) prevent the accumulation of dust or other particulate matter; and (ii) allow for easy and repeated cleaning and disinfection. For the same reasons, where walls and floors or ceilings meet, covings should be used.

A suitable flooring material is provided for by welded sheets of polyvinyl chloride (PVC); cracks and open joints, which may harbour dirt and microorganisms, must be eliminated. The preferred surface materials for walls are plastic, epoxy-coated plaster, plastic fibreglass or glass-reinforced polyester. Frequently, the final finish for floor, wall and ceiling is achieved using continuous welded PVC sheeting. False ceilings must be adequately sealed to prevent contamination from the space above them. Use should be made of well-sealed glass panels, especially in dividing walls, to ensure good visibility and satisfactory supervision. Doors and windows should fit flush with the walls. Windows should not be openable.

Internal fittings such as cupboards, drawers and shelves must be kept to a minimum. These may be made from stainless steel or a laminated plastic, which may be easily cleaned or disinfected; bare wood is to be avoided, although painted or otherwise sealed woodwork may be satisfactory. Stainless steel trolleys can be used to transport equipment and materials within the clean and aseptic areas but these must remain confined to their respective units. Equipment should be so designed as to be easily cleaned and sterilized (or disinfected).

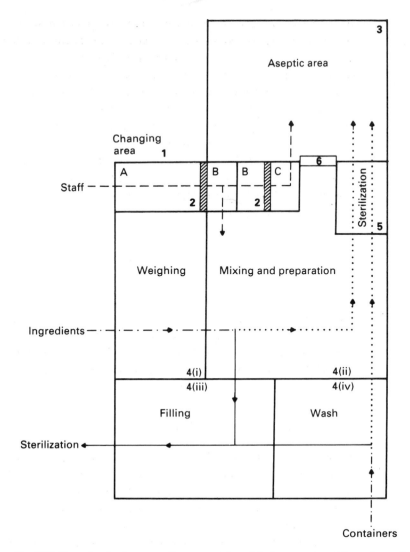

Fig. 22.1 Example of a diagrammatic representation of the layout and workflow of a sterile products manufacturing unit: **1**, The changing area in this example is built on the black (A)–grey (B)–white (C) principle; passage into the clean area is through A and B (see section 3.1.6) whereas entry to the aseptic area is first through A and B followed by C (see section 3.2.2). **2**, Dividing step-over sill. **3**, For details of aseptic area requirements, see text; a laminar airflow work station would be included in this area. **4i–4iv**, These areas are clean areas. In filling rooms for terminally sterilized products, care should be exercised to protect containers from airborne contamination. The final rinse point (i.e. where the containers are finally washed) should be sited as near as possible to the filling point. **5**, Articles which are to be transferred directly to the aseptic area from elsewhere must be sterilized by passage through a double-ended sterilizer. Solutions manufactured in the clean area may be brought into the aseptic area through a sterilizing-grade membrane filter. **6**, Double-doored hatchway through which presterilized articles may be passed into the aseptic area (see section 3.2.3).

Note: Inspection, holding and final packaging areas have been omitted. Direction of workflow: ——▶——, for terminally sterilized products; ···▶···, for aseptically prepared products; —·—▶—·—, shared stages of preparation.

Clean and aseptic areas must be adequately illuminated; lights are best housed above transparent panels set in a false ceiling. Electrical switches and sockets should fit flush to the wall. When required, gases should be piped into the area from outside the unit. Pipes and ducts, if they have to be brought into the clean area, must be effectively sealed through the walls. Additionally they must either be boxed in (which prevents dust accumulation) or readily cleanable. Alternatively, pipes and ducts may be sited above false ceilings.

Sinks supplied to clean areas should be made of stainless steel and have no overflow, and the water should be of at least potable quality. Wherever possible, drains in clean areas should be avoided. If installed, however, they should be fitted with effective, easily cleanable traps and with air breaks to prevent backflow. Any floor channels in a clean area should be open, shallow and cleanable and should be connected to drains outside the area. They should be monitored microbiologically. Sinks and drains should be excluded from aseptic areas except where radiopharmaceutical products are being processed when sinks are a requirement.

3.1.4   *Air supply*

Areas for the manufacture of sterile products are classified according to the required characteristics of the environment. Each manufacturing operation requires an appropriate level of microbial and particulate cleanliness; four grades (Table 22.1) are specified in the *Rules and Guidance for Pharmaceutical Manufacturers and Distributors* (1997), defined by measures of airborne contamination (Table 22.2). Environmental quality is substantially influenced by the air supplied to the manufacturing environment.

Filtered air (Chapter 17) is used to achieve the necessary standards; this should be maintained at positive pressure throughout a clean or aseptic area, with the highest

Table 22.1 Environmental grades and typical manufacturing operations

Environmental grade	Typical operations		Area designation in Fig. 22.1
	Aseptically prepared products	Terminally sterilized products (TSP)	
A	Aseptic preparation and filling in a protective work unit	Filling of products at particular microbiological risk	3
B	Background environment to grade A preparation areas	Background environment to grade A preparation areas	3
C	Preparation of solutions to be filtered	Preparation of 'at risk' solutions	4ii
		Filling of products	4ii
D	Handling of components after washing	Preparation of solutions and components for subsequent filling	4iv (aseptic)
			4ii (TSP)

Table 22.2 Basic operating standards for the manufacture of sterile products

| Environmental grade | Operating standards* | | Recommended limit of viable airborne microorganisms (cfu m^{-3}) |
| | Maximum permitted number of airborne particles/m^3 equal to or above specified size | | |
	0.5 μm	5 μm	
A	3 500	0	<1
B	350 000	2 000	10
C	3 500 000	20 000	100
D	ND	ND	200

* Particulate burdens for the manufacturing environment 'at rest' are more rigorous for grades B, C and D.
ND, not defined.

pressure in the most critical rooms (aseptic or clean filling rooms) and a progressive reduction through the preparation and changing rooms (Fig. 22.1); a minimum 10-kPa pressure differential is normally required between each class of room. A minimum of 20 air changes per hour is usual in clean and aseptic rooms. The air inlet points should be situated in or near the ceiling, with the final filters placed as close as possible to the point of input to the room.

The greatest risk of contamination of a pharmaceutical product comes from its immediate environment. Additional protection from particulate and microbial contamination is therefore essential in both the filling area of the clean room and in the aseptic unit. This can be provided by a protective work station supplied with a unidirectional flow of filtered sterile air. Such a facility is known as a laminar airflow unit in which the displacement of air is either horizontal (i.e. from back to front) or vertical (i.e. from top to bottom) with a minimum homogenous airflow rate of 0.45 m s^{-1} at the working position. Thus, airborne contamination is not added to the work space and any generated by manipulations within that area is swept away by the laminar air currents.

The efficacy of the filters through which the air is passed should be monitored at predetermined intervals (Chapter 17).

3.1.5 Clothing

Cotton material is comfortable to wear but because of the possibility of the shedding of fibres it is regarded as being unsuitable in the present context. Terylene, which sheds virtually no fibres, is suitable. Airborne particulate and microbial contamination is reduced when trouser suits, close-fitting at the neck, wrists and ankles, are worn. Clean suits for clean areas should be provided at least once daily, but fresh headwear, overshoes and powder-free gloves are necessary for each working session. Special laundering facilities for this clothing is desirable. Additional requirements for clothing worn in grade A/B areas are considered in section 3.2.1.

Changing facilities

Entry to clean or aseptic areas should be through a changing room fitted with interlocking doors; this acts as an airlock to prevent the influx of air from outside. This access route is intended for personnel only and does not constitute a means for regularly transferring materials and equipment into these areas. Staff entering the changing rooms should already be clad in the standard factory or hospital protective garments.

For a clean area, passage through the changing room should be from a 'black' area to a 'grey area', via a dividing step-over sill (Fig. 22.1). Movement through these areas and finally into the clean room is permitted only on observance of a strict protocol. In this, outer garments are removed in the 'black' area and clean-room trouser suits donned in the 'grey' area. After handwashing in a sink fitted with hand or foot-operated taps the operator may enter the clean room.

The changing procedure for personnel entering an aseptic area is dealt with in section 3.2.2.

Cleaning and disinfection

A strict cleaning and disinfection policy is essential if microbial contamination is to be kept to a minimum. Cleaning agents include alkaline detergents and ionic and non-ionic surfactants. A wide range of disinfectants is available commercially (Chapter 10) and a selection of those suitable for use in the sterile product manufacturing environment is given in Table 22.3. Different types of disinfectants should be employed in rotation to help prevent the development of resistant strains of microorganisms. In-use dilutions should not be stored unless sterilized. Disinfectants and detergents for use in grade A/B areas must be sterile prior to use.

As already mentioned, smooth, polished surfaces are cleaned most easily. Floors and horizontal surfaces should be cleaned and disinfected daily, walls and ceilings as often as required, but the interval should not exceed 1 month. Regular microbiological monitoring should be carried out to determine the efficacy of disinfection procedures. Records should be kept and immediate remedial action taken should normal levels for that area be exceeded.

Operation

The number of persons involved in sterile manufacturing should be as small as possible

Table 22.3 Disinfectants used during the manufacture of sterile products

Disinfectant	Application
Clear soluble phenols	Interior surfaces and fittings
Halogens, e.g. sodium hypochlorite	Working surfaces (limited use)
Alcohols: ethanol or isopropanol (usually as 70% solutions)	Working surfaces, equipment, gloved hands (rapid action)
Cationic agents (usually in 70% alcohol), e.g. cetrimide, chlorhexidine	Skin, gloved hands (rapid action with residual activity)

so as to avoid the inevitable turbulence and shedding of particles and organisms associated with operatives. All operations should be undertaken in a controlled and methodical manner as excessive activity may also increase turbulence and shedding of particles and organisms.

Containers made from fibrous materials such as paper, cardboard and sacking, are generally heavily contaminated (especially with moulds and bacterial spores) and should not be taken into clean or aseptic areas where fibres or microorganisms shed from them could contaminate the product. Ingredients which must be brought into clean areas must first be transferred to suitable metal or plastic containers.

Containers and closures for terminally sterilized products must be thoroughly cleaned before use and should undergo a final washing and rinsing process in apyrogenic distilled water (which has been passed through a bacteria-proof membrane filter) immediately prior to filling. Those containers and closures destined for use in aseptic manufacture must, in addition, be sterilized after washing and rinsing in preparation for aseptic filling.

3.2   Aseptic areas: additional requirements

Additional requirements for aseptic areas, over and above those discussed in sections 3.1.1–3.1.8, are considered below.

3.2.1   *Clothing*

Section 3.1.5 considered the general requirements for clothing. Additional requirements are demanded for aseptic areas. Since the operative is a potential source of contamination, it is axiomatic that steps must be taken to minimize this. Accordingly, the operative must wear sterile protective clothing including headwear (which should totally enclose hair and beard), powder-free rubber or plastic gloves, a non-fibre-shedding facemask (to prevent the release of droplets) and footwear. A suitable garment is a single or two-piece trouser suit. Fresh sterile clothing should normally be provided each time a person enters an aseptic area.

3.2.2   *Entry to aseptic areas*

Entry to an aseptic suite is usually by a 'black–grey–white' changing procedure. In this scheme, progress through from 'black' to 'white' represents passage into areas of increasing cleanliness, with the 'grey' area acting as an intermediate stage before entry to the 'white' (aseptic) changing area. Movement from 'black' to 'white' is generally through two changing rooms, the 'grey' area also serving as an entry to the clean room (Fig. 22.1 and section 3.1.6). In the 'black' area, the operative removes outer shoes and clothing, swings the legs over a dividing sill and dons slippers. He or she then enters the 'grey' area where, after washing, hands and forearms are dried, a sterile hood and mask donned, and the hands and forearms rewashed and redried. The operative next enters the 'white' area where a sterile-area suit, overboots and gloves are put on; the gloved hands are rinsed in a disinfectant solution. The aseptic area may then be entered and work commenced.

Equipment and operation

Articles which are to be discharged from the clean room (or elsewhere) to the aseptic area must be sterilized. To achieve this they should be transferred via a double-ended sterilizer (i.e. with a door at each end). If it is not possible, or required, that they be discharged directly to the aseptic area, they should be (i) double-wrapped before sterilization; (ii) transferred immediately after sterilization to a clean environment until required; and (iii) transferred from this clean environment via a double-doored hatch (where the outer wrapping is removed) to the aseptic area (where the inner wrapper is removed at the workbench). Hatchways and sterilizers should be arranged so that only one side of the entry into an aseptic area may be opened at any one time. Solutions manufactured in the clean room may be brought into the aseptic area through a sterile 0.22-μm bacteria-proof membrane filter.

Workbenches, including laminar airflow units, and equipment, should be disinfected immediately before and after each work period. Equipment used should be of the simplest design possible commensurate with the operation being undertaken.

Aseptic manipulations should be performed in the sterile air of a laminar airflow unit. Speed, accuracy and simplicity of movement, in accordance with a complete understanding of what is required, are essential features of a good aseptic technique.

Under no circumstances should living cultures of microorganisms, whether they be for vaccine preparation (Chapter 16) or for use in monitoring sterilization processes (Chapter 23), be taken into aseptic areas. As already pointed out, separate premises are needed for the aseptic filling of live or of attenuated vaccines.

3.2.4 *Isolator and blow/fill/seal technology*

Advances in technology now permit self-contained work stations to be created which incorporate many of the design principles of clean rooms and laminar air flow units. Isolators are designed to minimize direct human interventions in processing areas by internally providing grade A positive-pressure zoned laminar air flow and transfer devices accessed by means of a glove/sleeve system. As the name suggests, the work area can be isolated from the surrounding environment and a controlled background of grade D is usually adequate for aseptic processing in an isolator. Blow/fill/seal units are purpose-built machines providing, in one continuous operation, the automated formation of containers from thermoplastic granules, their subsequent filling and heat sealing. For aseptic production, these are fitted with a grade A air shower and operated in a grade C environment; for products subject to terminal sterilization a background grade D environment is sufficient.

4 Guide to Good Pharmaceutical Manufacturing Practice

Between 1971 and 1983 the essential features of GMP were covered in the UK by three editions of the *Guide to Good Pharmaceutical Manufacturing Practice*. This guide was prepared by the UK Medicines Inspectorate in consultation with industrial, hospital, professional and other interested parties. The principles of this national guide were subsequently assimilated into the *EC Guide to Good Manufacturing Practice for*

Medicinal Products in 1989 and are now published in the UK as *Rules and Guidance for Pharmaceutical Manufacturers and Distributors* (1997) by the Medicines Control Agency, Department of Health.

Compliance with the principles of GMP is one of the major factors considered by the Licensing Authority when examining an application for a licence to manufacture under the Medicines Act (1968). Similar codes exist in the USA and other countries.

5 Conclusions

The sole objective of all hygiene and manufacturing controls is to ensure the quality of the pharmaceutical product for the safety and protection of the patient. The manufacture of non-sterile pharmaceutical products requires that certain criteria of cleanliness, personal hygiene, production methods and storage must be met. Many such products are for oral and topical use and the question may fairly be posed as to the point of what are now quite stringent conditions. Nevertheless, some carefully controlled hospital studies have indeed shown that both types of medicine may be associated with nosocomial (hospital-acquired) infections and this risk can be minimized by the application of GMP principles.

A greater degree of stringency is required for the production of terminally sterilized products. Again, as the final product is subjected to a sterilization process (usually thermal), it may be asked why so much emphasis is placed upon process and environmental controls. The single most important reason is to ensure the lowest possible microbial burden to the sterilizer, thereby ensuring the highest sterility assurance levels attainable (Chapter 20). It must also be realized (as reiterated in Chapter 23) that it is far better to control a process from beginning to end, i.e. with frequent checks all along the line, than to rely solely on tests which can only determine whether a small proportion of the final products in a batch are satisfactory.

Even further criteria must be satisfied when products are being prepared aseptically where microbiological quality is entirely dependent upon observance of the highest possible production standards. It is essential that operatives have a sound working knowledge of the properties of microorganisms, and that they appreciate the importance of personal hygiene, of the techniques that will be adopted, and of the possible sources of contamination and error. In this respect, it is a sobering thought to realize that the great majority of reported defective medicinal products has resulted from human error or carelessness, not from technology failure.

6 Further reading

Denyer S.P. (1988) Clinical consequences of microbial action on medicines, In: *Biodeterioration* (eds D.R. Houghton, R.N. Smith & H.O W. Eggins), vol. 7, pp. 146–151. London: Elsevier Applied Science.

Denyer S.P. (1992) Filtration sterilization. In: *Principles and Practice of Disinfection, Preservation and Sterilization*, 2nd edn (eds A.D. Russell, W.B. Hugo & G.A.J. Ayliffe), pp. 573–604. Oxford: Blackwell Science.

Denyer S.P. & Baird R.M. (eds) (1990) *Guide to Microbiological Control in Pharmaceuticals*. Chichester: Ellis Horwood. (Chapters 4 and 5 provide additional information.)

Neiger J. (1997) Life with the UK pharmaceutical isolator guidelines: a manufacturer's viewpoint. *Eur J Parenteral Sci*, **2**, 13–20.

Ringertz O. & Ringertz S.H. (1982) The clinical significance of microbial contamination in pharmaceutical and allied products. *Adv Pharm Sci*, **5**, 201–226.

Rules and Guidance for Pharmaceutical Manufacturers and Distributors (1997) London: HMSO.

Spooner D.F. (1996) Hazards associated with the microbiological contamination of cosmetics, toiletries and non-sterile pharmaceuticals. In: *Microbial Quality Assurance in Cosmetics, Toiletries and Non-sterile Pharmaceuticals*, 2nd edn (eds R.M. Baird & S.F. Bloomfield), pp. 9–27. London: Taylor & Francis.

Underwood E. (1992) Good manufacturing practice. In: *Principles and Practice of Disinfection, Preservation and Sterilization*, 2nd edn (eds A.D. Russell, W.B. Hugo & G.A.J. Ayliffe), pp. 274–291. Oxford: Blackwell Science.

United States Pharmacopeia (1995) 23rd revision. Rockville, MD: US Pharmacopeial Convention. (Note the section dealing with microbial limit tests.)

23 Sterilization control and sterility assurance

1   Introduction

2   Bioburden determinations

3   Environmental monitoring

4   Sterilization monitors
4.1 Physical indicators
4.2 Chemical indicators
4.3 Biological indicators

5   Sterility testing
5.1 Methods
5.2 Antimicrobial agents

5.2.1 Specific inactivation
5.2.2 Dilution
5.2.3 Membrane filtration
5.3   Positive controls
5.4   Specific cases
5.5   Sampling

6   Conclusions

7   Acknowledgements

8   Further reading

1 Introduction

A product to be labelled 'sterile' must be free of viable microorganisms. To achieve this, the product, or its ingredients, must undergo a sterilization process of sufficient microbiocidal capacity to ensure a minimum level of sterility assurance (Chapter 20). It is essential that the required conditions for sterilization be achieved and maintained through every operation of the sterilizer.

Historically, the quality control of sterile products consisted largely, or, in some cases, even exclusively, of a sterility test, to which the product was subjected at the end of the manufacturing process. However, a growing awareness of the limitations of sterility tests in terms of their ability to detect low concentrations of microorganisms, has resulted in a shift in emphasis from a crucial dependence on end-testing to a situation in which the conferment of the status 'sterile' results from the attainment of satisfactory quality standards throughout the whole manufacturing process. In other words, the quality is 'assured' by a combination of process monitoring and performance criteria; these may be considered under four headings:

Bioburden determinations (section 2)
Environmental monitoring (section 3)
In-process monitoring of sterilization procedures (section 4)
Sterility testing (section 5).

In well-understood and well-characterized sterilization processes (e.g. heat and irradiation), where physical measurements may be accurately made, sterility can be assured by ensuring that the manufacturing process as a whole conforms to the established protocols for the first three of the above headings. In this case the process has satisfied the required parameters thereby permitting *parametric release* of the product without recourse to a sterility test.

This chapter will discuss briefly the principles and applications of the various methods of monitoring and validating sterilization processes.

2 Bioburden determinations

The term 'bioburden' is used to describe the concentration of microorganisms in a material; this may be either a total number of organisms per millilitre or per gram, regardless of type, or a breakdown into such categories as aerobic bacteria or yeasts and moulds. Bioburden determinations are normally undertaken by the supplier of the raw material, whose responsibility it is to ensure that the material supplied conforms to the agreed specification, but they may also be checked by the recipient. The maximum permitted concentrations of contaminants may be those specified in various pharmacopoeias or the levels established by the manufacturer during product development.

The level of sterility assurance which is achieved in a terminally sterilized product is dependent upon the design of the sterilization process itself and upon the bioburden immediately prior to sterilization (see Chapter 19). However, the adoption of high standards for the quality of the raw materials is not, in itself, a strategy which will ensure that the product has an acceptably low bioburden immediately prior to sterilization. It is necessary also to ensure that the opportunities for microbial contamination during manufacture are restricted (see below), and those organisms that *are* present initially do not normally find themselves in conditions conducive to growth. It is for these reasons that manufacturing processes are designed to utilize adverse temperatures, extreme pH values and organic solvent exposures in order to prevent an increase in the microbial load. For example, water is the most common, and potentially the most significant, source of contamination in the manufactured product, and maintenance of water at elevated temperatures is commonly employed as a means of limiting the growth of organisms such as *Pseudomonas* spp. which can proliferate during storage, even in distilled or deionized water. Precautions such as these ensure that chemically synthesized raw materials have bioburdens which are generally much lower than those found in 'natural' products of animal, vegetable or mineral origin.

3 Environmental monitoring

The levels of microbial contamination in the manufacturing areas (Chapter 22) are monitored on a regular basis to confirm that the numbers do not exceed specified limits. The concentrations of bacteria and of yeasts/moulds in the atmosphere may be determined either by use of 'settle plates' (Petri dishes of suitable media exposed for fixed periods, on which the colonies are counted after incubation) or by use of air samplers which cause a known volume of air to be passed over the agar surface. Similarly, the contamination on surfaces, including manufacturing equipment, may be measured using swabs or contact plates (also known as Rodac—replicate organism detection and counting—plates) which are specially designed Petri dishes slightly overfilled with agar, which, when set, projects very slightly above the plastic wall of the dish. This permits the plate to be inverted onto, or against, any solid surface, thereby allowing transfer of organisms from the surface onto the agar.

Less commonly, environmental monitoring can extend also to the operators in the manufacturing area whose clothing, e.g. gloves or face masks, may be sampled in order to estimate the levels and types of organisms which may arise as product contaminants from those sources.

4 Sterilization monitors

Monitoring of the sterilization process can be achieved by the use of physical, chemical or biological indicators of sterilizer performance. Such indicators are frequently employed in combination.

4.1 Physical indicators

In heat-sterilization processes, a temperature record chart is made of each sterilization cycle with both dry and moist heat (i.e. autoclave) sterilizers; this chart forms part of the batch documentation and is compared against a master temperature record (MTR). It is recommended that the temperature be taken at the coolest part of the loaded sterilizer. Further information on heat distribution and penetration within a sterilizer can be gained by the use of thermocouples placed at selected sites in the chamber or inserted directly into test packs or bottles. Since autoclaving depends also upon steam under pressure as well as temperature, pressure measurements form an essential part of the physical monitoring of this process. In addition, periodic leak tests are performed on prevacuum steam sterilizers to assess the efficiency of air removal prior to the introduction of steam.

For gaseous sterilization procedures, elevated temperatures are monitored for each sterilization cycle by temperature probes, and routine leak tests are performed to ensure gas-tight seals. Pressure and humidity measurements are recorded. Gas concentration is measured independently of pressure rise, often by reference to weight of gas used.

In radiation sterilization, a plastic (often perspex) dosimeter which gradually darkens in proportion to the radiation absorbed gives an accurate measure of the radiation dose and is considered to be the best technique currently available for following the radiosterilization process.

Sterilizing filters are subject to a bubble point pressure test, which is a technique employed for determining the pore size of filters, and may also be used to check the integrity of certain types of filter device (membrane and sintered glass; see Chapter 20) immediately after use. The principle of the test is that the wetted filter, in its assembled unit, is subjected to an increasing air or nitrogen gas pressure differential. The pressure difference recorded when the first bubble of gas breaks away from the filter is related to the *maximum* pore size. When the gas pressure is further increased slowly, there is a general eruption of bubbles over the entire surface. The pressure difference here is related to the *mean* pore size. A pressure differential below the expected value would signify a damaged or faulty filter. A modification to this test for membrane filters involves measuring the diffusion of gas through a wetted filter at pressures below the bubble point pressure (diffusion rate test); a faster diffusion rate than expected would again indicate a loss of filter integrity. In addition, a filter is considered ineffective when an unusually rapid rate of filtration occurs.

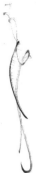

Efficiency testing of high-efficiency particulate air (HEPA) filters used for the supply of sterile air to aseptic workplaces (Chapter 22) is normally achieved by the generation upstream of dioctylphthalate (DOP) or sodium chloride particles of known dimension, followed by detection in downstream filtered air. Retention efficiency is recorded as the percentage of particles removed under defined test conditions. Microbiological tests are not normally performed.

4.2 Chemical indicators

Chemical monitoring of a sterilization process is based on the ability of heat, steam, sterilant gases and ionizing radiation to alter the chemical and/or physical characteristics of a variety of chemical substances. Ideally, this change should take place only when satisfactory conditions for sterilization prevail, thus confirming that a sterilization cycle has been successfully completed. In practice, however, the ideal indicator response is

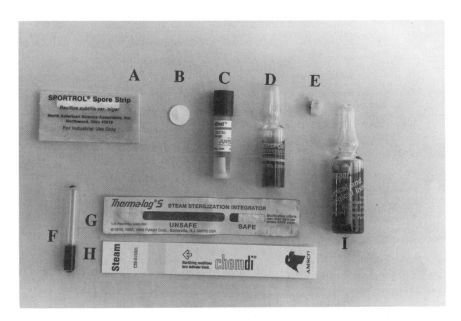

Fig. 23.1 Examples of biological and chemical indicators used for monitoring sterilization processes. (A and B) A spore strip (in a glassine envelope) and a spore disc, respectively; the spores are dried onto absorbent paper or fabric. (C) Attest™ indicator comprising a plastic vial containing a spore strip together with a sealed glass ampoule of culture medium; the ampoule is crushed after exposure and the medium immerses the strip. (D) Chemspor™ indicator in which bacterial spores are suspended in culture medium; the horizontal band on the ampoule also darkens on autoclaving to enable steam-exposed and non-exposed ampoules to be distinguished. (E) Plastic carrier with dried *Bacillus stearothermophilus* spores designed for monitoring low-temperature steam and formaldehyde cycles. (F) Browne's tube™; the liquid within the tube changes colour on heat exposure. (G) Thermalog™ strip in which a blue dye progresses from left to right during heat exposure. (H) Chemdi™ displays colour change in arrowed section of the strip after heating. (I) Chemspor™ which is a combined chemical and biological indicator; the ampoule contains a spore suspension in culture medium together with a second, smaller ampoule which contains a chemical indicator.

not always achieved and so a necessary distinction is made between (i) those chemical indicators which integrate several sterilization parameters (i.e. temperature, time and saturated steam) and closely approach the ideal; and (ii) those which measure only one parameter and consequently can only be used to distinguish processed from unprocessed articles. Thus, indicators which rely on the melting of a chemical substance show that the temperature has been attained but not necessarily maintained.

Chemical indicators generally undergo melting or colour changes (some examples are given in (Fig. 23.1)), the relationship of this change to the sterilization process being influenced by the design of the test device (Table 23.1). It must be remembered, however, that the changes recorded do not necessarily correspond to microbiological sterility and consequently the devices should never be employed as sole indicators in a sterilization process. Nevertheless, when included in strategically placed containers or packages, chemical indicators are valuable monitors of the conditions prevailing at the coolest or most inaccessible parts of a sterilizer.

4.3 Biological indicators

Biological indicators (BIs) for use in thermal, chemical or radiation sterilization processes consist of standardized bacterial spore preparations which are usually in the form either of suspensions in water or culture medium or of spores dried on paper, aluminium or plastic carriers. As with chemical indicators, they are usually placed in dummy packs located at strategic sites in the sterilizer. Alternatively, for gaseous sterilization these may also be placed within a tubular helix (Line–Pickerill) device. After the sterilization process, the aqueous suspensions or spores on carriers are aseptically transferred to an appropriate nutrient medium which is then incubated and periodically examined for signs of growth. Spores of *Bacillus stearothermophilus* in sealed ampoules of culture medium are used for steam sterilization monitoring, and these may be incubated directly at 55°C; this eliminates the need for an aseptic transfer.

Table 23.1 Examples of chemical indicators for monitoring sterilization processes

Sterilization method	Principle	Device	Parameter(s) monitored
Heat Autoclaving or dry heat	Temperature-sensitive coloured solution	Sealed tubes partly filled with a solution which changes colour at elevated temperatures; rate of colour change is proportional to temperature, e.g. Browne's tubes	Temperature, time
Dry heat only	Temperature-sensitive chemical	Usually a temperature-sensitive white wax concealing a black marked or printed (paper) surface; at a predetermined temperature the wax rapidly melts exposing the background mark(s)	Temperature

Continued on p. 444

Table 23.1 *Continued*

Sterilization method	Principle	Device	Parameter(s) monitored
Heating in an autoclave only	Steam-sensitive chemical	Usually an organic chemical in a printing ink base impregnated into a carrier material. A combination of moisture and heat produces a darkening of the ink, e.g. autoclave tape. Devices of this sort can be used within dressings packs to confirm adequate removal of air and penetration of saturated steam (Bowie–Dick test)	Saturated steam
	Capillary principle (Thermalog S)	Consists of a blue dye in a waxy pellet, the melting-point of which is depressed in the presence of saturated steam. At autoclaving temperatures, and in the continued presence of steam, the pellet melts and travels along a paper wick forming a blue band the length of which is dependent upon both exposure time and temperature	Temperature, saturated steam, time
Gaseous sterilization Ethylene oxide (EO)	Reactive chemical	Indicator paper impregnated with a reactive chemical which undergoes a distinct colour change on reaction with EO in the presence of heat and moisture. With some devices rate of colour development varies with temperature and EO concentration	Gas concentration, temperature, time (selected devices); NB a minimum relative humidity (rh) is required for device to function
	Capillary principle (Thermalog G)	Based on the same 'migration along wick' principle as Thermalog S. Optimum response in a cycle of 600 mg l^{-1} EO, temperature 54°C, rh 40–80%. Lower EO levels and/or temperature will slow response time, blue colour of band is fugitive at rh <30%	Gas concentration, temperature, time (selected cycles)
Low temperature steam and formaldehyde	Reactive chemical	Indicator paper impregnated with a formaldehyde-, steam- and temperature-sensitive reactive chemical which changes colour during the sterilization process	Gas concentration, temperature, time (selected cycles)
Radiation sterilization	Radiochromic chemical	Plastic devices impregnated with radiosensitive chemicals which undergo colour changes at relatively low radiation doses	Only indicate exposure to radiation
	Dosimeter device	Acidified ferric ammonium sulphate or ceric sulphate solutions respond to irradiation by dose-related changes in their optical density (see also section 2.1.3)	Accurately measure radiation doses

Aseptic transfers are also avoided by the use of self-contained units where the spore strip and nutrient medium are present in the same device ready for mixing after use.

The bacterial species to be used in a BI must be selected carefully, since it must be non-pathogenic and should possess above-average resistance to the particular sterilization process. Resistance is adjudged from the spore destruction curve obtained upon exposure to the sterilization process; recommended BI spores and their decimal reduction times (*D*-values; Chapter 20) are shown in Table 23.2. Great care must be taken in the preparation and storage of BIs to ensure a standardized response to sterilization processes. Indeed, while certainly offering the most direct method of monitoring sterilization processes, it should be realized that BIs may be less reliable monitors than physical methods and are not recommended for routine use, except in the case of gaseous sterilization.

One of the long-standing criticisms of BIs is that the incubation period required in order to confirm a satisfactory sterilization process imposes an undesirable delay on the release of the product. This problem has been overcome, with respect to steam sterilization at least, by the use of a detection system in which a spore enzyme, α-glucosidase (reflective of spore viability), converts a non-fluorescent substrate into a fluorescent product in as little as 1 hour.

Filtration sterilization requires a different approach from biological monitoring, the test effectively measuring the ability of a filter to produce a sterile filtrate from a culture of a suitable organism. For this purpose, *Serratia marcescens*, a small Gram-negative rod-shaped bacterium (minimum dimension 0.5 μm), has been recommended in the *Pharmaceutical Codex* (1979). The bacterial challenge test is the most severe to which a filter of any construction can be subjected. In the membrane-filter industry, the test using *Ser. marcescens* is usually reserved for filters of 0.45-μm pore size, and a more rigorous test involving *Brevundimonas diminuta*—formerly *Pseudomonas diminuta*—having a minimum dimension of 0.3 μm is applied to filters of 0.22-μm

Table 23.2 Biological indicators for monitoring sterilization processes*

Sterilization process	Species	Inoculum size	*D*-value
Heating in an autoclave (121°C)	*Bacillus stearothermophilus*	>10^5	1.5 min
	Clostridium sporogenes	>10^5	0.8 min
Dry heat (160°C)	*Bacillus subtilis* var. *niger*	>10^5	5–10 min
Ethylene oxide (EO)† (EO 600 mg l^{-1}, temperature 54°C and 60% relative humidity)	*Bacillus subtilis* var. *niger*	>5 × 10^5	2.5 min
Low temperature steam (73°C) and formaldehyde (12 mg l^{-1})‡	*Bacillus stearothermophilus*	—	5 min
Ionizing radiation	*Bacillus pumilus*	10^7–10^8	3 kGy (0.3 Mrad)

* *British Pharmacopoeia* (1993).
† *European Pharmacopoeia* (1997).
‡ Soper & Davies (1990).

pore size. The latter filters are defined as those capable of completely removing *Brev. diminuta* from suspension. In this test, using this organism, a realistic inoculum level must be adopted, since the probability of bacteria appearing in the filtrate rises as the number of *Brev. diminuta* cells in the test challenge increases; a standardized inoculum size of 10^7 cells cm^{-2} is normally employed. The extent of the passage of this organism through membrane filters is enhanced by increasing the filtration pressure. Thus, successful sterile filtration depends markedly on the challenge conditions.

5   Sterility testing

A sterility test is basically a test which assesses whether a sterilized pharmaceutical or medical product is free from contaminating microorganisms, by incubation of either the whole or a part of that product with a nutrient medium. It thus becomes a destructive test and raises the question as to its suitability for testing large, expensive or delicate products or equipment. Furthermore, by its very nature such a test is a statistical process in which part of a batch is randomly* sampled and the chance of the batch being passed for use then depends on the sample passing the sterility test.

A further limitation is that which is inherent in a procedure intended to demonstrate a negative. A sterility test is intended to demonstrate that no viable organisms are present, but failure to detect them could simply be a consequence of the use of unsuitable media or inappropriate cultural conditions. To be *certain* that no organisms are present it would be necessary to use a universal culture medium suitable for the growth of *any* possible contaminant and to incubate the sample under an infinite variety of conditions. Clearly, no such medium, or combination of media, are available, and, in practice, only media capable of supporting non-fastidious bacteria, yeasts and moulds are employed. Furthermore, in pharmacopoeial tests, no attempt is made to detect viruses, which , on a size basis, are the organisms most likely to pass through a sterilizing filter. Nevertheless, the sterility test does have an important application in monitoring the microbiological quality of filter-sterilized, aseptically filled products and does offer a final check on terminally sterilized articles. In the UK, test procedures laid down by the *European Pharmacopoeia* must be followed; this provides details of the sample sizes to be adopted in particular cases. The principles of these tests are discussed in brief below.

5.1   Methods

There are three alternative methods available when conducting sterility tests.

1   The direct inoculation procedure involves introducing test samples directly into nutrient media. The *British Pharmacopoeia* recommends two media: (i) fluid mercaptoacetate medium, which contains glucose and sodium mercaptoacetate (sodium thioglycollate) and is particularly suitable for the cultivation of anaerobic organisms (incubation temperature 30–35°C); and (ii) soyabean casein digest medium, which will support the growth of both aerobic bacteria (incubation temperature 30–35°C) and

* It has been proposed that random sampling be applied to products which have been processed and filled aseptically. With products sterilized in their final containers, samples should be taken from the potentially coolest or least sterilant-accessible part of the load.

fungi (incubation temperature 20–25°C). Other media may be used provided they can be shown to be suitable alternatives.

2   Membrane filtration is the technique recommended by most pharmacopoeias and involves filtration of fluids through a sterile membrane filter (pore size ≤0.45 μm), any microorganism present being retained on the surface of the filter. After washing *in situ*, the filter is divided aseptically and portions transferred to suitable culture media which are then incubated at the appropriate temperature for the required period of time. Water-soluble solids can be dissolved in a suitable diluent and processed in this way.

3   A sensitive method for detecting low levels of contamination in intravenous infusion fluids involves the addition of a concentrated culture medium to the fluid in its original container, such that the resultant mixture is equivalent to single strength culture medium. In this way, sampling of the entire volume is achieved.

With the techniques discussed above, the media employed should previously have been assessed for nutritive (growth-supporting) properties and a lack of toxicity using specified organisms. It must be remembered that any survivors of a sterilization process may be damaged and thus must be given the best possible conditions for growth.

As a precaution against accidental contamination, product testing must be carried out under conditions of strict asepsis using, for example, a laminar airflow cabinet to provide a suitable environment (Chapter 22).

Both the British and European pharmacopoeias indicate that it is necessary to conduct control tests which confirm the adequacy of the facilities by sampling of air and surfaces and carrying out control tests using samples 'known' to be sterile. In reality, this means

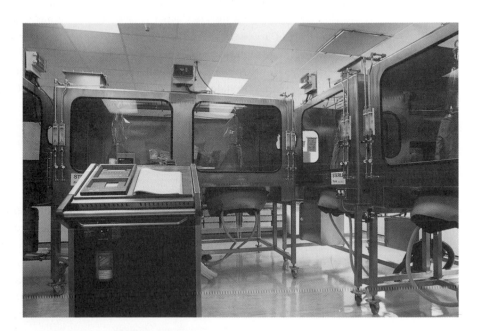

Fig. 23.2 Isolators used for sterility testing. The operator works within the hood which is suspended inside the cubicle; the hydrogen peroxide generator which is used to sterilize the isolators is shown in the left foreground. (Courtesy of SmithKline Beecham Pharmaceuticals.)

samples that have been subjected to a very reliable sterilization process, e.g. radiation, or samples that have subjected to a sterilization procedure more than once. In order to minimize the risk of introducing contaminants from the surroundings or from the operator during the test itself, isolators are often employed which physically separate the operator from the materials under test. These are designed on the same principle as a glove box, but on a much larger and more sophisticated scale, so the operator works inside a sterile cubicle but is separated from the atmosphere within it by a flexible moulded covering (rather like a space suit) which is an integral part of the cubicle base (Fig. 23.2).

5.2 Antimicrobial agents

Where an antimicrobial agent comprises the product or forms part of the product, for example as a preservative, its activity must be nullified in some way during sterility testing so that an inhibitory action in preventing the growth of any contaminating microorganisms is overcome. This is achieved by the following methods (sections 5.2.1–5.2.3).

5.2.1 *Specific inactivation*

An appropriate inactivating (neutralizing) agent (Table 23.3) is incorporated into the culture media. The inactivating agent must be non-toxic to microorganisms as must any product resulting from an interaction of the inactivator and the antimicrobial agent.

Although Table 23.3 lists only benzylpenicillin and ampicillin as being inactivated by β-lactamase (from *B. cereus*), other β-lactams may also be hydrolysed by their appropriate β-lactamase. Other antibiotic-inactivating enzymes are also known (Chapter 9) and have been considered as possible inactivating agents, e.g. chloramphenicol acetyltransferase (inactivates chloramphenicol) and enzymes that modify aminoglycoside antibiotics. In addition, encouraging results have been obtained by the use of antibiotic-absorbing resins.

Table 23.3 Inactivating agents*

Inhibitory agents	Inactivating agents
Phenols, cresols	None (dilution)
Alcohols	None (dilution)
Parabens	Dilution and Tween
Mercury compounds	-SH compounds
Quaternary ammonium compounds	Lecithin + Lubrol W; Lecithin + Tween (Letheen)
Benzylpenicillin† Ampicillin	} β-Lactamase from *Bacillus cereus*
Other antibiotics†	None (membrane filtration)
Sulphonamides	*p*-Aminobenzoic acid

* Neutralizing agents; see also Table 11.4 (Chapter 11).
† See text.

Dilution

The antimicrobial agent is diluted in the culture medium to a level at which it ceases to have any activity, for example phenols, cresols and alcohols (see Chapter 11). This method applies to substances with a high dilution coefficient, η.

Membrane filtration

This method has traditionally been used to overcome the activity of antibiotics for which there are no inactivating agents, although it could be extended to cover other products if necessary, e.g. those containing preservatives for which no specific or effective inactivators are available. Basically, a solution of the product is filtered through a hydrophobic-edged membrane filter which will retain any contaminating microorganisms. The membrane is washed *in situ* to remove any traces of antibiotic adhering to the membrane and is then transferred to appropriate culture media.

5.3 Positive controls

It is essential to show that microorganisms will actually grow under the conditions of the test. For this reason positive controls have to be carried out; in these, the ability of small numbers of suitable microorganisms to grow in media in the presence of the sample is assessed. The microorganism used for positive control tests with a product containing or comprising an antimicrobial agent must, if at all possible, be sensitive to that agent, so that growth of the organism indicates a satisfactory inactivation, dilution or removal of the agent. The *British Pharmacopoeia* suggests the use of appropriate strains of *Staphylococcus aureus*, *Cl. sporogenes* and *Candida albicans* for aerobic, anaerobic and fungal positive controls, respectively.

In practice, a positive control (media with added test sample) and a negative control (media without it) are inoculated simultaneously, and the rate and extent of growth arising in each should be similar. However, the negative control without the test sample, is, in effect, exactly the same as the nutritive properties control which is also described in the test procedure, so, for the organisms concerned, it is not necessary to do both.

All the controls may be conducted either before, or in parallel with, the test itself, providing that the same batches of media are used for both. If the controls are carried out in parallel with the tests and one of the controls gives an unexpected result, the test for sterility attempt is recorded as invalid, and, when the problem is resolved, the test is 'recommended' *as if for the first time*. It is important to recognize that the terms 'recommended' and 'retest' have different meanings. A 'retest' may, under certain circumstances, be performed when the first (and, exceptionally, even the second) *valid* test shows signs of product contamination.

5.4 Specific cases

Specific details of the sterility testing of parenteral products, ophthalmic and other non-injectable preparations, catgut, surgical dressings and dusting powders will be found in the British and European pharmacopoeias.

Sampling

A sterility test attempts to infer the state (sterile or non-sterile) of a batch from the results of an examination of part of a batch, and is thus a statistical operation.

Suppose that p represents the proportion of infected containers in a batch and q the proportion of non-infected containers. Then, $p + q = 1$ or $q = 1 - p$.

Suppose also that a sample of two items is taken from a large batch containing 10% infected containers. The probability of a single item taken at random being infected is $p = 0.1$ (10% = 0.1), whereas the probability of such an item being non-infected is given by $q = 1 - p = 0.9$.

The probability of both items being infected is $p^2 = 0.01$, and of both items being non-infected, $q^2 = (1 - p)^2 = 0.81$. The probability of obtaining one infected item and one non-infected item is $1 - (0.01 + 0.81) = 0.18 = 2pq$.

In a sterility test involving a sample size of n containers, the probability p of obtaining n consecutive 'steriles' is given by $q^n = (1 - p)^n$. Values for various levels of p (i.e. proportion of infected containers in a batch) with a constant sample size are given in Table 23.4 which shows that the test cannot detect low levels of contamination. Similarly, if different sample sizes are employed (based also upon $(1 - p)^n$) it can be shown that as the sample size increases, the probability of the batch being passed as sterile decreases.

The *British Pharmacopoeia* makes an allowance for accidental contamination which may arise during the execution of a sterility test by allowing the test to be repeated. Under these circumstances the following rules apply.

1 If no growth occurs with fresh samples, the batch passes the test.

2 If growth occurs, but the organism differs from that found previously, the test is repeated on a third sample from the batch using double the number of containers of product.

3 If no growth occurs with the third sample, the batch passes the sterility test; if, however, any microorganism is found, the batch is treated as non-sterile, unless or until the material has been resterilized and has passed the above tests.

In actual fact, however, these additional tests increase the chances of passing a batch containing a proportion of infected items (Table 23.4, first retest). This may be

Table 23.4 Sampling in sterility testing

	Infected items in batch (%)					
	0.1	1	5	10	20	50
p	0.001	0.01	0.05	0.1	0.2	0.5
q	0.999	0.99	0.95	0.9	0.8	0.5
Probability P, of drawing 20 consecutive sterile items:						
First sterility test*	0.98	0.82	0.36	0.12	0.012	<0.00001
First retest†	0.99	0.99	0.84	0.58	0.11	0.002

* Calculated from $P = (1 - p)^{20} = q^{20}$.
† Calculated from $P = (1 - p)^{20} [2 - (1 - p)^{20}]$.

deduced by using the mathematical formula

$$(1 - p)^n[2 - (1 - p)^n]$$

which gives the chance in the first retest of passing a batch containing a proportion p of infected containers.

It can be seen from the above that a sterility test can only show that a proportion of the products in a batch is sterile. Thus, the correct conclusion to be drawn from a satisfactory test result is that the batch has passed the sterility test *not* that the batch is sterile.

6   Conclusions

The techniques discussed in this chapter comprise an attempt to achieve, as far as possible, the continuous monitoring of a particular sterilization process. The sterility test *on its own* provides no guarantee as to the sterility of a batch; however, it is an additional check, and continued compliance with the test does give confidence as to the efficacy of a sterilization or aseptic process. Failure to carry out a sterility test, despite the major criticism of its inability to detect other than gross contamination, may have important legal and moral consequences.

7   Acknowledgements

We are grateful to SmithKline Beecham Pharmaceuticals for permission to use Fig. 23.2.

8   Further reading

Baird R.M. & Bloomfield S.F. (eds) (1996) *Microbial Quality Assurance in Cosmetics, Toiletries and Non-sterile Pharmaceuticals.* London: Taylor & Francis.

British Pharmacopoeia (1993) London: HMSO.

Denyer S.P. (1982) In-use contamination in intravenous therapy—the scale of the problem. In: *Infusions and Infection. The Hazards of In-use Contamination in Intravenous Therapy* (ed. P.F. D'Arcy), pp. 1–16. Oxford: Medicine Publishing Foundation.

Denyer S.P. (1992) Filtration sterilization. In: *Principles and Practice of Disinfection, Preservation and Sterilization*, 2nd edn. (eds A.D. Russell, W.B. Hugo & G.A.J. Ayliffe), pp. 573–604. Oxford: Blackwell Science.

Denyer S.P. & Baird R.M. (eds) (1990) *Guide to Microbiological Control in Pharmaceuticals.* Chichester: Ellis Horwood. (Chapters 7, 8 and 9 provide additional information).

European Pharmacopoeia, 3rd edn. (1997) Maisonneuve: SA.

Gardner J.F. & Peel M.M. (1991) *Introduction to Sterilisation, Disinfection and Infection Control*, 2nd edn. Melbourne: Churchill Livingstone.

Greene V.N. (1992) Control of sterilization processes. In: *Principles and Practice of Disinfection, Preservation and Sterilization*, 2nd edn. (eds A.D. Russell, W.B. Hugo & G.A.J. Ayliffe), pp. 605–624. Oxford: Blackwell Scientific Publications.

Gilbert P. & Allison D. (1996) Redefining the 'sterility' of sterile products. *Eur J Parenteral Sci*, **1**, 19–23.

Health Technical Memorandum (1994) *Sterilisers.* HTM 2010. London: Department of Health.

Hodges, N.A. (1995) Reproducibility and performance of endospores as biological indicators. In: *Microbiological Quality Assurance: a Guide Towards Relevance and Reproducibility of Inocula* (eds M.R.W. Brown & P. Gilbert), pp. 221–234. New York: CRC Press.

Hoxey E.V., Soper C.J. & Davies D.J.G. (1984) The effect of temperature and formaldehyde concentration on the inactivation of *Bacillus stearothermophilus* spores by LTSF. *J Pharm Pharmacol*, **36**, 60.

Line S.J. & Pickerell J.K. (1973) Testing a steam-formaldehyde sterilizer for gas penetration efficiency. *J Clin Pathol*, **26**, 716–720.

Pharmaceutical Codex (1994) London: Pharmaceutical Press.

Soper C.J. & Davies D.J.G. (1990) Principles of sterilization. In: *Guide to Microbiological Control in Pharmaceuticals* (eds S.P. Denyer & R.M. Baird), pp. 157–181. Chichester: Ellis Horwood.

United States Pharmacopoeia (1995) 23rd revision. Rockville, MD: US Pharmacopeial Convention.

24 Production of therapeutically useful substances by recombinant DNA technology

1   Introduction

2   The basic principles of recombinant
     DNA technology
2.1 Introduction to cloning
2.2 Expression of cloned genes
2.2.1 Transcription
2.2.2 Translation
2.2.3 Post-translational modification
2.3 Maximizing gene expression
2.4 Choice of cloning host

3   Production of medically important
     polypeptides and proteins

4   Authenticity and efficacy of drugs
     produced by recombinant DNA
     technology

5   Future trends with protein
     pharmaceuticals
5.1 Small-molecule drugs
5.2 Anti-sense agents
5.3 Gene therapy and gene repair

6   Glossary

7   Further reading

1   Introduction

Natural products of pharmaceutical interest are synthesized by a wide variety of organisms, ranging from prokaryotes such as bacteria to eukaryotes such as yeast, other fungi, flowering plants, animals and man. The commercial production of compounds from microbes is relatively simple since the organism in question can be grown on a large scale and high-yielding variants can be isolated following many successive rounds of mutation and selection. A good example is penicillin production by *Penicillium chrysogenum* (Chapter 7), where the wild strain yield of a few milligrams per litre has been raised to over $20\,g\,l^{-1}$. Commercial production of compounds from plants is less easy since synthesis may be tissue or organ specific and may only occur at a certain developmental stage. If the genetics of the producing organism have not been studied then selection of high-yielding variants is extremely difficult. Molecules of pharmacological interest from higher animals are by definition extremely potent, for example hormones, and so are synthesized in relatively minute quantities. This is a serious limitation if the producing organisms are animals such as cattle or pigs, as in the case of insulin, but production is well nigh impossible if the only source is man himself, as with human growth hormone.

In order that demand should meet supply, or to reduce production costs, it would be of great benefit if microorganisms could be induced to synthesize pharmacologically active molecules whose production is normally limited to higher plants and animals. With the advent of recombinant DNA technology, often called genetic engineering, this is now possible and synthesis no longer is restricted to polypeptides.

The advantages of recombinant DNA technology are enormous, as the following example shows. Somatostatin is a hormone that inhibits the secretion of pituitary growth hormone. The researchers who first isolated somatostatin required nearly half a million sheep brains to produce 5 mg of the substance. Using a chemically synthesized gene, 9 litres of bacterial culture, costing just a few pounds or dollars, produced the same amount. Development work has already led to the production of numerous biologically active human agents in clinically significant amounts, and a number of them are commercially available (see Table 24.2, pp. 463–464).

2   The basic principles of recombinant DNA technology

2.1   Introduction to cloning

Let us suppose that we wish to construct a bacterium which produces human insulin. Naively, it might be thought that all that is required is to introduce the human insulin gene into its new host. The fallacy with this idea is that foreign genes are not maintained in cells, since they are not replicated. With recombinant DNA technology this problem is solved by inserting the insulin gene into a cloning vector. The latter is simply a DNA molecule that can replicate *in vivo*. Cloning vectors are usually plasmids (Chapter 9), which are extrachromosomal, autonomously replicating DNA molecules (Fig. 24.1).

In order to insert foreign DNA into a plasmid, use is made of special enzymes known as restriction endonucleases. These enzymes cut large DNA molecules into shorter fragments by cleavage at specific recognition sites (Fig. 24.2), i.e. they are highly specific deoxyribonucleases (DNases). Some of these enzymes generate fragments with single-strand protrusions called 'sticky-ends' because their bases are complementary. Fragments of the foreign DNA are inserted into plasmid vectors cut

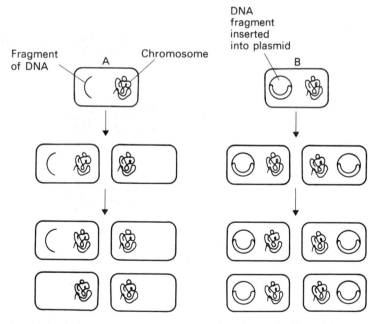

Fig. 24.1 The requirement for a cloning vector: (A) fragments of DNA introduced into the bacterium by transformation do not undergo replication and gradually are diluted out of the population; (B) DNA fragments introduced into plasmids are inherited by both daughter progeny at cell division.

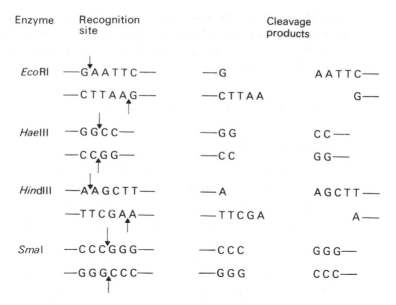

Enzyme	Recognition site	Cleavage products	
*Eco*RI	—G A A T T C—	—G	A A T T C—
	—C T T A A G—	—C T T A A	G—
*Hae*III	—G G C C—	—G G	C C —
	—C C G G—	—C C	G G—
*Hind*III	—A A G C T T—	—A	A G C T T —
	—T T C G A A—	—T T C G A	A—
*Sma*I	—C C C G G G—	—C C C	G G G—
	—G G G C C C—	—G G G	C C C—

Fig. 24.2 The recognition sites of some common restriction endonucleases. The arrows indicate the cleavage points.

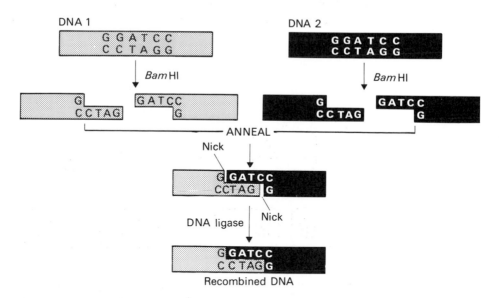

Fig. 24.3 The construction of a chimeric (or recombinant) DNA molecule by joining together two DNA fragments produced by cleavage of different parental DNA molecules with the same restriction endonuclease.

open with the same enzyme, which therefore have matching ends (Fig. 24.3). The resulting recombinants or *chimeras* are transformed into the new host microbe. Since each transformant may contain a different fragment of the foreign genome it is necessary to select those with the desired gene. In practice this can be the most difficult step, but the screening methods used are outside the scope of this chapter. Suffice to say that a necessary prerequisite usually is a sensitive test for the desired protein product.

Theoretically, it is possible to clone any desired gene by 'shotgunning'. This is done by inserting into plasmids a random mixture of fragments from total human DNA, in the case of the insulin gene, and then selecting the appropriate clone. However, if introduced into a bacterium this clone would not make human insulin. The reason for this is that many genes of eukaryotes, including the human insulin gene, are a mixture of coding regions (called *exons*) and non-coding regions (called *introns*). In eukaryotes, genes containing introns are transcribed into messenger RNA (mRNA) in the usual manner but then the corresponding intron sequences are spliced out (Fig. 24.4). Unfortunately not all bacteria can splice out introns.

A solution to the problem of introns is to isolate mRNA extracted from the human pancreas cells that make insulin. These cells are rich in insulin mRNA from which introns have already been spliced out. Using the enzyme *reverse transcriptase* it is possible to convert this spliced mRNA into a DNA copy. This copy DNA (cDNA), which carries the uninterrupted genetic information for insulin can be cloned. Although yeast cells (*Saccharomyces*) can splice out introns it is normal practice to eliminate them anyway by cDNA cloning.

An alternative approach is to synthesize an artificial gene in the test-tube starting with the appropriate deoxyribonucleotides. This approach, which demands that the entire amino acid sequence be known, has been used to clone genes encoding proteins 200 amino acids long.

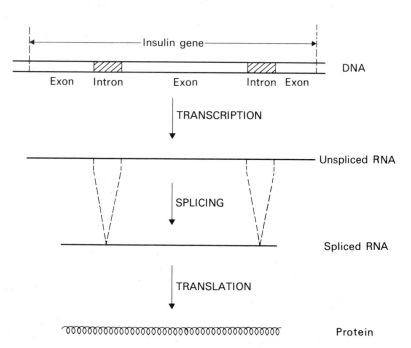

Fig. 24.4 Splicing of a messenger RNA molecule transcribed from a hypothetical insulin gene containing two introns.

2.2   Expression of cloned genes

Once a gene is cloned it is necessary to convert the information contained in it into a functional protein. There are a number of steps in gene expression: (i) transcription of DNA into mRNA; (ii) translation of the mRNA into a protein sequence: and (iii) in some instances, post-translational modification of the protein. In discussing these steps in more detail, expression of a cloned insulin gene will be used as an example.

2.2.1   *Transcription*

Transcription of DNA into mRNA is mediated by the enzyme RNA polymerase. The first stage is binding of the RNA polymerase to recognition sites on the DNA which are called *promoters*. After binding, the RNA polymerase proceeds along the DNA molecule until a termination signal is encountered. It follows that a gene which does not lie between a promoter and a termination signal will not be transcribed. This would be the case with a cloned insulin gene, since neither a cDNA gene nor an artificially synthesized gene will carry a promoter. The solution is to clone the gene into a vector close to a bacterial promotor. An example is shown in Fig. 24.5.

2.2.2   *Translation*

Translation of mRNA into protein is a complex process which involves interaction of the messenger with ribosomes. One prerequisite for this is that the mRNA must carry a ribosome binding site (RBS) in front of the gene to be translated. After binding, the ribosome moves along the mRNA and initiates protein synthesis at the first AUG codon it encounters. A synthetic insulin gene will lack an RBS and if a cDNA is used as the starting material the RBS may be lost in the process of cloning. The solution is to

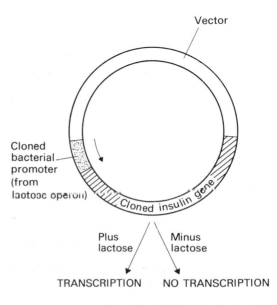

Fig. 24.5 Insertion of a cloned insulin gene into a vector carrying a bacterial promoter. The arrow indicates the direction of transcription. If we suppose the bacterial promoter is derived from the lactose operon then transcription will be initiated only in the presence of lactose.

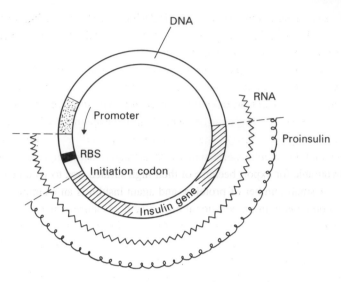

Fig. 24.6 The use of a vector carrying a promoter and adjacent ribosome binding site (RBS) and initiation codon to obtain synthesis of proinsulin from a synthetic gene. The arrow indicates the direction of transcription.

utilize a vector in which the insulin gene can be inserted downstream from a promoter and RBS (Fig. 24.6).

Post-translational modification

A number of proteins undergo post-translational modifications and insulin is one of these. Proteins which are to be secreted are synthesized with an extra 15–30 amino acids at the N-terminus. These extra amino acids are referred to as a *signal sequence* and a common feature of these sequences is that they have a central core of hydrophobic amino acids flanked by polar or hydrophilic residues. During passage through the membrane the signal sequence is cleaved off (Fig. 24.7). If the insulin gene were cloned by the cDNA method then the signal sequence would be present and, in *Escherichia coli* at least, the insulin would be transported through the cytoplasmic membrane (*exported*). Using the synthetic gene approach, a signal sequence would be present on the protein only if the corresponding coding sequence had been incorporated at the

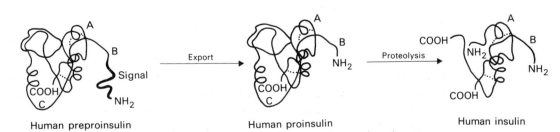

Fig. 24.7 The conversion of preproinsulin to insulin by sequential removal of the signal peptide and the C fragment.

time of construction. Sometimes it is desirable for the bacterium to export the protein, in which case a signal sequence is incorporated; with other proteins it may be desirable that they are retained within the cell.

In *E. coli* cells, the presence of a signal sequence usually results in export of a protein into the periplasmic space rather than into the growth medium. Unfortunately, many recombinant proteins are rapidly and extensively degraded in the periplasmic space because of the presence there of numerous proteases. In Gram-positive bacteria and eukaryotic microorganisms, signal sequences direct proteins into the growth medium. Filamentous organisms such as fungi or actinomycetes might be particularly favourable for export because of their high surface area to volume ratio.

A small number of proteins, and again insulin is an example, are synthesized as pro-proteins with an additional amino acid sequence which dictates the final three-dimensional structure. In the case of proinsulin, proteolytic attack cleaves out a stretch of 35 amino acids in the middle of the molecule to generate insulin. The peptide that is removed is known as the C chain. The other chains, A and B, remain crosslinked and thus locked in a stable tertiary structure by the disulphide bridges formed when the molecule originally folded as proinsulin. Bacteria have no mechanism for specifically cutting out the folding sequences from pro-hormones and the way of solving this problem is described in a later section.

Another modification which can be made *in vivo* is glycosylation, for example that of β and γ interferons, although the biological role of the sugar residues is not known. Bacteria cannot glycosylate the products of cloned mammalian genes. These non-glycosylated proteins retain their pharmacological activity but their pharmacokinetics and *in vitro* stability may be different. Yeast cells can glycosylate proteins but the pattern of glycosylation may well be different from that seen in the normal host of the gene. Non-glycosylated or wrongly glycosylated proteins may provoke the formation of antibodies following administration.

2.3 Maximizing gene expression

From a commercial point of view it is desirable to maximize the yield of protein in a fermentation. This means maximizing gene expression and important factors are:
1 the number of copies of the plasmid vector per unit cell (*copy number*);
2 the strength of the promoter;
3 the sequences of the RBS and flanking DNA;
4 proteolysis.

The limiting factor in expression is the initiation of protein synthesis. Increasing the copy number of the plasmid increases the number of mRNA molecules transcribed from the cloned gene and this results in increased protein synthesis. Similarly, the stronger the promoter (see Fig. 24.5), the more mRNA molecules are synthesized. The base sequence of the RBS (see Fig. 24.6) and the length and sequence of the DNA between the RBS and the initiating AUG codon are so important that a single base change, addition or deletion, can affect the level of translation up to 1000-fold.

Proteolysis does not affect transcription and translation but by degrading the desired product it influences the apparent rate of gene expression. Although proteolysis can be reduced it is difficult to eliminate it completely. One approach is to use protease-deficient

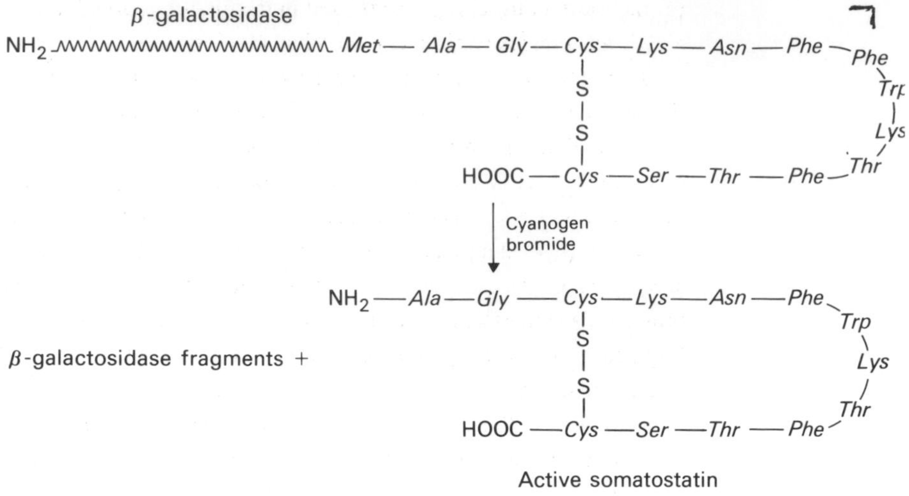

β-galactosidase

NH₂ ⎰⎰⎰⎰⎰⎰⎰⎰⎰⎰⎰⎰⎰⎰⎰⎰⎰ Met —— Ala —— Gly ——Cys——Lys —— Asn ——Phe ——Phe
                                                              | \
                                                              S   Trp
                                                              | |
                                                              S   Lys
                                                              | /
                                              HOOC —— Cys ——Ser ——Thr ——Phe ——Thr

Cyanogen bromide

β-galactosidase fragments +

NH₂ ——Ala ——Gly —— Cys——Lys ——Asn ——Phe
                                  | \
                                  S   Trp
                                  | \
                                  S   Lys
                                  | /
                 HOOC ——Cys ——Ser ——Thr ——Phe ——Thr

Active somatostatin

Fig. 24.8 Release of somatostatin from a hybrid protein by cyanogen bromide cleavage. Somatostatin can be purified free of cyanogen bromide and fragments of β-galactosidase.

mutants and another is to protect the desired protein by fusion to an *E. coli* protein (see below).

Somatostatin was the first human peptide to be synthesized in a bacterial cell. It is only 14 amino acids long and genes for polypeptides of this size are very amenable to direct chemical synthesis. However, small peptides are rapidly degraded in *E. coli* and for this reason the synthetic gene was fused to the 5' end of the β-galactosidase gene. This results in the synthesis of a fusion protein which is relatively stable in *E. coli*. Somatostatin does not contain any methionine residues, so the synthetic gene was constructed in such a way that a methionine was incorporated at the junction of the fusion peptide. By treatment with cyanogen bromide, which breaks proteins into polypeptide fragments at methionine residues, authentic somatostatin could be recovered (Fig. 24.8). Although in this particular instance, and in the case of insulin and β-endorphin, the fusion protein contained a remnant of the *E. coli* β-galactosidase gene at the N-terminus, other bacterial proteins have been used, for example tryptophan synthetase, β-lactamase, etc.

2.4   **Choice of cloning host**

A number of cloning hosts are in widespread use. *Escherichia coli* is still the most popular organism for initial genetic manipulations and is used for the commercial production of a number of therapeutic proteins. *Bacillus subtilis* has not lived up to its initial promise of high-level protein secretion and interest in it is declining. *Saccharomyces cerevisiae* is widely used but faces competition from recombinant animal cells: progress with the latter has been impressive and high-level expression and secretion systems are available. Good progress has also been made in developing cloning systems for filamentous fungi and actinomycetes, two groups of organisms which have long been used in the production of low molecular weight pharmaceuticals. More recently, there has been growing interest in the development of cloning systems for the more unusual organisms used in the pharmaceutical industry. The advantages and disadvantages of the main microbial cloning systems are shown in Table 24.1.

Recombinant proteins can be produced in plants and animals as well as microbes. For example, a number of important human proteins, e.g. α_1-antitrypsin, have been produced in rats and mice and in some instances can be engineered to be secreted in the breast milk. Clearly, small mammals are not desirable as production vehicles. However, good expression can also be obtained with animals such as sheep and goats. Given the history of large mammals as sources of antitoxins for human therapy they also may be acceptable for the production of recombinant proteins. A large number of recombinant proteins also have been produced in plants, e.g. proteins toxic to insect larvae, antibody fragments, etc. Already some of these recombinant plants are grown commercially, and are being consumed, so there is no reason why they cannot be sources of protein drugs as well. In this context it is worth noting that the pharmaceutical industry is used to manufacturing drugs from plants, as plants are the source of many of the older medicines still in use.

3   Production of medically important polypeptides and proteins

The overproduction of a wide variety of proteins has now been achieved in *E. coli* and other cloning hosts. Many of these proteins are in clinical trials and, as indicated earlier, over a dozen are already on the market. The current status of many of these proteins is summarized in Table 24.2. The efficacy of many of the proteins listed remains to be determined because until the advent of recombinant DNA technology sufficient quantities were not available to enable clinical trials to be undertaken. It should be noted that clinical efficacy alone is not sufficient. Market size is just as important since it can cost up to £50 million to bring a new drug to the market place and company shareholders expect a good return on their investment.

One of the advantages of recombinant DNA technology is that is enables *analogues* of human proteins to be produced. Thus, numerous groups have produced α–α and α–β hybrid interferons. Some of these hybrids have altered properties *in vitro* but whether this will translate into a clinical benefit remains to be determined. In some instances the analogues have only a single amino acid change. Thus, changing cysteine residue 17 in interferon-β to a serine residue yields a protein with improved half-life and *in vitro* stability. Changing methionine residue 358 in α_1-antitrypsin to valine yields a more oxidation-resistant enzyme.

4   Authenticity and efficacy of drugs produced by recombinant DNA technology

To demonstrate the safety and efficacy of any polypeptide drug, regardless of whether it is made by recombinant DNA technology, organic synthesis or extraction from a natural source, a number of quality criteria need to be met. Not only must the protein be produced in accordance with good manufacturing practice but it must also meet specification. Although the absolute specification will vary depending on the identity of the protein, the therapeutic target and the route and period of administration, certain

Table 24.1 Comparison of different organisms as cloning hosts

Organism	Advantages	Disadvantages
Escherichia coli	Ease of manipulation Promoters and gene regulation well understood Easy to culture on large scale Already used in manufacture of insulin, interferon and human somatotrophin	Do not usually get export of proteins into growth medium Over-expressed foreign proteins often form aggregates ('inclusions') of denatured protein Many foreign proteins rapidly degraded Many post-translational modifications do not occur
Bacillus subtilis	Many proteins naturally exported into growth medium Non-pathogenic Easy to culture Some *Bacillus* enzymes excreted at high level (>5 g l^{-1})	Still not much known about gene regulation Good, high-level expression vectors lacking High-level export of heterologous proteins not achieved
Saccharomyces cerevisiae	Widely used industrial organism which is easy to culture Glycosylates proteins Can get export into growth medium of heterologous proteins High-level expression systems developed Heterologous proteins inside cell do *not* form inclusions	Much still to be learned about control of gene expression Post-translational modifications of proteins not necessarily the same as those in the animal cell
Filamentous fungi	Large surface area to volume ratio should favour protein export Have been used in industrial microbiology for over 40 years	Promoters/gene regulation poorly understood but may be similar to yeast Good expression systems lacking Rheology of fermentations important
Actinomycetes	Large surface area to volume ratio should favour protein export Widely used in industrial microbiology Good expression systems being developed	Promoters/gene regulation still poorly understood Rheology of fermentations important
Mammalian cells	Get export of proteins Get desired post-translational modifications and products not likely to be immunogenic to humans Good expression systems available	Large-scale growth of animal cells costly Great care needed to avoid contamination of cultures

Table 24.2 Current status of selected recombinant proteins

Protein	Size/structure	Expression system	Clinical indications	Comments
Human insulin	Two peptide chains: A, 21 amino acids long, and B, 30 amino acids long	E. coli	Juvenile onset diabetes	Approved for sale A and B chains made separately as fusion proteins and joined in vitro Compared with animal insulins some undesirable side-effects have been noted
Human somatotrophin	191 amino acids	E. coli	Pituitary dwarfism	Approved for sale If useful in treatment of osteoporosis then market size will be much larger Has additional methionine residue at N-terminus, but technology for removing this now available
Interferon-α_{2a} Interferon-α_{2b}	166 amino acids	E. coli	Various cancers and viral diseases	Approved for sale Over 80% success in treatment of hairy cell leukemia; success with other cancers lower and more variable Market size may be limited Unpleasant ('flu-like') side-effects
Interferon-γ	143 amino acids, glycosylated	E. coli	Chronic granulomatous disease	Approved for sale In clinical trials for treatment of cancer and viral diseases
Tissue plasminogen activator	530 amino acids, glycosylated	E. coli Yeast Animal cells	Acute mycocardial infarct Pulmonary embolism	Approved for sale Animal cell culture most effective way of producing active enzyme
Relaxin	53 amino acids; insulin-like (two protein chains)	E. coli	Facilitates childbirth	Prepares endometrium for parturition and reduces fetal distress Pig relaxin shown to be clinically effective
α-Antitrypsin	394 amino acids, glycosylated	E. coli Yeast	Treatment of emphysema	Prevents cumulative damage to lung tissue caused by leucocyte elastase In clinical trials

Continued on p. 464

Table 24.2 Continued

Protein	Size/structure	Expression system	Clinical indications	Comments
Interleukin-2	133 amino acids	E. coli Animal cells	Treatment of cancer	Approved for sale Very toxic and side-effects severe
Tumour necrosis factor	157 amino acids	E. coli Animal cells	Treatment of cancer	
Human serum albumin	582 amino acids; 17 disulphide bridges	Yeast	Plasma replacement therapy	Normally obtained from plasma but now concern over potential contamination with AIDS virus
Factor VIII	2332 amino acids	Mammalian cells	Treatment of haemophilia	Normally obtained from plasma but now concern over potential contamination with AIDS virus
Factor IX	415 amino acids glycosylated; modified residues	Mammalian cells	Treatment of Christmas disease	Approved for sale Must be made in mammalian cells since glycosylation and conversion of first 12 glutamate residues to pyroglutamate essential for activity
Erythropoietin	166 amino acids glycosylated	Mammalian cells	Treatment of anaemia associated with dialysis and AZT/AIDS	Approved for sale Without glycosylation protein is cleared very quickly from plasma
Hepatitis B surface antigen	Monomer has 226 amino acids	Yeast Mammalian cells	Vaccination	Approved for sale Monomer self-assembles into structure resembling virus particles
Granulocyte colony stimulating factor	127 amino acids	E. coli	Adjunct to cancer chemotherapy	Approved for sale By stimulating white blood cell formation, aids recovery
Granulocyte–macrophage colony stimulating factor	127 amino acids	E. coli	Improved bone marrow transplant	Approved for sale

Table 24.3 Specification of therapeutic proteins to be administered parenterally

Criterion	Appropriate analytical methods
Greater than 95% pure	Gel electrophoresis; HPLC
Microheterogeneity below specified level	Polyacrylamide gel electrophoresis C- and N-terminal analysis. Amino acid composition
Endotoxin below specified level	Limulus amoebocyte lysate method (see also Chapter 18)
Contaminating DNA below specified level (<10 pg dose^{-1})	Hybridization
Toxic chemicals used in purification below specified level	Appropriate methods
IgG below specified limit (if monoclonal antibodies used in purification)	ELISA or RIA
Absence of microorganisms	Sterility test (see also Chapter 23)

HPLC, high-performance liquid chromatography; ELISA, enzyme-linked immunosorbent assay method; RIA, radioimmunoassay method.

quality guidelines have been adopted by most countries. This core specification is shown in Table 24.3.

Although many of the quality control tests used are designed to assess *purity* they often give data which confirms the *identity* of the protein, e.g. chromatographic behaviour (high-performance liquid chromatography), electrophoretic mobility and amino acid composition. However, most of the analytical techniques in current use give no indication of the three-dimensional structure of the protein and hence no indication of biological activity. Thus, the absolute specific activity of the protein needs to be determined in a biological test. Determination of the specific activity is particularly important with proteins overproduced in *E. coli*, for such proteins exist in aggregates with nucleic acid often called 'inclusions'. The protein in these aggregates has to be extracted with denaturing agents such as urea, sodium dodecyl sulphate or guanidinium hydrochloride and then renatured, a process akin to recreating native egg white from a meringue.

As indicated earlier, recombinant DNA technology can be used to deliberately produce desired analogues of natural proteins. However, undesirable analogues may also be produced inadvertently during the production process. For example, when the human somatotrophin gene is expressed in *E. coli*, the resultant protein has an additional methionine residue at the N-terminus. Other foreign gene products may or may not carry this additional methionine residue. Recently, methods have been developed for enzymatically removing this N terminal methionine and for mediating another post-translational modification, C-terminal amidation.

Another undesirable modification is removal of some amino acids residues from the C-terminus and/or the N-terminus by microbial exoproteases. Care needs to be taken during the fermentation and extraction stages to minimize proteolytic damage, and any 'nibbled' molecules should be removed during purification.

5 Future trends with protein pharmaceuticals

Already over a dozen recombinant-derived therapeutically useful proteins are being marketed and at least as many more are in clinical trials. So, what of the future? There are two disadvantages with developing proteins as therapeutic entities. First, most of them are not active when given orally, and parenteral administration is almost *de rigeur*. Some proteins can be administered in other ways, e.g. insulin can be given *per rectum* but this is not a route which is favoured in many countries outside of France and Japan. Other proteins may be active if given sublingually or if administered by aerosol. Clearly, much work needs to be done in developing new dosage forms particularly suited to the administration of proteins. Second, most of the proteins being marketed or currently in clinical trials were obvious candidates for development, e.g. insulin and interferons. Identifying the next generation of therapeutically useful proteins will be much more difficult. There are hundreds of human proteins of which relatively little is known but only a few are likely to be worth developing. For example, a factor which promotes bone growth would have many clinical benefits but the candidate proteins have yet to be identified.

5.1 Small-molecule drugs

One trend which has become obvious is that many pharmaceutical companies are turning their attention to the application of recombinant DNA technology in the production of small molecules. Microorganisms are widely used in the production of drugs, e.g. antibiotics and steroid transformations. Where the rate-limiting step in production has been identified, cloning the relevant gene could well facilitate synthesis and give increased yields and/or decreased production times. In addition, novel metabolic pathways can be introduced into microorganisms and this could eliminate more conventional but complex production processes involving plants.

5.2 Anti-sense agents

Many drugs treat the *symptoms* of a disease rather than the *cause* of the disease, e.g. the different classes of drug for the treatment of hypertension. Where the primary cause of the disease is overexpression then anti-sense agents may be of value. These are nucleic acids which are complementary to the $5'$ region of a mRNA molecule and bind to it. In this way the translation of the mRNA into protein is reduced or eliminated and hence the anti-sense molecule modulates expression. There are two major problems with anti-sense nucleic acids as therapeutic entities. First, small single-stranded nucleic acids are rapidly degraded inside cells. The solution to this problem is to use modified nucleic acids, e.g. ones in which the phosphodiester backbone is replaced with a peptide chain ('peptide nucleic acids'). The second issue is delivering enough of the anti-sense molecules to the target cells. This can be achieved with proper formulation, and a number of anti-sense drugs are in clinical trials.

5.3 Gene therapy and gene repair

There are many inherited diseases where the genetic basis for the disorder is known but for which no effective drug therapy exists. For example, Lesch–Nyhan disease is caused by a deficiency in hypoxanthine–guanine phosphoribosyl transferase and adenosine deaminase deficiency causes severe immunodeficiency disease. One way of treating these diseases is to take cells from the patient and transfect them *in vitro* with a vector molecule carrying a normal gene and a selectable marker. Those cells carrying the selectable marker are checked to see that they carry the gene of interest, cultured, and then re-introduced into the patient where they provide the missing function. This is known as *gene therapy*.

There are a number of problems with gene therapy. First, it is restricted to those diseases which can be treated by manipulating skin cells or stem cells since these are the only cells which can be cultured outside the body for any length of time. Second, the vectors used are derived from viruses and there is a risk, albeit very small, that the vector virus could recombine with an endogenous virus and cause cancer. Third, the normal gene which has been introduced does not replace the defective gene. Rather, it is inserted elsewhere in the genome as an additional gene copy. Thus, gene therapy is only of use for treating disorders which display homozygous recessive inheritance. An alternative approach is to use *gene repair*. In this case a single-stranded nucleic acid, complementary to the region around the defect, is introduced into the target cells. By stimulating recombination the defect can be repaired. One advantage of gene repair over gene therapy is that the former can be used to treat disease caused by dominant mutations.

6 Glossary

Clone (Noun)   A group of cells all descended from a common ancestor: in genetic engineering, usually refers to a cell carrying a foreign gene. (Verb) To use the techniques of gene manipulation *in vitro* to transfer a gene from one organism to another.

Cloning vector   Plasmid (*vide infra*) into which a foreign gene is placed to ensure its replication in a new host cell.

Exon   Portion of DNA that codes for the final mRNA.

Fusion protein   Covalent linkage of two distinct protein entities, e.g. β-galactosidase and somatostatin. A fusion protein need not retain the different biological properties of its two components.

Genome   Haploid sets of chromosomes with their associated genes.

Intron   An intervening sequence in DNA.

Operon   Two or more genes subject to coordinate regulation by an operator and a repressor.

Plasmid   An extrachromosomal circular DNA molecule in bacteria. Often used as cloning vector.

Promoter   Region of a DNA molecule at which RNA polymerase binds and initiates transcription.

Restriction endonuclease   A deoxyribonuclease which cuts DNA at specific sequences which exhibit twofold symmetry about a point. Name derives from the fact that their presence in a bacterial cell prevents (restricts) the growth of many infecting bacteriophages.

Reverse transcriptase   An enzyme coded by certain RNA viruses which is able to make complementary single-stranded DNA chains from RNA templates and then to convert these DNA chains to double-helical form.

'Sticky-ends'   Complementary single-stranded tails projecting from otherwise double-helical nucleic acid molecules.

'Shotgunning'   Cloning of a complete set of DNA fragments from a particular genome.

Signal sequence Amino acid sequence in protein, whose function is to direct its final intracellular or extracellular location.

Splicing (1) Gene splicing: manipulations, the object of which is to attach one DNA molecule to another; (2) RNA splicing; removal of introns from mRNA precursors.

Vector *See* Cloning vector.

7 Further reading

Bollon A.P. (1984) *Recombinant DNA Products: Insulin, Interferon and Growth Hormone*. Boca Raton, Florida: CRC Press.

Bonnen E.M. & Spiegel R.J. (1984) Interferon-alpha: current status and future promise. *J Biol Resp Mod*, **3**, 580–598.

Courtney M., Jallat S., Tessier L-H., Benavente A., Crystal R.G. & Lecocq J-P. (1985) Synthesis in *E. coli* of alpha$_1$-antitrypsin variants of therapeutic potential for emphysema and thrombosis. *Nature*, **313**, 149–151.

Glick B.R. & Pasternak J.J. (1994) *Molecular Biotechnology: Principles and Applications of Recombinant DNA*. Washington, D.C.: American Society for Microbiology.

Goeddel D.V., Heyneker H.L., Hoxumi T., Arentzen R., Itakura K., Yansura D.G., Ross M.J., Miozzari G., Crea R. & Seeburg P.H. (1979) Expression in *Escherichia coli* of a DNA sequence coding from human growth hormone. *Nature*, **281**, 544–548.

Goeddel D.V., Kleid D.G., Bolivar F., Heyneker H.L., Yansura D.G., Crea R., Hirose T., Kraszewski A., Itakura K. & Riggs A.D. (1979) Expression in *Escherichia coli* of chemically synthesised genes for human insulin. *Proc Natl Acad Sci USA*, **76**, 106–110.

Goeddel D.V., Yelverton E., Ullrich A., Heyneker H.L., Miozzari G., Holmes W., Seeburg P.J., Dull T., May L., Stebbing N., Crea R., Maeda S., McCandliss R., Sloma A., Tabor J.M., Gross M., Familletti P.C. & Pestka S. (1980) Human leukocyte interferon produced by *E. coli* is biologically active. *Nature*, **287**, 411–416.

Guerigan J.L. (Ed.) (1982) *Insulins, Growth Hormone and Recombinant DNA Technology*. New York: Raven Press.

Guerigan J.L., Bransome E.D. & Outschoorn A.S. (1981) *Hormone Drugs*. Rockville: US Pharmacopeial Convention, Inc.

Itakura K., Hirose T., Crea R., Riggs A.D., Heyneker H.L., Bolivar F. & Boyer H.W. (1977) Expression in *Escherichia coli* of a chemically synthesised gene for the hormone somatostatin. *Science*, **198**, 1056–1063.

Madigan M.T., Mastinks J.M. & Parker J. (1997) Genetic Engineering and Biotechnology. *Brock's Biology of Microorganisms*, 8th edn. London: Prentice Hall.

Old R.W. & Primrose S.B. (1989) *Principles of Gene Manipulation: An Introduction to Genetic Engineering*, 4th edn. Oxford: Blackwell Scientific Publications.

Primrose S.B. (1991) *Molecular Biotechnology*, 2nd edn. Oxford: Blackwell Scientific Publications.

Shine J., Fettes I., Lan N.C.Y., Roberts J.L. & Baxter J.D. (1980) Expression of cloned β-endorphin gene sequences by *Escherichia coli*. *Nature*, **285**, 456–461.

Tomlinson E. (1991) Impact of the new biologies on the medical and pharmaceutical sciences. *Pharm J*, **247**, 335–344.

25 Additional applications of microorganisms in the pharmaceutical sciences

1 Introduction
1.1 Early treatment of human disease
1.2 Present-day exploitation

2 Pharmaceuticals produced by microorganisms
2.1 Dextrans
2.2 Vitamins, amino acids and organic acids
2.2.1 Vitamins
2.2.2 Amino acids
2.2.3 Organic acids
2.3 Iron-chelating agents
2.4 Enzymes
2.4.1 Streptokinase and streptodornase
2.4.2 L-Asparaginase
2.4.3 Neuraminidase
2.4.4 β-Lactamases

3 Applications of microorganisms in the partial synthesis of pharmaceuticals
3.1 Production of antibiotics
3.2 Streroid biotransformations

3.3 Chiral inversion

4 Use of microorganisms and their products in assays
4.1 Antibiotic bioassays
4.1.1 Microbiological assays
4.1.2 Radioenzymatic (transferase) assays
4.2 Vitamin and amino acid bioassays
4.3 Phenylketonuria testing
4.4 Carcinogen and mutagen testing
4.4.1 Mutations at the gene level
4.4.2 The Ames test
4.5 Use of microbial enzymes in sterility testing
4.6 Immobilized enzyme technology

5 Use of microorganisms as models of mammalian drug metabolism

6 Insecticides

7 Concluding remarks

8 Further reading

1 Introduction

There has long been a tendency, especially in medical and pharmaceutical circles, to regard microbes as harmful entities to be destroyed. However, as will be described in this chapter, the exploitation of microorganisms and their products has assumed an increasingly prominent role in the diagnosis, treatment and prevention of human diseases. Non-medical uses are also of significance, e.g. the use of bacterial spores (*Bacillus thurungiensis*) and viruses (baculoviruses) to control insect pests, the fungus *Sclerotinia sclerotiorum* to kill some common weeds, and improved varieties of *Trichoderma harzianum* to protect crops against fungal infections.

1.1 Early treatment of human disease

The earliest uses of microorganisms to treat human disease can be traced to the belief that formation of pus in some way drained off noxious humours responsible for systemic conditions. Although the spontaneous appearance of pus in their patients' wounds satisfied most physicians, deliberate contamination of wounds was also practised. Bizarre concoctions of bacteria such as 'ointment of pigs' dung and 'herb sclerata' were favoured during the Middle Ages. Both early central European and South

American civilizations cultivated various fungi for application to wounds. In the nineteenth century, sophisticated concepts of microbial antagonism were developed following Pasteurs's experiments demonstrating inhibition of anthrax bacteria by 'common bacteria' simultaneously introduced into the same culture medium. Patients suffering with diseases such as diphtheria, tuberculosis and syphilis were treated by deliberate infection with what were then thought to be harmless bacteria such as staphylococci, *Escherichia coli* and lactobacilli. Following their discovery in the early part of this century, bacterial viruses (bacteriophages) were considered as potential antibacterial agents, an idea that soon fell into disuse. This idea has recently been revived but has been criticized because of the possibility of transferring antibiotic resistance genes from phage to host bacteria.

<table>
<tr><td>1.2</td><td>

Present-day exploitation

Some of the most important and widespread uses of microorganisms in the pharmaceutical sciences are the production of antibiotics, vaccines and the use of microorganisms in the recombinant DNA industry. These are described in Chapters 7, 15 and 24. However, there are a variety of other medicinal agents derived from microorganisms including vitamins, amino acids, dextrans, iron-chelating agents and enzymes. Microorganisms as whole or subcellular fractions, in suspension or immobilized in an inert matrix are employed in a variety of assays. Microorganisms have also been used in the pharmaceutical industry to achieve specific modifications of complex drug molecules such as steroids, in situations where synthetic routes are difficult and expensive to carry out.</td></tr>
</table>

2   Pharmaceuticals produced by microorganisms

2.1   Dextrans

Dextrans are polysaccharides produced by lactic acid bacteria, in particular members of the genus *Leuconostoc* (e.g. *L. dextranicus* and *L. mesenteroides*) following growth on sucrose. These polymers of glucose first came to the attention of industrial microbiologists because of their nuisance in sugar refineries where large gummy masses of dextran clogged pipelines. Dextran is essentially a glucose polymer consisting of $(1 \rightarrow 6)$-α-links of high but variable molecular weight (15 000–20 000 000; Fig. 25.1). Growth of the dextran producer strain is carried out in large fermenters in media with a low nitrogen but high carbohydrate content. The average molecular weight of the dextrans produced will vary with the strain used. This is important because dextrans for clinical use must have defined molecular weights which will depend on their use. Two main methods are employed for obtaining dextrans of a suitable molecular weight. The first involves acid hydrolysis of very high molecular weight polymers, whilst the second utilizes preformed dextrans of small size which are added to the culture fluid. These appear to act as 'templates' for the polymerization, so that the dextrans are produced with much shorter chain lengths. Once formed, dextrans of the required molecular weight are obtained by precipitation with organic solvents prior to formulation.

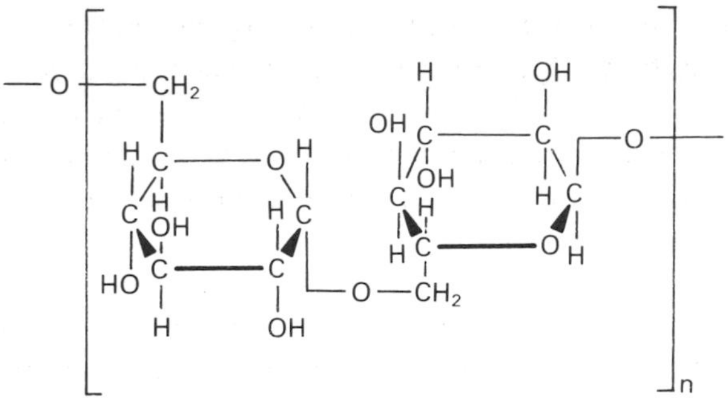

Fig. 25.1 Structure of dextran showing $(1 \rightarrow 6)$-α-linkage.

Dextrans are produced commercially for use as plasma substitutes (plasma expanders) which can be administered by intravenous injection to maintain or restore the blood volume. They can be used in applications to ulcers or burn wounds where they form a hydrophilic layer which absorbs fluid exudates.

A summary of the properties of the different types of dextrans available is presented in Table 25.1. Dextrans for clinical use as plasma expanders must have molecular weights between 40 000 (= 220 glucose units) and 300 000. Polymers below the minimum are excreted too rapidly from the kidneys, whilst those above the maximum are potentially dangerous because of retention in the body. In practice, infusions containing dextrans of average molecular weights of 40 000, 70 000 and 110 000 are commonly encountered.

Iron dextran injection contains a complex of iron hydroxide with dextrans of average molecular weight between 5000 and 7000, and is used for the treatment of iron-deficiency anaemia in situations where oral therapy is ineffective or impractical. The sodium salt of sulphuric acid esters of dextran, i.e. dextran sodium sulphate, has anti-coagulant properties comparable with heparin and is formulated as an injection for intravenous use.

2.2 Vitamins, amino acids and organic acids

Several chemicals used in medicinal products are produced by fermentation (Table 25.2).

2.2.1 *Vitamins*

Vitamin B_2 (riboflavin) is a constituent of yeast extract and incorporated into many vitamin preparations. Vitamin B_2 deficiency is characterized by symptoms which include an inflamed tongue, dermatitis and a sensation of burning in the feet. In genuine cases of malnutrition, these symptoms will accompany those induced by other vitamin deficiencies. Riboflavin is produced commercially in good yields by the moulds *Eremothecium ashbyii* and *Ashbya gossypii* grown on a protein-digest medium.

Pernicious anaemia was a fatal disease first reported in 1880. It was not until 1926 that it was discovered that eating raw liver effected a remission. The active principle was later isolated and called vitamin B_{12} or cyanocobalamin. It was initially obtained

Table 25.1 Properties and uses of dextrans

Type of dextran*	Molecular weight (average)	Product	Sterilization method	Clinical uses
Dextran 40	40 000	10% w/v in 5% w/v glucose injection or 0.9% w/v sodium chloride injection	Autoclave	IV infusion: improves blood flow and tissue function in burns and conditions associated with local ischaemia
Dextran 70	70 000	6% w/v in 5% w/v glucose injection or 0.9% w/v sodium chloride injection	Autoclave	IV: used to produce an expansion of plasma volume in conditions associated with loss of plasma proteins
Dextran 110	110 000	6% w/v in 5% w/v glucose injection or 0.9% w/v sodium chloride injection	Autoclave	IV: as for dextran 70
Iron Dextran	5000–7500 (complex with ferric chloride)	Colloidal solution In 0.9% w/v sodium chloride injection	Autoclave	Deep IM: non-deficiency anaemia (oral therapy ineffective or impractical) IV (slow infusion): non-deficiency anaemia (oral therapy ineffective or impractical)
Dextran sodium sulphate		Powder for preparing solution	Autoclave	Anticoagulant (intravenous use of solution
Chemically cross-linked dextrans		—	—	Water-insoluble: chromatographic techniques (fractionation and purification

* In the USA, dextran injections with average molecular weights of about 75 000 are also available.
IV, intravenous; IM, intramuscular.
The current *British Pharmacopoeia* and *British National Formulary* should be consulted for further information, including toxic manifestations.

from liver but during the 1960s it was noted that it could be obtained as a by-product of microbial metabolism (Table 25.1). Hydroxycobalamin is the form of choice for therapeutic use and can be derived either by chemical transformation of cyanocobalamin or directly as a fermentation product.

Biotin is a member of the vitamin B family and is an essential factor in the processes and maintenance of normal metabolism in human beings. It is an essential growth factor for some bacteria. Its chemical structure was established in the early 1940s and a practical, highly stereospecific, chemical synthesis enabled D-biotin, identical to that found in yeasts and other cells, to be produced.

2.2.2 Amino acids

Amino acids find applications as ingredients of infusion solutions for parenteral nutrition and individually for treatment of specific conditions. They are obtained either by fermentation processes similar to those used for antibiotics or in cell-free extracts employing enzymes isolated from bacteria (Table 25.1). Details of the many and varied

Table 25.2 Examples of vitamins, amino acids, antibiotics and organic acids produced by microorganisms

Pharmaceutical	Producer organism	Use
Riboflavin (vitamin B$_2$)	*Eremothecium ashbyii* *Ashbya gossypii*	Treatment of vitamin B$_2$ deficiency disease
Cyanocobalamin (vitamin B$_{12}$)	*Propionibacterium freudenreichii* *Propionibacterium shermanii* *Pseudomonas denitrificans*	Treatment of pernicious anaemia
Amino acids, e.g. glutamate, lysine	*Corynebacterium glutamicum* *Brevibacterium flavum*	Supplementation of feeds/food; intravenous infusion fluid constituents
Antibiotics*, e.g. Benzylpenicillin	*Penicillin notatum, P. chrysogenum*	Antibacterial drug
Gentamicin	*Micromonospora purpurea*	Antibacterial drug
Nystatin	*Streptomyces noursei*	Antifungal drug
Organic acids Citric acid	*Aspergillus niger*	Effervescent products; sodium citrate used as an anticoagulant; potassium citrate used to treat cystitis
Lactic acid	*Lactobacillus delbrueckii* *Rhizopus oryzae*	Calcium lactate is a convenient source of Ca^{2+} for oral administration; constituent of intraperitoneal dialysis solutions
Gluconic acid	*Gluconobacter suboxydans* *Aspergillus niger*	Calcium gluconate is a source of Ca^{2+} for oral administration; gluconates are used to render bases more soluble, e.g. chlorhexidine gluconate

* For further information, see Chapters 5, 6 and 7.

processes reported in the literature will be found in the appropriate references at the end of the chapter.

2.2.3   *Organic acids*

Examples of organic acids (citric, lactic, gluconic) produced by microorganisms, together with pharmaceutical and medical uses, are depicted in Table 25.2. Citric and lactic acids also have widespread uses in the food and drink and plastics industries, respectively. Gluconic acid is also used as a metal-chelating agent in, for example, detergent products.

2.3   **Iron-chelating agents**

Growth of many microorganisms in iron-deficient growth media results in the secretion of low molecular weight iron-chelating agents called siderophores, which are usually phenolate or hydroxamate compounds. The therapeutic potential of these compounds has generated considerable interest in recent years. Uncomplicated iron deficiency can be treated with oral preparations of ferrous (iron II) sulphate but such treatment is not without hazard and iron salts are common causes of poisoning in children. The accidental consumption of around 3 g of ferrous sulphate by a small child leads to acidosis, coma and heart failure amongst a variety of other symptoms which, if untreated, are fatal. Desferrioxamine B (Fig. 25.2), the deferrated form of a siderophore produced by

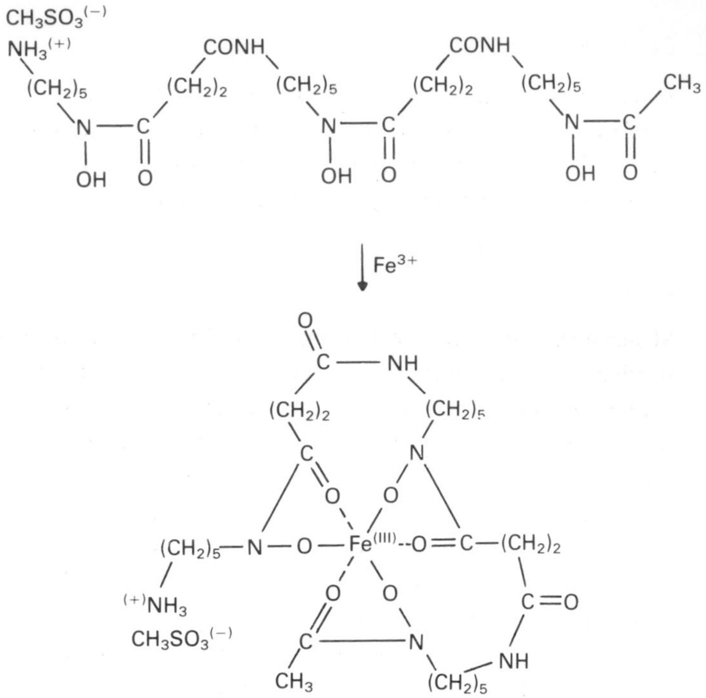

Fig. 25.2 Structure of desferrioxamine B (Desferal) and its corresponding iron chelate.

Streptomyces pilosus, is a highly effective antidote for the treatment of acute iron poisoning. Desferrioxamine owes its effectiveness both to its high affinity for ferric iron (its binding constant is in excess of 10^{30}) and because the iron–desferrioxamine complex is highly water-soluble and is readily excreted through the kidneys. In haemolytic anaemias such as thalassaemia, desferrioxamine is used together with blood transfusions to maintain normal blood levels of free iron and haemoglobin. Desferrioxamine is prepared as a sterile powder for use as an injection, but it is also administered orally in acute iron poisoning to remove unabsorbed iron from the gut. Patients with iron overload disorders treated with desferrioxamine may, however, have increased susceptibility to infections.

The important role played by iron availability during infections in vertebrate hosts has only been recognized relatively recently. The ability of the host to withhold growth-essential iron from microbial and, indeed, neoplastic invaders whilst retaining its own access to this metal has led to suggestions that microbial iron chelators or their semisynthetic derivatives may be of use in antimicrobial and anticancer chemotherapy. Preliminary work has shown some encouraging results. The bacterial siderophores parabactin and compound II secreted by *Paracoccus denitrificans* have been shown to inhibit the growth of leukaemia cells in culture and in experimental animals. They also appear capable of inhibiting the replication of RNA viruses.

Siderophores like desferrioxamine may, therefore, find increasing applications not only in the treatment of iron poisoning and iron-overloaded disease states but also as chemotherapeutic agents, although the possible problems noted above cannot be ignored.

2.4 Enzymes

Several enzymes have important therapeutic and other medical or pharmaceutical uses (Table 25.3). In this section, those enzymes used therapeutically will be described, with section 4 discussing the applications of microbially derived enzymes for antibiotic inactivation in sterility testing and diagnostic assays.

2.4.1 Streptokinase and streptodornase

Mammalian blood will clot spontaneously if allowed to stand: however, on further standing, this clot may dissolve as a result of the action of a proteolytic enzyme called plasmin. Plasmin is normally present as its inactive precursor, plasminogen. Certain strains of streptococci were found to produce a substance which was capable of activating plasminogen (Fig. 25.3), a phenomenon that suggested a potential use in liquefying clots. This substance was isolated, found to be an enzyme and called streptokinase.

Streptokinase is administered by intravenous or intra-arterial infusion in the treatment of thrombo-embolic disorders, e.g. pulmonary embolism, deep-vein thrombosis and arterial occlusions. It is also used in acute myocardial infarction.

A second enzyme, streptodornase, present in streptococcal culture filtrates, was observed to liquefy pus. Streptodornase is a deoxyribonuclease which breaks down deoxyribonucleoprotein and DNA, both constituents of pus, with a consequent reduction in viscosity. Streptokinase and streptodornase together have been used to facilitate

Table 25.3 Clinical uses and other applications of enzymes

Enzyme	Source	Clinical and/or other use	Section
Streptokinase	Certain streptococcal strains	Liquefying blood clots	2.4.1
Streptodornase	Certain streptococcal strains	Liquefying pus	2.4.1
L-Asparaginase	*E. coli* or *Erwinia carotovora*	Cancer chemotherapy	2.4.2
Neuraminidase	*Vibrio cholerae*	Possible: increase immunogenicity of tumour cells	2.4.3
β-Lactamases	*Bacillus cereus* (or other bacteria, as appropriate)	Sterility testing, treatment of penicillin-induced allergic reaction	2.4.4, 4.5
Other antibiotic-modifying or -inactivating enzymes	Some AGAC-resistant bacteria	Sterility testing, assay	4,1,2, 4.5
	Some CMP-resistant bacteria	Sterility testing	4.5
Glucose oxidase	*Aspergillus niger*	Blood glucose analysis	4.6

AGAC, aminoglycoside–aminocyclitol antibiotics (see Chapter 5); CMP, chloramphenicol.

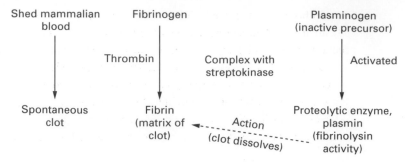

Fig. 25.3 Action of streptokinase.

drainage by liquefying blood clots and/or pus in the chest cavity. The combination can also be applied topically to wounds which have excessive suppuration.

Streptokinase and streptodornase are isolated following growth of non-pathogenic streptococcal producer strains in media containing excess glucose. They are obtained as a crude mixture from the culture filtrate and can be prepared relatively free of each other. They are commercially available as either streptokinase injection or as a combination of streptokinase and streptodornase.

2.4.2 L-Asparaginase

L-Asparaginase, an enzyme derived from *E. coli* or *Erwinia carotovora*, has been employed in cancer chemotherapy where its selectivity depends upon the essential requirement of some tumours for the amino acid L-asparagine. Normal tissues do not require this amino acid and thus the enzyme is administered with the intention of depleting tumour cells of asparagine by converting it to aspartic acid and ammonia. Whilst L-asparaginase showed promise in a variety of experimentally induced tumours, it is only useful in humans for the treatment of acute lymphoblastic leukaemia, although it is sometimes used for myeloid leukaemia.

2.4.3 Neuraminidase

Neuraminidase derived from *Vibrio cholerae* has been used experimentally to increase the immunogenicity of tumour cells. It appears capable of removing *N*-acetylneuraminic (sialic) acid residues from the outer surface of certain tumour cells, thereby exposing new antigens which may be tumour specific together with a concomitant increase in their immunogenicity. In laboratory animals administration of neuraminidase-treated tumour cells was found to be effective against a variety of mouse leukaemias. Preliminary investigations in acute myelocytic leukaemia patients has suggested that treatment of the tumour cells with neuraminidase in combination with conventional chemotherapy may increase remission rates.

2.4.4 β-Lactamases

β-Lactamase enzymes, whilst being a considerable nuisance because of their ability to confer bacterial resistance by inactivating penicillins and cephalosporins (see Chapter 9), are useful in the sterility testing of certain antibiotics (see section 4.5) and, prior to culture, in inactivating various β-lactams in blood or urine samples in patients undergoing therapy with these drugs. One other important therapeutic application is in the rescue of patients presenting symptoms of a severe allergic reaction following administration of a β-lactamase-sensitive penicillin. In such cases, a highly purified penicillinase obtained from *Bacillus cereus* is administered either intramuscularly or intravenously and in combination with other supportive measures such as adrenaline or antihistamines.

3 Applications of microorganisms in the partial synthesis of pharmaceuticals

Whole microbial cells as well as microbially derived enzymes have played a significant role in the production of novel antibiotics. The potential of microorganisms as chemical catalysts, however, was first fully realized in the synthesis of industrially important steroids. These reactions have assumed increasing importance following the discovery that certain steroids such as hydrocortisone have anti-inflammatory activity, whilst derivatives of the steroidal sex hormones are useful as oral contraceptive agents. More recently, chiral inversion of non-steroidal anti-inflammatory drugs (NSAIDs) has been demonstrated.

3.1 Production of antibiotics

In the antibiotics industry, the hydrolysis of benzylpenicillin to give 6-aminopenicillanic acid by the enzyme penicillin acylase is an important stage in the synthesis of many clinically useful penicillins (see Chapters 5 and 7). The combination of genetic engineering techniques to produce hybrid microorganisms with significantly higher acylase levels, together with their entrapment in gel matrices (which appears to improve the stability of the hybrids), has resulted in considerable increases in 6-aminopenicillanic acid yields.

A second example is provided by the production by fermentation of cephalosporin C, which is used solely for the subsequent preparation of semisynthetic cephalosporins (Chapters 5 and 7).

Furthermore, antibiotics produced by fermentation of various moulds or, especially, *Streptomyces* spp. can be employed by medicinal chemists as starting blocks in the production of what might be more effective antimicrobial compounds.

3.2 Steroid biotransformations

Since steroid hormones can only be obtained in small quantities directly from mammals, attempts were made to synthesize them from plant sterols which can be obtained cheaply and economically in large quantities. However, all adrenocortical steroids are characterized by the presence of an oxygen at position 11 in the steroid nucleus. Thus, although it is easy to hydroxylate a steroidal compound it is extremely difficult to obtain site-specific hydroxylation, so that many of the routes used for synthesizing the desired steroid are lengthy, complex and consequently expensive. This problem was

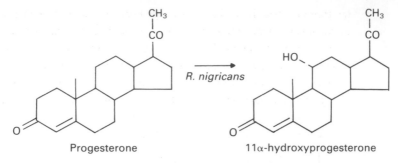

Fig. 25.4 Conversion of progesterone to 11α-hydroxyprogesterone by *Rhizopus nigricans*.

overcome when it was realized that many microorganisms are capable of performing limited oxidations with both stereo- and regio-specificity. Thus, by simply adding a steroid to growing cultures of the appropriate microorganism, specific site-directed chemical changes can be introduced into the molecule. In 1952, the first commercially employed process involving the conversion of progesterone to 11α-hydroxyprogesterone by the fungus *Rhizopus nigricans* was introduced (Fig. 25.4). This reaction is an important stage in the manufacture of cortisone and hydrocortisone from more readily available steroids. Table 25.4 gives several other examples of microbially directed oxidations employed in the manufacture of steroidal drugs.

More recent advances involving the employment of microorganisms in biotransformation reactions utilize immobilized cells (both living and dead). Immobilization of microbial cells, usually by entrapment in a polymer gel matrix, has several important advantages. Whole microbial cells contain complex multistep enzyme systems and there is therefore no longer a need to extract enzymes or enzyme systems which may be inactivated during purification procedures. It also increases the stability of membrane-associated enzymes which are unstable in the solubilized state, as well as permitting the conversion of water-insoluble compounds like steroids in two-phase water–organic solvent systems.

3.3   **Chiral inversion**

Several clinically used drugs, e.g. salbutamol (a β-adrenoceptor agonist), propanol (a β-adrenoceptor antagonist) and the 2-arylpropionic acids (NSAIDs) are employed in

Table 25.4 Examples of biological transformations of steroids

Starting material	Product	Type of reaction
Progesterone	11α-hydroxyprogesterone	Hydroxylation
Compound S*	Hydrocortisone	Hydroxylation
11α-hydroxyprogesterone	Δ-11α-hydroxyprogesterone	Dehydrogenation
Hydrocortisone	Prednisolone	Dehydrogenation
Cortisone	Prednisone	Dehydrogenation

* Derived from diosgenin by chemical transformation.

the racemic form. In the last series, e.g. ibuprofen, activity resides almost exclusively in the S(+) isomers; chiral inversion, in the undirectional manner R(–) → S(+), occurs *in vivo* over a 3-hour period. The S(+) form is a more effective inhibitor of prostaglandin synthesis, and enzymes from some fungal enzymes convert a racemic mixture into the S(+) isomer *in vitro*. It has thus been suggested that the enantiomerically pure S(+) form could be administered clinically to give a reduced dosage and possible less toxicity.

COOH   COOH

   ---H R(–) form   ---Ar S(+) form

CH₃   Ar   CH₃   H

4   Use of microorganisms and their products in assays

Microorganisms have found widespread uses in the performance of bioassays for:

1   determining the concentration of certain compounds (e.g. amino acids, vitamins, some antibiotics) in complex chemical mixtures or in body fluids;

2   diagnosing certain diseases;

3   testing chemicals for potential mutagenicity or carcinogenicity;

4   monitoring purposes involving the use of immobilized enzymes;

5   sterility testing of antibiotics.

4.1   Antibiotic bioassays

Antibiotics may be assayed by a variety of methods (see Chapter 8, pages 166–188, in *Pharmaceutical Microbiology*, 5th edition 1992). Only microbiological and radio-enzymatic assays will be considered briefly here: see Figs 25.5 and 25.6 and sections 4.1.1 and 4.1.2.

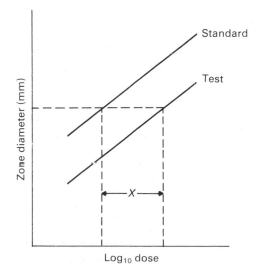

Fig. 25.5 Graphical representation of a two-by-two assay response. *X* is the horizontal distance between the two lines. The antilog of *X* gives the relative potency of the standard and test.

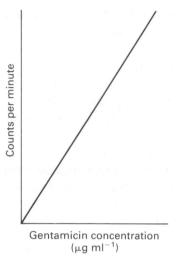

Fig. 25.6 Relationship between concentration of aminoglycoside antibiotic and the transfer of radioactivity from adenosine triphosphate to phosphocellulose.

4.1.1 Microbiological assays

In microbiological assays the response of a growing population of microorganisms to the antimicrobial agent is measured. The usual methods involve agar diffusion assays, in which the drug diffuses into agar seeded with a susceptible microbial population and produces a zone of growth inhibition.

In the commonest form of microbiological assay used today, samples to be assayed are applied in some form of reservoir (porcelain cup, paper disc or well) to a thin layer of agar seeded with indicator organism. The drug diffuses into the medium and after incubation a zone of growth inhibition forms, in this case as a circle around the reservoir. All other factors being constant, the diameter of the zone of inhibition is, within limits, related to the concentration of antibiotic in the reservoir.

During incubation the antibiotic diffuses from the reservoir, and that part of the microbial population away from the influence of the antibiotic increases by cell division. The edge of a zone is formed when the minimum concentration of antibiotic which will inhibit the growth of the organism on the plate (critical concentration) reaches, for the first time, a population density too great for it to inhibit. The position of the zone edge is thus determined by the initial population density, growth rate of the organism and the rate of diffusion of the antibiotic.

In situations where the likely concentration range of the tests will lie within a relatively narrow range (e.g. in determining potency of pharmaceutical preparations) and high precision is sought, then a Latin square design with tests and calibrators at two or three levels of concentration may be used. For example an 8×8 Latin square can be used to assay three samples and one calibrator, or two samples and two calibrators at two concentrations each (over a two- or fourfold range), with a coefficient of variation of around 3%. Using this technique, parallel dose–response lines should be obtained for the calibrators and the tests at the two dilutions (Fig. 25.5). Using such a method, potency can be computed or determined from carefully prepared nomograms.

Conventional plate assays require several hours' incubation and consequently the possibility of using rapid microbiological assay methods has been studied. Two such methods are:

1 Urease assay. When *Proteus mirabilis* grows in a urea-containing medium it hydrolyses the urea to ammonia and consequently raises the pH of the medium. This production of urease is inhibited by aminoglycoside antibiotics (inhibitors of protein synthesis; Chapter 8). In practice, it is difficult to obtain reliable results by this method.

2 Luciferase assay. In this technique, firefly luciferase is used to measure small amounts of adenosine triphosphate (ATP) in a bacterial culture, ATP levels being reduced by the inhibitory action of aminoglycoside antibiotics. This method may find more application in the future as more active and reliable luciferase preparations become available.

4.1.2   *Radioenzymatic (transferase) assays*

These depend on the fact that bacterial resistance to aminoglycosides (Chapter 9), such as gentamicin, tobramycin, amikacin, netilmicin, streptomycin, spectinomycin, etc., and chloramphenicol is frequently associated with the presence of specific enzymes (often coded for by transmissible plasmids) which either acetylate, adenylylate or phosporylate the antibiotics, thereby rendering them inactive (Chapter 9). Aminoglycosides may be susceptible to attack by aminoglycoside acetyltransferases (AAC), aminoglycoside adenylyltransferases (AAD), or aminoglycoside phosphotransferases (APH). Chloramphenicol is attacked by chloramphenicol acetyltransferases (CAT). Acetyltransferases attack susceptible amino groups and require acetyl coenzyme A, while AAD or APH enzymes attack susceptible hydroxyl groups and require ATP (or another nucleotide triphosphate).

Several AAC and AAD enzymes have been used for assays. The enzyme and the appropriate radiolabelled cofactor ([1-^{14}C] acetyl coenzyme A, or [2-^{3}H] ATP) are used to radiolabel the drug being assayed. The radiolabelled drug is separated from the reaction mixture after the reaction has been allowed to go to completion; the amount of radioactivity extracted is directly proportional to the amount of drug present. Aminoglycosides are usually separated by binding them to phosphocellulose paper, whereas chloramphenicol is usually extracted using an organic solvent. An example of a standard curve (for gentamicin) is provided in Fig. 25.6.

These types of assay are rapid, taking approximately 2 hours, show good precision and are much more specific than microbiological assays.

4.2   Vitamin and amino acid bioassays

The principle of microbiological bioassays for growth factors such as vitamins and amino acids is quite simple. Unlike antibiotic assays (see section 4.1) which are based on studies of growth inhibition, these assays are based on growth exhibition. All that is required is a culture medium which is nutritionally adequate for the test microorganism in all essential growth factors except the one being assayed. If a range of limiting concentrations of the test substance is added, the growth of the test microorganism will

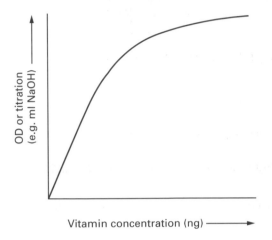

Fig. 25.7 Standard curve in a vitamin assay.

Assay microorganism	Vitamin or amino acid
Lactobacillus casei	Biotin
L. arabinosus	Calcium pantothenate
L. leichmannii	Cyanocobalamin
L. casei	Folic acid
Saccharomyces uvarum	Inositol
L. arabinosus	Nicotinic acid
Acetobacter suboxydans	Pantothenol
L. casei	Pyridoxal
Neurospora crassa or *S. carlsbergiensis*	Pyridoxine
L. casei	Riboflavine
L. viridans	Thiamine

Table 25.5 Some examples of microorganisms used as bioassays for vitamins and amino acids

be proportional to the amount added. A calibration curve of concentration of substance being assayed against some parameter of microbial growth, e.g. cell dry weight, optical density or acid production, can be plotted. An example of a standard curve is presented in Fig. 25.7 and from this the concentration of growth factor in the unknown solution can be determined. One example of this is the assay for pyridoxine (vitamin B_6) which can be assayed using a pyridoxine-requiring mutant of the mould *Neurospora*. Lactic acid bacteria have extensive growth requirements and are often used in bioassays. It is possible to assay a variety of different growth factors with a single test organism simply by preparing a basal media with different growth-limiting nutrients. Table 25.5 summarizes some of the vitamin and amino acid bioassays currently available. In practice, only vitamins are assayed by bioassay procedures, because most amino acids are currently determined chemically.

4.3 Phenylketonuria testing

Phenylketonuria (PKU) is an inborn error of metabolism by which the body is unable to convert surplus phenylalanine (PA) to tyrosine for use in the biosynthesis of, for

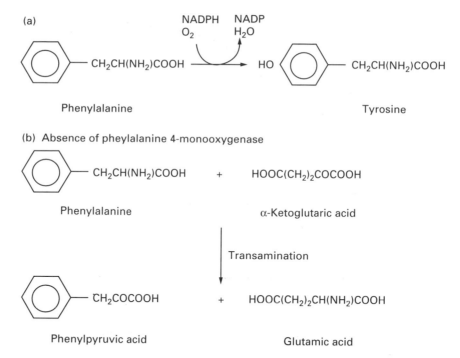

(a)

Phenylalanine

Tyrosine

(b) Absence of pheylalanine 4-monooxygenase

Phenylalanine

α-Ketoglutaric acid

Transamination

Phenylpyruvic acid

Glutamic acid

Fig. 25.8 (a) Normal metabolism, in which phenylalanine is converted by phenylalanine 4-mono-oxygenase to tyrosine. (b) Phenylketonuria, in which there is a transamination reaction between phenylalanine and α-ketoglutaric acid. Phenylalanine 4-mono-oxygenase is absent in about 1 in every 10 000 human beings because of a recessive mutant gene.

example, thyroxine, adrenaline and noradrenaline. This results from a deficiency in the liver enzyme phenylalanine 4-mono-oxygenase (phenylalanine hydroxylase). A secondary metabolic pathway comes into play in which there is a transamination reaction between PA and α-ketoglutaric acid to produce phenylpyruvic acid (PPVA), a ketone and glutamic acid. Overall, PKU may be defined as a genetic defect in PA metabolism such that there are elevated levels of both PA and PPVA in blood and excessive excretion of PPVA (Fig. 25.8).

Control of PKU can be achieved simply by resorting to a low PA-containing diet. Failure to diagnose PKU, however, will result in mental deficiency, and early diagnosis is essential. In 1968, the UK Medical Research Council Working Party on PKU recommended the adoption of the Guthrie test as a convenient method for screening newborn infants. This assay employs *Bacillus subtilis* as the test organism. In minimal culture media, growth of this bacterium is inhibited by β-2-thienylalanine (Fig. 25.9a) and its competitive reversal in the presence of PA (Fig. 25.9b) or PPVA. The use of filter-paper discs impregnated with blood or urine permits the detection of elevated levels of PA and PPVA. The test can be quantitated by the measurement of the diameter of the growth zone around the filter-paper disc and comparing it with a calibration curve constructed from known concentrations of PA or PPVA (Fig. 25.9c).

If positive, the Guthrie test provides presumptive evidence for the presence of PKU. It should be confirmed by other, chemical, means.

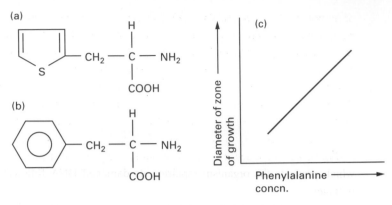

Fig. 25.9 (a) β-Thienylalanine, (b) phenylalanine, (c) standard curve in Guthrie test.

4.4   **Carcinogen and mutagen testing**

A carcinogen is a substance which causes living tissues to become carcinomatous (to produce a malignant epithelial tumour). A mutagen is a chemical (or physical) agent which induces mutation in a human (or other) cell.

Mutagenicity tests are used to screen a wide variety of chemicals for their ability to cause a mutation in the DNA of a cell. Such mutations can occur at:

1   gene level (a 'point' mutation);
2   individual chromosome level;
3   chromosome set level, i.e. a change in the number of chromosomes (aneuploidy).

Some compounds are only mutagenic or carcinogenic after metabolism (often in the liver). This aspect must, therefore, be considered in designing a suitable test method (see section 4.4.2).

4.4.1   *Mutations at the gene level*

Forward mutation refers to mutation of the natural ('wild-type') organism to a more stringent organism. By contrast, reverse (backward) mutation is the return of a mutant strain to the wild-type form, i.e. it is a heritable change in a previously mutated gene that restores the original function of that gene.

There are two types of reverse mutation:

1   frame-shift: in these mutants, the gene is altered by the addition or deletion of one or more basis so that the triplex reading frame for RNA is modified;
2   base-pair: in these mutants, a single base is altered so that the triplex reading frame is again modified.

These principles of reverse mutation are utilized in one important method, the Ames test (section 4.4.2), which is used to detect compounds that act as mutagens or carcinogens (most carcinogens are mutagens).

4.4.2   *The Ames test*

The Ames test is used to screen a wide variety of chemicals for potential carcinogenicity or as potential cancer chemotherapeutic agents. The test enables a large number of compounds to be screened rapidly by examining their ability to induce mutagenesis in several specially constructed bacterial mutants derived from *Salmonella typhimurium*. The test strains contain mutations in the histidine operon so that they cannot synthesize the amino acid histidine. Two additional mutations increase further the sensitivity of the system. The first is a defect in their lipopolysaccharide structure (Chapter 1) such that they are in fact deep rough mutants possessing only 2-keto-3-deoxyoctonate (KDO) linked to lipid A. This mutation increases the permeability of the mutants to large hydrophobic molecules. The second mutation concerns a DNA excision repair system which prevents the organism repairing its damaged DNA following exposure to a mutagen.

The assay method involves treatment of a large population of these mutant tester strains with the test compound. Histidine-requiring mutants are used to detect mutagens capable of causing base-pair substitutions (in some strains) or frame-shift mutations (other strains). This can be carried out by incorporating both the test strain and test compound in molten agar (at 45°C), which is then poured onto a minimal glucose agar plate. Alternatively, the mutagens can be applied to the surface of the top agar as a liquid or as a few crystals. The medium used for the top agar contains a trace of histidine which permits all the bacteria on the plate to undergo several divisions, since for many mutagens some growth is a necessary prerequisite for mutagenesis to occur. After incubation for 2 days at 37°C the number of revertant colonies can be counted and compared with control plates from which the test compound has been omitted. Each revertant colony is assumed to be derived from a cell which has mutated back to the wild type and thus can now synthesize its own histidine: see Fig. 25.10 for a summary.

A further refinement to the Ames test permits screening of agents which require metabolic activation before their mutagenicity or carcinogenicity is apparent. This is achieved by incorporating into the top agar layer, along with the bacteria, homogenates of rat (or human) liver whose activating enzyme systems have been induced by exposure to polychlorinated biphenyl mixtures. This test is sometimes referred to as the *Salmonella*/microsome assay since the fraction of liver homogenate used, called the S9 fraction, contains predominantly liver microsomes.

It is important to realize that this test is flexible and is still undergoing modification and development. Almost all the known human carcinogens have been tested and shown

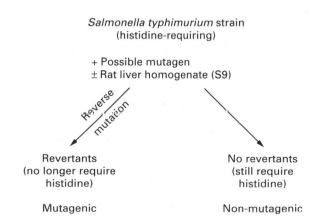

Salmonella typhimurium strain
(histidine-requiring)

+ Possible mutagen
± Rat liver homogenate (S9)

Reverse mutation

Revertants
(no longer require
histidine)

Mutagenic

No revertants
(still require
histidine)

Non-mutagenic

Fig. 25.10 Summary of the
Ames test.

to be positive. These include agents such as β-naphthylamine, cigarette smoke condensates, aflatoxin B and vinylchloride, as well as drugs used in cancer treatment such as adriamycin, daunomycin and mitomycin C. Whilst the test is not perfect for the prediction of mammalian carcinogenicity or mutagenicity and for making definitive conclusions about potential toxicity or lack of toxicity in humans, it nevertheless represents a significant advance providing useful information rapidly and cheaply. The Ames test forms an important part of a battery of tests, the others of which are non-microbial in nature, for detecting mutagenicity or carcinogenicity.

4.5 Use of microbial enzymes in sterility testing

Sterile pharmaceutical preparations must be tested for the presence of fungal and bacterial contamination before use (see Chapters 18 and 23). If the preparation contains an antibiotic, it must be removed or inactivated. Membrane filtration is the usual recommended method. However, this technique has certain disadvantages. Accidental contamination is a problem, as is the retention of the antibiotic on the filter and its subsequent liberation into the nutrient medium.

Enzymic inactivation of the antibiotic (see also Chapter 9) prior to testing would provide an elegant solution to this problem. Currently, the only pharmacopoeial method permitted is that of using an appropriate β-lactamase to inactivate penicillins and cephalosporins. Other antibiotics which are susceptible to inactivating enzymes are chloramphenicol (by chloramphenicol acetyltransferase) and the aminoglycosides, e.g. gentamicin, which can be inactivated by phosphorylation, acetylation or adenylylation. A method for acetylating and consequently inactivating aminoglycosides prior to testing and using 3-N-acetyltransferase (an enzyme with wide substrate specificity) in combination with acetyl coenzyme A has been described, but this method has yet to be adopted.

4.6 Immobilized enzyme technology

The therapeutic uses of microbially derived enzymes have already been examined (section 2.4). However, enzymes also form the basis of many diagnostic tests used in clinical medicine. For example, glucose oxidase, an enzyme used in blood glucose analysis, is obtained commercially from *Aspergillus niger*. Future development and improvement of such diagnostic tests is likely to involve the immobilization of enzymes in enzyme electrodes. Several types of glucose oxidase electrodes have been developed, although none is yet in clinical use. One basic system employs glucose oxidase layered over a platinum electrode. As the reaction proceeds and oxygen is consumed, i.e. glucose + oxygen $\rightarrow$ gluconic acid + hydrogen peroxide, the reduction in oxygen levels is detected by the underlying electrode. However, problems of enzyme inactivation *in vivo*, competition between glucose and oxygen in body fluids and calibration have prevented the adoption of this system as an implantable glucose monitor in diabetic patients. However, there are currently a number of major research efforts in this area and it is likely that biosensors employing immobilized enzymes which are potentially useful for monitoring many substances of clinical importance will become readily available in the not-too-distant future.

5 Use of microorganisms as models of mammalian drug metabolism

The safety and efficacy of a drug must be exhaustively evaluated prior to its approval for use in the treatment of human diseases. Investigations of the manner in which a drug is metabolized are extremely valuable since they provide information on its mode of action, why it exhibits toxicity and how it is distributed, excreted and stored in the body. Traditionally, drug metabolism studies have relied on the use of animal models and, to a lesser extent, liver microsomal preparations, tissue culture and perfused organ systems. Each of these models has certain advantages and disadvantages. Animals in particular are expensive to purchase and maintain and there is considerable pressure from animal welfare groups to curb the use of animals in scientific research.

The use of microbial systems as *in vitro* models for drug metabolism in humans has been proposed since there are many similarities between certain microbial enzyme systems and mammalian liver enzyme systems. The major advantages of using microorganisms is their ability to produce significant quantities of metabolites that would otherwise be difficult to obtain from animal systems or by chemical synthesis, and the considerable reduction in operating costs compared with animal studies.

Microbial drug metabolism studies are usually carried out by firstly screening a large number of microorganisms for their ability to metabolize a drug substrate. The organism is usually grown in a medium such as peptone glucose in flasks which are shaken to ensure good aeration. Drugs as substrates are generally added after 24 hours of growth and are then sampled for the presence of metabolites at intervals up to 14 days after substrate addition. Once it has been determined that a microorganism can metabolize a drug, the whole process can be scaled up for the production of large quantities of metabolites for the determination of their structure and biological properties.

As an example of this the metabolism of the antidepressant drug imipramine can be considered. In mammalian systems, this is metabolized to five major metabolites: 2-hydroxyimipramine, 10-hydroxyimipramine, iminodibenzyl, imipramine-*N*-oxide and desipramine (Fig. 25.11). For microbial metabolism studies, a large number of fungi are screened, from which several are chosen for the preparative scale production of imipramine metabolites. *Cunninghamella blakesleeana* produces the hydroxylated metabolites 2-hydroxyimipramine and 10-hydroxyimipramine; *Aspergillus flavipes* and *Fusarium oxysporum* f. sp. *cepae* yield the *N*-oxide derivative and iminodibenzyl, respectively; whilst the pharmacologically active metabolite desipramine is produced by *Mucor griseocyanus* together with the 10-hydroxy and *N*-oxide metabolites. By scaling up this procedure, significant quantities of the metabolites that are formed during the mammalian metabolism can be obtained.

Microorganisms thus have considerable potential as tools in the study of drug metabolism. Whilst they cannot completely replace animals they are extremely useful as predictive models for initial studies.

6 Insecticides

Like animals, insects are susceptible to infections which may be caused by viruses, fungi, bacteria or protozoa. The use of microorganisms to spread diseases to particular

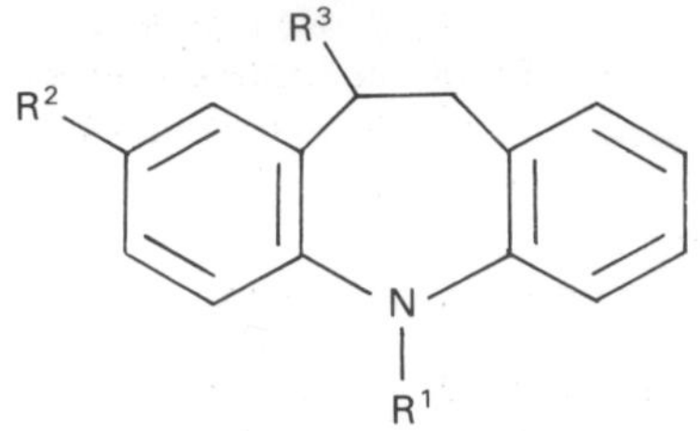

Imipramine	$R^1 = (CH_2)_3N(CH_3)_2; R^2 = R^3 = H$
Desipramine	$R^1 = (CH_2)_3NHCH_3; R^2 = R^3 = H$
2-hydroxyimipramine	$R^1 = (CH_2)_3N(CH_3)_2; R^2 = OH; R^3 = H$
10-hydroxyimipramine	$R^1 = (CH_2)_3N(CH_3)_2; R^2 = OH; R^3 = H$
Iminodibenzyl	$R^1 = R^2 = R^3 = H$
Imipramine-N-oxide	$R^1 = (CH_2)_3N(CH_3)_2; R^2 = R^3 = H$

$$\downarrow$$
$$O$$

Fig. 25.11 Structure of imipramine and its metabolites.

insect pests offers an attractive method of bio-control, particularly in view of the ever-increasing incidence of resistance to chemical insecticides. However, any micro-organism used in this way must be highly virulent, specific for the target pest but non-pathogenic to animals, man or plants. It must be economical to produce, stable on storage and preferably rapidly acting. Bacterial and viral pathogens have so far shown the most promise.

Perhaps the best studied, commercially available insecticidal agent is *B. thuringiensis*. This insect pathogen contains two toxins of major importance. The δ-endotoxin is a protein present inside the bacterial cell as a crystalline inclusion within the spore case. This toxin is primarily active against the larvae of lepidopteran insects (moths and butterflies). Its mechanism of action is summarized in Fig. 25.12. Commercially available preparations of *B. thuringiensis* are spore-crystal mixtures prepared as dusting powders. They are used primarily to protect commercial crops from destruction by caterpillars and are surprisingly non-toxic to man and animals. Although the currently available preparation has a rather narrow spectrum of activity, a variant *B. thuringiensis* strain has recently been isolated and found to produce a different δ-endotoxin with activity against coleopteran insects (beetles) rather than lepidopteran or dipteran (flies and mosquitoes) insects.

The second *B. thuringiensis* toxin, the β-exotoxin has a much broader spectrum encompassing the Lepidoptera, Coleoptera and Diptera. It is an adenine nucleotide, probably an ATP analogue which acts by competitively inhibiting enzymes which catalyse the hydrolysis of ATP and pyrophosphate. This compound, however, is toxic when administered to mammals so that commercial preparations of the *B. thuringiensis* δ-endotoxin are obtained from strains which do not produce the β-exotoxin.

Strains of *B. sphaericus* pathogenic to mosquitoes were isolated several years ago. More recently, strains of this organism with increased toxicity to mosquitoes have been isolated and might have considerable potential as control agents.

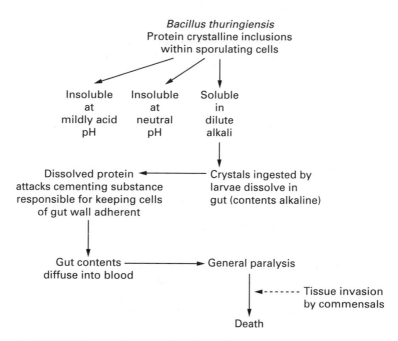

Fig. 25.12 Mechanism of action of δ-endotoxin from *B. thuringiensis*.

Other insect pathogens are currently being evaluated for activity against insects which are vectors for diseases such as sleeping sickness, as well as those which cause damage to crops. Viruses may well have the greatest potential for insect control since they are host-specific and highly virulent, and one infected insect can release vast numbers of virus particles into the environment. They have already been used with considerable success against the spruce sawfly and pine moth.

7 Concluding remarks

Microorganisms are not always the killers they are made out to be. In fact, mankind has been remarkably adept at harnessing microbes for a variety of purposes. In many instances, e.g. antibiotics by whole or partial synthetic production (Chapter 7) and various forms of vaccines, products have been obtained to turn the tables on infecting organisms. Other products have been used for a variety of purposes (including many non-pharmaceutical or non-medical ones, outside the scope of this chapter). Microorganisms have also been employed for specific assay purposes and different types of chemical transformations, as well as in genetic engineering (Chapter 24). Immobilized microorganisms have now been used with considerable success in the partial synthesis of steroids and antibiotics and in the production of the antiviral compound adenine arabinoside (Chapter 5).

There are reports of the benefits of botulinum toxin in the treatment of cerebral palsy in children. The toxin, produced by *Clostridium botulinum*, is a powerful and deadly poison, but is also an effective muscle relaxant. It is not licensed for use as such in the UK but is undergoing clinical trials. Current evidence suggests that repeat injections are necessary some 4–6 months after the first.

Recent studies on the therapeutic uses of toxins have demonstrated also that:

1 botulinum toxin can be used to study synapse remodelling and that enzyme-inactivated toxin can be employed to deliver other molecules into motor nerve ending.

2 *Pseudomonas* cytotoxin hybrids destroy cancer cells and have given promising results in tumour destruction.

3 Cholera toxin and related toxins act as immune modulators, with potential use as adjuvants and as therapeutic agents in the treatment of immunologically mediated human disease.

A cautionary note must still be added, however: problems of toxicity remain and these must be overcome before widespread therapeutic usage is feasible.

The beneficial harnessing of microbes is likely to continue well into the next century.

8   Further reading

Ames B.N., McCann J. & Yamasaki E. (1975) Methods for detecting carcinogens and mutagens with the *Salmonella*/mammalian microsome mutagenicity test. *Mutat Res*, **31**, 347–364.

Breeze A.S. & Simpson A.M. (1982) An improved method using acetyl-coenzyme A regeneration for the enzymic inactivation of aminoglycosides prior to sterility testing. *J Appl Bacteriol*, **53**, 277–284.

Clark A.M., McChesney J.D. & Hufford C.D. (1985) The use of microorganisms for the study of drug metabolism. *Med Res Rev*, **5**, 231–253.

Conference (1973) Streptokinase in clinical practice. *Postgrad Med J*, **49**, 3–142.

Data J.L. & Nies A.S. (1974) Dextran 40. *Ann Intern Med*, **81**, 500–504.

Davis G., Green M.J. & Hill H.A.O. (1986) Detection of ATP and creatinine kinase using an enzyme electrode. *Enzyme Microb Tech*, **8**, 349–352.

Demain A.L., Somkuti G.A., Hunter-Cevera J.C. & Rossmore H.W. (1989) *Novel Microbial Products for Medicine and Agriculture*. Amsterdam: Elsevier.

Doenicke A., Grote B. & Lorenz W. (1977) Blood and blood substitutes. *Br J Anaesth*, **49**, 681–688.

Fukui S. & Tanaka A. (1982) Immobilized microbial cells. *Annu Rev Microbiol*, **36**, 145–172.

Harvey A. (ed.) (1993) *Drugs from Natural Products. Pharmaceuticals and Agrochemicals*. Chichester: Ellis Horwood.

Hewitt W. & Vincent S. (1989) *Theory and Application of Microbiological Assay*. London: Academic Press.

Hutt A.J., Kooloobandi A. & Hanlon G.W. (1993) Microbial metabolism of 2-arylpropionic acids: Chiral inversion of ibuprofen and 2-phenylpropionic acid. *Chirality*, **5**, 596–601.

Jones R.L. & Grady R.W. (1983) Siderophores as antimicrobial agents. *Eur J Clin Microbiol*, **2**, 411–413.

Kier D.K. (1985) Use of the Ames test in toxicology. *Reg Toxicol Pharmacol*, **5**, 59–64.

Mackowiack P.A. (1979) Clinical uses of microorganisms and their products. *Am J Med*, **67**, 293–306.

Priest F.G. (1992) Biological control of mosquitoes and other biting flies by *Bacillus sphaericus* and *Bacillus thuringiensis*. *J Appl Bacteriol*, **72**, 357–369.

Queener S.W. (1990) Molecular biology of penicillin and cephalosporin biosynthesis. *Antimicrob Agents Chemother*, **34**, 943–948.

Reid E. & Wilson D. (eds) (1990) *Analysis for Drugs and Metabolites including Anti-infective Agents*. Methodological Surveys in Biochemistry and Analysis, vol. 20. Royal Society of Chemistry.

Scientific American (1981) Issue on industrial microbiology, vol. 245, No. 3. (An excellent series of papers describing the manufacture by microorganisms or products useful to mankind.)

Smith R.V. & Rosazza J.P. (1975) Microbial models of mammalian metabolism. *J Pharm Sci*, **64**, 1737–1759.

Turner A.P.F. & Pickup J.C. (1985) Diabetes mellitus: biosensors for research and management. *Biosensors*, **1**, 85–115.

Verall M.S.(1985) *Discovery and Isolation of Microbial Products*. Chichester: Ellis Horwood.

Weinberg E.D. (1984) Iron withholding: a defence against infection and neoplasia. *Physiol Rev*, **64**, 65–107.

White L.O. & Reeves D.S. (1983) Enzymatic assay of aminoglycoside antibiotics. In: *Antibiotics: Assessment of Antimicrobial Activity and Resistance* (eds A.D. Russell & L.B. Quesnel), pp. 199–210. Society for Applied Bacteriology Technical Series No. 18. London: Academic Press.

White R.J. (1982) Microbiological models as screening tools for anticancer agents: potentials and limitations. *Annu Rev Microbiol*, **36**, 415–433.

Index

Note: page numbers in *italics* refer to
figures, those in **bold** refer to tables

[A_w] *see* water activity
abortion
  brucellosis   29
  listeriosis   28
abscesses, fibrin deposition   83–4
acanthamoeba keratitis   207
Acanthamoeba spp.   207
accelerated electron radiation   401,
    403, 405
acetic acid   235
N-acetyl-3-*O*-1-carboxyethyl-
    glucosamine   5
N-acetylglucosamine   5
acetyltransferases   188
acid-fast stain for bacterial spores   12
Acinetobacter   30
acquired immune deficiency syndrome
    see AIDS
Acremonium chrysogenum   157, 158
acridine dyes   174, 226
acriflavine   226, 249
actinomycetes
  cloning host   **462**
  industrial water supplies   342
active immunity   304–5, 328–9
acute phase proteins   281
acycloguanosine *see* acyclovir
acyclovir (acycloguanosine)   70,
    126–7, 130, 174
adaptation, drug resistance   133
additive effects of drug
    combinations   128
adenosine arabinoside   125
adenosine deaminase deficiency
    467
adenosine triphosphatase   258
adenosine triphosphate (ATP)   17
  firefly light-emitting system   25
  microbial   372
  non-microbial   25
adenovirus   57, **63**
  oncogenic   72
adenyl cyclase   86
adenylyltransferases   188
adhesins, antibodies against   79
adult T-cell leukaemia/lymphoma
    syndrome   72
adverse drug reactions   135–6
aflatoxins   49, 372
agglutinins   79
  B. pertussis   81
AIDS
  Candida albicans infection   44
  cryptococcal meningitis   47
  fungal infections   114
  Mycobacterium avium intracellulare
    276

Pneumocystis carinii pneumonia
    117, 178
  secondary infections   72
  trimetrexate treatment   178
air, filtered   432–3
air supply for clean areas   432–4
air-filtration systems   341, 433
air-sampling machine   340
albumin, human serum   **464**
Alcaligenes spp.   342, 346
alcohols   **210**, 213–14
  aliphatic   213
  aralkyl   213–14
  fusel   40
  membrane-active agents   178
  preservatives   213–14
  properties   **209**
aldehydes   **210**, 214–16
  antiviral activity   57
  properties   **209**
  sporicidal action   204
  toxicity   208
alexidine   216–17
alkyl polyguanides   204
alkyl quaternaries   204
allergies   279
allografts   301
allylamines, synthetic   122
Alternaria spp.   347
alveolar region, macrophages   78
amantadine hydrochloride   124, *125*
Ames test   484–5
6-β-amidinopenicillanic acid   93, *94*,
    95
amikacin   106, *107*, 108
aminacrine   226
D-amino acids   163
amino acids   472–3
  bioassays   481–2
amino groups   259
aminoacyl-tRNA   172
aminoglycoside–aminocyclitol
    antibiotics   106–8, 169, 171
  active uptake   171
  energy-dependent phase of uptake
    171
  energy-independent phase of uptake
    171
  resistance   188–9, **190**
  ribosomal target site alteration   189
aminoglycoside-modifying enzymes
    189, **190**
aminoglycosides   131, 133, 481
  burn wounds   144
  cystic fibrosis infections   140
  enzymatic inactivation   133
  toxicity   135
6-aminopenicillanic acid (6-APA)   92,
    93
amoebiasis, intestinal   108
cyclic AMP   86

amphoterocin B   114, *115*
  action   179
  combination with 5-flucytosine
    134
ampicillin   93, *94*, **95**
  candidiasis superinfection   136
  Gram-negative bacteria lysis   167
  Haemophilus influenzae resistance
    145
  kidney infection   141
  typhoid fever   142
n-amyl alcohol   40
amylase   83
anaphylactic reactions   299
anaphylaxis   135
anaphylotoxins   292
anionic surfactants   357
ankylosing spondylitis   301
antagonism   128
anthelmintics, imidazole derivatives
    120, 121
anthrax   27
  vaccine   **311**
anti-inflammatory drugs   301
anti-sense agents   466
antibacterial agents, non-antibiotic
  cell wall targetting   256
  cellular targets   **260**, *261*
  cytoplasm effects   258–9
  cytoplasmic membrane activity
    257–8
  mode of action   256–9, **260**, *261*,
    262
  multitarget reactors   259, 262
antibacterial agents, semi-solid
    248–9
antibiotic policies   145–7
  costs   146
  drug resistance   146
  free prescribing   146–7
  restricted dispensing/reporting
    147
antibiotic resistance *see* resistance
antibiotics
  activity spectrum   **182**
  aminoglycoside–aminocyclitol
    106–8, 170, 171, 188–9, **190**
  antifungal   114, *115*
  assays   479–81
  β-lactams   92–3, *94*, 95–8, *99*,
    100–4
  combination   134–5
  definition   91–2
  enzymic inactivation   486
  glycopeptide   111–12
  macrolides   108–11
  manufacture   149–50
    benzylpenicillin   149, 150–8
    cephalosporin C   149, 158, *159*,
    160
  fermentation   149, 150

β-lactams 149–50
penicillin V 149, 158
mechanisms of action 162–79
chromosome function/replication
173–6
protein synthesis 169–70, **163**,
171–6
microorganisms in partial synthesis
477
polypeptide 111
production from microorganisms
470, **473**
rifamycins 106
semisynthesis 92
sources 92
synthesis 92
tetracyclines 104–6
antibodies 283
binding 80
feedback 296
maternally-acquired 327
passive acquired immunity 303
pre-formed 328
secretory 327
transplacental passage 302
antibody-dependent cell-mediated
cytotoxicity (ADCC) 297
antifungal agents 114, *115*
disinfectant powders 249
antigen 283
antigen-antibody complexes 86
antigen-presenting cells 294
antigens 284
cross-reactive 298
antilymphocyte serum 301
antimessages 69
antimicrobial action, target sites **163**
antimicrobial agents/drugs
acid **210**, 212–13
adverse reactions 135–6
anatomical site of infection 133
chemoprophylaxis 136–7
choice 202–8
chemical agent properties 203
microbial challenge 203
vegetative bacteria 204
clinical use 130–1, 137–45
combinations 226–7
dilution 449
distribution 133
environmental factors 208
generic substitution 146
host factors 131
intended application 207–8
lipid solubility 133
liquid
antifungal activity 244–5
bacteriostasis estimation 242–4
virucidal activity testing 245–8
membrane filtration 449
neutralizing agents **240**
non-antibiotic 229–32
bacterial spore resistance 270–2
fungal resistance 274–5
protozoal resistance 275
resistance 263–4, **265**, 266–76
viral resistance 275, *276*
see also biocides
organism susceptibility 131, *132*
pharmacological factors 131, 133

preservatives 365–8
properties **209**
resistance 133–4
selection 131, 133
semi-solid *243*
specific inactivation 448
sterility testing 448–9
superinfection 136
synergism 227
synthetic 115–22, *123*
therapeutic concentrations 133
toxicity 208
types of compound 208, **210–11**,
212–21, **222**, 223–7
antimycobacterial drugs, resistance
196–7
antiseptics 202, 230
antibacterial activity **205**
antifungal activity 205, **206**
α-antitrypsin 461, **463**
antitubercular drugs 117–18
antiviral drugs 124–8, 174
API system 20
arabinogalactan 168
arabinose 168
arabinosyl transferase enzyme 168
Archaebacteria 4
Arthus reaction 300
2-arylpropionic acid 478
ascospores 40, 41
Neurospora crassa 48
aseptic areas for manufacture of sterile
products 435–6
Ashbya gossypii 471
L-asparaginase 476
Aspergillus flavipes 487
Aspergillus flavus 49
Aspergillus fumigatus 49
Aspergillus niger 205, 486
Aspergillus oryzae 49
Aspergillus parasiticus 49
Aspergillus spp. 49–50
building contamination 349
glass container contamination 348
isolated from air 340
packaging contamination 348
assay methods
plate 481
urease 371
asthma, extrinsic 291
athlete's foot 51
atmosphere
chemical disinfection 341, 342
compressed air 342
disinfection 250–1
filtration 341
microbial content 340–1
microbial count reduction 341–2
microbiological quality checking
340
microbiological standard
requirements 341
microorganism fall-out in
manufacturing process 428
suspended particles 340
ultraviolet irradiation 341, 342
attenuation 279
Aurebasidium pullulans 351
Aurebasidium spp. 349
autoclave *see* steam sterilizer

autoclaving, instruments 425
autografts 301
autoimmune destruction 86
autoimmunity 279, 298–9
autolysins 167
avoparcin 198–9
azalides
action on ribosomes 169
protein synthesis inhibition 172
azathioprine 301
azidothymidine *see* zidovudine (AZT)
azithromycin 110, 118, 172
AZT *see* zidovudine (AZT)
aztreonam 102, *103*

B cells 285, 296
baby hamster kidney (BHK) cell
monolayers 246
bacillary dysentery 29, 57
bloody flux 82
MacConkey's medium 18
bacille Calmette–Guérin (BCG)
vaccine 297, 306, **311**, 333,
336
efficiency 326
potency 316
sterility tests 317
Bacillus anthracis 10, 27
Bacillus brevis 27
Bacillus cereus 27, 76
biocide resistance 264
emetic toxin 85
penicillinase production 477
Bacillus licheniformis 27
Bacillus megaterium 342
Bacillus polymyxa 27
Bacillus pumilus 386
Bacillus sphaericus 488
Bacillus spp.
antibiotic source 92
isolated from air 340
packaging contamination 348
properties 27
raw materials for manufacturing
process 347
spore 11
transfer from manufacturing process
operators 346
Bacillus stearothermophilus 386,
387, 443
Bacillus subtilis 27
biocide resistance 264
cloning host 460, **462**
contamination of non-sterile
products during manufacture
380
PKU screening 483
sterilization reference organism
386, 388
water supply 342
Bacillus thuringiensis 488, *489*
bacitracin 27, 92, 111
resistance 196
bacteraemia 84, 282
bacteraemic shock 376
see also endotoxic shock
bacteria 3–4
acid-fast organisms 32
acquired resistance to biocides
272–4

adaptation to intrinsic resistance 272
aerobes 16
aggregates 4
anaerobes 16, 17
binary fission 14, 21, 22
biochemical tests 20
bioluminescence 25
bond energy 17
carbohydrate metabolism 17
cell counts 20–1
cell envelope 86
colony-forming units (CFU) 21
conjugation 14–15
culture media 17
direct epifluorescent filtration technique (DEFT) 23
DNA 14
electric conductivity 24–5
energy storage 17
facultative 16
flow cytometry 23–4
growth 15–25
  consumable determinants 15–16
  curves 22–3
  energy provision 17–18
  environmental determinants 16–17
  gas requirements 15, 16
  inhibition 16–17
  mean generation time 21–2
  measurement 20–2
  media 16, 17
  pH 16
  requirements 15–17
  temperature 16
  water requirement 15–16
identification 18–20
isolated from air 340
light-scattering/-absorbing units 21
luminous 25
media 16, 17, 18–20
metabolic pathways 18
micro-calorimetry 24
microaerophilic 16
microscopy 23
oxygen requirement 16
quick detection methods 23–5
reproduction 14–15
resistance to biocides 264, **265**, 266
sexual reproduction 10
toxins 14
transduction 15
transformation 14, 15
vegetative 204
viable counts 21
water storage 343
see also Gram-negative bacteria; Gram-positive bacteria
bacterial cell
  appendages 10
  capsules 10
  envelope 266
  pigment 10
  polysaccharide backbone 5
  proteins of outer layer 8
  shape 4
  size 4
  slime 10

structure 4–5, 6, 7–10
  wall 164–8
    crosslinking 166
    peptide bond formation 166
bacterial cell wall 4
  lysis by disinfectants 256
  non-antibiotic antibacterial agent activity 256
bacterial chromosome 9–10
bacterial culture
  death curve 230, 231
  growth curve 230, 231
  pH effects on growth 235
bacterial infections
  epithelial tissue 80
  gastrointestinal 141–3
  systemic 80
bacterial spores 11–13
  acid-fast stain 12
  antimicrobial agent choice 204
  biocide resistance 270–2
  coat 12
  dehydration 11–12
  development 271
  formation process 11–12
  germination 12–13, 271
  heat resistance 11–12, 13, 397
  mature 271
  outgrowth 12–13, 271
  susceptibility 271
bacterial vaccines 307–8, **311–12**
  combined 310
  fermentation 307–8
  processing of bacterial harvest 308
  safety tests 316
  seedlot system 307
  single component 310, **311–12**
bactericidal activity of semi-solid antibacterials 248–9
bactericides 131, 229
  multidose injections 414
  quantitative suspension tests 239
bacteriophages see phages
bacteriostasis
  cup-plate technique 243
  ditch-plate technique 242–3
  estimation 242–4
  gradient-plate technique 244
  serial dilution 242
  solid dilution method 243
bacteriostats 229
  semi-solid antibacterial agents 248
bacteriuria 140, 141
Bacteroides fragilis 30
  aztreonam resistance 102
  phages 248
Bacteroides spp. 30
Baird-Parker medium 19
baker's yeast 35
base-pair mutation 484
BCG vaccine see bacille Calmette–Guérin (BCG) vaccine
benzalkonium chloride 417, 419
benzoic acid **210**, 212
benzyl alcohol 213
D-benzylpenicillenic acid 104
benzylpenicillin 92, 93
  brain abscess 145
  degradation products 96
  Gram-negative bacteria

lysis 167
  protection 7
hydrolysis 477
manufacture 149
  carbon source 155
  cell removal 157
  contaminants 155–6
  crude extract treatment 157–8
  defoaming agents 153–4
  extraction 157–8
  fed nutrients 155–6
  fermentation control 154–7
  fermenter 152–4
  GMP 158
  inoculum preparation 151
  inoculum transfer to vessel 154
  instrumentation 154
  isolation 157
  lactose 155
  media additions 154
  nitrogen source 155
  organism 150–1
  oxygen supply 152–3
  PAA stimulation 156–7
  pH 156
  production strains 151
  sampling 154
  sulphate supply 155
  temperature control 153, 156
  termination of fermentation 157
biguanides **210**, 216–17
  mycobacterial resistance 269
  properties **209**
biliary excretion 133
binary fission of bacteria 14
bio-control 488–9
bioburden
  determination 440
  measurement 372
  reduction in pharmaceutical products 371
biocide-degrading enzymes, constitutive 266
biocides 230
  bacterial resistance 10, 264, **265**
    intrinsic 264, **265**, 266
  cationic 268, 269
  insusceptibility 263
  relative microbial responses 263–4
  see also antimicrobial agents/drugs, non-antibiotic
biofilms 77
  physiological (phenotypic) adaptation to intrinsic resistance 272
  production 264
biological indicators of sterility 442, 443, 445–6
bioluminescence 25
  preservatives 254
biotin 472
bisbiguanides 178
  see also chlorhexidine
bismuth sulphite agar 19
bisphenols 222, 224
bisulphites 262
Black Death 28
black fluids 222, 223
blepharitis 79
blood substitute, dextran 10, 471

blow/fill/seal units 436
blue–green algae 3, 4
boils 26, 143
bone marrow 284
    multipotential cells 285
    suppression 135–6
Bordetella pertussis 28–9, 80, 334
    non-invasive pathogen 81–2
    vaccine production 308
    see also pertussis; whooping cough
Borrelia burgdorferi 32
Borrelia recurrentis 32
Borrelia vincenti 32
botulinum
    antitoxin **318**
    toxin in medical use 489, 490
botulism 27, 76, 85
bovine spongiform encephalopathy
    (BSE) 73, 207, 323–4
    sterilization 386
    see also prions
brain abscess 145
Branhamella catarrhalis 26
Branhamella spp. 26
Brevundimonas diminuta 445–6
brewer's yeast 35
brilliant green 226
β-bromopenicillanic acid 103
bronchiectasis 138
bronchitis 138
    chronic 29
bronchodilators 416
bronchopneumonia 30
bronchoscope, disinfection 276
bronopol 214
    thiol group reaction 259
Brucella abortus 29, 80, 81
Brucella melitensis 29
Brucella suis 29
buildings 349–50
Burkitt's lymphoma 72
burns, infected wounds 144

cadexomer-I₂ 220
calcium alginate 422
campylobacter
    antimicrobial agent choice 204
    gastrointestinal infections 142
Campylobacter jejuni 31
Campylobacter spp. 30–1
cancer chemotherapy 476
Candida albicans 35, 44–7
    amphoterocin B activity 114
    antimicrobial agent choice 205
    cell wall 44–5
    flucytosine activity 122
    gene isolation 45
    germ tube formation 46, 47
    HO gene 47
    hyphal form 45
    mating type switching 46, 47
    morphological switching 45–6
    mutants 45
    phenotypic switching 45
    positive control for sterility testing
        449
Candida parapsilosis 44
Candida spp., contaminated medicines
    356
candidiasis

intestinal 114
    ketoconazole 122
    superinfection 136
candidosis, vaginal 44, 46
capacity use–dilution test 238
capreomycin 111, 118
capsids 54, 57
    assembly 69
capsomeres 54–6, 57
1-carbacephems *101*, 102
1-carbacephems 101–2
    see also carbapenems
carbapenems 167
    see also 1-carbacephems
carbenicillin 93, *94*, **95**
    burn wounds 144
    gentamicin combination 108
carbohydrate metabolism 17
carbolic acid *see* phenol
carboxypeptidase 167
carbuncle 143
carcinogen screening 62, 484–6
catgut, sterilized surgical 423
cationic compounds 268, 269
cationic surfactants 224–5, 358
    pH effects on antibacterial activity
        236
CD4+ cells 72, 73
CD8 expression 296
cefacetrile *98*, **99**
cefaclor 97, *98*, **100**
cefamandole 97, *98*, **100**
cefibuten 97, *99*, **100**
cefixime 97
cefotaxime 96, 97, *99*, **100**
    kidney infection 141
    PBP binding 167
cefoxitin 97, *98*, **100**
cefpodixime 97, *99*, **100**
ceftazidime 96, *99*, **100**
    PBP binding 167
ceftizoxime 96, *99*, **100**
ceftriaxone 96, *99*, **100**
cefuroxime 96, 97, *98*, **100**
ceilings 349
    clean areas 430, 434
cell membrane *see* cytoplasmic
    membrane
cell surface, pH effects on antibacterial
    activity 236
cell wall *see* bacterial cell wall
cell-mediated immunity 283, 293–6
cellulitis 143
cellulose, oxidized 422
central nervous system
    infections 144–5
    secondary disease 86
cephalexin 97, *98*, **100**
    PBP binding 167
cephaloridine 167
cephalosporin C 477
    manufacture 149, 158, *159*, 160
cephalosporins 92, 93–7, 131
    activity spectrum 97
    β-lactam ring interaction with
        transpeptidases 167
    β-lactamase susceptibility 97
    biosynthetic genes 156–7
    enzymatic inactivation 133
    half-life 97

PBP binding 167
    peptidoglycan crosslinking 166–8
    pharmacokinetic properties 97
    resistance 192
    structure–activity relationships 96–
        7
cephamycins 157
cephapirin 97, *98*
cephradine 97, *98*, **100**
changing facilities, clean areas 433
cheese ripening 49
chemical indicators of sterility 442–3,
    444
chemoprophylaxis 136–7
Chick–Martin test 237, 238
chickenpox outbreaks 88, 325
chimeras 455
chiral inversion 478–9
chitin
    Candida albicans 44
    S. cerevisiae cell wall 43, 44
Chlamydia psittaci 31
Chlamydia spp. 31
Chlamydia trachomatis 31
chloramine 218
chloramphenicol 91, 92, 112, *113*,
    133, 190–1
    action on ribosomes 170
    bone marrow suppression 135–6
    drug-resistant ribosomes 190
    efflux proteins 190
    enzymatic inactivation 133
    mammalian cell penetration 172
    protein synthesis inhibition 171–2
    ribosome effects 172
    typhoid fever treatment 137
chloramphenicol acetyltransferases
    (CATs) 112, 190
chlorbutol 213–14
    ophthalmic preparations 419
chlorhexidine **210**, 216–17, 258
    bacterial spore activity 271
    cytoplasm coagulation 259
    E. coli sensitivity 267
    mechanism of action 258, **260**
    microbial attack 359
    microorganism sensitivity **265**
    mycobacterial resistance 269
    ophthalmic preparations 417, 419
    properties **209**
    Proteus resistance 268
    S. marcescens resistance 268
    Sacch. cerevisiae sensitivity 274
chlorine 217–18
    antiviral activity 57
    compounds **209**, **210**
    gas 345
    thiol group reaction 259
chlorine-releasing agents, thiol group
    reaction 259
chlorocresol *222*, 224, 253
chloroform 219, 367–8
p-chloromercuribenzoate 259
chloroxylenol **209**, *211*, *222*, 224,
    268
    potentiators 258
chlortetracycline 105
cholera 28, 283
    antibiotic treatment 142
    contaminated medicine 356

toxin in medical use 490
vaccine 306, 308
Chromobacter spp. 342
chromosomal mutations, acquired
resistance 182–3
chromosomes
bacterial 9–10
function/replication 173–6
selective inhibition 173–5
supercoiling 173, 175
unwinding 174
ciprofloxacin 118, 120, *121*, 188
kidney infection 141
typhoid fever 142
Cladosporium spp. 348
building contamination 349
filters 351
isolated from air 340
raw materials for manufacturing
process 347
clarithromycin 110, 118
clavams 97–8, 100, *101*
clavulanic acid *101*
combination therapy 98, 100
cleanliness, pharmaceutical
manufacture 427–8, 433
clindamycin 112, *113*
protein synthesis inhibition 172
wound infections 144
clomocycline 104
clonal deletion, tolerance 298
cloned gene expression 457–9
post-translational modification
458–9
transcription 457
translation 457–8
cloning 454–6
host choice 460–1
shotgunning 456
systems 461, **462**
Clostridium botulinum 76
medical use of toxin 489
toxin 14, 85
Clostridium difficile 27
pseudomembranous colitis 136
Clostridium novyi 27
Clostridium perfringens 27, 282
toxin production 83
Clostridium septicum 27
Clostridium spore 11
Clostridium sporogenes 27, 499
Clostridium spp.
isolated from air 340
properties 27
transfer from manufacturing process
operators 346
water supply 342
Clostridium tetani 27
exotoxin 283
medicament-borne infection 382
non-sterile pharmaceutical products
376
tissue damage 85
clotrimazole 120, *123*
clumping 239, 240
cluster of differentiation 294
co-trimoxazole 117
gastrointestinal infections 142, 143
typhoid fever treatment 137
coagulase 282

coccoid bacteria 4
colistin 111
see also polymyxins
collagenase 83, 282
colony-forming units (CFU) 21
colostrum, secretory antibodies 327
colouring agents 358–9
common cold 62
partially invasive pathogens 82
common-source outbreaks 87, 88
community protection against
epidemics 322
community-acquired pathogens 198
complement
cascade 293
fixation 80
system 87, 281, 291–3
complement activation
alternative pathway 293
classical pathway 291–3
regulation 293
complex-mediated reactions 300
compound II 474
compressed air 342
concentration exponent 233–4
congenital rubella syndrome 332
conjugation
bacterial 14–15
plasmid transfer 183
resistance plasmid transfer 133
conjunctiva 79
conjunctivitis 26, 29, 31
contact lenses 79
disinfection 419
solutions 418–19
contact plates 440
corn starch liquor 155
cortisone manufacture 478
Corynebacterium diphtheriae 27, 80,
82
β-phage 62
tissue damage 85
Corynebacterium spp.
isolated from air 340
properties 27
cosmetic preparations, preservatives
251, 252
cotrimoxazole 178
Coulter counter 23, *24*
cowpox 322
Coxiella burnetti 31
cresol 222, 223
Creutzfeldt–Jakob disease (CJD) 73,
207, 323–4, 356
sterilization 386
CRM197 335
crop pest control 488
Cryptococcus neoformans 35, 47
amphoterocin B activity 114
meningitis treatment with drug
combination 134
crystal violet 226
Cunninghamella blakesleeana 487
cup-plate method 243, 248, 249
cyanocobalamin 472
cycloserine 118
see also D-cycloserine
D-cycloserine 165
mechanism of action **163**, 164
see also cycloserene

cyclosporin A 301
cystic fibrosis 138, 139
cystitis 29
cytarabine 125, *126*
cytokines 295
cytolytic reactions 299
cytomegalovirus **63**, 127
HIV infection 72
interferons 70
cytopathic effect (CPE) 66, *67*
Cytophaga spp. 342
cytoplasm 4, 9–10
coagulation 259
non-antibiotic antibacterial agent
activity 258–9
cytoplasmic membrane 4, 8–9, 178–9
active transport system 9
antibacterial agent penetration
pathways 267–8
non-antibiotic antibacterial agent
activity 257–8
porins 185
selective disruption 178
cytotoxic reactions 299
cytotoxic T cells 296

D-biotin 472
D-value 13, 387, 389, 391, 403
Dane particles 246–7
dapsone *116*, 117
ddI 73, 126
decaprenyl-arabinose 168
defence mechanisms, specific 283–4
Deinococcus (Micrococcus)
radiodurans 403
deletions 183
demethylchlortetracycline 105
deoxyribonuclease (DNase) 83, 454
deoxyribonucleic acids 258
dequalinium chloride 226
dermatophytes 50
desferrioxamine 473–4
dextrans 10, 470–1, **472**
dextrose agar 20
di-(5-chloro-2-hydroxyphenyl)
sulphide 257
diabetes, infection of islets of
Langerhans 86
diamidines 226
Gram-negative bacteria sensitivity
267
diaminopyrimidine derivatives *116*,
117
diarrhoea, traveller's 143
dibromopropamidine 226
dichloroisocyanurate, HIV
disinfection 207
dichloroisocyanuric acid 218
dideoxycytidine (DDC) 125–6
dideoxyinosine *see* ddI
dihydrofolate reductase (DHFR) 176
inhibitors 174, 177–8
dihydrofolic acid 176
dihydropteroate synthetase (DHPS)
187
dihydropteroic acid 176
dihydrostreptomycin 106
diphosphatidyl glycerol 8
diphtheria 27, 82
antitoxin **318**

tetanus 334
tissue damage 85
toxin
  non-toxic derivative 335
  production 62
toxoid 334
vaccination 333–4
  efficiency 326
vaccine 304, 308, **311**, 314, 315
diphtheria, tetanus and pertussis
    (DTP) immunization 333,
    334–5
dipicolinic acid (DPA) *see* pyridine
    2,6-dicarboxylic acid
diplococci, aggregates 4
Diplococcus pneumoniae see
    Streptococcus pneumoniae
direct epifluorescent filtration
    technique (DEFT) 23
disease
  common-source outbreaks 87, 88
  early treatment 469–70
  epidemiology 87–8
  immunity 278–9
  infectious 305
  manifestation 81–4
  propagated-source outbreaks 87,
    88
  severity 325–6
  slow virus 73, 276
  transmission *76*
  see also infection
disinfectants 201–2, 230
  acid 267
  air 250–1
  antibacterial activity **205**
  cell wall lysis 256
  concentration for virucidal activity
    247
  contamination 370
  factors affecting disinfection
    process 232–7
  Gram-negative bacteria protection
    7
  in vivo tests 241–2
  liquid 237–48
    quantitative suspension
      tests 239–40
    suspension tests 237–8
  microbial attack 359
  mycobactericidal activity 241
  powders 249
  skin tests 241–2
  solid 249–50
  sporicidal activity 241
  storage 353
  types 201–28
    see also individual compounds
  viable airborne microorganism
    determination 250–1
disinfection
  aseptic areas 436
  atmosphere 250–1
  attainable level **203**
  clean areas for pharmaceutical
    manufacture of sterile
    products 433
  concentration exponent 233–4
  contact lenses 419
  dilution effect 233–4

dynamics 230–2
equipment **424**
hepatitis B virus 206
high level 201, 202
HIV 206–7
inoculum size 236, *237*
instruments 207
interfering substances 236
intermediate level 201–2
low level 202
manufacturing equipment 352
pH effects 234–6
policies 227–8
potency/concentration relationship
    233–4
rate of kill 231
surface activity effects 236
survivor/time curve *232*
temperature effects 232–3
viable counts 239
virus 57
water 345
ditch-plate technique 242–3, 248
DNA
  bacterial 14
  viral 15
DNA gyrase 173, 174
  inhibition by quinolones 175
  quinolone binding 187
DNA ligase 174
DNA polymerase 173, 174, 246
DNA strand replication 174
doors 349–50
doxycycline 105
drains 349
dressings 419–21
  packaging 420–1
  spray-on 421
  sterilization 419–20
drug
  efficacy 487
  fever 135
  safety 487
  see also resistance
drug combinations 128–9, 134–5
  indications 128–9
  justifications for use 128
  resistance prevention 135
  responses 128
dry heat sterilizer 397–8
duck hepatitis B virus (DHBV) 246
dyes 226

early proteins 59
Ebola virus **65**, 205
econazole 120, *123*
EDTA 8, 258, 267, 268
  contact-lens solutions 419
efflux 134
efflux proteins
  chloramphenicol 190
  tetracycline resistance 196
  tetracyclines 190
egg inoculation for virucidal activity
    245
electron accelerators 401, 403, 405
electron transport chain 9
  inhibition 257
elongation factors 172–3
Embden–Meyerhof pathway 18

S. cerevisiae 42
emulsions
  breakdown 372, 374
  preservative evaluation 252
encephalitis 144
endocarditis prevention 136–7
endospore 11
endothelial cells 285
endotoxic shock 372
  see also bacteraemic shock
endotoxins 86, 282, 283
energy
  reactions producing 17–18
  storage 17
enteric fever 84
enteritis 29
Enterobacter cloacae 342
Enterobacteriaceae, biocide
    resistance 266–9
enterococci
  biocide sensitivity 263
  multi-drug resistance 134
  resistance 183
  transfer from manufacturing process
    operators 346
  see also vancomycin-resistant
    enterococci (VRE)
enterotoxins 283
Enterotube 20
enterovirus infection 62
environment, contamination sources for
    non-sterile products 377
environmental monitoring, sterility
    assurance 441
enzymes 475–7
  microbial in sterility testing 486
  plasmid mediated inactivation
    133–4
eosinophils 285
epidemics 88, 325
  community protection 322
Epidermophyton floccosum 50, 51
Epidermophyton spp. 346
epifluorescence, preservatives 254
episomes 9
Epstein–Barr virus **63**, 72
equipment
  aseptic areas 436
  sterilization 423–5
Eremothecium ashbyii 471
ergosterol synthesis 179
ermA gene 191
ermB gene 191
ermC gene 191
Erwinia carotovora 476
Erwinia spp. 347
erythrogenic toxin, *Streptococcus
    pyogenes* 26
erythromycin 108, 109
  gastrointestinal infections 142
  legionnaire's disease treatment
    131, 139
  mycoplasma infections 139
  new derivatives 109–10
erythropoietin **464**
Escherichia coli 29
  ampicillin resistance 181
  L-asparaginase production 476
  biocide resistance 266–7, 268
  bismuth sulphite agar 19

cloning host   460, **462**
deep rough mutants   267
enteropathic strains   82
enterotoxigenic   143
exotoxins   86
K-antigens   80
lux cluster insertion   25
MacConkey's medium   18
macrolide resistance   191
meningitis   144, 145
multidrug resistance pumps (MDR)
      196
multiple antibiotic resistance (MAR)
      196
multiple resistance   197
peptidoglycan   6
phages   58, 248
phospholipid structure   8
signal sequence   458, 459
somatostatin synthesis   460
toxin production   82
water supply   342
Escherichia coli 0157 infection
      outbreak   323
Escherichia coli K12(lambda)   60
ester antimicrobials   **210**, 212–13
ethambutol   168
   M. tuberculosis resistance   196, 197
ethanol   **210**, 213
   formation   42
   properties   **209**
ethionamide   118
ethylene oxide   262
   antiviral activity   57
   toxicity   399–400
ethylene oxide sterilization   **400**, 399
   operating cycle   *401*
   sterilizer design/operation   400–1
ethylenediamine tetraacetic acid *see*
      EDTA
ethylphenols   *222*, *223*
eukaryotes   4
exaltation   279
exons   456
exopolymer matrix   77
exotoxins   86, 282, 283
expanded cortex theory   12
eye preparations
   drops   417–18
   lotions   418
   ointments   418
   preservatives   359
eye-drops   417–18
   preservatives   417
   Ps. aeruginosa contamination   382
   sterilization   419
   storage temperature   364

F_0 value   13, 392
F-pili   10
   conjugation   14
F-value   391, 392, 398
Fab fragments   286
Factor VIII   356, **464**
Factor IX   **464**
famciclovir   127
fansidar   178
fats, microbial attack   358
Fc fragments   286
fentichlor   257

fever   282
fibrin
   deposition   281
      around abscesses   83–4
   foam   422
fibrinolysins   83
filters, manufacturing process   351
filtration sterilization   405–7
   biological monitoring   445–6
   gases   407
   liquids   406
   see also membrane filtration
fimbriae   10, 79
fire fly light-emitting system *see*
      luciferase
fittings, clean areas   430
flagella   10
flaviviruses   **65**
Flavobacterium spp.   30, 342
flavouring agents   358–9
floors   349
   clean areas   430, 434
flow cytometry, bacteria   23–4
flucytosine   122, *123*
5-flucytosine   134
5-fluoridine phosphates   122
5-fluorocytosine   174, 176
fluoroquinolones   120
5-fluorouracil   122, 174
folate
   antagonists   176–8
   metabolism in microbial/mammalian
         cells   176, *177*
   utilization   176
food, microbial growth   76
food industry, *D*-value   13
food poisoning   27
   Campylobacter jejuni   31
   contaminated medicines   356–7
   staphylococcal   26
   Vibrio parahaemolyticus   28
   see also salmonellosis
formaldehyde   215–16
   amino group reaction   259
   low temperature steam (LTSF)
         process   399, **400**, 401
   plasmid-mediated resistance   279
   sterilization   399, 401–2
   toxicity   399
foscarnet *see* sodium phosphoformate
fosfomycin resistance   195
frameshift mutations   182, 183, 484
framycetin   106, 108
Francisella tularensis   28
fungal infections, imidazole
         derivatives   120, 122
fungi
   antimicrobial agent choice   204–5
   azole actions om membrane   179
   biocide resistance   274–5
   dimorphic   35
   filamentous   **462**
   media   20
   polarity   37–8
fungicides   230
   activity testing   245
   quantitative suspension tests   239
fungistats   230
   activity testing   245
furaltadone   *119*

furazolidone   *119*
Fusarium oxysporum f. sp. *cepae*
      487
Fusarium spp.   347
fusel alcohols   40
fusidic acid   112, *113*, 172–3
   action on ribosomes   170
   resistance   191
fusion protein   460

gamma-irradiation   401, 403
   sterilizer   403, *404*, 405
   see also ionizing radiation; radiation
         sterilization
ganciclovir   126–7
Gardnerella vaginalis   27
gas gangrene   27
gas sterilization   399–401
   monitoring   441, **444**
gastrointestinal infections   141–3
gastrointestinal tract
   commensal microorganisms   78
   vascular permeability   82, 86
gelatin foam, absorbable   422
gene therapy   467
gene transfer, drug resistance   133
general protoplasmic poison   259
generic substitution of drugs   146
genes
   biosynthetic   156–7
   cloned   457–9
   expression maximization   459–60
   light-emitting   25
   repair   467
genetic code   10
genetic engineering *see* recombinant
         DNA technology
gentamicin   92, 106, *107*, 108
gentian violet   226
Germall   115, 252
German measles vaccine   304
glass containers   348
β-glucan, *Candida albicans*   44–5
glucan, *S. cerevisiae* cell wall   43
Gluconobacter spp.   92
glucose oxidase production   486
glucose-6-phosphate dehydrogenase
         deficiency   136
glutaraldehyde   **210**, 214–16
   amino group reaction   259
   cell wall activity   256
   HIV disinfection   207
   mycobacterial resistance   270
   properties   **209**
   toxicity   208
glycerol teichoic acid   6
glycocalyx   10, 77
glycolytic pathway, *S. cerevisiae*   42
glycopeptide antibiotics *see*
         glycopeptides
glycopeptides   111–12, 165–6
   multi-drug resistance   134
   resistance   194–5
   see also teicoplanin; vancomycin
glycosylation   459
glycylcyclines   105–6
gonorrhoea   26
good manufacturing practice (GMP)
      158, 427, 428
good pharmaceutical manufacturing

practice (GPMP) 368, 370–1,
  436–7
hospital pharmacies 381
validation 371, 372
gradient-plate technique 244
graft rejection 301
Gram-negative bacteria 5, 7
  aminoglycoside-modifying
    enzymes 189
  antimicrobial agent choice 204
  biocide resistance 266–9
  contaminated medicines 356
  cytoplasmic membrane 185
  endotoxins 282
  envelope 7
  fusidic acid resistance 191
  industrial water supplies 342
  outer membrane 267
  porins 185
Gram-negative cocci 26
Gram-negative rods 28–32
Gram-positive bacteria 5, 7
  aminoglycoside-modifying
    enzymes 189
  biocide sensitivity 263
  cytoplasmic membrane 185
  fusidic acid resistance 191
Gram-positive cocci 26
  biocide resistance 266
Gram-positive rods 27–8
granulocyte colony stimulating
    factor 464
granulocyte-macrophage colony
    stimulating factor 464
griseofulvin 92, 114, *115*
growth hormone, contaminated 356
Guthrie test 483
gyrA gene 187

H-2 complex 301
H-antigens 284
haemagglutination, bacterial 10
haemodialysis solutions 416
haemolysins 83, 283
haemophiliacs, HIV infection 356
Haemophilus influenzae 29
  ampicillin resistance 145
  erythromycin activity 108
  meningitis 144
  respiratory tract infection 82
  transfer from manufacturing process
    operators 346
  upper respiratory tract infections
    137
  vaccine 307, **311**
Haemophilus influenzae Type B (HiB)
    immunization 335
Haemophilus pneumoniae 139
haemorrhagic fever 205
haemostats, absorbable 421–2
halazone 218, *219*
halogens 217–20
  sporicidal action 204
hand disinfection
  hygienic 241
  surgical 242
hand washing 428
  nurses 378
hapten–protein conjugates 104
HAT medium 288

hay fever 291
Hazard Analysis of Critical Control
    Points (HACCP) 339
health hazards, non-sterile
    pharmaceutical
    products 375–6
heat, disinfection process 232–3
heat sterilization 390–9
  monitoring 441, **443–4**
heat transfer, dry heat sterilizer 397–8
heavy metals 220–1
  Saccharomyces cerevisiae
    effects 275
HeLa cell lines 66
Helicobacter pylori 31
helper T cells 295
helplessness, tolerance 298
HEPA filters 407, 442
hepatitis
  environment specificity 208
  viruses **63**
hepatitis A
  vaccine **313**
  virus **65**
hepatitis B
  immunoglobulins **319**
  surface antigen (HBsAg) 247, 307,
    464
  vaccine 307, **313**
hepatitis A virus **65**
hepatitis B virus
  animal model 246
  disinfection 206
    policies 227
  interferons 70
  oncogenic 72
  see also duck hepatitis B virus
    (DHBV)
hepatitis C virus **65**
hepatocellular carcinoma 49
herd immunity 88
herpes infection, acyclovir 126
herpes keratitis 125
herpes simplex 321
  encephalitis 144
  phosphonoacetic acid activity 127
  virus **63**
herpes virus **63**
  interferons 70
  plaque assays 245, 246
herpes zoster 321
hexachlorophane 222, 224, 257
  Gram-negative bacteria
    sensitivity 267
hexose monophosphate pathway,
    S. cerevisiae 42
high-efficiency particulate air (HEPA)
    filters 407, 442
histamine 281, 291, 293
HIV **65**, 72–3
  AZT activity 125
  contaminated Factor VIII products
    356
  disinfection 206–7
    policies 227
  glutaraldehyde sterilization 215
  immune system effects 294
  Kaposi's sarcoma 72
  protease inhibitors 127
  reactivation 127

reverse transcriptase 174, 247
  TIBO activity 127
  viral protein production 70
HLA-B27 301
HO gene 47
hospital patients
  compromised 382
  resistance to medicament-borne
    infection 383
hospital-acquired infection 77
hospitals
  disinfection policies 227
  environment as contamination
    source 379
  pharmacies 380–1
host
  autoimmune destruction 86
  damage 282–3
host factors, antimicrobial drugs 131
human immunodeficiency virus *see*
    HIV
human immunoglobulins 304, 305,
    318–19
human leucocyte antigen (HLA) 294,
    301
human papilloma virus 72
human serum, pooled 328
human T-cell lymphotrophic virus type
    I (HTLV-1) **65**, 72
humectants 358
humoral antigen–antibody
    reactions 291
humoral immune response 283
humoral immunity 285–6
hyaluronidase 83, 282
hybridoma 288–9
hydrochloric acid 280
hydrocortisone manufacture 478
hydrogen peroxide **211**, 221
  ribosome effects 259
p-hydroxybenzoic acid *see* parabens
hygiene 346–7
  personal 428
  pharmaceutical manufacture 427–8
hyperglycaemia 86
hypersensitivity 135, 299–302
  delayed 299, 300
  immediate 291, 299
  stimulatory 300
  types I-V reactions 299–300
hypochlorite **210**, 218
  antiviral activity 57
  properties **209, 210**, 218
  thiol group reaction 259
hypoxanthine-guanine phosphoribosyl-
    transferase (HGPRT) 287,
    288, 467

ibuprofen 479
idiotypic determinants 296–7
idoxuridine 125, *126*, 174
imidazole derivatives 120, 122, *123*
imidazoles 178, 179
imipenem 101, 102
imipramine 487
immobilized enzyme technology 486
immune response 283
  magnitude 328
  specificity 328
  tumours 301–2

immune system
  adaptive 283–4
  innate 280–3
  recovery from infection 87
immunity 302–3
  acquired 302–3
    active 328–9
    passive 327–8
  active 304–5
  cells involved 284–99
  classes 326–9
  generation strategies 321
  humoral 285–6
  longevity 327
  natural 302
immunization 321–2
  antibody response 286
  cost 327
  juvenile schedule 335–6
  programme objectives 325–7
  routine against infectious disease
    330–5
  safety 326
  special risk groups 336
  travelling 326
immunogens 283
  effectiveness 326
  non-replicating 328
immunoglobulin A (IgA) 290
immunoglobulin D (IgD) 290
immunoglobulin E (IgE) 290–1
immunoglobulin G (IgG) 286, 287,
  290, 318
  transplacental 327
immunoglobulin M (IgM) 289–90
immunoglobulins 285–6
  classes 289–91
  globular domains 286
  human 304, 305, 318–19
  quality control 319
immunological memory 324
immunological products 304–5
  see also vaccines
immunological tolerance 297–8
immunology 278–9
immunoregulation 296–7
immunosera 304, 305, 317–18
immunosuppression
  fungal infections 114, 144
  Pneumocystis carinii pneumonia
    117
immunosuppressive drugs 301
impetigo 26, 143
implants 421
in-process control 427
inactivating agents 240, 448
  see also neutralizing agents
inactivation factor (IF) 388, 389, 393
incubators, chemical sterilization 425
infection
  anatomical site 133
  bacterial 80, 141–3
  common source 323–4
  establishment 75
  fungal 120, 122
  gastrointestinal 141–3
  intracellular 131
  iron availability 474
  manifestations 81
  medicament-borne 381–3

administration route 382–3
  microbial contamination
    type/degree 382
  patient resistance 383
  prevention 136–7
  propogated source 324–5
  recovery 87
  respiratory tract 137–9
  routes 76
  skin 143–4
  spread 323–5
  time–concentration profile 328
  viral 143, 356
  wound 28, 30, 144
  see also candidiasis; candidosis
infective agents, obligate pathogens
  87
inflammation 281–2
inflammatory response modulation 80
influenza
  partially invasive pathogens 82
  vaccine 307, 310, 313, 326
influenza A virus 124
influenza virus 62, 64
  chick embryo cell system for
    growing 66–7
  combat of herd immunity 88
  enveloped particles 70
  viral protein production 70
inhA gene mutations 197
inhaler solutions 416
initiation codon 458
injectable products 411–15
  autoclaving 413
  design 411–12
  drug stability 415
  intravenous infusions 412–14
  isotonicity adjustment 412
  multidose 412, 414
  packaging 413
  single-dose 414
  small-volume aqueous 414–15
  small-volume oily 415
  total parenteral nutrition 414
inoculum size 236, 237
insecticides 487–9
instruments
  disinfection 207
  sterilization 423–5
insulin 463
  cloned gene 456, 457, 458
alpha-interferon 297
interferons 70–1, 128, 281, 463
  antitumour effect 71
  recombinant DNA technology 461
interleukin-1 (IL-1) 282
interleukin-2 (IL-2) 296, 297, 464
intoxication 81, 85
intracellular pathogens 131, 172
intravenous infusions 412–14
  additives 413–14
introns 456
iodine 217, 219, 220
  antiviral activity 57
  compounds 211
    properties 209
  thiol group reaction 259
iodophors 219–20
ionizing radiation see radiation
  sterilization

iron dextran injection 471
iron poisoning 474
iron-chelating agents 473–4
isoamyl alcohol 40
isografts 301
isolators
  pharmaceutical manufacture of
    sterile products 436
  sterility testing 447, 448
isoleucyl tRNA 173
  synthetase 192
isoniazid 117, 118, 168
  M. tuberculosis resistance 168,
    196–7
isopropanol 213
itraconazole 122

joints, artificial 425

kanamycin 106, 107, 108
Kaposi's sarcoma 72
KatG catalase-peroxidase enzyme
  system 168
katG gene 197
Kelsey–Sykes test 238
keratin 11
  fungal utilization 50
ketoconazole 120, 122, 123
kidney
  infection 141
  inflammation 26
  malfunction 86
Klebsiella aerogenes 342
Klebsiella pneumoniae 346
Klebsiella pneumoniae subsp.
  aerogenes 30
MacConkey's medium 18
Klebsiella spp.
  medicament-borne infection 382
  multiple resistance 197
  urinary tract infections 140
Krebs citric acid cycle 18

β-lactam antibiotics 92–3, 94, 95–8,
  99, 100–4
  bacterial cell wall crosslinking
    block 165–7
  manufacture 149–50
  resistance 192–4
β-lactam bond 165
β-lactamase 93, 192, 476–7
lactic acid, vaginal 79
lactobacilli 79
Lactobacillus spp. 347
lactose 155
laminar airflow unit 433, 436
lanosterol 179
latamoxef 100, 101
latent heat 393
lecithinase 282
Legionella pneumophila 31–2
  erythromycin activity 108
  pneumonia 138, 139
  roxithromycin activity 110
Legionella spp., environment
  specificity 208
legionellosis 31–2, 138–9
  antimicrobial agent choice 204
  intracellular infection 131
lens disinfection 207

leprosy 32
  dapsone therapy 117
Leptospira icterohaemorrhagiae 33
Lesch–Nyhan disease 467
leucocidins 81, 282
leucocytes, toxicity of
    antimicrobials 242
Leuconostoc dextranicum 10
Leuconostoc mesenteroides 10
Leuconostoc spp.
  dextran production 470
  intravenous infusions 412
leucovorin 178
leukotrienes 281, 291
ligatures 422–3
light emitting genes 25
Limulus test 372
lincomycin 112, *113*
  protein synthesis inhibition 172
lincosamide resistance 191
lipid A 339
lipid carrier molecule 165
lipid solubility of drugs 133
lipopolysaccharide 7, 8, 178, 267,
  268
  aminoethanol/aminocarabinose
    incorporation 195
  polyclonal activation 298
  polymyxin activity 179
  Ps. aeruginosa 269
Listeria monocytogenes 27–8
Listeria spp.
  antimicrobial agent choice 204
  environment specificity 208
  lux cluster insertion 25
listeriosis 28
lockjaw *see* tetanus
lomefloxacin 120
loracarbef *101*
low temperature steam formaldehyde
  (LTSF) process 215, **394**, 399,
  400–1
luciferase 25, 372
luciferin 25
lung abscess 138, 139
lux cluster 25
Lyme disease 32
lymph nodes 285
lymph system 84
lymphocytes 283
  cell-mediated immunity 294
lymphokines 281, 298
lymphoreticular organs 284
lysogenic cells 59
Lysol 223
lysozyme 59, 280
  Gram-negative bacteria protection
    7

MacConkey's medium 18
macrolesions 183
macrolide, lincosamide and
  streptogramin (MLS)
    antibiotics, resistance 191
macrolides 108–11
  action on ribosomes 170
  efflux 133
  protein synthesis inhibition 172
  resistance 191
macrophage activating factor 295

macrophage chemotactic factor 295
macrophage migration inhibitory
  factor 295
macrophages 280, 285
  alveolar region 78
  endogenous pyrogen release 86
major histocompatibility complex
  (MHC) 294, 296, 301
malachite green 226
malaria, Epstein–Barr virus infection
  72
mammalian cells, cloning host 461,
  462
mammalian drug metabolism models
  487
mannitol salt medium 19
mannoproteins
  Candida albicans 44
  S. cerevisiae cell wall 43–4
Mantoux skin test 333
Marburg virus, disinfection 205
mast cells 285
master temperature record (MTR)
  441
MDRTB 118, 134, 196–7
measles
  immunoglobulins **319**
  outbreaks 88, 325
  vaccination 331
  vaccine 304, **313**
  virus **64**
measles, mumps and rubella (MMR)
  vaccination 331–2
  juvenile immunization
    schedule 336
measles, mumps and rubella vaccine
  (MMR Vac) 310
mebendazole 120
mec gene 194
mecillinam 92–3, *94*, **95**
  PBP binding 167
medical devices 77
medicines, contaminated 356–7
Medicines Act (1968) 380
membrane attack complex 292
membrane enzymes 257–8
  thiol-containing 258
membrane filters **406**, 407
membrane filtration
  antimicrobial agents 449
  sterility testing 447
  water disinfection 345
membrane permeability 258
membrane potentials 257
membrane-active agents 178
  resistance 195–6
meningitis
  bacterial 26, 144, 145
  cryptococcal 47, 122
  drug combinations 134
  infantile 29
  meningococcal 26
    secondary case prevention 137
    sulphonamide activity 116–17
  pneumococcal 145
  viral 144
mepacrine 174
mercuric chloride 234
mercury
  inducible resistance 273

salts in cytoplasm coagulation 259
meropenem *101*, 102
messenger RNA (mRNA) 58
  copying 174
  early molecules 59
  late 69
  translation into protein 457
metabisulphites 212
methacycline 105
methicillin-resistant *Staphylococcus
  aureus* (MRSA) 134, 194, 197
  antimicrobial agent choice 204
  biocide resistance 263, 273–4
  mupirocin 113
  phenol disinfection 223
methisazone 125
methotrexate 178
metronidazole 120, *123*
  brain abscess 145
  DNA strand breakage 175
  wound infections 144
MIC 242, **243**
miconazole 120, *123*
micro-calorimetry, bacteria 24
microbial cell, antigenic structure 284
microbial challenge 203–7
microbial growth on food 76
microbial spoilage 355–65
  types 356–60
microbial toxin detection 372
microbiological assay 480–1
Micrococcus spp.
  contamination sources for non-sterile
    products 378
  industrial water supplies 342
  packaging contamination 348
microcolonies 77
microflora, commensal 77, 78
Micromonospora purpurea 92
microorganisms
  antibiotic assays 479–81
  attachment 79
  human disease treatment 469–70
  models of mammalian drug
    metabolism 487
  portals of entry 77–9
  raw materials for manufacturing
    process 347–8
  survival 79
  transfer from operators 346
  viable airborne determination
    250–1
Microsporon spp. 346
Microsporum spp. 50
Mima spp. 346
minimum infective number (MIN) 76
minimum inhibitory concentration
  (MIC) 242, **243**
minocycline 105
monobactams 92, 102, 167
monoclonal antibodies 286–9
  production 287–8
  uses 289
monocytes 280, 285
Morganella 30
mosquito control 488
moulds 35
  antibiotic production 477
  biocide response 264
  incubation temperature 20

isolated from air 340
raw materials for manufacturing
process 347
MRSA *see* methicillin-resistant
Staphylococcus aureus
msrA gene 191
mucociliary blanket of respiratory
tract 78
mucopeptide 5, 80
slime layers 79
see also peptidoglycan
mucopolysaccharide slime layers 79
Mucor griseocyanus 487
Mucor sp. 340
mucous membranes 77–8, 280
commensal microflora 78
multidose products, contamination
sources 377, 379
multidrug export genes 274
multidrug resistance 134
multidrug resistance pumps
(MDR) 196
multiple antibiotic resistance
(MAR) 196
mumps
vaccination 331
vaccine 306, **313**
virus **64**
mupirocin 112–13
protein synthesis inhibition 173
resistance 192
murein 5
see also mucopeptide; peptidoglycan
mutagenicity testing 484–6
mutation
acquired resistance to biocides 272
drug resistance 133
reverse 484
mycobacteria
arabinogalactan synthesis 168
biocide resistance 264, 266,
269–70
mycolic acid synthesis 168
non-tuberculous infection 106
survival following phagocytosis 81
mycobactericides 241
Mycobacterium avium intracellulare
276
antimicrobial agent choice 204
biocide resistance 269
Mycobacterium bovis 332
Mycobacterium chelonae 270
Mycobacterium leprae 32, 269
Mycobacterium smegmatis 25
Mycobacterium terrae 241
Mycobacterium tuberculosis 32
antimicrobial agent choice 204
biocide resistance 269, 270
chlorehexidine insusceptibility 217
glutaraldehyde sterilization 215
HIV infection 72
human infection 332
intermediate level disinfection 202
isoniazid resistance 168
multiple drug-resistant (MDRTB)
strains 118, 134, 196–7
mycobactericidal activity 241
rifampicin activity 106
streptomycin activity 107
survival following phagocytosis 81

transmission 276
tuberculin test 300
mycolic acid 270
synthesis 168
Mycoplasma pneumoniae
antibody production 86
pneumonia 138, 139
mycotoxins 49
myxoedema 298
myxoviruses **64**

naftidine 178, 179
nalidixic acid 120, 133
pseudomonad selective media 19
nasopharynx, colonization 346
National Health Service
Crown immunity removal 380–1
purchasing policy 380
natural immunity 302
natural killer (NK) cells 297, 298
nebulizer device 417
necrotising fasciitis 26, 143
necrotoxins 283
Neisseria gonorrhoeae 26, 75
biocide sensitivity 268
plasmid transfer by transformation
183
sulphonamide resistance 181
transmission 87
Neisseria meningitidis 26
meningitis 144–5
respiratory tract infection 82
vaccine 307, **311**
Neisseria pharyngis 346
Neisseria spp.
erythromycin activity 108
properties 26
neomycin 106, 108
netilmicin 106, 108
neuraminidase 476
Neurospora crassa 35, 47–9
trichogyne 48
neurotoxins 14
neutralizing agents 240, 448
neutrophils 280
nitrofurans 119, 175
nitrofurantoin 119, 133
DNA strand breakage 175
nitrofurazone 119
nitroimidazoles 175
nocardicins 102, *103*
non-ionic surfactants 358
non-nucleoside antiviral compounds
127
norA and *norB* gene mutants 188
norfloxacin 120, *121*
gastrointestinal infections 143
noxythiolin 216
nucleic acid synthesis inhibitors 186–8
nucleic acids 259
nucleoside analogues 125–7
nucleoside triphosphate synthesis
173–4
nystatin 114, *115*, 179

O-antigens 284
occupational risks 336
oestradiol implants 421
ofloxacin 118
oils, microbial attack 358

oleandomycin 108, 109
olivanic acid 101, 102
ophthalmia, purulent 26
ophthalmic preparations 417–19
contact-lens solutions 418–19
design 417
eye drops 417–18
lotions 418
ointments 418
solutions 356
see also eye-drops
opsonization, pathogenesis 80
organic acids 473
organic chlorine compounds 218–19
organic polymers, microbial
attack 358
organomercury compounds
microbial attack 359
mycobacterial resistance 269
ornithosis 31
osteomyelitis, staphylococcal 26
overkill for virucidal activity 247
1-oxaphems 100–1
oxygen utilization pathway 18
oxyribonucleic acids 258

PAA *see* phenylacetic acid
p-aminobenzoic acid (PABA) 176,
177
hyperproduction 187
sulphonamide activity 177
p-aminosalicylic acid (PAS) 117
packaging
contamination sources for non-sterile
products 377
dressings 420–1
injectable products 413
materials 348–9
microbial spoilage 364
pharmaceutical manufacture 429
polymers 358
preservatives 267–8
pandemics 88
papilloma virus **64**
parabactin 474
parabens **210**, 212–13, 267
bacterial spore activity 271
Paracoccus denitrificans 474
paramyxovirus **64**
parasites
elimination 279
immunity 291
paratyphoid fever 29, 283
antibiotic treatment 142
MacConkey's medium 18
parenteral nutritional fluids
contaminated 356
see also total parenteral nutrition
paromomycin 108
passive immunity 327–8
Pasteurella pestis see Yersinia pestis
Pasteurella tularensis see Francisella
tularensis
pathogenesis
conjunctiva 79
consolidation 79–81
contact 78
intestinal tract 78
opsonization 80
phagocytosis avoidance 80–1

physico-chemical barriers   78
respiratory tract   78
urogenital tract   78–9
pathogenicity   75–7
pathogens   279
active spread   83–4
invasive   83–4
non-invasive   81–2
obligate   87
partially invasive   82
passive spread   84
primary defence strategies   282
PBPs *see* penicillin-binding proteins
penicillanic acid   102–3
derivatives   102–3
sulphone   103
penicillin G *see* benzylpenicillin
penicillin V *see*
phenoxymethylpenicillin
penicillin-binding proteins (PBPs)   97,
98, 167, 192, 193
penicillinase   477
penicillins   92–3, *94*, **95**
antigens   104
β-lactam ring interaction with
transpeptidases   167
broad spectrum   131
enzymatic inactivation   133
hypersensitivity   103–4
meningitis treatment   145
naturally occurring   92
peptidoglycan crosslinking   165–7
production from *Penicillium
chrysogenum*   453
resistance   192, 193–4
Streptococcus pneumoniae   198
semisynthetic production   92–3
structure   *92*
synthesis   477
Penicillium camembertii   49
Penicillium chrysogenum   92, 150,
158, 453
Penicillium digitatum   35
Penicillium marneffei   50
Penicillium notatum   92, 150
Penicillium roquefortii   49
Penicillium spp.   49–50
building contamination   349
glass container contamination   348
isolated from air   340
packaging contamination   348
penicilloic acid   192
pentachlorophenol   257
peptic ulcer   31
peptidase   83
peptide nucleic acids   466
peptidoglycan   5, *6*, 80, 266
assembly disruption   168
biosynthesis   164–8
inhibition   164–8
network expansion   12
synthesis inhibitor resistance   192–5
see also mucopeptide; murein
peptidyl transferase   171, 172
peracetic acid   221
peritoneal dialysis solutions   416
peritonitis, bacterial   26
pernicious anaemia   471–2
peroxygen compounds   221
sporicidal action   204

personal hygiene   428
pertussis
vaccination   334
safety   326
vaccine   304, 306, 308, **312**, 315
see also Bordetella pertussis;
whooping cough
Peyer's patches   285
phages   15, 57–62, 470
epidemiological uses   62
indicator organisms for virucidal
activity testing   247–8
induction   61
lambda of *E. coli*   60
lysogeny   60–2
lytic growth cycle   59–60, *61*
temperate   59, 60–2
therapy   58
transduction   62
virulent   59–60
plaque formation   60
phagocytes
endogenous pyrogen release   86
killing   81
phagocytic cells   131, 293
phagocytic system, recovery from
infection   87
phagocytosis   280–1
avoidance   80–1
protection   77
survival   81
phagolysosome   281
phagosome   281
pharmaceutical manufacture
atmosphere   340–2
bioburden   440
measurement   372
reduction   371
contamination
non-sterile products   376, 380–1
removal   370–1
definition   426–7
documentation   429
endotoxin levels   372
environmental cleanliness   427–8
hygiene   345–6, 427–8
microbial contamination control
426, 427–9
microbial transfer from operators
346
microorganisms in partial synthesis
477–9
packaging   429
post-market surveillance   373
process
buildings   349–50
cleaning equipment/utensils   353
cleansing   352
critical control points   349
design   429
disinfection   352
equipment   350–3
filters   351
glass containers   348
microbial checks   352–3
packaging   348–9
raw materials   347–8
validation   349
pyrogen testing   372
quality control   429

procedures   371–2
quality of materials   428–9
respiratory tract flora   345–6
sampling time   371
skin flora   345–6
spoilage detection   372
sterile products   429–30, *431*,
432–6
storage   429
transport   429
validation procedures   371
water supply   342–5
pharmaceutical products
chemical deterioration   357
formulation design/development
368–70
microbial attack
observable signs   359–60
susceptible ingredients   357–9
microbial risk control   368–73
microbial spoilage   360–5
contaminant inoculum   361
moisture content   362–3
nutritional factors   361–2
packaging design   364
pH   364
protection of microorganisms
365
redox potential   363
storage temperature   364
microbiological quality   339
parametric release   439
physico-chemical deterioration   357
physico-chemical parameter
manipulation   369
potency determination   480
preservation   365–8
preservatives   369
quality assurance   368–73
pharmaceutical products, non-sterile
contamination   374–6
control   383
environment   377, 379
equipment sources   379
extent   379–81
human sources   378–9
manufacture   380–1
packaging   377
prevention   383
sources   376–9
in use   377–9, 381
water supply   376
health hazards   375–6
spoilage   374–5
pharmaceutical products, sterile
410–11
absorbable haemostats   421–2
aseptic areas   430, *431*, 432–5,
435–6
blow/fill/seal units   436
clean areas   430, *431*, 432–5
cleaning   434
containers   435
disinfection   434
dressings   419–21
environmental contamination   433
GPMP   437
implants   421
injections   411–15
isolators   436

504   *Index*

ligatures 422–3
microbiological monitoring 434
non-injectable 416
operation of clean area 434–5
ophthalmic preparations 417–19
sterilization methods 410–11
sutures 422–3
terminal sterilization 429–30
vaccine preparation 430
pharyngitis, acute 137
phenolics 211
properties 209
phenols 221, 222, 223–4
bacterial spore activity 271
black fluids 222, 223
coefficient tests 237–8
cytoplasm coagulation 259
dilution 234
E. coli sensitivity 267
interaction with packaging
materials 367
minimum inhibitory
concentration 243
mycobacterial resistance 269–70
pH effects 235
white fluids 222, 223
phenoxyacetic acid 158
phenoxyethanol 214
2-phenoxyethanol 257
phenoxymethylpenicillin 92
manufacture 149, 158
phenylacetic acid (PAA) 92, 93, 156
phenylalanine 483
phenylethanol 214
phenylketonuria (PKU) testing 482–3
phenylmercuric acetate 253, 417, 419
phenylmercuric nitrate 417, 419
phenylmercuric salts 220
pheromones, oligopeptide 36
phosphatidyl ethanolamine 8
phosphatidyl glycerol 8
phospholipase 83
phospholipid 7, 8
arrangement in cytoplasmic
membrane 8
bilayer 9
phosphonoacetic acid 127
phosphotransferases 188
Photobacterium fischeri 25
phthalylsulphathiazole 116
physical indicators of sterility 441–2
picornaviruses 64–5
pigment, bacterial cell 10
pili 10, 79
pinocytosis 82
pipleines 351
Pityrosporum spp. 346
pivmecillinam 93, 94, 95
plague 28, 283
plant matter, decaying 342
plaque assays for virucidal
activity 245–6
plasma substitutes 471
plasmid-coded acquired resistance to
biocides 272–4
plasmids
enzyme inactivation 133–4
foreign DNA insertion 454–5
resistance 133, 187, 273
acquired 183–4

transposons 183
pneumococcal polysaccharide
vaccine 307, 311
Pneumocystis carinii 72
Pneumocystis carinii pneumonia
co-trimoxazole activity 117
trimetrexate therapy 178
pneumonia 138–9
bacterial 26
pneumococcal 139
staphylococcal 139
polarity 37–8
polio vaccine 304, 306, 309, 310,
314, 315
inactivated (IPV) 330, 331
live oral (OPV) 330, 331
juvenile immunization schedule
335
poliomyelitis
paralytic 330
vaccination 326, 330–1
effects on incidence 322
killed (Salk) 330
live (Sabin) 330
see also polio vaccine;
poliovirus
poliovirus 57, 62, 64, 69
faecal excretion of vaccine
virus 330–1
plaque assays 245
types 330, 331
polyclonal activation 298
polyenes 114, 115, 178, 179
antibiotic-resistance 43
polyglycerol-phosphate 5
polyhexamethylene biguanide 207,
217
polyhydroxybutyric acid 9
polymers, packaging 358
polymyxins 27, 92, 111, 178–9
resistance 195–6
polynoxylin 216
polypeptide antibiotics 111, 461
polyphosphate 9
polyribitol 5
polyvinylchloride, plasticized 413
porins 8, 270
cell membrane 185
channels 267, 268
potassium monoperoxysulphate 221
povidone–iodine 219, 220
poxviruses 63, 69
pregnancy, urinary tract infections
140
preservatives 202, 251–4, 365–8
availability 366–8
bioluminescence 254
challenge tests 369
combinations 252–4
concentration 366
containers 367–8
efficacy 252
epifluorescence 254
evaluation 252
eye-drops 417
inoculum size 366
microbial attack 359
multiphase systems 367
packaging 267–8
performance criteria 252

pH effects 367
rapid methods of evaluation 254
synergy 253–4
temperature 366
water activity [AUwu] 366
prions 73
antimicrobial agent choice 207
biocide activity 276
pro-drugs 93
proflavine 174, 226
proguanil 216
bacterial DHFR inhibition 177–8
proinsulin 459
prokaryotes 4
prokaryotic nucleus 9
promoters 457
prontosil 115, 116
propamidine 226
propanol 478
prophage 59, 61, 62
β-propiolactone 262
propogated-source outbreaks 87, 88
FIP 88
proproteins 459
propylene glycol 342
prostaglandins 281
prostate infections 141
proteases 77
protective clothing 346–7, 428
aseptic areas 435
clean areas 433
protein A 81
protein A–IgG complexes 81
protein drugs 461
protein synthesis inhibition
azalides 172
chloramphenicol 171–2
clindamycin 172
lincomycin 172
macrolides 172
mupirocin 173
resistance 188–92
streptomycin 169
proteins
administration route 466
fusion 460
glycosylation 459
identity 465
medically important 461, 463–4
recombinant 461, 466
synthesis 169–70, 163, 171–6
proteolysis 459–60
Proteus mirabilis 188
Proteus morganii 29–30
Proteus spp.
biocide resistance 264
transfer from manufacturing process
operators 346
water supply 342
Proteus vulgaris 29–30
prothionomide 118
protonmotive force 257
Protozoa
antimicrobial agent choice 207
metronidazole activity 120
resistance to biocides 275
Providencia spp. 30
Providencia stuartii 264
provirus 71
pseudomembranous colitis 27

superinfection 136
vancomycin therapy 111
pseudomonads
  biocide resistance 269
  selective media 19
Pseudomonas acidophila 92
Pseudomonas aeruginosa 28, 75
  antimicrobial agent choice 204
  biocide resistance 264, 269
  burn colonization 144
  cephalosporin activity 96, 97
  chlorhexidine sterilization 217
  clavulanic acid activity 100
  contaminated medicines 356, 382
  contamination of non-sterile
    products 376, 377
    during manufacture 380
    sources 378, 379
    in use 381
  cystic fibrosis infections 139
  EDTA sensitivity 269
  eye-drop contamination 417
  gentamicin activity 108
  medicament-borne infection 356,
    382
  membrane permeabilization
    evaluation 258
  phages 248
  polymyxin
    activity 178, 179
    resistance 195–6
  QAC activity 225
  tetracycline activity 105
  transfer from manufacturing process
    operators 346
  urinary tract infections 140
Pseudomonas cytotoxin 490
Pseudomonas spp.
  contamination of
    sweetening/flavouring
    agents 359
  indigenous to fresh water 342
  raw materials for manufacturing
    process 347
pseudomonic acid A *see* mupirocin
psittacosis 31
  pneumonia 138
public health measures 322
puerperal sepsis 26
purine synthesis 173–4
pus 84
pustules 143
pyelitis 29
pyelonephritis 29
pyrazinamide 118
  M. tuberculosis resistance 196,
    197
pyridine 2,6-dicarboxylic acid 11, *12*
pyridoxine assay 482
pyrimidine synthesis 173–4
pyrogens
  bacterial 348
  testing in pharmaceutical
    manufacture 372
pyruvil transferase 195

Q-fever 31, 138
*qac*A, *qac*B and *qac*C genes 274
QACs *see* quaternary ammonium
  compounds

quality assurance 368–73, 427
quality control 368, 427
  GPMP 370
  pharmaceutical manufacture 429
quaternary ammonium compounds
  (QACs) 207, **211**, 224–5
  atmospheric disinfection 342
  bacterial spore activity 271
  BS specification 240
  cell membrane effects 268
  clumping 240
  E. coli sensitivity 267
  Gram-negative bacteria
    sensitivity 267
  interaction with packaging
    materials 367
  membrane-active agents 178
  microbial attack 359
  mycobacterial resistance 269
  properties **209**
  viable counts 240
4-quinolone antibacterials 120
  see also quinolones
quinolones 131
  derivatives 226
  DNA gyrase
    inhibition 175
    site of action 173
  resistance 187–8

rabies 62
  immunoglobulins **319**
  vaccine 306, 309, **314**
  virus **64**
radiation sterilization 401–3, *404*,
  405
  monitoring 441, **444**
  sterilizer design 403, *404*, 405
radioenzymatic assays 481
rainfall 342
rate of kill 231
recombinant animal cells 460
recombinant DNA technology 453–4,
  470
  cloning 454–6
  drug authenticity/efficacy 461, 465
  medically important
    polypeptide/protein
    production 461
  natural protein analogue
    production 465
  principles 454–61
  proteolytic damage 465
  small molecule production 466
recombinant proteins 466
  production from mammals 461
redox potential 363
relapsing fever 32
relaxin **463**
replica plating 41–2
resistance 181
  access prevention to target sites
    185
  acquired 181–4
    chromosomal mutations 182–3
    genetic basis 182–4
    plasmids 183–4
    transposons 184
  aminoglycoside-aminocyclitol
    group 188–9, **190**

antibiotic policies 146
antimicrobial drugs 133–4
antimycobacterial drugs 196–7
β-lactam antibiotics 192–4
bacitracin 196
bacterial conjugation 15
biochemical mechanisms 184–97
cephalosporins 192
fusidic acid 191
genetic determinants **184**
glycopeptides 194–5
intrinsic 181–2
membrane-active antibiotics 195–6
multidrug 134
mupirocin 192
penicillins 192, 193–4
peptidoglycan synthesis inhibitors
  192–5
plasmid-acquired 133, 183–4, 187
plasmid-mediated 273
polymyxins 195–6
problem 197–9
protein synthesis inhibitors 188–92
sterilization 387–8
super-infection 131
target sites 185–6
teicoplanin 194, 195
tetracyclines 190, 196
urinary tract infections 140
vancomycin 195
respiratory tract 78
  flora 346–7
  infections 137–9
restriction endonuclease 454, *455*
reticuloendothelial system 280
retroviruses **65**
reverse transcriptase 125, 456
  activity assay 247
  inhibitiors 127
rheumatic fever 26
rheumatoid arthritis 299
rhinovirus 62, **65**, 82
  infection 70
  receptors 69
Rhodotorula spp. 340
ribavirin 125, *126*
riboflavin 471
ribosome binding site 457–8, 459
ribosomes
  bacterial 169, 170
  non-antibiotic antibacterial agent
    activity 258, 259
  streptomycin action 170, 171
rickettsia, chloramphenicol activity
  112
Rickettsia prowazeki 31
Rickettsia quintana 31
Rickettsia spp. 31
Rickettsia typhi 31
Rideal–Walker test 221, 237, 238
rifabutin 106
rifampicin 106, 118
  chemoprophylaxis 137
  legionnaires' disease
    treatment 131, 139
  resistance 106, 188
  structure *106*
  transcription effects 175–6
rifamycin 106
  resistance 188

ringworm 50, 51, 77
  griseofulvin 114
risk categories for equipment in contact
  with patient 227–8
risk control, microbial 368–73
RNA methylase genes 191
RNA polymerase 174, 457
rod-shaped bacteria 4
rotavirus 64
  plaque assays 245
roxithromycin 110
rubella
  vaccination 331–2
  vaccine 306, **314**
  virus **65**

Sabouraud maltose 20
Saccharomyces cerevisiae 35, 36–
  44
  ascus formation 40, 42
  bud scar 44
  budding pattern 38–9
  cell ageing 44
  cell polarity 37–8, *39*
  cell wall 43–4
  chitin ring *38*, 44
  chlorhexidine sensitivity 274
  cloning host 460, **462**
  developmental switch 40–1
  diploid 36, *37, 39*
  diplophase 40
  ethanol formation 42
  fusel alcohol effects 40
  genetic manipulation 36
  glycolytic pathway 42
  haploid 36, *37, 39*
  haplophase 40
  heavy metal activity 275
  hyphal growth *40*
  invasive filaments 38, 40
  life cycle 36–42
    comparison with *N. crassa* 48–9
  meiosis 40–2
  metabolism 42–3
  morphological change 37
  mutants 36
  mutation combinations 42
  oligopeptide pheromones 36
  physiology 42–3
  polyene antibiotic-resistant mutants
    43
  pseudohyphae 38, 39–40
  replica plating 41–2
  schmoos 36
  spore formation 40–2
  sporulation 40–1, 43
  sterol requirement 43
  trehalose production 42–3
  unsaturated fatty acid requirements
    43
  vegetative cell cycle 36–40
salbutamol 478
Salmonella enteritidis 29
Salmonella paratyphi 29
  exotoxin production 84
  subepithelial tissue penetration 84
Salmonella spp.
  medicament-borne infection 382
  partially invasive pathogens 82
  phenol disinfection 223

Salmonella typhi 29, 80
  bismuth sulphite agar 19
  chloramphenicol activity 172
  drug sensitivity 137
  exotoxin production 84
  K-antigens 80
  phage typing 62
  phenol coefficient tests 237
  subepithelial tissue penetration 84
  survival following phagocytosis 81
  vaccine production 308
Salmonella typhimurium 29
  Ames test 485
  deep rough mutants 267
  exotoxin production 84
  lux cluster insertion 25
  subepithelial tissue penetration 84
Salmonella/microsome assay 485
salmonellosis 82, 84
  antibiotic treatment 142
  contamination of non-sterile
    products during manufacture
    380
sanitizer 230
Sarcina spp. 346
sarcinae, aggregates 4
scarlet fever 26, 85
Schick test toxin 334
self antigens, tolerance evasion 298
serial dilution 242
serotonin 281
Serratia marcescens 30
  chlorhexidine resistance 268
  filtration sterilization biological
    monitoring 445
  formaldehyde resistance 273
  pigment 10
Serratia spp.
  indigenous to fresh water 342
  medicament-borne infection 382
serum sickness 300
services, clean areas 432
sewage contamination 342
sex strands 10
Shigella boydii 29
Shigella flexneri 29
Shigella shiga 29, 57–8
Shigella sonnei 29
Shigella spp
  gastrointestinal infections 142
  partially invasive pathogens 82
  phenol disinfection 223
shotgunning 456
siderophores 77, 473, 474
signal sequence 458
silver salts, plasmid-mediated
  resistance 273
sisomicin 106
skin 280
  commensal microflora 77
  eruptions 135
  flora 143, 346–7
    contamination sources 378
  infections 143–4
  tests
    disinfectants 241–2
    semi-solid antibacterial agents
    249
  trauma 77
slime 10

mucopeptide/mucopolysaccharide
  layers 79
slit sampler 250–1
slow virus diseases 73, 276
smallpox 279
  chick embryo cell system for
    growing virus 67
  control 321
  vaccination 326
  vaccine 304, 305–6
sodium hypochlorite 345
sodium phosphonoformate 127
soft tissue infections 143–4
soil erosion 342
solid dilution method 243
somatostatin 460
somatotrophin **463**
sorbic acid 212
sparfloxacin 120
spermine 280
spiramycin 108, 109
spirochaetes 4, 32–3
spleen 285
spoilage, non-sterile pharmaceutical
  products 374–5
spores, biocide resistance 266
sporicides 229, 241
  quantitative suspension tests 239
sporulation 271
squalene epoxidase 122
Stachybotrys spp., filters 351
Staphylococcus albus 346, 380
Staphylococcus aureus 4, 26
  bacitracin resistance 196
  brain abscess 145
  chlorehexidine sterilization 217
  contamination sources for non-sterile
    products 378
  cystic fibrosis infections 139
  enterotoxin 85
  erythromycin resistance 109
  lung abscess 139
  msrA gene 191
  penicillin resistance 181
  phage 58
    typing 62
  pigment 10
  pneumonia 139
  positive control for sterility testing
    449
  prophages 61
  protein A 81
  quinolone resistance 188
  skin flora 143
  skin infections 143–4
  tetracycline-resistant 105
  topoisomerase mutations 187
  transduction 183
  transfer from manufacturing process
    operators 346
  virulent strains 80
  see also methicillin-resistant
    Staphylococcus aureus (MRSA)
Staphylococcus epidermidis 77
Staphylococcus spp.
  aggregates 4
  burn colonization 144
  contamination sources for non-sterile
    products 378
  isolated from air 340

properties 26
selective media 19
steam sterilization 392, 393–5
  superheated steam 393–5
steam sterilizer 394–7
  design 394–7
  operation 395–7
  temperature monitoring 395
sterile fluids, non-injectable 415–16
sterile pharmaceutical products 416
  absorbable haemostats 421–2
  dressings 419–21
  implants 421
  injections 411–5
  instruments and equipment 423–5
  non-injectable sterile fluids 415–6
  opthalmic preparations 417–9
  surgical ligatures and sutures 422–3
sterility assurance 388–9, 439
bioburden determination 440
  environmental monitoring 440–1
sterility testing 446–51
  accidental contamination 450
  antimicrobial agents 448–9
  direct inoculation 446–7
  inactivating agents 240, 448
  isolators *447*, 448
  low level contamination 447
  membrane filtration 447
  methods 446–8
  microbial enzymes 486
  neutralizing agents
  positive controls 449
  random sampling 446
  sampling 450–1
sterilization 385, 399–401
  catgut 423
  conditions **408**
  control 439–40
  D-value 370
  dressings 420
  equipment 423–5
  ethylene oxide **400**
  eye-drops 419
  filtration 405–7
    biological monitoring 445–6
  formaldehyde 401–2
  gas 399–401, 441, **444**
  heat 390–9, 441, **443–4**
    dry 397–8
    moist 392–7
    process 390–2
    temperature profile *391*
    temperature/time cycles 393
  injectable products 413, 415
  instruments 423–5
  manufacturing equipment 352
  methods 389–90
  microorganism sensitivity 386–9
  monitors 441–3, **444**, 445–6
    biological indicators *442*
    chemical indicators 442–3, **444**
    physical indicators 441–2
  radiation 401–3, *404*, 405, 441,
    444
  raw materials for manufacturing
    process 348
  reference organisms 386
  resistance 387–8
  steam 392, 393–5

superheated 393–5
steam sterilizer design/operation
  395–7
sterility assurance 388–9, **390**
survivor curves 386, *387*, 388
  terminal 429–30
steroids 301
  biotransformations 477–8
  inhaler preparations 416
  synthesis 470
sterol 43
sticky-ends 454
storage, pharmaceutical manufacture
  429
Streptococcus faecalis 342
Streptococcus pneumoniae 4, 26
  penicillin resistance 198
  pneumonia treatment 138, 139
  transformation 14
  upper respiratory tract infections
    137
Streptococcus pyogenes 4, 26, 80
  burn colonization 144
  erythrogenic toxin 26
  penicillin susceptibility 181
  pH of antibacterial agent 235–6
  skin infections 143
  toxin 83, 85
  transduction 183
  transfer from manufacturing process
    operators 346
  upper respiratory tract infections
    137
Streptococcus salivarus 346
Streptococcus spp.
  aggregates 4
  isolated from air 340
  properties 26
  raw materials for manufacturing
    process 347
streptodornase 475–6
streptogramins, resistance 191
streptokinase 282, 475–6
Streptomyces aureofaciens 158
Streptomyces clavuligerus 98, 157
Streptomyces olivaceus 102
Streptomyces spp., antibiotic
  source 92
streptomycin 92, 106, 107–8
  action on ribosomes 170, 171
  tuberculosis therapy 117, 118
styes 26
succinylsulphathiazone 116
sulbactam 103
sulphadiazine 116
sulphadimidine 116
sulphites 212, 262
sulphonamides 115–17, 177
  DHFR inhibitor combination 178
  resistance to 187
  thymine production blocking 174
sulphur dioxide 212, 262
  amino group reaction 259
supercoiling regions, chromosomal
  173, 175
superinfection 131, 136
suppressor T cells 295–6
surface activity, antibacterial action
  236
surface adhesins 78

surface antigens 284
surfactants 224–5
  anionic 224
  cationic 224–5, 236, 358
  microbial attack 357–8
  non-ionic 358
  potentiation of antibacterial
    agent 236
surgical prophylaxis 130–1, 136
survivor curves, sterilization 386,
  387, 388
survivor/time curve *232*
swabs 440
sweetening agents 358–9
synergism 128
syphilis 33
systemic lupus erythematosus 299

T cell receptors 294, 296
T cells 285
  activation 298
  classes 295–6
  suppression 297
    absence 298
T-even phage DNA 59
T-even phages 69
tar acids **211**, 223
taurolidine 216
tazobactam 103
teichoic acids 6, 7, 266
  bacterial cell wall 167
teicoplanin 112
  pentapeptide binding 165–6
  resistance 194, 195
  use in multi-drug resistance 134
temafloxacin 120
temocillin 93, *94*, **95**
temperature
  coefficient 232–3, 366
  record chart 441
terbinafine 122, *123*
testosterone implants 421
tetanus 27, 283
  antitoxin 304, **318**
  immunoglobulins **319**
  tissue damage 85
  vaccination 334
    efficiency 326
  vaccine 304, 308, **311**, 314, 315
tetrachlorosalicylanilide (TCS) 257
tetracycline 104–5
  candidiasis superinfection 136
  group 104–6
  mycoplasma infections 139
  resistance and efflux proteins 196
tetracyclines 92
  action on ribosomes 169
  bacteriostatic action 171
  efflux 133
  efflux proteins 190
  protein synthesis effects 171
  resistance 190
tetrahydrofolate 176, *177*
tetrahydroimidazobenzodiazepinone
  (TIBO) 127
tetroxoprim *116*, 117
thiacycline 105
thiatetracyclines 105
iso-thiazolones 259
thienamycine 101, 102

thiocarbamates, synthetic   122
thiol groups   258, 259
thiomersal   220–1
    ophthalmic preparations   417, 419
thromboxanes   281
thrush
    oral   44, 114
    vaginal   44, 46
thymidine kinase   126
thymidylate synthetase   174, 176
thymidylic acid   174, 176
thymine production blocking   173
thymus   284
thyroiditis   298
thyrotoxicosis   298, 300
ticarcillin, burn wounds   144
tinea   50
    tolnaftate activity   122
tissue culture for virucidal activity
        245
tissue damage   84–7
    direct   84–6
    indirect   86–7
    membrane function interference   85
    secondary disease   86
    target cells   85
tissue fluid loss   86
tissue plasminogen activator   **463**
tissue transplantation   301–2
tobacco mosaic virus (TMV)   56
tobramycin   106, 108
tolerance   297–8
    mechanism breakdown   298
tolnaftate   122, *123*
tonsillitis   26
tonsils   285
topoisomerase   173, 175
    mutations   187
total parenteral nutrition   414
    storage temperature   364
    see also parenteral nutritional fluids
toxaemia, generalized   84
toxins   77
    ingestion   76
    see also endotoxins; exotoxins;
        pyrogens
trachoma   31
transcription   174
transduction
    bacterial   15
    plasmid transfer   183, 184
transformation
    bacterial   15
    plasmid transfer   183, 184
transpeptidases   166–8
transplantation   301–2
    organ rejection   279
transport, pharmaceutical
        manufacture   429
transposons
    acquired resistance   184
    conjugative   184
    glycopeptide resistance   194–5
    plasmids   183
transversions   182, 183
travelling
    immunization   326
    risks   336
trehalose   42–3
Treponema pallidum   33, 87

Treponema pertenue   33
tricarbanilide   257
triacetyloleandomycin   108
triazoles   179
tricarboxylic acid cycle, *S. cerevisiae*
        42
trichlorocarbanilide (TCC)   257
Trichophyton mentagrophytes   77, 205
Trichophyton spp.   50–1
    griseofulvin activity   114
    transfer from manufacturing process
        operators   346
triclosan   224, 267
trimethoprim   *116*, 117, 187
    bacterial DHFR inhibition   177
    prostate infections   141
    resistance   187
trimetrexate   178
triphenylmethane dyes   226
tuberculin test   300
tuberculosis   32
    disinfection of equipment   204
    drug therapy   117–18
    drug resistance   134
    incidence   276, 332–3
    MDRTB   118, 134, 196–7
    streptomycin activity   107
    vaccination   332–3
tularaemia   28
tumour
    destruction   490
    immune response   301–2
    necrosis factor   **464**
    recognition   279
    viruses   71–2
typhoid fever   29, 84, 283
    antibiotic treatment   142
    chloramphenicol therapy   172
    drug sensitivity   137
    MacConkey's medium   18
    phenol coefficient tests   237
    vaccination immunity longevity
        327
    vaccine   306, 307, 308, **312**
typhus infection   31
tyrothricin   27

UDP-*N*-acetylmuramic acid   165
ultraviolet irradiation sterilization
        401, 405
uncoupling agents   257
undecaprenyl phosphate   174
undulant fever   29
unsaturated fatty acids, *S. cerevisiae*
        requirements   43
URA3 gene   45
urethritis, non-gonococcal   31
urinary bladder
    catheterization   139
    irrigation solutions   416
urinary tract infections   78–9, 139–41
    community-acquired   141
    drug resistance   140
    drug therapy   140–1
    recurrent   141
urogenital tract   78–9
urological irrigation solutions   416

vaccination   279, 321–2
    active acquired immunity   302

cost   327
    effectiveness   326
    immunity longevity   327
    programmes   88
        objectives   325–7
        routine against infectious disease
            330–5
    safety   326
vaccine production
    aluminium testing   317
    bacterial   307–8
    calcium presence testing   317
    final product control   315–17
    free formalin   317
    from microorganisms   470
    in-process control   312, 314, 315
    manufacturing   430
    phenol concentration   317
    potency   315–16
    quality control   312, 314–17
    safety tests   316
    seed lot system   307
    sterility tests   317
    toxicity testing   317
    viral   309–10, 312, **313**, 314–17
vaccines   304, 305–10, **311**, 312, **313**,
        314–17
    aseptic filling   436
    bacterial   307–8, 310, **311–12**, 316
    bacterial cell component   306–7
    classes   329–30
    component   329–30
    costs   320
    killed   306, 329–30
    larger organisms   320
    live   305–6, 329
    toxoid   306
    viral   309–10, 312, **313**, 314–17
    subunit   307
vaccinia virus   **63**, 69
vaginal pH   79
vaginitis   27
vaginosis, bacterial   120
VanA phenotype   194, 195
vancomycin   111
    pentapeptide binding   165
    resistance   194
    rifampicin combination   106
    use in multi-drug resistance   134
vancomycin-resistant enterococci
        (VRE)   197, 199
VanH phenotype   194, 195
varicella
    immunoglobulins   **319**
    vaccine   **314**
variola major   321
variola virus   **63**
variolation   279, 321
vascular permeability, histamine   293
venereal infection   79
viable airborne microorganism
        determination   250–1
viable counting   239, 240
Vibrio cholerae   28, 80
    exotoxin   86, 203
    neuraminidase production   476
    toxin production   82
    vaccine production   308
Vibrio parahaemolyticus   28
vibrios   4

Vincent's angina   32
viomycin   111
viral chemotherapy   70–1
viral DNA replication   69
  inhibition   174
viral genome   55
viral infection
  contaminated medicines   356
  skin   143
viral protein production   69–70
viral vaccines   309–10, 312, **313**,
    314–17
  attentuated   316
  blending   309–10
  combined   310
  drying   310
  filling   310
  safety tests   316
  single-component   310, **313–14**
  viral harvest processing   309
  virus growth   309
virion   69
virucidal activity testing   245–8
  animal model   246
  egg inoculation   245
  endogenous reverse transcriptase
    247
  hepatitis B virus   246
  immune reaction   246–7
  phages   247–8
  plaque assays   245–6
  tissue culture   245
  virus morphology   247
virucide   230
virulence   75, 279
  definition   79
virulence factors   75
  extracellular   77
virus–host cell interactions   57
viruses˜   53
  antimicrobial agent choice   205–7
  capsid   54, 57
    assembly   69, 70
  capsomeres   54–6, 57
  chemical agent effects   57
  cytopathic effect (CPE)   66, *67*
  degree of virulence   75
  DNA   69
  endocytosis   69
  general properties   53–4
  HeLa cell lines   66
  helical symmetry   56
  hexon   57

human   62, **63–5**, 66–70
  attachment   68–9
  cell culture   66
  chick embryo cell system for
    growing   66–8
  cultivation   66–8
  multiplication   68–70
  non-enveloped   70
  penetration   69
  uncoating   69
  viral protein production   69–70
icosahedral symmetry   57
lipoprotein envelope   55
membrane glycoprotein receptors
    68–9
metabolic capabilities   54
morphology   *55*, 247
nucleic acid content   54
nucleocapsid release   69
oncogenic   71
penton   57
physical agent effects   57
protein coat   54
replication   66, *67*
resistance to biocides   275, *276*
RNA   69–70
  oncogenic   71
size   54
slow   73
structure   54–6
subunit structure   54–6
temperate   15
upper respiratory tract infections
    137
see also antiviral drugs; phage;
    prions
vitamin B   471, 472
vitamin B$_6$ assay   482
vitamins   471–2, **473**
  bioassays   481–2
Vogel-Johnson medium   19
volutin granules   9
vomiting   76
VRE   197, 199

walls   349
  clean areas   430, 434
water
  chlorine gas disinfection   345
  deionized   343
  demineralized   343
  disinfection   345
  distilled   344

distribution system   344–5
mains supply   343
membrane filtration   345
microbial ecology   342–5
microbial flora growth
    reduction   344
microbial quality checking   345
non-injectable   416
raw   343
reservoir storage   343
reverse osmosis production   344
sodium hypochlorite disinfection
    345
softened   343
ultraviolet irradiation   345
water activity [AUwu]   362–5, 369
  preservatives   366
water supply contamination   376
water systems, storage tanks   32
water vapour, phase diagram   *394*
Weil's disease   33
white fluids   *222*, 223
  Kelsey–Sykes test   238
whooping cough   28–9, 81, 283
  epidemics   326
  see also Bordetella pertussis;
    pertussis
windows   349–50
wound infections   30
  burn   144
  postoperative   144
  secondary   28

xenografts   301
xylenols   *222*, 223

yaws   33
yeasts   35
  biocide response   264
  industrial water supplies   342
  isolated from air   340
yellow fever
  vaccination immunity longevity
    327
  vaccine   306, **314**
  virus   **65**
Yersinia pestis   28

z-value   13, 387–8
zidovudine (AZT)   73, 125, 130, 174
zinc-based products   378